Core Concepts in Dialysis and Continuous Therapies

Colm C. Magee • J. Kevin Tucker
Ajay K. Singh
Editors

Core Concepts in Dialysis and Continuous Therapies

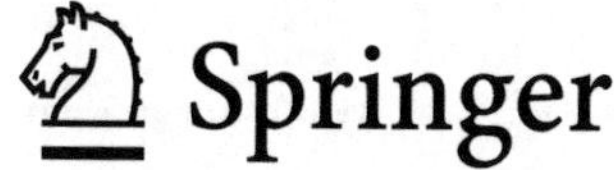

Editors
Colm C. Magee, MD, MPH, FRCPI
Department of Nephrology
Beaumont Hospital
Dublin, Ireland

Ajay K. Singh, MBBS, FRCP, MBA
Global and Continuing Education
Harvard Medical School
Boston, MA, USA

J. Kevin Tucker, MD
Department of Medicine/Renal Division
Brigham and Women's Hospital
Harvard Medical School
Boston, MA, USA

ISBN 978-1-4939-7943-1 ISBN 978-1-4899-7657-4 (eBook)
DOI 10.1007/978-1-4899-7657-4

Springer Boston, MA, Heidelberg New York Dordrecht London

Softcover reprint of the hardcover 1st edition 2016

Printed on acid-free paper

Springer Science+Business Media LLC New York is part of Springer Science+Business Media (www.springer.com)

Foreword

Dialysis from its earliest days had its foundations in both science and clinical medicine. The Scottish chemist Thomas Graham, known as the "Father of Dialysis" provided a scientific description of solute diffusion. Georg Haas, at the University of Giessen near Frankfurt am Main, performed the first (albeit clinically unsuccessful) dialysis treatments involving humans. Later, Willem Kolff, working under extraordinary conditions in the Netherlands, pioneered the first clinically successful dialytic treatment of a patient with acute kidney injury. A half century ago, Belding Scribner and colleagues pioneered the wider application of dialysis as a therapy for irreversible kidney failure, by providing a means for repetitive access to the circulation without the destruction of blood vessels. In the past five decades, the use of dialysis as a life sustaining therapy has expanded both in the USA and globally, to a degree likely beyond the comprehension of the early pioneers. Today over 60 nations provide universal access to maintenance dialysis, and more than a million people receive dialysis each year worldwide. Truly clinical necessity has been the mother of dialysis invention and innovation.

There exist many tomes that comprehensively cover the technical aspects of delivering dialysis therapy, along with the clinical care of patients on dialysis. Additionally, there are handbooks on dialysis which now cover all of the "how-to" practical aspects needed for immediate management decisions. Yet there remains a gap in information that this book covers—namely this text fills a need for a succinct coverage of the core concepts around renal replacement therapy inclusive of hemodialysis, peritoneal dialysis, and continuous therapies. Moreover this book provides timely and authoritative reviews from leading experts in the field. It also brings an international flavor by recruiting authors from around the world, reflecting global issues and needs. The target audience? Nephrologists and informed generalists. I congratulate the editors and authors for covering the clinical art and techne of dialysis, and for a job well done.

Jonathan Himmelfarb, MD

Contents

Contributors

Manoj Bhattarai University of Pittsburgh, Pittsburgh, PA, USA

Katrina Campbell Department of Nutrition & Dietetics, Princess Alexandra Hospital, Woollongabba, QLD, Australia

Juan Jesus Carrero Department of Renal Medicine, Karolinska Institute, Huddinge, Sweden

Elliot Charen Department of Medicine and Division of Nephrology and Hypertension, Mount Sinai Beth Israel/Icahn School of Medicine at Mount Sinai, New York, NY, USA

Paul Cockwell Department of Renal Medicine, Queen Elizabeth Hospital Birmingham, Birmingham, UK

Andrew Davenport Royal Free Hospital, University College Medical School, London, UK

Clara J. Day Department of Renal Medicine, Queen Elizabeth Hospital Birmingham, Birmingham, UK

Thomas A. Depner University of California—Davis, Sacramento, CA, USA

Ken Farrington Department of Renal Medicine, Lister Hospital, Stevenage, Hertfordshire, UK

Seth B. Furgeson University of Colorado-Anschutz Medical Campus, Aurora, CO, USA

Helen C. Gallagher School of Medicine & Conway Institute of Biomolecular and Biomedical Research, University College Dublin, Dublin, Ireland

Joel D. Glickman Hospital of the University of Pennsylvania, Philadelphia, PA, USA

Roger Greenwood Department of Renal Medicine, Lister Hospital, Stevenage, Hertfordshire, UK

Nikolas B. Harbord Department of Medicine and Division of Nephrology and Hypertension, Mount Sinai Beth Israel/Icahn School of Medicine at Mount Sinai, New York, NY, USA

James Harms Division of Nephrology, Department of Medicine, University of Alabama at Birmingham, Birmingham, AL, USA

Carmel M. Hawley Department of Nephrology, Princess Alexandra Hospital, Brisbane, QLD, Australia

Olof Heimbürger Department of Renal Medicine, Department of Clinical Science, Intervention and Technology, Karolinska University Hospital, Karolinska Institutet, Stockholm, Sweden

David W. Johnson Department of Nephrology, Princess Alexandra Hospital, Brisbane, QLD, Australia

Jameela Kari Department of Pediatrics, King Abdulaziz University, Jeddah, Saudi Arabia

Alice Kennard Department of Nephrology, Princess Alexandra Hospital, Brisbane, QLD, Australia

Claire Kennedy Department of Nephrology, Beaumont Hospital, Dublin, Ireland

Timmy Lee Department of Medicine, University of Alabama, Birmingham, AL, USA

Amanda K. Leonberg-Yoo Division of Nephrology, Tufts Medical Center, Boston, MA, USA

Colm C. Magee Department of Nephrology, Beaumont Hospital, Dublin, Ireland

Sandip Mitra Department of Renal Medicine, Manchester Academic Health Science Centre, University of Manchester & Central Manchester Foundation Trust, Manchester, UK

Nicos Mitsides Department of Renal Medicine, University of Manchester and Devices for Dignity Healthcare Technology Co-operative, Central Manchester University Hospitals NHS Foundation Trust, Manchester, Lancashire, UK

Patrick T. Murray School of Medicine, University College Dublin, Dublin, Ireland

Federico Nalesso Department of Nephrology, Dialysis, Transplant, San Bortolo Hospital, Vicenza, Italy

Sagar U. Nigwekar Department of Internal Medicine/Nephrology, Harvard Medical School, Massachusetts General Hospital, Boston, MA, USA

Paul M. Palevsky VA Pittsburgh Healthcare System, Pittsburgh, PA, USA

Ridhmi Rajapakase University of Pittsburgh, Pittsburgh, PA, USA

Claudio Ronco Department of Nephrology, Dialysis, Transplant, San Bortolo Hospital, Vicenza, Italy

Megan Rossi School of Medicine, University of Queensland, Brisbane, QLD, Australia

Keia Sanderson Division of Nephrology, Children's Mercy Hospital, Kansas City, MO, USA

Rebecca Kurnik Seshasai Drexel University College of Medicine, Philadelphia, PA, USA

Roman Shingarev Department of Nephrology, Memorial Sloan Kettering Center, Birmingham, AL, USA

Ajay K. Singh Global and Continuing Education, Harvard Medical School, Boston, MA, USA

Sivakumar Sridharan Department of Renal Medicine, Lister Hospital, Stevenage, Hertfordshire, UK

David J. R. Steele Department of Medicine, Massachusetts General Hospital, Boston, MA, USA

Dirk Gijsbert Struijk Department of Nephrology, Dianet, Academic Medical Center, Amsterdam, The Netherlands

Scott M. Sutherland Department of Pediatrics, Lucile Packard Children's Hospital, Stanford University Medical Center, Stanford, CA, USA

Isaac Teitelbaum Department of Medicine, University of Colorado Hospital, Aurora, CO, USA

Ashita Tolwani Division of Nephrology, Department of Medicine, University of Alabama at Birmingham, Birmingham, AL, USA

Bradley A. Warady Division of Nephrology, Children's Mercy Hospital, Kansas City, MO, USA

University of Missouri–Kansas City School of Medicine, Kansas City, USA

Daniel E. Weiner Tufts Medical Center, Tufts University School of Medicine, Boston, MA, USA

Keith Wille Division of Pulmonary, Allergy, and Critical Care Medicine, Department of Medicine, University of Alabama at Birmingham, Birmingham, AL, USA

James F. Winchester Department of Medicine and Division of Nephrology and Hypertension, Mount Sinai Beth Israel/Icahn School of Medicine at Mount Sinai, New York, NY, USA

Jonathan Wong Department of Renal Medicine, Lister Hospital, Stevenage, Hertfordshire, UK

Joshua Zaritsky Department of Pediatrics, Division of Nephrology, A. I. duPont Hospital for Children, Wilmington, DE, USA

Nicholas A. Zwang Department of Nephrology, Massachusetts General Hospital, Boston, MA, USA

Part I
Hemodialysis

Epidemiology of End-Stage Renal Disease

1

Amanda K. Leonberg-Yoo and Daniel E. Weiner

1.1 Introduction/Impact on Global Care

End-stage renal disease (ESRD) represents the final stage of what often, although not always, is a gradual progression through the stages of chronic kidney disease (CKD). The operative definition of ESRD is based on receipt of kidney replacement therapy to supplant the function of an irreversibly failing kidney. Worldwide, particularly in developed countries, the most common kidney replacement modality is hemodialysis; however, ESRD also refers to other dialysis modalities, kidney transplantation, and, depending on the perspective, kidney failure in individuals who either by choice or by circumstance do not receive kidney replacement therapy.

The current prevalence and projected growth in the ESRD population worldwide reflects the increasing burden of CKD and the conditions that cause CKD. The Global Burden of Disease study ranked CKD as the 19th leading cause of global years of life lost in 2013, an increase from 36th in 1990 [1]; notably, diabetic kidney disease saw the largest rise in age-standardized death rate of any of the 235 conditions classified in this study. Both improved survival associated with management of associated diseases, such as diabetes and cardiovascular disease, as well as increasing prevalence of CKD likely accounts for this concerning trend.

While the number of individuals treated with dialysis and kidney transplant is widely reported in many countries, limited patient access to kidney replacement therapy, particularly in developing countries, and a lack of systematic reporting of people with kidney failure who are not initiated on kidney replacement therapy likely results in a marked underestimation of the true incidence of kidney failure. There is no systematic reporting of those with kidney failure who prefer to forgo kidney replacement therapies or for whom kidney replacement therapy is unavailable, thus highlighting a preference bias in truly interpreting epidemiologic trends and the impact of ESRD on health-care worldwide.

Potentially modifiable risk factors exist along the spectrum of CKD that, if identified and treated, could reduce the incidence and prevalence of kidney failure. For example, diabetes and hypertension remain the leading cause of CKD both in developed and in developing countries [2]. In 2008, the global prevalence of hypertension in the population over the age of 25 was 40 % with similar prevalence rates across different strata of income [3], while the prevalence of diabetes among men worldwide has risen from 6.4 % in 2000 to 8.3 % in 2011 [4]. Other causes of CKD, such as IgA nephropathy and Balkan nephropathy, may be more related to regional influences, including genetic predisposition and exposure to nephrotoxic agents, respectively. With progressive global shifts toward urbanization, it is likely that diabetes, hypertension, and other lifestyle conditions like obesity will increasingly contribute to CKD development and progression. Concurrently, in developing countries, modifiable factors, such as infections, unregulated pharmaceutical administration, and other environmental factors, continue to contribute to CKD and therefore ESRD prevalence [2].

1.2 Provision of Dialysis Care

In the USA, the development of a delivery system for care for people with ESRD was born out of a necessity of acute treatment of victims of acute kidney injury (AKI) during combat during the Korean War, with additional attempts to treat AKI at a handful of hospitals across the USA. Subsequently, following the development of the Scribner shunt, the first maintenance dialysis facility opened in 1962 and, within a few years, the US Veterans Administration introduced a national, organized, population-based maintenance hemodialysis program. This was controversial at the time as

D. E. Weiner (✉)
Tufts Medical Center, Tufts University School of Medicine, Boston, MA, USA
e-mail: dweiner@tuftsmedicalcenter.org

A. K. Leonberg-Yoo
Division of Nephrology, Tufts Medical Center, Boston, MA, USA

A. K. Singh et al. (eds.), *Core Concepts in Dialysis and Continuous Therapies*, DOI 10.1007/978-1-4899-7657-4_1

dialysis was not thought to be the standard of care for individuals with chronic kidney failure. The explicit goal of these early maintenance dialysis programs was to save and rehabilitate individuals suffering from kidney failure, thus allowing these individuals to contribute to society [5]. Dialysis care was delivered in-center, typically 1–2 times per week either all day or all night. Demand for this therapy soon outgrew the capacity of these small programs. Interestingly, there was a large emphasis on home hemodialysis in the 1970s with 40 % of the dialysis-dependent population performing home hemodialysis.

Reflecting the high demand for maintenance dialysis and the fact that the only limitation to successful living for many people with kidney failure was financial, the US government implemented the Medicare entitlement for ESRD in 1973, thus establishing a federal program to provide dialysis for all Medicare eligible people in the USA. The Medicare ESRD program established hemodialysis as a nonexperimental therapy, legitimizing maintenance dialysis therapies.

While many countries today fund dialysis largely through governmental programs, some countries have adopted public–private partnerships and have emphasized the role of philanthropic organizations for providing dialysis care. These organizations play a role in the availability of kidney replacement therapy either by providing financial assistance with public and corporate donations or by organizing hemodialysis centers independent from hospital-based dialysis clinics. In particular, several Southeast Asian countries rely on these nongovernment organizations. For example, both Malaysia and Singapore who have ESRD prevalence rates of 980 and 1661 per million population, respectively, have experienced growth in their ESRD population over the past two decades, with a rate of change in prevalence rates in Malaysia of 51 % and in Singapore of 16 %. Growth in this population has occurred likely because of improved access to dialysis or transplantation. For example, in Malaysia, kidney replacement was virtually inaccessible until the 1980s, while, since the 1990s, hemodialysis treatment rates have increased eightfold [6]. This increase has occurred in a time of economic growth, increased partnership with nongovernmental organizations, and changes in health-care laws allowing such partnerships independent of government and hospitals to exist. The Malaysian government has also provided grant matching for all nongovernmental organizations performing subsidized treatments.

1.3 Prevalence of ESRD and ESRD Modalities

The prevalence of ESRD is rising rapidly, in large part reflecting aging populations in developed countries and an increase in the prevalence of comorbid conditions that lead to kidney disease, including diabetes, hypertension, and obesity. Prevalence rates can be also correlated to access to kidney replacement therapies, in part explaining recent rises in ESRD prevalence seen in lower income countries, although in many lower income countries availability of kidney replacement therapy remains limited due to a lack of financial resources. In both higher and lower income countries, regardless of financial resources, there may also be a substantial number of people who do not opt for kidney replacement therapy due to personal preference or cultural beliefs.

Prevalence rates are reported by multiple registries worldwide. One of the most mature data collection systems is the United States Renal Data System (USRDS), which was established in 1988 to characterize the US ESRD population and provide insights into patient care for individuals with kidney failure. In recent years, the USRDS data reports have been expanded to include international comparisons, with data from individual nations similarly drawn from local registries. Figure 1.1 presents worldwide prevalence data for treated ESRD patients in 2011, including those receiving dialysis therapies as well as kidney transplant. Prevalence rates of ESRD are consistently highest in Taiwan and Japan, with 2584 and 2309 per million population, respectively. The USA prevalence rates in 2011 are 1924 per million population.

The preferred modality for kidney replacement therapy may differ by region, and, even within the hemodialysis subset, there are numerous strategies for providing therapy. In the USA, for example, most hemodialysis is provided in-center at free-standing dialysis facilities. In contrast, the uptake of home dialysis has been higher in Canada, Australia, and New Zealand, while Australia has experimented with novel delivery strategies such as independent community house hemodialysis. In Europe, hemodiafiltration is common. Utilization of peritoneal dialysis (PD) also varies tremendously, likely reflecting economic incentives, national policies, availability of hemodialysis and PD, and experience with PD among providers. For example, Hong Kong has a PD first policy, such that nearly all patients with kidney failure initiate with PD and only transition to hemodialysis in the case of treatment failure. Even so, hemodialysis comprises the vast majority of kidney replacement therapy offered worldwide (Fig. 1.2).

Worldwide, use of PD is below 20 % in almost all countries that provided data to the USRDS for their 2013 data report. Major exceptions to this trend are Hong Kong and Mexico (Jalisco). In Hong Kong, PD is the preferred method for initiation of kidney replacement therapy. The history of Hong Kong's development of a dialysis program highlights an infrastructure that promotes a "PD first" policy. In the 1980s, community-level experience with PD showed that it was a safe, feasible, and cost-effective modality. The Central Renal Committee of Hong Kong devoted resources to expand continuous ambulatory PD across the city and implemented their PD-first strategy in 1985. This resulted in a

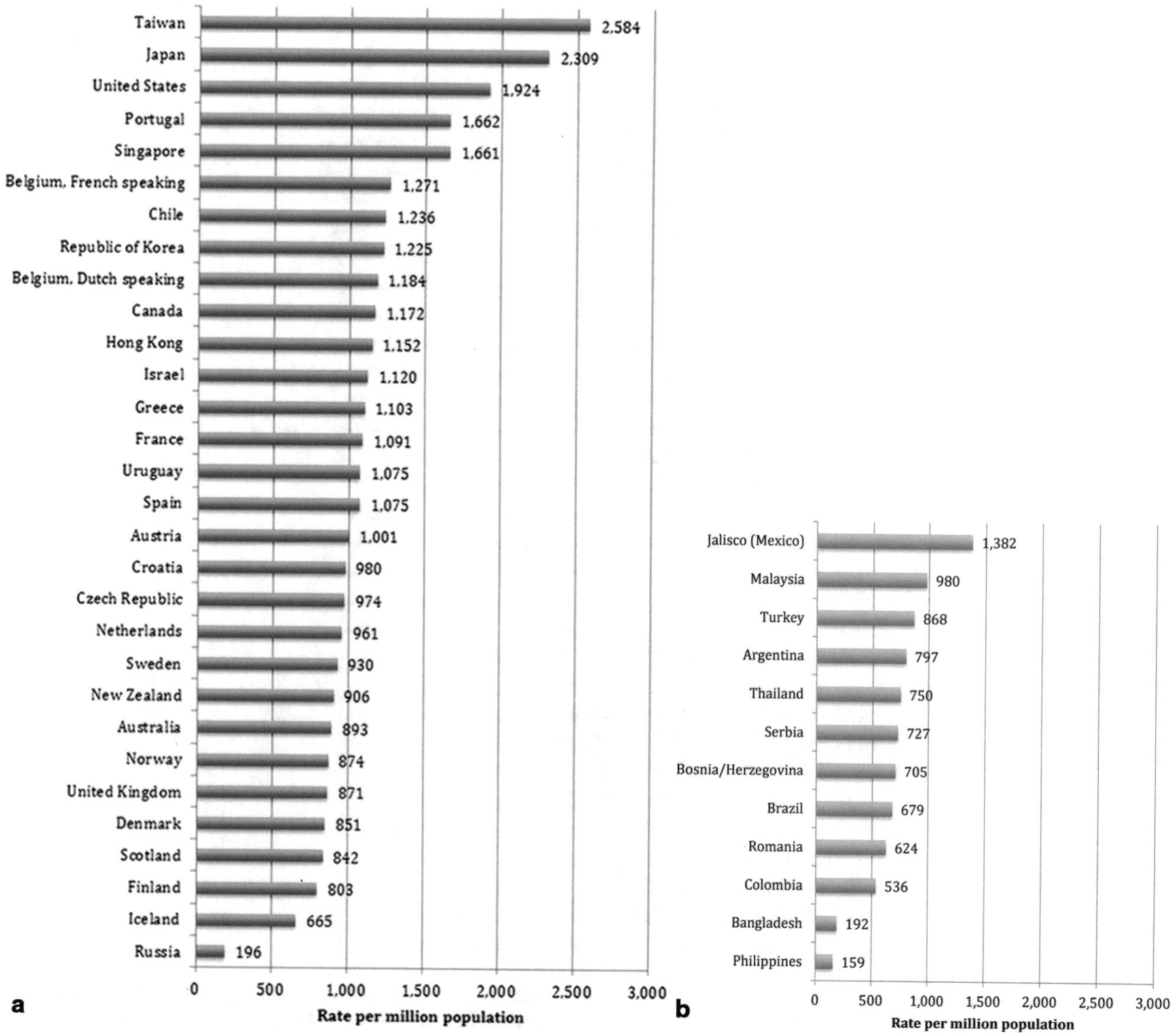

a

	Rate per million population
Taiwan	2,584
Japan	2,309
United States	1,924
Portugal	1,662
Singapore	1,661
Belgium, French speaking	1,271
Chile	1,236
Republic of Korea	1,225
Belgium, Dutch speaking	1,184
Canada	1,172
Hong Kong	1,152
Israel	1,120
Greece	1,103
France	1,091
Uruguay	1,075
Spain	1,075
Austria	1,001
Croatia	980
Czech Republic	974
Netherlands	961
Sweden	930
New Zealand	906
Australia	893
Norway	874
United Kingdom	871
Denmark	851
Scotland	842
Finland	803
Iceland	665
Russia	196

Axis: 0, 500, 1,000, 1,500, 2,000, 2,500, 3,000 — Rate per million population

b

	Rate per million population
Jalisco (Mexico)	1,382
Malaysia	980
Turkey	868
Argentina	797
Thailand	750
Serbia	727
Bosnia/Herzegovina	705
Brazil	679
Romania	624
Colombia	536
Bangladesh	192
Philippines	159

Axis: 0, 500, 1,000, 1,500, 2,000, 2,500, 3,000 — Rate per million population

Fig. 1.1 Prevalence of ESRD worldwide in 2011, with **a** high-income countries and **b** low- and middle-income countries. Gross national income values were derived from 2011 World Bank data. High-income economies are defined as GNI $12,746 or more. Prevalence for Taiwan, Japan, and the Philippines include only dialysis data

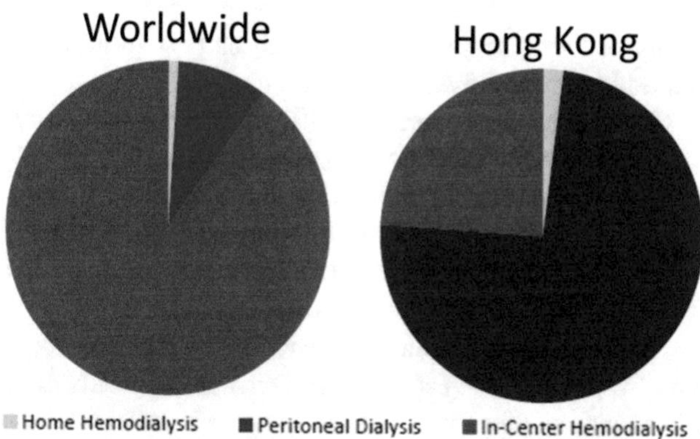

Fig. 1.2 Dialysis modality use worldwide among prevalent dialysis and in Hong Kong, where a peritoneal dialysis (PD) first policy is in place

robust infrastructure for care of PD patients, funded through government spending and charitable organizations. Currently, PD comprises approximately three quarters of maintenance dialysis in Hong Kong is PD, and hemodialysis is only pursued if there is a contraindication to PD [7].

Kidney transplantation is the other major kidney replacement modality, and, on average, is associated with better clinical outcomes than dialysis. There are multiple barriers that impact kidney transplant rates, including health-related concerns for acceptance of living kidney donors, infection risks and other sequelae of life-long immunosuppression, costs associated with transplant and transplant medications, cultural preferences and religious beliefs, and national policies regarding donor payment as well as opt-in versus opt-out donation policies for deceased donors. For example, Japan,

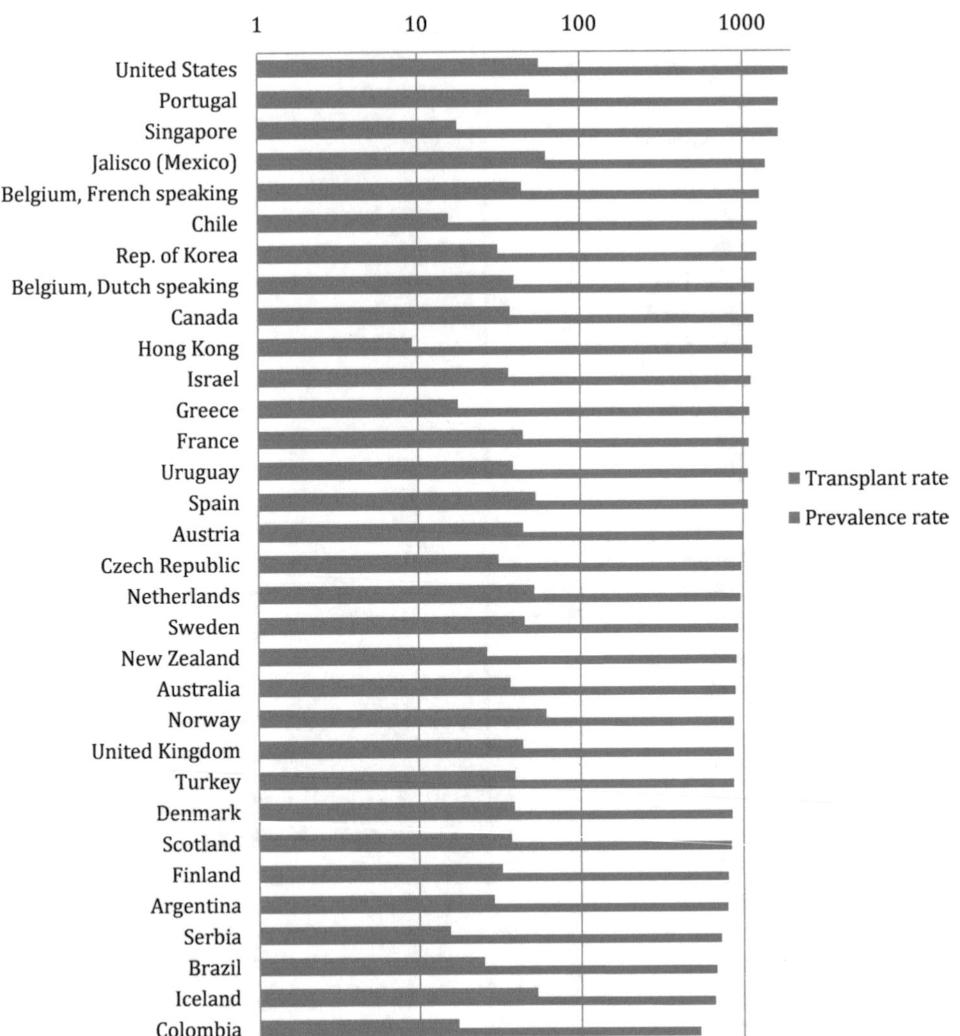

Fig. 1.3 Percentage of transplant relative to prevalence of ESRD worldwide. Values represent the rate per million population of transplant recipients relative to the prevalence rate per million population of ESRD. (Data are derived from the 2013 USRDS annual data report)

which has one of the highest prevalence rates of dialysis, has one of the lowest rates of transplantation. Less than 5 % of the population is registered for Japan's Kidney Transplant Network, which may reflect a cultural bias against transplantation of organs in general. Major variability exists in transplant rates worldwide (Fig. 1.3).

Comprehensive care for individuals with end-stage kidney disease is a large financial burden, and a higher prevalence of kidney failure leads to higher total cost of care. Nearly universal availability of treatments for end-stage kidney disease remains in the realm of high-income countries, and the reduced prevalence in lower-income countries likely stems from challenges in initiating and sustaining kidney replacement therapy programs. International population differences may highlight financial factors that impact the accessibility of kidney replacement therapy (Fig. 1.4). As outlined by White et al., in their publication discussing global equity in kidney replacement therapy availability, there is clearly a disparity between high-income countries versus low- and middle-income countries with regard to kidney replacement therapy prevalence [8]. This relates to the disease burden of dialysis equipment, associated support staff, and also access to care. Other factors including patient education and suitability of living environment for dialysis (PD specifically) can lead to lower prevalence rates of dialysis.

Overall, the prevalence of ESRD mirrors the prevalence of other comorbid conditions. As discussed earlier, chronic diseases and comorbid conditions like diabetes, hypertension, and obesity, all predispose to kidney failure. Already common in wealthier nations, the prevalence of these risk factors is rising more rapidly in developing nations, such that diabetes prevalence and affluence are no longer synonymous. Diabetes is the cause of ESRD in approximately 60 % of patients in Singapore, Jalisco (Mexico), and Malaysia, while other countries, including the USA, Japan, New Zealand, and the Republic of Korea, name diabetes as a cause of ESRD in over 40 % of the ESRD population.

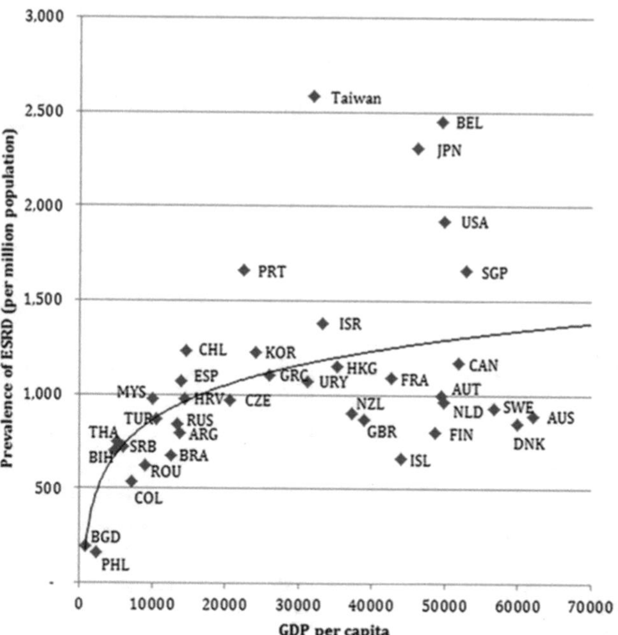

Fig. 1.4 Kidney replacement therapy rates in 2011 as a function of per capita gross domestic product (GDP). (Data on GDP per capita obtained from World Bank, 2011. Data on kidney replacement therapy prevalence from the USRDS 2013 Annual Data Report (www.usrds.org))

1.4 Incidence of ESRD

CKD, including kidney failure, is a worldwide health concern. Incidence rates have shown variable patterns of change over the past several years, with exponential growth in some countries such as Bangladesh and Mexico (Jalisco), whereas other countries like the USA and China (Hong Kong) have shown relative stability in incident ESRD cases over the past 5 years. In countries where mature financing systems for dialysis care are in place, changes in the availability of kidney replacement therapy are unlikely to drive changes in incidence rates, whereas in developing economies, greater funding and therefore availability of dialysis care may promote rising incidence rates. Review of country-specific data from 2006 to 2011 shows that the USA has experienced little change in the reported incidence rate of end-stage kidney disease (Table 1.1). Similar high-economic countries such as Canada and 14 out of 18 European countries have shown little growth in incident cases of end-stage kidney disease. Other countries, including Mexico (Jalisco), the Philippines, Thailand, Malaysia, and Iceland have seen fairly large growth in incidence. In fact, 14 of 41 countries have shown a change greater than 10% in incidence rates of end-stage kidney disease. In many of these countries, such as the Philippines and Malaysia, this may reflect increasing availability of dialysis related to changes in funding mechanisms as described earlier. Countries with exponential increases in incident rates such as Bangladesh are likely inflated due to poor reporting mechanisms or unavailability of dialysis in earlier years.

The difference in rates of incident end-stage kidney disease can be explained by many mechanisms, such as economic differences, cultural values, medical resource allocation, and medical knowledge among populations in general and health-care workers including knowledge about the progression of CKD. Many feel that the 2002 CKD staging system introduced by the Kidney Disease Outcomes Quality Initiative (KDOQI), by defining CKD as something more than just a kidney failure, provided an important framework for discussion of disease progression and risk factors for progression, facilitating implementation of strategies to slow progression of kidney disease and providing a timeframe for preparing for kidney failure. Interestingly, cost-effectiveness models show that population-based screening of CKD is not cost effective overall, although it may be beneficial in certain subgroups including people with hypertension or the elderly [9, 10]. This reflects the low incidence of kidney failure in people without risk factors as well as limited therapies beyond renin–angiotensin–aldosterone system blockade to reduce progression in many patients. Japan is one of the few countries that has routine screening of children and adults, using urine dipstick testing to evaluate for hematuria and proteinuria; given the very high prevalence of IgA nephropathy, signs of which may be apparent at an early age, screening in this population may be cost-effective when the financial burden of dialysis care is incorporated into cost models [11].

1.5 Expansion of Kidney Replacement Therapy to the Elderly Populations

The elderly comprise a growing portion of the incident and prevalent ESRD population. The estimated lifetime risk based on models simulating kidney disease development shows a strong relationship between older age and incident CKD in the US population, independent of comorbid conditions like diabetes and hypertension [12, 13]. The risk of progression is heightened by physiologic changes related to aging leading to a decline in kidney function, increased risk of AKI due to medication effects and episodes of hypovolemia and hypotension, and increased use of medications and medical interventions that can be harmful to kidneys. Not surprisingly, octogenarians and nonagenarians have increasing incidence rates of treated ESRD while, in the USA, the population from 20 to 60 years old has remained relatively stable (Fig. 1.5).

Due to a higher burden of age-related comorbidity, the elderly may have a higher prevalence of associated comorbidities, including cardiovascular disease, cerebrovascular disease, and physical and cognitive impairment, to name a

Table 1.1 End-stage renal disease (ESRD) incidence rates in 2006 and 2011 (per million population). (Data are derived from the 2013 USRDS annual data report)

	2006	2011	Percent change from 2006 to 2011
Argentina	141	156	10.6
Australia	118	110	−6.8
Austria	160	137	−14.4
Bangladesh	8	32	300.0
Belgium, Dutch speaking	192	182	−5.2
Belgium, French speaking	187	188	0.5
Bosnia/Herzegovina	133	121	−9.0
Brazil	185	176	−4.9
Canada	166	161	−3.0
Chile	141	197	39.7
Colombia	126	93	−26.2
Croatia	142	119	−16.2
Czech Republic	186	172	−7.5
Denmark	119	111	−6.7
Finland	87	85	−2.3
France	144	149	3.5
Greece	198	203	2.5
Hong Kong	149	157	5.4
Iceland	69	103	49.3
Israel	192	188	−2.1
Jalisco (Mexico)	346	527	52.3
Japan	275	295	7.3
Republic of Korea	185	205	10.8
Malaysia	138	209	51.4
Netherlands	113	117	3.5
New Zealand	119	108	−9.2
Norway	100	102	2.0
Philippines	75	103	37.3
Portugal	232[a]	226	−2.6
Romania	75	127	69.3
Russia	28	43	53.6
Scotland	116	97	−16.4
Singapore	241	279	15.8
Spain	128	121	−5.5
Sweden	130	122	−6.2
Taiwan	418	361[b]	−13.6
Thailand	139	227	63.3
Turkey	192	238	24.0
UK	115	113	−1.7
USA	366	362	−1.1
Uruguay	138	177	28.3

[a] 2008 data
[b] 2010 data

few. This creates a complex subgroup of ESRD patients that requires additional advanced care planning and increased resources. Certain regional movements, including the Choosing Wisely campaign and the Renal Physicians Association in the USA, have started to address ethical issues surrounding the aging ESRD population, working to identify the optimal balance among aggressive medical care, quality of life and duration of life in this vulnerable population [14]. The decision to initiate or continue kidney replacement therapy in the elderly will need increasing attention given the aging ESRD population with an emphasis on balancing individualized risks and benefits of dialysis therapy with patients' values and goals.

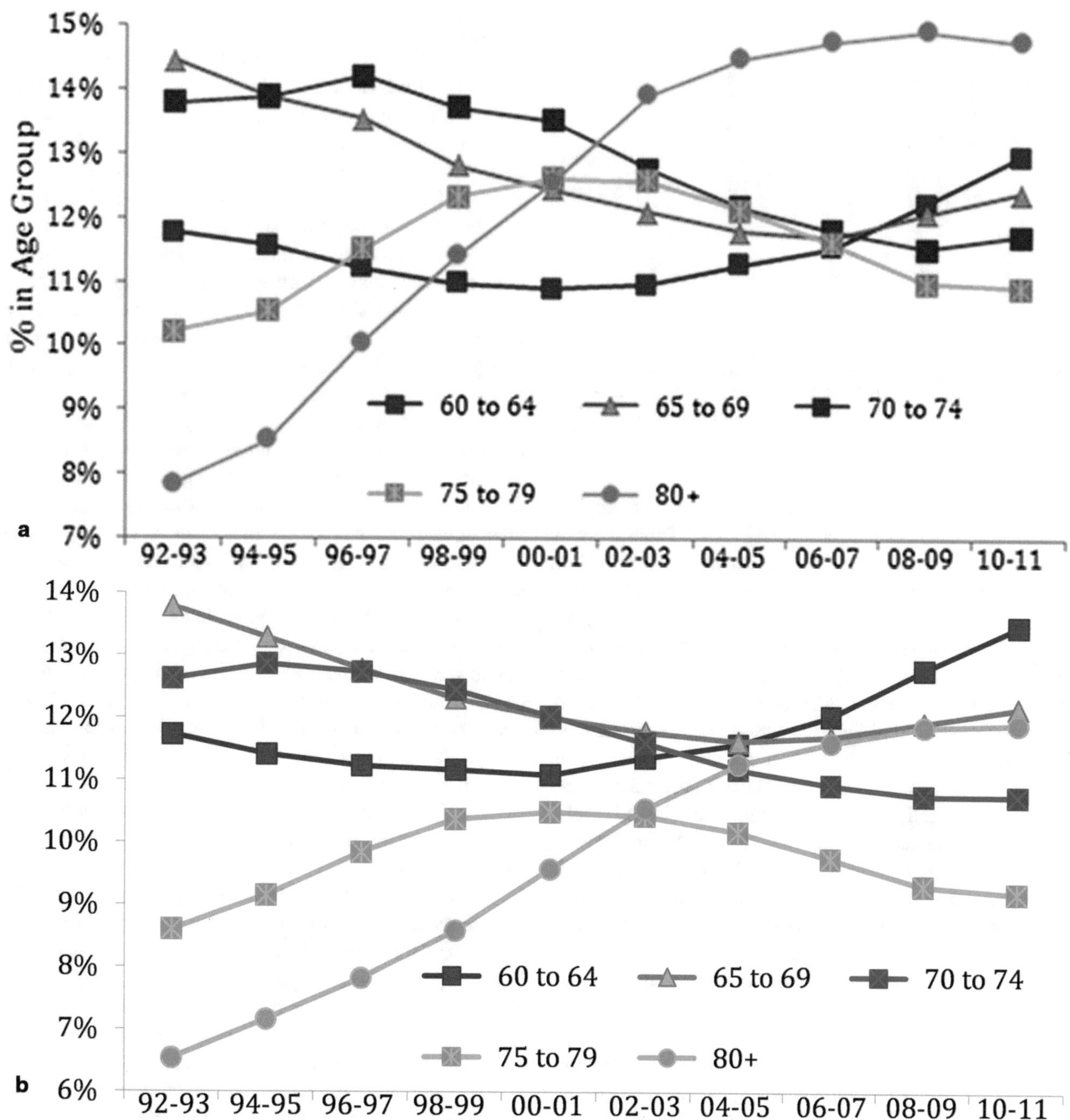

Fig. 1.5 CKD and ESRD. Incident (**a**) and prevalent (**b**) hemodialysis and peritoneal dialysis (PD) patients in the USA. (Data derived using data supplied by the USRDS RenDER)

1.6 Outcomes Among ESRD Patients

The purpose of dialysis and kidney transplantation can be considered broadly as replacement of kidney function to permit sufficient health to engage in activities and achieve life goals. These goals differ from person to person, making the decision to receive kidney replacement therapy and the choice of a specific modality very individualized. Across the ESRD spectrum, outcomes vary, based largely on preexisting comorbid conditions but perhaps also on treatment modality. Clinically relevant outcomes include readily measureable factors like mortality and hospitalization as well as outcomes that are more difficult to quantify, such as quality of life and symptom burden.

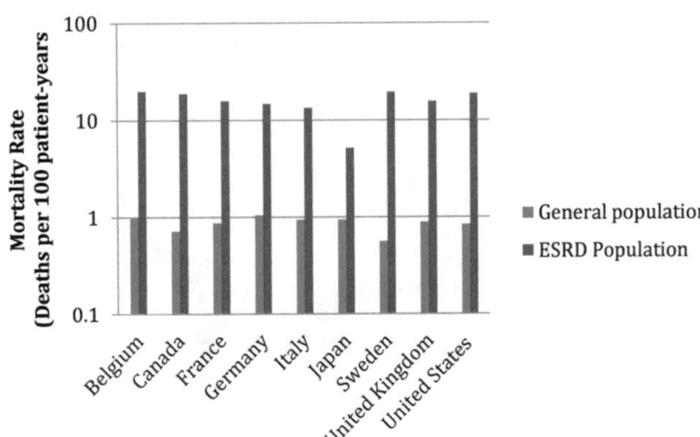

Fig. 1.6 Mortality rate of ESRD after 365 days of dialysis compared with country specific death rates. ESRD mortality rates from 2002 to 2004, 2005 to 2008 cohort (DOPPS data) and death rates from 2012 (WHO Life Tables)

One of the best resources for evaluating outcomes in ESRD is the Dialysis Outcomes and Practice Patterns Study (DOPPS), an international, longitudinal observational cohort study of hemodialysis patients that has studied patient outcomes and risk factors for outcomes, using differing practices among countries to highlight important clinical practices and risk factors [15]. DOPPS data suggest that there are substantial mortality differences as well as treatment and patient-specific differences across nations. In many of the DOPPS reports, outcome differences remain significant, even when adjusting for patient case mix [16]. Factors that vary internationally and may affect mortality include dialysis adequacy (including dosage and duration), ultrafiltration rates and volume management, vascular access, and anemia and bone mineral disorder management. In DOPPS data from 2002 to 2004 and 2005 to 2008, the overall mortality rate among DOPPS hemodialysis participants is 15 per 100 patient-years, with the plurality of these deaths occurring in the early phase of initiation of dialysis (less than or equal to 120 days after initiation (Fig. 1.6).

Mortality in ESRD has improved with time; however, mortality rates remain significantly higher than seen in many other chronic medical conditions. Unadjusted mortality rates for individuals in the USA with ESRD in 2011 were 246 per 1000 patient-years, actually reflecting substantial improvement (16% decreased mortality rate) over the past decade [17]. In comparison, when looking at other chronic medical conditions such as all cancers, mortality rates are approximately 137 deaths per 1000 patient years with an average decline of annual death rates by 13% per year from 2001 to 2010 [18]. Similarly, for cardiovascular disease, improvements in mortality in the dialysis population have not matched improvements seen in the general population [19].

Diabetes, the leading cause of ESRD worldwide, with up to 60% of kidney failure due to diabetes in countries like Singapore, Malaysia, and Mexico (Jalisco), remains an important predictor of poor outcomes in individuals receiving kidney replacement therapy. Five-year survival among individuals with diabetes receiving dialysis approximates 33%, which is far lower than for dialysis patients with hypertension (42%) and glomerulonephritis (53%) as the primary cause of kidney failure [14, 20]. This likely reflects additional complications of diabetes including systemic vascular disease. This survival disparity lessens among patients treated with kidney transplantation, potentially reflecting that only the healthiest patients with kidney failure receive a kidney transplant. Individuals with diabetes who received a transplant have 5-year survival rates of 75–83%, depending on cadaveric versus living donor kidney transplant [21].

Mortality rates are also affected by kidney replacement therapy modality. There are no generalizable clinical trials that compare outcomes associated with ESRD modalities, although data from cohort studies strongly suggest survival advantages with kidney transplant versus dialysis and likely similar survival among patients undergoing in-center hemodialysis versus PD. A systematic review of 110 studies showed that kidney transplantation was associated with lower mortality and other clinically relevant outcomes including reduced cardiovascular events and improved quality of life compared with dialysis and that the mortality benefit appeared to increase in magnitude over time, a finding that likely reflects higher short-term risk of death in per-transplant period [21]. Several studies also suggest that transplantation earlier in kidney failure may be associated with longer allograft survival, providing some support for preemptive transplantation.

Reported mortality differences across dialysis modalities are inconsistent, possibly reflecting baseline differences in study populations that affect who receive specific therapies. For example, in the USA, patients treated with PD have historically been younger and healthier than those treated with hemodialysis; additionally, socioeconomic status and education may be higher among PD patients, reflecting both patient self-selection and provider biases about ability to perform self-care. Within the ESRD population, short-term mortality rates show an early survival advantage for PD compared to hemodialysis [22]; however, this survival advantage over time wanes, leaving them with similar long-term mortality risk (see Table 1.2 for a summary of major studies evaluating survival by modality). Factors influencing this early survival advantage associated with PD may include fewer comorbid conditions, including diabetes, as well as the type of vascular access used for hemodialysis. One recent study suggested that higher early mortality risk among hemodialysis patients was driven by use of central vascular catheters for incident vascular access and that, when PD was compared to patients initiating hemodialysis with a functioning arteriovenous fis-

Table 1.2 Observational studies comparing mortality between incident hemodialysis and peritoneal dialysis (PD) patients

	Country	Cohort period	Sample size	Statistical approach	Follow-up	Key results
Asia	Taiwan [26]	1997–2006	HD 4271 PD 4271	Propensity score match with Cox proportional hazards	5 years	No significant overall difference; younger PD patients with better survival
	Republic of Korea [27]	2005–2008	HD 24,399 PD 7881	Cox proportional hazards and propensity score matching	Through December 2009	PD with 20 % higher risk of overall mortality; younger patients (<55) with equivalent survival
Australia/New Zealand	New Zealand and Australia [28]	1991–2005	HD 14,733 PD 10,554	Cox proportional hazards model including analyses in propensity-score quartiles	Through December 2005	11 % lower risk for death with PD in first year; 33 % higher risk with PD thereafter
Europe	Finland [29]	2000–2009	HD 3246 PD 1217	Cox proportional hazards model	10 years	No significant difference; trend towards lower risk in younger patients (<45) with PD
	Denmark [30]	1990–1999	HD 3281 PD 1640	Cox proportional hazards	Through December 1999	PD with 14 % lower risk of death within first 2 years, irrespective of diabetes or age
	Netherlands [31]	1987–2002	HD 10,841 PD 5802	Cox proportional hazards model	16 years	Lower mortality risk with younger, nondiabetic PD patients in first 15 months; no difference thereafter No difference in older nondiabetic PD patients in first 15 months, but higher risk after 15 months
	Scotland [32]	1982–2006	HD 2107 PD 1090	Cox proportional hazards model	Through December 2006	No survival difference in PD patients listed for transplant
	ERA-EDTA registry [33]	1998–2006	HD 12,731 PD 3097	Cox proportional hazards model	3 years	PD with 18 % lower mortality risk. Survival benefit was greater in individuals without comorbidity
North America	USA [34]	1995–1998	HD 767 PD 274	Cox proportional hazards model with propensity score adjustment	7 years	No significant difference in first year Higher mortality risk in second year with PD
	USA [35]	2001–2004	HD 22,360 PD 1358	Marginal structural model	2 years	Lower mortality risk with PD (48 %)
	USA [36]	1996–2004	HD 620,020 PD 64,406	Marginal structural model	5 years	No significant difference in 5 year adjusted survival of PD patients
	USA [37]	2003	HD 6337 PD 6337	Propensity-score matched cohort	4 years	Lower early mortality risk in PD patients; however similar late survival
	Canada [38]	1998–2006	HD 4538 PD 2035	Cox proportional hazard		No difference in early or late mortality with PD
	Canada [39]	1991–2004	HD 32,531 PD 14,308	Cox proportional hazards model	Through December 2007	PD with lower mortality risk in first 2 years. No difference after 2 years
South America	Colombia [40]	2001–2003	HD 437 PD 486	Cox proportional hazards model	Through December 2005	No difference in mortality. Lower risk of death for young, nondiabetic patients treated with PD

Table 1.3 Dialysis reimbursement policies in five European countries, the USA and one Canadian province. (Derived using data extracted from Vanholder et al. [41])

	Belgium	Germany	The Netherlands	UK	France	USA	Ontario, Canada
Reimbursement per week for dialysis services	HD > PD	Variable	HD > PD	HD > PD	HD > PD	HD = PD	HD > PD
Inclusive reimbursement package	No	No	Yes	No	No	Yes	No
Includes nephrologist fees	Yes	No	Yes	No	Yes[a]	No	No
Includes most oral medications	No	No	No	No	No	No	No
Three sessions per week	Yes[a]	Yes[a]	No	Yes	Yes[b]	Yes[c]	Yes
Case mix differential reimbursement							
Chronic viral infection	No	Yes	No	Yes	No	No	No
Vascular access	No	No	No	Yes	No	No	No
Quality metric scores linked to reimbursement	No	Yes	No	No	No	Yes	No

[a] Refers to in-hospital hemodialysis only
[b] Four sessions are allowed
[c] Requires medical justification

tula, hemodialysis patients actually fared slightly better [23, 24]. Studies suggest that patient quality of life may be better with PD. For example, a prospective cohort study involving 37 dialysis centers in the USA showed that PD patients were 1.5 times more likely to call their care excellent overall as compared to hemodialysis patients [25]. Given the lack of an obvious mortality difference, a practical approach to modality selection that incorporates resource availability, patient preference, and consideration of specific comorbid conditions that may favor one modality should be accounted for when evaluating treatment options.

Comparisons across international samples show important differences in patient outcomes, some of which reflect societal emphases, some of which represent population differences, and some of which may reflect different financial incentives. Among a sample of seven European and North American countries, reimbursement varies quite dramatically between modality of dialysis and inclusion of products or services in the reimbursement package (Table 1.3). In the majority of countries sampled, hospital/in-center hemodialysis was most highly reimbursed, with the exception of Germany, where reimbursement was higher for PD, and the USA, where there is similar reimbursement regardless of dialysis modality. Inclusion of different products, including physician fees, within a reimbursement package also differs among countries, with most countries excluding ESA therapy and nephrologists fees from the dialysis payment bundle. There also is a differential payment scale for clinically complex patients including individuals with certain infections, diabetes, or elderly age in Germany. Only two countries are reimbursed relative to clinical quality metrics of target hemoglobin and dialysis adequacy. This practice may change as cost-effective strategies and quality improvement are emphasized within dialysis practice patterns [41].

1.7 Conclusion

The prevalence and incidence of ESRD continues to rise worldwide. Given the increasing burden of conditions that cause kidney failure, such as diabetes and hypertension, this pattern is likely to persist. In developing nations, where dialysis may become increasingly available, tremendous increases in the treated ESRD population are possible, and coping with the costs associated with ESRD therapies will be challenging. Mortality rates remain high among dialysis patients, although recent data suggest some improvement in outcomes. While transplant appears to be the optimal form of kidney replacement therapy for many younger patients with longer life expectancy, there appears to be little difference in survival between in-center hemodialysis and PD, making individualized patient preference paramount in deciding between these modalities. Future research is needed to evaluate the optimal role for more frequent hemodialysis modalities, fusion modalities (concurrent hemodialysis and PD) and newer hemodialysis strategies like hemodiafiltration. Outcomes-based measures on a global perspective will be helpful in determining the focus of research and optimal clinical management to ensure best-practice for this population.

References

1. GBD 2013. Mortality and Causes of Death Collaborators. Global, regional, and national age-sex specific all-cause and cause-specific mortality for 240 causes of death, 1990–2013: a systematic analysis for the Global Burden of Disease Study 2013. Lancet. 2015;385:117–71.
2. Jha V, Garcia-Garcia G, Iseki K, Li Z, Naicker S, Plattner B, et al. Chronic kidney disease: global dimension and perspectives. Lancet. 2013;283(9888):260–72.

3. Ikeda N, Sapienza D, Guerrero R, Aekplakorn W, Naghavi M, Mokdad AH, et al. Control of hypertension with medication: a comparative analysis of national surveys in 20 countries. Bull World Health Organ. 2014;92:10–9C.
4. Whiting DR, Guariguata L, Weil C, Shaw J. IDF diabetes atlas: global estimates of the prevalence of diabetes for 2011 and 2030. Diabetes Res Clin Pract. 2011;94(3):311–21.
5. Watnick S, Crowley ST. ESRD care within the US Department of Veterans Affairs: a forward-looking program with an illuminating past. Am J Kidney Dis. 2014;63(3):521–9.
6. Morad Z, Choong HL, Tungsanga K, Suhardjono A. Building philanthropic support for renal replacement services in Southeast Asia: lessons from Indonesia, Malaysia, Singapore and Thailand. Am J Kidney Dis. (Manuscript draft).
7. Li PK, Chow KM. Peritoneal-dialysis-first policy made successful: perceptions and actions. Am J Kidney Dis. 2013;62(5):993–1005.
8. White SL, Chadban SJ, Jan S, Chapman JR, Cass A. How can we achieve global equity in provision of renal replacement therapy? Bull World Health Organ. 2008;86(3):229–37.
9. Manns B, Hemmelgarn B, Tonelli M, Au F, Carter Chiasson T, Dong J, et al. Population based screening for chronic kidney disease: cost effectiveness study. BMJ. 2010;341:c5869.
10. Boulware LE, Jaar BG, Tarver-Car ME, Brancati FL, Powe NR. Screening for proteinuria in US adults: a cost-effectiveness analysis. JAMA. 2003;290(23):3101–14.
11. Kondo M, Yamagata K, Hoshi S-L, Saito C, Asahi K, Moriyama T, et al. Cost-effectiveness of chronic kidney disease mass screening test in Japan. Clin Exp Nephrol. 2012;16(2):279–97.
12. Grams ME, Chow EKH, Segev DL, Coresh J. Lifestime incidence of CKD stage 3–5 in the United States. Am J Kidney Dis. 2013;62(2):245–52.
13. Stevens LA, Viswanathan G, Weiner DE. Chronic kidney disease and end-stage renal disease in the elderly population: current prevalence, future projections, and clinical significance. Adv Chronic Kidney Dis. 2010;17(4):293–301.
14. Williams AW, Dwyer AC, Eddy AA, Fink JC, Jaber BL, Linas SL, et al. Critical and honest conversations: the evidence behind the "choosing wisely" campaign recommendations by the American Society of Nephrology. Clin J Am Soc Nephrol. 2012;7:1–12.
15. Young EW, Goodkin DA, Mapes DL, Port FK, Keen ML, Chen K, et al. The Dialysis Outcomes and Practice Patterns Study (DOPPS): an international hemodialysis study. Kidney Int. 2000;57:S74–81.
16. Robinson BM, Bieber B, Pisoni RL, Port FK. Dialysis Outcomes and Practice Patterns Study (DOPPS): its strengths, limitations, and role in informing practices and policies. Clin J Am Soc Nephrol. 2012;7:1897–905.
17. U.S. Renal Data System, USRDS 2013 Annual data report: atlas of chronic kidney disease and end-stage renal disease in the United States, National Institutes of Health, National Institute of Diabetes and Digestive and Kidney Diseases, Bethesda, MD, 2013.
18. SEER 9 incidence 1975–2011 & U.S. mortality 1975–2010, all races, both sexes. rates are age-adjusted.
19. Roberts MA, Polinghorne KR, McDonald SP, Ierino FL. Secular trends in cardiovascular mortality rates of patients receiving dialysis compared with the general population. Am J Kidney Dis. 2011;58(1):64–72.
20. Locatelli F, Pozzoni P, Vecchio LD. Renal replacement therapy in patients with diabetes and end-stage renal disease. J Am Soc Nephrol. 2004;15(Suppl 1):S25–9.
21. Tonelli M, Wiebe N, Knoll G, Bello A, Browne S, Jadhav D, et al. Kidney transplantation compared with dialysis in clinically relevant outcomes. Am J Transplant. 2011;11(10):2093–109.
22. McDonald SP, Marshall MR, Johnson DW, Polkinghorne KR. Relationship between dialysis modality and mortality. J Am Soc Nephrol. 2009;20:155–63.
23. Perl J, Wald R, McFarlane P, Bargman JM, Vonesh E, Na Y. Hemodialysis vascular access modifies the association between dialysis modality and survival. J Am Soc Nephrol. 2011;22(6):1113–21.
24. Mehrotra R, Chiu YW, Kalantar-Zadeh K, Bargman J, Vonesh E. Similar outcomes with hemodialysis and peritoneal dialysis in patients with end-stage renal disease. Arch Intern Med. 2011;171:110–8.
25. Rubin HR, Fink NE, Plantinga LC, Sadler JH, Kliger AS, Powe NR. Patient ratings of dialysis care with peritoneal dialysis vs hemodialysis. JAMA. 2004;291(6):697–703.
26. Chang YK, Hsu CC, Hwang SJ, Chen PC, Huang CC, Lit TC, Sung FC. A comparative assessment of survival between propensity score-matched patients with peritoneal dialysis and hemodialysis in Taiwan. Medicine (Baltimore). 2012;91(3):144–51.
27. Kim H, Kim KH, Park K, Kang SW, Yoo TH, Ahn SV. A population-based approach indicates an overall higher patient mortality with peritoneal dialysis compared to hemodialysis in Korea. Kidney Int. 2014;86(5):991–1000.
28. McDonald SP, Marshall MR, Johnson DW, Polkinghorne KR. Relationship between dialysis modality and mortality. J Am Soc Nephrol. 2009;20(1):155–63.
29. Haapio M, Helve J, Kyllonen L, Gronhagen-Riska C, Finne P. Modality of chronic renal replacement therapy and survival—a complete cohort from Finland, 2000–2009. Nephrol Dial Transplant. 2013;28(12):3072–81.
30. Heaf JG, Lokkegaard H, Madsen M. Initial survival advantage of peritoneal dialysis relative to haemodialysis. Nephrol Dial Transplant. 2002;17(1):112–7.
31. Liem YS, Wong JB, Hunink MG, de Charro FT, Winkelmayer WC. Comparison of hemodialysis and peritoneal dialysis survival in The Netherlands. Kidney Int. 2007;71(2):153–8.
32. Traynor JP, Thomson PC, Simpson K, Ayansina DT, Prescott GJ, Mactier RA. Comparison of patient survival in non-diabetic transplant-listed patients initially treated with haemodialysis or peritoneal dialysis. Nephrol Dial Transplant. 2011;26(1):245–52.
33. van de Luijtgaarden MW, Noordzij M, Stel VS, Ravani P, Jarraya F, Collart F, et al. Effects of comorbid and demographic factors on dialysis modality choic and related patient survival in Europe. Nephrol Dial Transplant. 2011;26(9):2940–7.
34. Jaar BG, Coresh J, Plantinga LC, Fink NE, Klag MJ, Levey AS, et al. Comparing the risk for death with peritoneal dialysis and hemodialysis in a national cohort of patients with chronic kidney disease. Ann Intern Med. 2005;143(3):174–83.
35. Lukowsky LR, Mehrotra R, Kheifets L, Arah OA, Nissenson AR, Kalantar-Zadeh K. Comparing mortality of peritoneal and hemodialysis patients in the first 2 years of dialysis therapy: a marginal structural model analysis. Clin J Am Soc Nephrol. 2013;8(4):619–28.
36. Mehrotra R, Chiu YW, Kalantar-Zadeh K, Bargman J, Vonesh E. Similar outcomes with hemodialysis and peritoneal dialysis in patients with end-stage renal disease. Arch Intern Med. 2011;171(2):110–8.
37. Weinhandl ED, Foley RN, Gilbertson DT, Ameson TJ, Snyder JJ, Collins AJ. Propensity-matched mortality comparison of incident hemodialysis and peritoneal dialysis patients. J Am Soc Nephrol. 2010;21(3):499–506.
38. Quinn RR, Hux JE, Oliver MJ, Austin PC, TOnelli M, Laupacis A. Selection bias explains apparent differential mortality between dialysis modalities. J Am Soc Nephrol. 2011;22(8):1534–42.
39. Yeates K, Zhu N, Vonesh E, Trpeski L, Blake P, Fenton S. Hemodialysis and peritoneal dialysis are associated with similar outcomes for end-stage renal disease treatment in Canada. Nephrol Dial Transplant. 2012;27(9):3568–75.
40. Sanabria M, Munoz J, Trillos C, Hernandez G, Latorre C, Diaz CS, et al. Dialysis outcomes in Colombia (DOC) study: a comparison of patient survival on peritoneal dialysis vs hemodialysis in Colombia. Kidney Int Suppl. 2008;108:S165–72.
41. Vanholder R, Davenport A, Hannedouche T, Kooman T, Kribben A, Lameire N, et al. Reimbursement of dialysis: a comparison of seven countries. J Am Soc Nephrol. 2012;23:1291–8.

2 Technical Aspects of Hemodialysis

Sandip Mitra and Nicos Mitsides

2.1 Introduction

The goal of renal replacement therapy is primarily to restore the chemical and fluid balance in uremia (milieu interior). In hemodialysis (HD), the processes of diffusion and convection are combined to achieve solute exchange and water removal across a semipermeable membrane to provide the necessary blood purification. Diffusion takes place through random movement of molecules that lead to a net solute transfer from higher to lower concentration between compartments separated by the semipermeable membrane. The diffusive capacity depends on the concentration gradient, the diffusive coefficient of the solute, and membrane properties [1]. Convection involves transfer of fluid volumes accompanied by the removal of dissolved larger solutes across the dialysis membrane (ultrafiltration). This process is dependent on the ultrafiltration rate and the solute sieving coefficient for the membrane [2]. In a typical HD session, both these exchange processes occur simultaneously and their contribution to overall purification can be difficult to quantify separately. The HD system is comprised of the blood compartment, the dialysate compartment, and the membrane interface. These components of dialysis technology and their application to renal replacement therapy are discussed below.

S. Mitra (✉)
Department of Renal Medicine, Manchester Academic Health Science Centre, University of Manchester & Central Manchester Foundation Trust, Oxford Road, Manchester M13 9WL, UK
e-mail: sandip.mitra@cmft.nhs.uk

N. Mitsides
Department of Renal Medicine, University of Manchester and Devices for Dignity Healthcare Technology Co-operative, Central Manchester University Hospitals NHS Foundation Trust, Manchester, Lancashire, UK

2.2 The Extracorporeal Blood Circuit

The extracorporeal circuit provides the necessary conduit for transporting blood from the patient's vascular system (via arteriovenous access) to the artificial kidney at a defined flow rate and then returning the dialyzed blood back to the patient. This must be achieved without damage to the blood cell components, coagulation of blood, or loss of integrity that can result in blood loss or contamination with microorganisms from the external environment. The closed extracorporeal setup consists of a blood access device (needles or catheter) connected by tubing to the dialyzer or the artificial kidney. All the circuit components in contact with blood are made of inert or highly biocompatible material and sterilized prior to packaging [3–5]. An extracorporeal blood volume of approximately 80–250 ml circulates outside an adult patient at any one time [6]. During HD, blood from the patient's vascular access (arterial needle) flows into the dialyzer and then back to the patient's access (venous needle). These afferent and efferent parts of the extracorporeal circuit are differentiated by color coding of two sections of the blood tubing: arterial (pre-dialyzer, red) and venous (post-dialyzer, blue).

2.2.1 Pre-dialyzer (Arterial Limb)

This entire part of the blood circuit (pre-dialyzer) constitutes the "arterial limb" of the circuit. The blood is propelled into the arterial tubing by a negative pressure (suction pressure) mechanically generated and maintained by a peristaltic blood pump (to draw the blood and propel it through the circuit). The pump could deliver blood to the dialyzer at rates that can vary from 0 to 600 ml/min but typically set between 300 and 550 ml/min, restricted by the pressures generated within the extracorporeal circuit. The machine displays the achieved blood flow rate (Qb, ml/min), calculated from the number of revolutions of the pump per minute and the volume of tubing segment within the pump [6]. The latter is

A. K. Singh et al. (eds.), *Core Concepts in Dialysis and Continuous Therapies*, DOI 10.1007/978-1-4899-7657-4_2

calculated from the predefined internal diameter of the blood pump segment. The arterial pump effect is measured as the "arterial pressure," which is a negative value. As the arterial pressure becomes more negative the tubing insert becomes flatter and the tubing calculated Qb is higher than the actual flow rate. Some machines automatically correct the displayed blood flow on the machine for the measured arterial pressure to derive the effective or delivered Qb (or effective blood flow rate (EBFR)) [7]. At pressures −150 mmHg or lower, EBFR deviates significantly from calculated Qb and can lead to loss of treatment efficiency. Excessive negative pressures could indicate poor arterial inflow due to vascular access problems and should be avoided [6].

The arterial pump rollers press against the blood column to drive the blood through the circuit; hence, tight rollers can damage blood cells causing hemolysis. If the rollers are too loose this may reduce the EBFR. Modern rollers use springs to create occlusion, so the pump tubing segment must be inserted properly. In case of emergency, all machines are provided with a handle to rotate the pump manually (hand cranking) and at a rate just fast enough to keep venous pressure in the distal circuit at the pre-alarm level.

While the blood circulates through the extracorporeal circuit and the artificial kidney, its natural disposition is to coagulate. Anticoagulation is necessary to prevent formation of microthrombi, blood coagulation, and resulting loss of circuit. A heparin-infusion driver, positioned after the blood pump and prior to the dialyzer inlet, adds a measured dose of the anticoagulant via an infusion port into the circulating blood. The location of the port facilitates the heparin to be pushed towards the dialyzer inlet and avoid the negative force of the blood pump drawing up air from the heparin line.

There is often an additional port for saline infusion, located on the arterial blood tubing in the pre-pump segment, so saline bags can be set up for priming or fluid infusions. If the saline infusion line is not clamped correctly, too much fluid or air can enter the extracorporeal blood circuit. Saline port connection errors between the arterial and venous part of the circuit can lead to potentially catastrophic consequences [8]. Traditionally, saline bags are set up to run fluid infusions. However, modern machines capable of producing ultrapure water enable the use of online-generated high-quality fluid to prime, rinse, and infuse a measured fluid bolus into the patient, obviating the need for saline bags.

The anticoagulated blood column is then propelled into the dialyzer via the mechanical force generated by the blood pump and a positive pressure inside the artificial kidney, which facilitates a hydrostatic gradient across the dialyzer membrane required for ultrafiltration.

Some machines can estimate the total blood volume processed (liters) within the dialyzer for a single treatment by count of blood pump turns. It is not a measure of delivered dialysis dose but can be a useful tool for quality assurance especially if there are significant treatment interruptions for a single session.

2.2.2 Post-dialyzer Venous Limb

After the blood is subjected to the processes of diffusion and convection within the dialyzer, it enters the "venous limb" of the circuit, returning blood back into the patient. Although the pressure in the venous limb distal to the dialyzer gradually falls, it remains sufficiently positive in order to enable return of the blood to the body. The pressure within this part of the circuit is monitored by the venous blood pressure monitor, which is located typically just before the air bubble chamber. High venous pressures indicate an obstruction in the venous limb distal to this point, and an alarm window can be set up to bring this to the attention of the dialysis staff. High-pressure alarms warrant, at first, a check of the lines for kinks and clamps. Additionally, venous needle blow out or clots in the air trap ought to be excluded. In the absence of any obvious cause, often the needle position may need to be adjusted or rotated [6]. Persistently high venous pressures, however, can be harmful and lead to potential loss of circuit. It could also indicate a stenosis within the vascular access [9]. Trends in such pressure changes can be employed as a screening tool for vascular access monitoring [10]. A low venous pressure is most commonly associated with low arterial pressure due to poor arterial flow or, alternatively, a wet venous isolator.

2.2.3 Air Trap (Bubble Chamber) and Air Detector

There is a distinct apparatus that sits in the venous limb between the dialyzer and the patient's venous access and acts as a gateway for safe return of the blood back into the patient. The air detector, an ultrasonic device, continuously checks for air or foam in the blood pathway at this location throughout the dialysis treatment by detecting changes to ultrasonic signal induced by the presence of air bubbles. The air trap will prevent entry of large air bubbles into the returning needle of the AV fistula.

An air detector's alarm sensitivity limits are preset by the manufacture but can be recalibrated by qualified technicians. When the air detector senses air, it will trigger audible and visual alarms, stop the blood pump, and clamp the venous blood tubing to stop return of the blood to the body and prevent air getting into the bloodstream. Of course, air leak beyond the detector can go undetected by this setup. The air detector and the venous line clamps must always be checked prior to the start of every dialysis session, as per manufacturer's instructions. The air trap chamber also serves to prevent blood clots (microthrombi) generated within the extracorporeal circuit from reaching the patient, by using a fine mesh screen.

Air in bloodlines and dialyzer typically occur due to underfilled air trap chamber, inadequate priming, empty saline bag, loose connections, or dialysis needle removal/dislodgement while blood pump is still running. Saline priming of the dialyzer and blood tubing and deaeration of the fluid pathway are important preparatory steps prior to each dialysis session to effectively remove trapped air from the circuit.

Extracorporeal circuit can also generate microbubbles [11]. The current trapping mechanism fails to recognize or limit transfer of such microemboli. In such cases, air emboli may cross through the shunt from venous to systemic circulation and cause varying degrees of damage to the brain and other organs (paradoxical embolism). Thus, it is reasonable to believe that a patient with a patent foramen ovale is at a higher risk for having neurologic morbidity as a result of recurrent venous air embolism during HD [12].

2.2.4 Transducer Protectors

Transducers are devices inside the machine that converts pressure into an electronic signal that can be displayed. They serve an important role in monitoring the pressures within arterial and venous circuit. Transducer protectors [13] act as a barrier between blood in the tube and the transducer in the machine. They connect to the machine's venous and/or arterial ports via a small tubing segment on top of the drip chamber. Transducer protectors use membranes with a nominal pore size of 0.2 μm that are hydrophobic when wetted, to stop fluid from passing through. Moisture would damage the transducer. If these filters get wet, they prevent airflow. Wet or clamped transducer protectors cause pressure-reading errors. On the other hand, a loose or damaged transducer protector on a pre-pump arterial drip chamber port could also allow air into the bloodline circuit. Wet transducer protectors must be changed immediately, and the machine side of the protector should be inspected for contamination or wetting [13]. If a fluid breakthrough is found on the removed transducer protector, the machine's internal transducer protector (backup) must be inspected by a qualified technician, for safety, quality, and infection control purposes.

2.2.5 Pressures in the Extracorporeal Circuit

The extracorporeal circuit can be viewed as an extension of the patients own circulation during the HD process, and its monitoring, therefore, is essential for patient safety. Pressure in the extracorporeal circuit is dependent on the blood flow rate and the resistance to flow which is primarily exerted at the levels of the arteriovenous fistula or catheters, dialysis needles, the dialyzer, and the tubing. Some machines may also have a dialysate compartment pressure monitor. These are more common for flow control-based ultrafiltration management systems. The pressure in the dialysate compartment should not exceed that of the blood compartment to prevent high levels of backfiltration throughout the dialyzer and risk of dialyzer membrane rupture. An outline of the pressure profiles through the different components of the extracorporeal circuit is provided in Fig. 2.1.

Minor changes in the geometry of tubing, for example, kinking can lead to very high pre-stenotic pressure leading to hemolysis [14]. This can be as a result of manufacturing or packing techniques. The site of kink determines which pressure alarms are affected and whether hemolysis ensues.

2.2.6 Blood Volume Monitor

Blood volume monitors (BVM) are continuous sensors built into specific blood lines for noninvasive monitoring of plasma volumes [15]. They use either ultrasound to measure density of plasma or optical scattering to measure the hematocrit. BVM can be used to guide ultrafiltration rates in individuals that are prone to intradialytic hypotension [16, 17]. Although BVM can be quite useful in some individuals with intradialytic blood pressure instability, its wider benefits in all types of patients including those with anemia and low serum albumin, require further clarification [15].

2.3 The Artificial Kidney (Dialyzer Membrane)

2.3.1 Structure and Setup

The artificial kidney (dialyzer) consists of a cylindrical rigid structure internally packed with the semipermeable membrane configured as hollow fibers (cellulose, modified cellulose, or synthetic polymers), which provide a blood channel and a separation barrier between the blood and dialysate compartment. They vary in size with a range of membrane surface area (0.8–2.2 m^2) and internal compartmental volumes [18]. There is a pair of inlet and outlet for each compartment.

Through its transit in the dialyzer, the blood comes in contact with the dialysate solution of a specified composition and experiences variable hydrostatic gradients. Typically for an average patient size of 70 kg with good vascular access, optimal performance of the dialyzer can be maintained with an EBFR of between 300 and 400 ml/min and a surface area of 1.8–2.0 (m^2) [19]. The blood and dialysate fluid columns

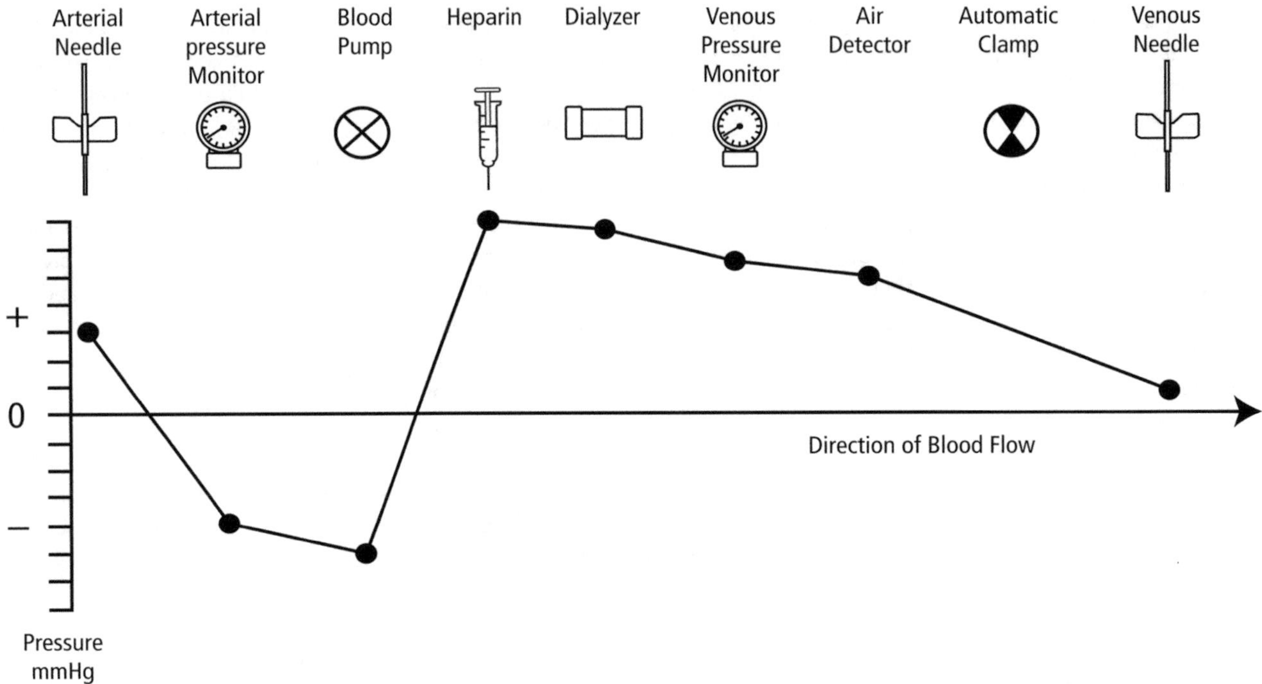

Fig. 2.1 Pressure profile within the extracorporeal circuit. The pressure profile is demonstrated at specified points in the circuit as indicated above the profile. The *horizontal axis* represents the direction of blood flow. The *vertical axis* represents the pressure generated within the circuit (mmHg millimetres of mercury)

can flow in the same direction within the dialyzer (concurrently) or in opposing directions (countercurrent). The latter provides a more uniform diffusive gradient across the whole length of the dialyzer compartment and is therefore preferred where less rapid shifts in toxins and electrolytes are required, for example, in those with extremely high urea levels, during first dialysis session, or in children. The pressure in the dialyzer is monitored by a dialysate inflow pressure monitor. Very high inflow pressures could mean a clotted dialyzer. Transmembrane pressure alarms are a measure of the altered pressure inside the dialyzer and maybe due to kinked lines, incorrect ultrafiltration, high venous pressure, or clotting. Although the rate at which the blood and dialysate pumps operate is a controlled variable, the distribution of blood and dialysate through the dialyzer can be uneven which can impact the efficiency of dialysis. The hollow fiber design offers the least resistance to the flow of both blood and dialysate, but the flow of blood tends to be higher in the centre of the cylindrical arrangement while that of dialysate higher in the periphery [20–22]. A more homogeneous flow distribution in the dialysate pathway has been achieved by using spacer yarns to separate the fibers or by the use of wave-patterned (Moiré structured) hollow fibers, which improve the fiber spacing within the device [22].

2.3.2 Dialyzer Efficiency

Dialyzer efficiency is denoted by its mass transfer coefficient (K_0A) for urea at infinite blood and dialysate flow, where K_0 is the transfer coefficient of the membrane and A is the surface area. K_0A is equivalent to the maximal clearance of urea (ml/min) that can be achieved [19]. High-efficiency dialyzers [19] can achieve greater urea clearances than low-efficiency dialyzers at comparable blood flow rates. Conventional cellulose, with good diffusive properties, have poor biocompatibility and limited pore size [23]. Modified cellulose and synthetic polymer microfibrils significantly enhance the efficiency and biocompatibility of the membrane. Ultrafiltration coefficient (K_{uf}) of the membrane is used to denote its permeability (ml of ultrafitrate/hr/mmHg) and high flux dialyzers typically have a K_{uf} between 20 and 80 ml/hr/mmHg [18, 24]. Factors such as entrapment of large negatively charged particles within the dialyzer could change its properties (Gibbs–Donan effect) [1, 25]. In addition to dialyzer properties, several other factors such as solute characteristics of the molecule, its charge, protein binding and patient hydration status, blood hematocrit, and viscosity may influence the overall performance of the system [1].

Super-high-flux and sorbent-coated membranes with very high cutoff (>60 kDa) provide an opportunity for enhanced removal of the uremic profile, but their clinical benefit and safety remain largely unproven [26, 27].

2.3.3 Dialyzer Biocompatibility and Reactions

Membrane incompatibility can result in either complement activation or activation of the coagulation cascade and cellular mediated pathways resulting in an acute phase reaction with pyrexia and hemodynamic instability or a chronic inflammatory state. The latter can lead to erythropoietin resistance, increased production of β2 microglobulin, and failure to thrive. Poor biocompatibility can also lead to procoagulability and clotting of both the dialyzer and blood circuit. Severe anaphylactic reactions to the artificial kidney have been reported especially during first use, typically manifested by wheezing, breathlessness, back pain, chest pain, hemolysis, or even sudden death [28]. These can be caused either by residual sterilant or the membrane material itself [5]. The use of gamma irradiation, steam sterilization, or electron-beam radiation and the use of materials with higher biocompatibility have reduced the incidence of anaphylactic reactions. A series of dialysis reactions, including deaths were reported due to heparin contaminated during the manufacturing process with oversulfated chondroitin sulfate [29]. New dialyzer materials or processing methods ought to be investigated in unexplained allergic reactions.

2.3.4 Dialyzer Reprocessing (Reuse) Systems

Dialyzer reuse over several treatment sessions for a particular patient has been a prevalent practice in some parts of the world for several years. Preparation of the dialyzer after each treatment session (dialyzer reprocessing) requires systems, which are effective and in good condition for optimum cleaning and maintenance of the dialyzer membrane surface area repeatedly used for HD. This optimizes the amount of useable membrane interface to come in contact with blood volume in order to provide adequate HD. Operational issues include scheduling and crucial quality-assurance procedures such as monitoring of applicable reuse chemicals, procedures for flushing and testing dialyzers for residual chemicals, rigorous monitoring on appropriate patient-specific dialyzer usage, and verification procedures for "volume pass" and "reuse number pass" [30, 31].

2.4 Dialysis Fluid and Its Pathway

This section of the dialysis machine has been the focus of major technological progress over the past few decades. The principle function of the dialysis fluid pathway is to prepare dialysate (combining treated water, acid concentrate, and a buffer) and deliver this fluid to the dialyzer at a prescribed flow rate under optimal conditions. Additionally, the circuit is designed to remove a prescribed amount of fluid from the patient (ultrafiltration). The spent dialysate with the removed fluid (effluent) is then drained out. The majority of this pathway is located inside the machine. The machine components that are reused and part of the fluid pathway must be sterilized as per manufacturer recommendations. The first step in the whole process, however, is dependent on treated water, prepared by water purification systems, being fed directly into the machine.

2.4.1 Water Treatment Systems

A single HD treatment can require upto 500 l of water. The water from the main supply goes through a series of steps of pre-filtration to remove particulate material, softening to remove calcium and magnesium, carbon filtration to remove chloramine, organic contaminants and chloride, and microfiltration followed by reverse osmosis. This involves the filtration of water through a membrane with pore size of 300 Da under high pressures. This could be done through single or a double reverse osmosis module and often coupled with electroionization or photoradiation treatment. The resultant water is devoid of most microorganisms and 90% of dissolved ions [32]. The water passes through cold sterilizing ultrafilters prior to its entry into the dialysate fluid pathway.

A standard HD session of three times weekly for 4 h at 500 ml/min dialysate flow could potentially expose a patient to 18,720 l of water contaminants per year. The quality of the water used for preparing the dialysate for HD must therefore meet recommended guidelines and standards [33–35]. Ultrapure water is defined as water with a bacterial count below 0.1 colony-forming unit/ml and endotoxin below 0.03 endotoxin unit/ml and is recommended for use in high-flux HD and hemodiafiltration. Both chemical and microbiological qualities are mandatory and provide an essential quality assurance of the treatment. An adequate water treatment system combined with ultrafilters at the inlet of the dialysis fluid pathway and a robust monitoring and governance process can help maintain high standards of water purity in HD.

2.4.2 Preparation of the Dialysate

Treated water enters the dialysis circuit and is heated to a specified temperature. Any air trapped in the water is removed by a deaerator unit where the water is submitted to negative pressures in a closed loop consisting of a pump, a

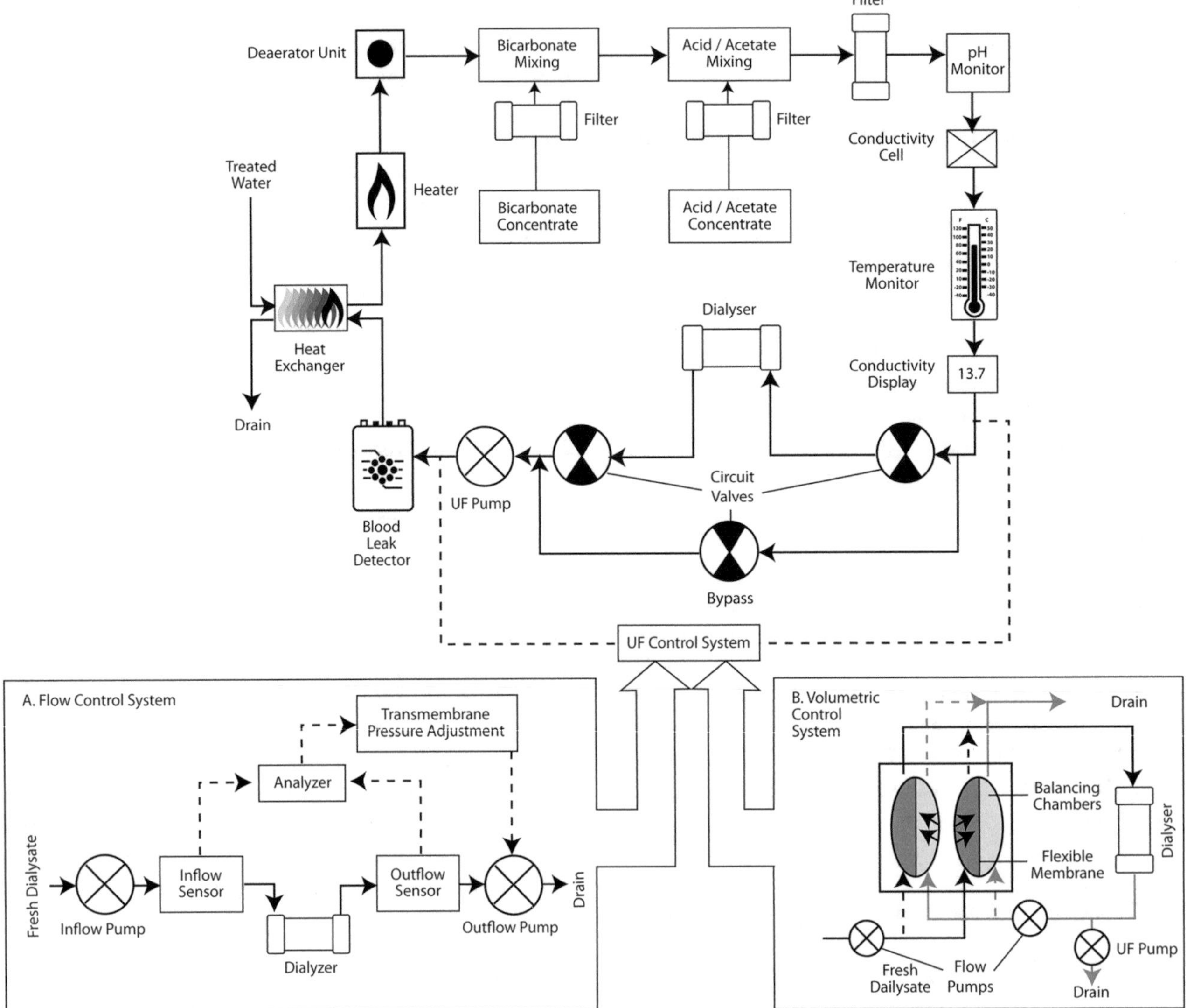

Fig. 2.2 Machine circuit for dialysate preparation and ultrafiltration. Inset pictures a and b represent the two commonly used automated ultrafiltration control systems, flow control, and volumetric control. *UF* Ultrafiltration

constricting valve, an air trap, and a vent. The proportioning chamber, at a specified ratio, mixes the purified water with the base and acid solutions. Although the pretreated water and acid component can be premixed to generate online dialysis fluid to be circulated in the main ring of the fluid distribution system in dialysis units, the base component (bicarbonate), supplied in powder cartridges, has to be freshly prepared and mixed at the point of treatment delivery to prevent bacterial growth [36].

The dialysate then undergoes self-check through a series of monitors and then enters the dialyzer compartment where the pressures are regulated by an automated ultrafiltration control system (UFCS). The dialysate effluent then passes through a deaeration system and blood leak monitor before providing further feedback to the UFCS. Both parts of UFCS form closed loops and aim to maintain an equal inflow and outflow of dialysate with a specific ultrafiltrate (UF) volume removed from the loop, the rate of which is determined by the UF prescription and the UF pump. Figure 2.2 provides an overview of a typical machine circuit for the preparation of dialysate demonstrating the two different automated UFCSs.

Variations to standard dialysate preparation include the single-pass batch system (Genius®) where a fixed volume of premixed dialysate (75 L) is typically utilized for the whole treatment session. Lack of need for water purification, ultrapure dialysate, and convenience are major advantages, especially in the intensive care setting and for home patients, although the fixed dialysate volume could limit HD efficiency for large patients.

2.4.3 Ultrafiltration Control system

Precise and automated regulation of fluid removal has enabled the safe performance of convective treatments during HD (ultrafiltration, high-flux HD, and hemodiafiltration). The two UF mechanisms typically employed are either volumetric or flow sensor control systems.

2.4.3.1 Volumetric Ultrafiltration Control System

Volumetric control systems [6, 37] are the most widely used and utilize balancing chambers located inside the machine. Each balancing chamber is split in half by a membrane. One half of each chamber gets filled by fresh dialysate en route to the dialyzer while the other by spent dialysate en route to the drain. The inlet and outlet of the chamber are controlled by two valves. As one half of the chamber fills with spent dialysate, it pushes an equal amount of fresh dialysate out of the chamber. Inversely as one half of the chamber fills with fresh dialysate, it forces an equal amount of spent dialysate out and towards the drain. There are two pumps controlling the inflow and outflow from the balancing chambers. The ultrafiltration pump removes fluid from the spent dialysis prior to it entering the balancing chamber (Fig. 2.2).

2.4.3.2 Flow Sensor Ultrafiltration Control System

A flow control system [6, 37] is based on flow sensors located on the inlet and outlet of the dialyzer to control the rate of inflow and outflow pumps to achieve balance. A separate analyzer system can guide an increase in the transmembrane pressure to act as a post-dialyzer ultrafiltration pump, which can remove excess fluid before the spent dialysate passes through the outflow sensor (Fig. 2.2). This system can limit the dialysate flow rates that can be applied.

2.4.4 Dialysate Composition

The dialysate is a combination of water mixed with specific portions of acid concentrate and a buffer solution to produce a near physiological solution to allow removal of soluble toxins and electrolytes form the bloodstream and replenish deficient electrolytes and buffer back into the circulation. The acid component, supplied directly to each machine from a central source or provided in individual containers, is a concentrate of acetate 5–6 mmol/l (or citrate 1 mmol/l), chloride salts of sodium, potassium, calcium, magnesium, and glucose. The salt concentrations can be varied for clinical use, particularly with regard to calcium and potassium. The final concentration of electrolytes is generated by a process of proportioning inside the machine. Several ratios of concentrate to water are in common use depending on the dialysis system to deliver a specified dialysate composition. Each proportioning ratio will therefore require its own particular acid and bicarbonate concentrates. Some machines are designed for use with a single proportioning ratio, whereas other machines can be set to use different proportioning ratios. Dialysate composition is monitored mainly by conductivity; hence, use of the wrong concentrates may lead to dialysate of the correct conductivity but the wrong composition. Failure to use the correct machine setting or appropriate concentrates with a given machine can lead to serious patient harm [6].

The typical dialysate sodium level is between 137 and 141 mmol/l to minimize diffusive sodium losses during UF. Low (<137) or high (>141) sodium setting on the machine are often used to achieve a net sodium gain or loss, respectively, but could be associated with osmotic symptoms during HD. Their long-term clinical benefit remains unproven. The usual dialysate potassium content is 2 mmol/l. Lower levels of dialysate K have been associated with increased mortality and should be avoided. Dialysate calcium levels are usually maintained at 1.25 or 1.5 mmol/l in standard HD. Glucose-free fluid may have less inflammatory effect but risk osmotic symptoms and hypoglycemia, particularly in diabetics on insulin therapy and in acute settings. Glucose-containing dialysates (100 mg/dl) are most widely used. Higher concentrations (200 mg/dl) are rarely used but may be beneficial in relieving headaches associated with osmotic shifts or to achieve enhanced fluid removal and caloric gain temporarily in specific patient groups. Additional phosphate supplementation in the fluid may be required in hyphosphatemia [38] (e.g., frequent nocturnal HD). Magnesium-containing fluids (5 mmol/l) are rarely used but may be required for patients with magnesium-losing states such as those with severe malabsorption syndrome, high-output stoma, or needing intravenous Mg supplementation.

2.4.5 Dialysate Circuit Monitoring

After dialysate mixing and proportioning, a series of monitoring checks are undertaken for the safety of the patient.

2.4.5.1 Dialysate Temperature Monitor

Temperatures of above 42 °C can cause hemolysis and protein degeneration in the blood compartment, as well as raising the temperature of the patient leading to vasodilatation and hemodynamic instability. Temperatures of 35 °C or lower may be too cold to be tolerated and cause shivering. Most dialysis units will set the dialysate temperature between 35 and 36.5 °C.

The HD process has been shown to increase body temperature and predispose to intradialytic hemodynamic instability. Using lower dialysate temperature (35–36 °C) improves hemodynamics and reduces cardiovascular strain [39, 40].

2.4.5.2 Conductivity Monitor

Conductivity is defined as the conductive potential of a solution to an electrical current and reflects the balance of positively charged to negatively charged particles in it. In dialysate fluid, this is made up of the electrolyte concentrations, and positively charged ions such as sodium, potassium, calcium, and magnesium are its main determinants. Conductivity can also be affected by temperature. Dialysate conductivity is typically maintained between 12 and 16 mS/cm (millisiemens per centimeter) [6]. The conductivity monitor remains in contact with the dialysate and consists of two electrodes placed 1 cm apart, across which a constant voltage is applied. Changes in electrolyte concentration therefore would cause changes in the voltage. The conductivity monitor is reasonably accurate but is reliant on successful calibration. However, the conductivity of a solution has a nonlinear relationship with temperature, salt concentration, and glucose composition of the fluid. The conductivity monitor is connected to an alarm, which is triggered when the fluid ionic composition has changed significantly outside the set limits. The type of concentrate and composition, the level of the probe in the fluid, the buffer cartridge, and temperature should be examined in these situations. If any significant alteration to the flow, pressure, or composition of the dialysate occurs the conductivity alarm would open the bypass valve to drain away the unsafe dialysate. After the necessary corrections are made, it may take several minutes for the conductivity readings to return to the normal range.

2.4.5.3 pH Monitor

The recommended dialysate pH is 6.8–7.6. Extremes in pH can lead to oxidative stress and hemolysis.

2.4.5.4 Blood Leak Detector

Blood should not be able to cross the dialysis membrane; any red cells present in the dialysate would alter the light signal in the sensor which might trigger an alarm that automatically stops the blood pump. The blood leak detector [6] is made up of an infrared or photoelectric sensor, and it is positioned immediately downstream of the dialysate outlet of the dialyzer. Persistent or severe blood leak alarms require cessation of the treatment, disconnection, and discard of the lines and dialyzer without washback.

2.5 Treatment Modes

The HD apparatus is configured not only to deliver a standard HD treatment session but also has design features that allow modifications to the treatment delivery under specific circumstances and clinical need.

2.5.1 Standard Hemodialysis Session

The steps for the initiation of HD involve a disinfection cycle taking approximately 40 min followed by compulsory test program. During this phase the machine will mix the dialysate fluid to achieve the correct concentration. The machine is then lined using the appropriate blood lines and the prescribed dialyzer. The line pack will contain arterial, venous, and, if appropriate, a substitution line if using HDF. Lines are also available for other modes, for example, single needle HD, or for specific monitoring purposes, such as the BVM. Priming of the blood circuit including the dialyzer is the next step (automated settings for priming cycles are inbuilt and vary according to the dialyzer and consumable in use for the treatment, for example, tubing volumes and pump speeds). The aim is to deaerate all lines and dialyzer and adjust any levels of fluid in the bubble trap. Once the required priming volume has been achieved most machines go into pre-circulation mode. Information can now be put into the machine, for example, the dialysate prescription and the UF volume, etc. Prescribed anticoagulation can now be drawn up. This may include not only a stat dose but also an infusion, which can now be attached to the infusion pump on the machine. A sterile area is prepared for vascular access preparation. Cannulation of the arteriovenous access follows a strict aseptic non-touch technique. Once the vascular access has been successfully cannulated, the next step is to connect this to the blood lines on the machine. Clinical observations (e.g., blood pressure) ought to be documented pretreatment, during treatment, and post-treatment. At completion of treatment, reinfusion takes place by choosing a preset method and pump speeds. Arteriovenous fistula needles can now be removed and hemostasis achieved. The machine can now be stripped down by removing the blood lines and dialyzer, followed by activation of the disinfection cycle as per manufacturer recommendations.

2.5.2 Profiled Dialysis

With the development of sensor capabilities, it is becoming increasingly possible to provide continuous, real-time monitoring of patients during HD treatment. This provides an opportunity to design a responsive mode that can detect the signals and, where clinically relevant, adjust or alter the dialysis prescription (biofeedback) to allow a more personalized treatment. The term profiled dialysis [41, 42] refers to the automated real-time adjustments to a specific prescription variable in order to match the patients changing biological parameters. It is aimed primarily at reducing circulatory stress and hemodynamic symptoms and is most beneficial in patients who suffer from repeated intradialytic hypotension and hemodynamic instability. The most widely used profile regimens [39, 41, 43, 44] are variations of the ultrafiltration rate (using BVM, to minimize sharp changes in blood volume), dialysate temperature (specific modules, thermoneutral or cool HD), or conductivity profiles (isonatric HD refers to maintaining a near constant conductivity gradient between blood and dialysate to minimize diffusive sodium losses). Biofeedback devices that vary the UF rate and conductivity in response to the relative BVM change may reduce serious hemodynamic instability on HD. However, the benefit and clinical impact of such technology are not yet fully understood [16, 41].

2.5.3 Single-Needle Hemodialysis (SNHD)

When difficult or inadequate vascular access does not allow two needle access (such as following repair surgery, incomplete maturation, or due to bruising from needle dislodgement), SNHD mode [45, 46] can allow continuation of dialysis treatment with a single needle, albeit with reduced HD efficiency. Specially adapted machines with dual blood pumps are required where both the arterial and venous tubing can be connected to a single vascular access needle. In SNHD, the arterial tubing carries blood to the dialyzer via the action of an arterial pump while a venous pump return the blood to the patient, coordinated in sequence to allow inflow and outflow from a single needle. SNHD will reduce the risk of blood loss in the event of needle dislodgement as both the arterial and venous ends would be disconnected and the blood pump would stop. Patients on frequent nocturnal home HD often utilize this mode for routine treatment.

2.5.4 Recirculation and Machine Bypass

HD machines offer a dialysate circuit bypass option. This allows dialysate flow to bypass the dialyzer (therefore not delivering fresh dialysate). During this time on bypass, the blood circuit can be isolated from the patient and allowed to circulate (recirculation) typically for 5–20 min. During this period staff can troubleshoot any problems with patient interruption or vascular access issues for a brief period of time without having to discontinue the entire setup and process. If blood is allowed to circulate on bypass mode for a long time, its composition might be altered significantly and not be safe to be returned to the patient.

2.5.5 Isolated Ultrafiltration (IsoUF)

The IsoUF mode is typically used for rapid or urgent fluid removal in emergencies such as pulmonary edema or refractory fluid overload states such as severe cardiac failure [47]. IsoUF used at the beginning of a dialysis session can be achieved by maintaining a transmembrane pressure gradient across the dialyzer generated by negative pressure in the dialysate compartment [48], while the dialysate delivery is in bypass mode. IsoUF preserves hemodynamic stability better during ultrafiltration.

2.6 Alarms and Treatment Hazards

HD is an invasive treatment process, and patient safety remains the most important consideration in the design of the technology. A variety of inbuilt monitors can detect faults and limit harm. Alarms are designed to alert users when a warning is needed or a fault has occurred and can be set to either shut down the dialysis circuit or alert the dialysis staff. Machines alarm configurations can vary.

For most alarms, a flashing light and an audible alarm usually accompanied by stoppage of the blood pump will occur. It is useful to remember that the "mute button" on the machine when pressed for silencing the alarms do not recommence the treatment. Most machines will have an emergency mode, which allows an automated switching off of the ultrafiltration pump and reduction of blood pump speed to 50 ml/min with or without an automatic bolus of fluid infusion.

The combination of integral safety features, adequate alarm settings or configurations and operator vigilance, are necessary to assure safety. Two groups of errors have been recognized (a) machine faults or parts malfunction or (b) user errors [49]. The majority of the hazards in the treatment today relate to user-related errors. It is therefore an integral part of the training accreditation that the operator is able to troubleshoot various components of safety and alarms. These individuals can be adequately trained dialysis staff, nephrologists, or technicians. Individual alarms in the blood and dialysate pathway and their troubleshooting has been discussed earlier in their respective sections.

2.6.1 Disconnection or Leakage

Dialysis systems are found lacking in the event of a disconnection or leakage from the bloodline [50, 51]. The lack of an alarm in this setting may be due to a complete or partial venous needle dislodgement, small pressure drops, incorrect alarm limits, or small leaks through faulty connectors. Extreme blood loss in HD is rare but can occur in venous needle dislodgement, rupture of access (aneurysm or anastomosis), and dialyzer crack or loose connections in circuit. For venous line dislodgement, back pressure created by the needle resistance prevents the machine's venous pressure monitors from sensing the loss of pressure created by the dislodgment. In this situation the venous pressure at the needle site will remain positive, and the alarm will not trigger. Smaller-gauge needles combined with high blood flows create significant back pressures, such that even if the needle is fully or partially dislodged from the patient, the venous pressure monitor continue sensing the pressure created by the needle's resistance, and the smaller drop in pressure associated with the disconnection may be insufficient in triggering an alarm.

The problem is exacerbated by the fact that users may sometimes widen the alarm limits to minimize nuisance alarms. These are usually caused by high venous pressures in the system due to roller pump generated oscillations in pressure and maneuvers that can naturally change the venous pressure such as coughing or even change in posture during HD. The resulting variations can often exceed even the customary ±50 mm Hg venous pressure monitor limits. All these limitations can make venous needle dislodgements and its life threatening consequences go undetected during HD. This problem is not unique to any specific machine model. Securement of access guided by a well-defined unit policy, avoidance of unnecessary widening of venous pressure alarm limits, and adequate visibility of the connection points for the extracorporeal circuit with greater vigilance can minimize risks significantly. Although efforts have been made to design innovative solutions to address this problem, detection of blood loss that can activate the venous clamp and stop the blood pump is not yet available in routine clinical practice.

2.6.2 Air Embolism

Air embolism [11, 52] is a rare event but may occur when a bolus of air enters the venous blood line below the air trap. This can lead to symptoms of chest pain, breathlessness, confusion, and headaches with potentially fatal consequences. If an air bolus is suspected, the venous line should be clamped and the patient turned onto the left side with feet elevation and seek further help.

2.6.3 Hemolysis

Hemolysis can occur either through mechanical (shear forces through kinks and obstructions to the circuit, defective blood pump, high negative pressure in the circuit), chemical (contaminated dialysate with disinfectant such as chlorine, bleach, formaldehyde, copper, nitrates, nitrites, or low-osmolar dialysate), or thermal factors (dialysate temperature >42 C) [4, 14, 36, 52].

2.6.4 Power Failure or Disruption

Power failure or disruption will set the machine alarms off and trigger venous line clamp. The backup battery will allow some time (approx 15–20 min) to reinfuse and terminate the treatment. Beyond this time period, manual intervention of freeing up the venous line and hand cranking the blood pump will be required (according to specified machine policy). If the water pressure falls or is turned off, the machine will not be able to prepare the dialysate and the treatment will have to be terminated.

In the event of any crisis on HD, where the etiology is unclear, in addition to all the necessary supportive measures the following steps should be undertaken: (a) stop dialysis, (b) take samples from venous and arterial lines and disconnect the patient, (c) collect dialysate sample and the used dialyzer, and (d) remove the machine from further use so that all evidence is well preserved for further investigation.

2.7 Configuration and Connectivity

The goal of technological reliability is primarily to avoid treatment disruptions related to technical faults, quick turnaround, and restoration of such faults and robust governance around safety checks and monitoring procedures.

The treatment parameters for each session can be captured electronically in modern machines through USB, Ethernet, and a variety of serial interfaces. Wireless interfaces may also be available for direct connection to hospital networks. Data card slots on some machines allow personal medical information and dialysis prescription to be stored on it to allow automatic setup of the machine parameters.

Dialysis machines are medical equipment regulated by the Food and Drug Administration (FDA). Complex design and manufacturing of dialysis machines incorporate pumps and multiple valves with electronic actuation to allow different mixing ratios, and employ sensors for monitoring pressure, temperature, pump speed, and transmembrane pressure gradient at specified points in the blood extracorporeal and dialysate circuits, during routine treatment. Advanced features, such as comprehensive self-test and fault-indication capabilities, require additional circuits and components. The technical governance of such complex life-saving technology requires a rigorous schedule of maintenance, hardware support, and software updates.

Dialysis equipment is powered [6] by AC but may also include batteries (or ultracapacitors), for example, to supplement the power supply's output when heating water for sterilization in home-use machines. Safety regulations require power supply self-monitoring for voltage, temperature, and current flow.

2.8 Technology and Human Factor Limitations

The advances in HD technology have significantly improved its performance and reliability but remains limited nevertheless by the need for a skilled operator, a dedicated setting, and restrictions imposed on the patient lifestyle. The cliché of an HD machine is based predominantly on the financial criteria and performance characteristics, as defined by effectiveness and efficiency. In future, user acceptance (staff and patients) and integration with different care delivery models could significantly enhance the value and differentiation of the technology.

The improved reliability and safety features may have desensitized us from the clinical dangers of the HD process itself [52], particularly factors that govern the interaction of the patient with the machine. The HD treatment could be viewed as single system that integrates the patient's cardiovascular system and the extracorporeal circuiting series and facilitates interaction with the dialysis technology across the membrane interface. With an increased number of elderly and frail individuals commencing HD, it is apparent that we need technology to address such patient complexities. Hemodynamic stability and intradialytic hypotension have been identified as significant factors that need to be addressed to improve outcomes [41]. Vascular access is another major factor that affects outcomes and remains the commonest cause of HD treatment failure [53, 54]. The treatment of uremia and removal of a range of uremic toxins is critically reliant on our understanding of the equilibration of the circulatory system with the toxin reservoirs (total body water and circulatory compartments) and its implications in various disease states and comorbidities.

Technological progress in dialysis is necessary but one that aims for paramount clinical safety combined with simplicity and reliability for the user. Capabilities of self-use of the technology will allow for wider adoption of the technology outside traditional settings such as in patient homes or self-care units. This will enable greater user engagement and empowerment, which has been linked to better outcomes in chronic illnesses. Adapting the technology to allow patients to participate or self-manage their treatment will be a major advancement in the adoption of extended dialysis schedules.

Future innovations will need to address technological and human factor limitations in HD therapy to bring about improvements in both the quantity and quality of life for the patient.

References

1. Huang Z, Gao D, Letteri JJ, Clark WR. Blood-membrane interactions during dialysis. Semin Dial. 2009;22(6):623–8. doi:10.1111/j.1525-139X.2009.00658.x.
2. Ledebo I. Principles and practice of hemofiltration and hemodiafiltration. Artif Organs. 1998;22(1):20–5.
3. Galli F. Vitamin E-derived copolymers continue the challenge to hemodialysis biomaterials. World J Nephrol. 2012;1(4):100–5. doi:10.5527/wjn.v1.i4.100.
4. Ghezzi PM, Bonello M, Ronco C. Disinfection of dialysis monitors. Contrib Nephrol. 2007;154:39–60. doi:10.1159/000096813.
5. Uda S, Mizobuchi M, Akizawa T. Biocompatible characteristics of high-performance membranes. Contrib Nephrol. 2011;173:23–9. doi:10.1159/000328941.
6. Misra M. The basics of hemodialysis equipment. Hemodial Int. 2005;9(1):30–6. doi:10.1111/j.1492-7535.2005.01115.x.
7. Kimata N, Wakayama K, Okano K, et al. Study of discrepancies between recorded and actual blood flow in hemodialysis patients. ASAIO J. 59(6):617–21. doi:10.1097/MAT.0b013e3182a708b9.
8. Allcock K, Jagannathan B, Hood CJ, Marshall MR. Exsanguination of a home hemodialysis patient as a result of misconnected blood-lines during the wash back procedure: a case report. BMC Nephrol. 2012;13(1):28. doi:10.1186/1471-2369-13-28.
9. Basile C, Ruggieri G, Vernaglione L, Montanaro A, Giordano R. A comparison of methods for the measurement of hemodialysis access recirculation. J Nephrol. 2003;16(6):908–13. http://www.ncbi.nlm.nih.gov/pubmed/14736020. Accessed 30 Mar 2015.
10. Kumbar L, Karim J, Besarab A. Surveillance and monitoring of dialysis access. Int J Nephrol. 2012;2012.
11. Stegmayr B, Forsberg U, Jonsson P, Stegmayr C. The sensor in the venous chamber does not prevent passage of air bubbles during hemodialysis. Artif Organs. 2007;31(2):162–6. doi:10.1111/j.1525-1594.2007.00358.x.
12. Forsberg U, Jonsson P, Stegmayr C, Stegmayr B. Microemboli, developed during haemodialysis, pass the lung barrier and may cause ischaemic lesions in organs such as the brain. Nephrol Dial Transplant. 2010;25(8):2691–5. doi:10.1093/ndt/gfq116.
13. Finelli L, Miller JT, Tokars JI, Alter MJ, Arduino MJ. National surveillance of dialysis-associated diseases in the United States, 2002. Semin Dial. 18(1):52–61. doi:10.1111/j.1525-139X.2005.18108.x.
14. Malinauskas RA. Decreased hemodialysis circuit pressures indicating postpump tubing kinks: a retrospective investigation of hemolysis in five patients. Hemodial Int. 2008;12(3):383–93. doi:10.1111/j.1542-4758.2008.00285.x.
15. Raimann J, Liu L, Tyagi S, Levin NW, Kotanko P. A fresh look at dry weight. Hemodial Int. 2008;12(4):395–405. doi:10.1111/j.1542-4758.2008.00302.x.
16. Locatelli F, Buoncristiani U, Canaud B, Köhler H, Petitclerc T, Zucchelli P. Haemodialysis with on-line monitoring equipment: tools or toys? Nephrol Dial Transplant. 2005;20(1):22–33. doi:10.1093/ndt/gfh555.
17. Santoro A, Mancini E, Basile C, et al. Blood volume controlled hemodialysis in hypotension-prone patients: a randomized, multicenter controlled trial. Kidney Int. 2002;62(3):1034–45. doi:10.1046/j.1523-1755.2002.00511.x.
18. Clark WR, Ronco C. Determinants of haemodialyser performance and the potential effect on clinical outcome. Nephrol Dial Transplant. 2001;16(Suppl 5):56–60.
19. Chelamcharla M, Leypoldt JK, Cheung AK. Dialyzer membranes as determinants of the adequacy of dialysis. Semin Nephrol. 2005;25(2):81–9. http://www.ncbi.nlm.nih.gov/pubmed/15791559. Accessed 30 March 2015.
20. Ronco C, Brendolan A, Crepaldi C, Rodighiero M, Scabardi M. Blood and dialysate flow distributions in hollow-fiber hemodialyzers analyzed by computerized helical scanning technique. J Am Soc Nephrol. 2002;13(Suppl 1):S53–S61. http://www.ncbi.nlm.nih.gov/pubmed/11792763. Accessed 11 Jan 2015.
21. Ronco C. Fluid mechanics and crossfiltration in hollow-fiber hemodialyzers. Contrib Nephrol. 2007;158:34–49. doi:10.1159/0000107233.

22. Ronco C, Scabardi M, Goldoni M, Brendolan A, Crepaldi C, La Greca G. Impact of spacing filaments external to hollow fibers on dialysate flow distribution and dialyzer performance. Int J Artif Organs. 1997;20(5):261–6. http://www.ncbi.nlm.nih.gov/pubmed/9209926. Accessed 11 Jan 2015.
23. Boure T. Which dialyser membrane to choose? Nephrol Dial Transplant. 2004;19(2):293–6. doi:10.1093/ndt/gfg508.
24. Eknoyan G, Beck GJ, Cheung AK, et al. Effect of dialysis dose and membrane flux in maintenance hemodialysis. N Engl J Med. 2002;347(25):2010–9. doi:10.1056/NEJMoa021583.
25. Nguyen MK, Kurtz I. Physiologic interrelationships between Gibbs–Donnan equilibrium, osmolality of body fluid compartments, and plasma water sodium concentration. J Appl Physiol. 2006:1–9. doi:10.1152/japplphysiol.00505.2006.
26. Van Tellingen A, Grooteman MP, Bartels PC, et al. Long-term reduction of plasma homocysteine levels by super-flux dialyzers in hemodialysis patients. Kidney Int. 2001;59(1):342–7. doi:10.1046/j.1523-1755.2001.00496.x.
27. Santoro A, Guadagni G. Dialysis membrane: from convection to adsorption. Clin Kidney J. 2010;3(Suppl 1):i36–i9. doi:10.1093/ndtplus/sfq035.
28. Ebo DG, Bosmans JL, Couttenye MM, Stevens WJ. Haemodialysis-associated anaphylactic and anaphylactoid reactions. Allergy. 2006;61(2):211–20. doi:10.1111/j.1398-9995.2006.00982.x.
29. Blossom DB, Kallen AJ, Patel PR, et al. Outbreak of adverse reactions associated with contaminated heparin. N Engl J Med. 2008;359(25):2674–84. doi:10.1056/NEJMoa0806450.
30. Brown C. Current opinion and controversies of dialyser reuse. Saudi J Kidney Dis Transpl. 2001;12(3):352–63. http://www.ncbi.nlm.nih.gov/pubmed/18209382. Accessed 30 March 2015.
31. Lowrie EG, Li Z, Ofsthun N, Lazarus JM. Reprocessing dialysers for multiple uses: recent analysis of death risks for patients. Nephrol Dial Transplant. 2004;19(11):2823–30. doi:10.1093/ndt/gfh460.
32. Damasiewicz MJ, Polkinghorne KR, Kerr PG. Water quality in conventional and home haemodialysis. Nat Rev Nephrol. 2012;8(12):725–34. doi:10.1038/nrneph.2012.241.
33. Penne EL, Visser L, van den Dorpel MA, et al. Microbiological quality and quality control of purified water and ultrapure dialysis fluids for online hemodiafiltration in routine clinical practice. Kidney Int. 2009;76(6):665–72. doi:10.1038/ki.2009.245.
34. Nystrand R. Microbiology of water and fluids for hemodialysis. J Chin Med Assoc. 2008;71(5):223–9. doi:10.1016/S1726-4901(08)70110–2.
35. Canaud B, Lertdumrongluk P. Ultrapure dialysis fluid: a new standard for contemporary hemodialysis. Nephrourol Mon. 2012;4(3):519–23. doi:10.5812/numonthly.3060.
36. Ledebo I. On-line preparation of solutions for dialysis: practical aspects versus safety and regulations. J Am Soc Nephrol. 2002;13(90001):78–83. http://jasn.asnjournals.org/content/13/suppl_1/S78.full. Accessed 16 Jan 2015.
37. Ronco C. Hemodiafiltration: evolution of a technique towards better dialysis care. Contrib Nephrol. 2011;168:19–27. doi: 10.1159/000321741.
38. Ebah LM, Akhtar M, Wilde I, et al. Phosphate enrichment of dialysate for use in standard and extended haemodialysis. Blood Purif. 2012;34(1):28–33. doi:10.1159/000339818.
39. Selby NM, McIntyre CW. A systematic review of the clinical effects of reducing dialysate fluid temperature. Nephrol Dial Transplant. 2006;21(7):1883–98. doi:10.1093/ndt/gfl126.
40. Selby NM, Burton JO, Chesterton LJ, McIntyre CW. Dialysis-induced regional left ventricular dysfunction is ameliorated by cooling the dialysate. Clin J Am Soc Nephrol. 2006;1(6):1216–25. doi:10.2215/CJN.02010606.
41. Davenport A. Using dialysis machine technology to reduce intradialytic hypotension. Hemodial Int. 2011;15:S37–S42. doi:10.1111/j.1542-4758.2011.00600.x.
42. Oliver MJ, Edwards LJ, Churchill DN. Impact of sodium and ultrafiltration profiling on hemodialysis-related symptoms. J Am Soc Nephrol. 2001;12(1):151–6. http://jasn.asnjournals.org/content/12/1/151.full. Accessed 18 Jan 2015.
43. Mercadal L, Piékarski C, Renaux J-L, Petitclerc T, Deray G. Isonatric dialysis biofeedback in hemodiafiltration with online regeneration of ultrafiltrate (HFR): rationale and study protocol for a randomized controlled study. J Nephrol. 25(6):1126–30. doi:10.5301/jn.5000084.
44. Agarwal R. How can we prevent intradialytic hypotension? Curr Opin Nephrol Hypertens. 2012;21(6):593–9. doi:10.1097/MNH.0b013e3283588f3c.
45. Rostoker G. La technique d'hémodialyse transitoire en uniponcture sur fistules natives: intérêts, limites, risques et précautions. Néphrol Thér. 2010;6(7):591–6. doi:10.1016/j.nephro.2010.05.004.
46. Trakarnvanich T, Chirananthavat T, Maneerat P, Chabsuwan S, Areeyakulnimit S. Is single-needle hemodialysis still a good treatment in end-stage renal disease? Blood Purif. 2007;25(5–6):490–6. doi:10.1159/000113008.
47. Canaud B, Lertdumrongluk P. Ultrapure dialysis fluid: a new standard for contemporary hemodialysis. Nephrourol Mon. 2012;4(3):519–23. doi:10.5812/numonthly.3060.
48. Ing TS. Isolated ultrafiltration: its origin and early development. Artif Organs. 2013;37(10):841–7. doi:10.1111/aor.12212.
49. Garrick R, Kliger A, Stefanchik B. Patient and facility safety in hemodialysis: opportunities and strategies to develop a culture of safety. Clin J Am Soc Nephrol. 2012;7:680–8. doi:10.2215/CJN.06530711.
50. Delfosse F, Boyer J, Lemaitre V, Inghels Y. [Disconnection of arteriovenous fistula: standardize the coverage of the hemorragic risk]. Néphrol Thér. 2012;8(1):23–34. doi:10.1016/j.nephro.2011.04.004.
51. Ross EA, Briz C, Sadleir RJ. Method for detecting the disconnection of an extracorporeal device using a patient's endogenous electrical voltages. Kidney Int. 2006;69(12):2274–7. doi:10.1038/sj.ki.5001508.
52. Davenport A. Intradialytic complications during hemodialysis. Hemodial Int. 2006;10(2):162–7. doi:10.1111/j.1542-4758.2006.00088.x.
53. Hakim R, Himmelfarb J. Hemodialysis access failure: a call to action. Kidney Int. 1998;54(4):1029–40. doi:10.1046/j.1523-1755.1998.00122.x.
54. Ng LJ, Chen F, Pisoni RL, et al. Hospitalization risks related to vascular access type among incident US hemodialysis patients. Nephrol Dial Transplant. 2011;26(11):3659–66. doi:10.1093/ndt/gfr063.

3 Hemodialysis Dose

Thomas A. Depner

3.1 Historical Perspective

Evidence that equilibration of the blood with an isotonic salt solution across a semipermeable membrane as a potential method for removing unwanted substances from the body including drugs and uremic toxins dates back many years [1–3]. However, it was not until Dr. Willem J. Kolff successfully applied hemodialysis (HD) to treat a patient with acute kidney failure that the hypothesized benefit for patients suffering from uremia was proven [4]. This landmark event also confirmed the previous logical hypothesis that the cause of the immediate life-threatening aspect of uremia is from accumulation of small (dialyzable) solutes that normally appear in the urine. The reversal of a previously fatal disease was considered miraculous (patients sometimes awakened from uremic coma during the procedure), so little thought was given to measuring the treatment or determining its adequacy. Perhaps because of its complexity, physicians at the time, including its inventor, also felt that its application should be limited to management of reversible acute kidney disease, serving to allow time for the native kidneys to recover. Not until 1960, with the development of a permanent vascular access device, was management of chronic kidney disease accepted, and a quest for measurement of the dose and its adequacy begun [5, 6].

3.2 Measuring Diffusion, the Basic Principle of Dialysis

How does the patient and family know that he/she had a good dialysis? Probably after a poor dialysis the patient might feel better, having avoided the symptoms of clinical disequilibrium that often follow significant solute and fluid removal.

T. A. Depner (✉)
University of California—Davis, 4406 Valmonte Dr., Sacramento, CA 95864, USA
e-mail: tadepner@ucdavis.edu

A. K. Singh et al. (eds.), *Core Concepts in Dialysis and Continuous Therapies*, DOI 10.1007/978-1-4899-7657-4_3

How does one measure the effect of dialysis? Simply keeping the patient alive is not enough, and one can argue further that even if the patient reports feeling well, the caregiver should not be satisfied. Measuring the dialysis dose and assessment of its adequacy should be anticipatory, identifying inadequacies at an early stage to allow corrections before the symptomatic stage. To answer the patient's question, the focus should be on the dialysis objective: removal of solute by simple diffusion across a semipermeable membrane.

Since the pioneering work of Thomas Graham [7] and Adolph Fick [8] in the mid to late 1800s, the driving force for diffusion of solutes and gases has been recognized as the concentration of the gas or solute. Most importantly, the rate of diffusion (e.g., bulk movement of solute) is directly proportional to the concentration gradient. Fick's first law of diffusion has been adapted to dialysis [8]:

$$Js = KoA(\Delta C), \quad (3.1)$$

Js is the rate of solute movement or flux (e.g., mg/min), Ko is a membrane-specific and solute-specific constant (e.g., cm/min), A is the membrane area (e.g., cm^2), ΔC is the solute concentration gradient across the membrane (e.g., mg/mL).

The proportionality constant KoA in Eq. 3.1 is defined as the ratio of flux (Js) to the concentration gradient (ΔC) across the membrane, which is essentially the definition of dialysance: a measurement similar to clearance that takes into consideration solute concentrations on both sides of the membrane. For a hollow-fiber kidney, KoA can be considered the initial clearance at the proximal end of the fibers before any buildup of solute on the dialysate side. When the dialysate concentration is zero, the denominator is simply the blood concentration, and clearance is then equal to dialysance. KoA can also be considered the dialyzer's maximum clearance at infinite blood and dialysate flow rates. It is a dialyzer-specific measure used to compare the effectiveness of different hollow-fiber dialyzers, but it is also solute-specific (e.g., KoA values for urea and creatinine are different for the same dialyzer). Similar to clearance, which is determined by, but independent of either solute concentrations or flux, KoA is also independent of blood and dialysate flow rates. Its value can be determined by measuring the cross-dialyzer clearance at specified blood and dialysate flow rates [9]:

$$K_0A = \frac{Q_b Q_d}{Q_b - Q_d} \ln\left(\frac{Q_d (Q_b - K_d)}{Q_b (Q_d - K_d)}\right), \quad (3.2)$$

Q_b and Q_d are effective blood and dialysate flow rates respectively, and K_d is the dialyzer solute clearance. Equation 3.2, known as the Michael's equation after its developer [9], is based on an exponential decline in solute concentration along the membrane as blood and dialysate flow in opposite directions for maximum efficiency.

More importantly, once the dialyzer KoA has been determined, a rearrangement of Eq. 3.2 can be used to predict the clearance for any blood and dialysate flow rate:

$$K_d = Q_{bw}\left[\frac{e^{K_0A\left(\frac{Q_d - Q_b}{Q_d Q_b}\right)} - 1}{e^{K_0A\left(\frac{Q_d - Q_b}{Q_d Q_b}\right)} - \frac{Q_b}{Q_d}}\right]. \quad (3.3)$$

3.3 Intermittent Dialysis is Self-Limiting

Despite the constant nature of KoA and the constancy of clearance during a single HD at fixed Q_b and Q_d, intermittent dialysis is intrinsically self-limiting. For peritoneal dialysis (PD), the clearance (but not the dialysance) gradually falls with time and will eventually extinguish during a single exchange of fluid as solute concentrations in the dialysate completely equilibrate with the patient's blood concentrations. For intermittent HD, clearances remain constant during the treatment because fresh dialysate is constantly supplied, but the treatment's effectiveness falls as concentrations in the patient's blood fall. In the absence of replenishment (G), removal of solute during HD would also extinguish with time (despite a constant Kt/V). This self-limiting feature of dialysis results both from solute buildup on the dialysate side (PD) and from reduction in solute concentrations on the blood side. In other words, for intermittent dialysis, the more one dialyzes the less solute is removed. Fortunately, uremic toxicity is also concentration-dependent, such that dialysis is more effective for the more toxic patient.

3.4 Diffusion in a Flowing Circuit

Figure 3.1 shows what happens inside the dialyzer as blood flows from inlet to outlet and dialysate flows in the countercurrent direction. Solute transfer from blood to dialysate depends on both flow rates and the membrane permeability to each solute. The gradient across the membrane diminishes with time and with distance along the membrane. For solutes with high membrane permeability, the gradient diminished more rapidly with distance as shown in Fig. 3.1a. The downstream dissipation of the gradient is correctable by increasing the blood flow, which explains the flow dependency of clearance. For solutes with low permeability, distance along the membrane has less impact, so solute removal is more dependent on membrane permeability and less dependent on flow as shown in Fig. 3.1b. For patients dialyzed intermittently (e.g., three times weekly) the gradient also diminishes with time and would eventually extinguish in the absence of new solute generation. This accounts in part for the inefficiency of intermittent dialysis as discussed below.

Within the hollow fiber, solutes diffuse across the membrane only from the water fraction of the blood. Because macromolecules like serum lipids and proteins occupy space that excludes water-soluble molecules, they reduce the effective blood flow to about 93 % of the whole blood flow. The role of larger blood components such as erythrocytes depends on the solute. For solutes like urea that diffuse rapidly across red cell membranes the patient's hematocrit has little influence on clearance, so solute delivery to the membrane is essentially a function of blood water flow, including erythrocyte water [10, 11]. For solutes like creatinine, phosphorus, and uric acid with negligible diffusion from red cells during the 10–20 s transit through the dialyzer, effective flow is restricted to plasma water, which must be used to measure clearances (Table 3.1) [12, 13]. However, red cells contain significant amounts of these solutes that eventually equilibrate with the plasma after leaving the dialyzer. This phenomenon explains in part why creatinine clearances have not been popular as a measure of dialysis adequacy; the post-dialyzer plasma creatinine concentration is spuriously low and may require several hours to equilibrate with red cells in the same blood sample.

Between dialyses, in addition to solutes, the patient accumulates water. Removal is easily accomplished during dialysis by applying hydrostatic pressure across the dialysis

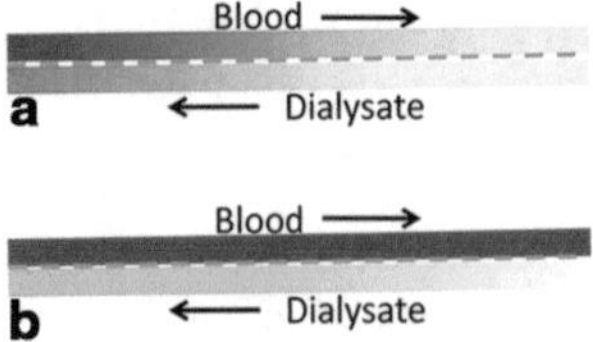

Fig. 3.1 Hollow-fiber solute gradients. **a** An easily dialyzed solute with blood flow-dependent clearance. **b** Solutes less well dialyzed; clearance is membrane-dependent, less dependent on blood flow

Table 3.1 Effective dialyzer blood compartment flow [12, 13]

Solute	Effective flow
Urea	Whole blood water
Creatinine	Plasma water
Phosphate	Plasma water

membrane. Since the resulting convective loss of fluid and solute is in the same direction as diffusive solute movement, it adds to the effectiveness of the dialysis. However, the augmenting effect of filtration is less than might be expected because convective transfer of solute across the membrane diminishes the gradient for diffusion, and in contrast to diffusive loss of easily dialyzed solutes like urea, convective losses occur along the entire length of the hollow fiber [14]. At the distal end where urea concentrations may be reduced by 70–80 %, convective transfer of solute is greatly diminished. Equation 3.4 is used to quantify instantaneous solute removal by convection, and illustrates the dilution effect.

$$K_d = Q_b\left(\frac{C_{in} - C_{out}}{C_{in}}\right) + Q_f\left(\frac{C_{out}}{C_{in}}\right), \qquad (3.4)$$

K_d is the dialyzer clearance, Q_b is the dialyzer blood outflow, C_{in} and C_{out} are the inflow and outflow solute concentrations respectively, and Q_f is the ultrafiltration flow rate. Note that if C_{out} is zero, that is, solute removal is complete, Q_f adds nothing to dialyzer clearance.

For high-flux dialyzers where filtration rates are typically an order of magnitude greater than for conventional-flux dialyzers, convective fluid removal at the proximal end of the hollow fiber is much greater than at the distal end where oncotic effects may cause filtration to move in the opposite direction, so-called back-filtration [15]. This effect counteracts the negative effect of filtration on diffusion and may contribute to the higher clearances achieved by high-flux dialyzers [16, 17]. For all modes of dialysis, contraction of blood and extracellular fluid volume due to solute-deprived fluid removal helps to maintain the concentration at the blood inlet for a longer time, and thereby increases the effectiveness of the dialysis. This phenomenon highlights the importance of including fluid volume shifts in the mathematical models of dialysis urea kinetics (see below).

3.5 Origin of Kt/V

The concentration of solute is the driving force for diffusion, and the rate of diffusion is directly proportional to the concentration as noted in Eq. 3.1. Ignoring the effects of volume changes and solute generation, the change in concentration (C) with time (t) can be simplified and expressed mathematically as:

$$dC/dt = -kC. \qquad (3.5)$$

The symbol k is the elimination constant, similar to that of an injected drug, and indicates that the fractional change in concentration (dC/C)/dt is constant during the treatment. When expressed as a fraction of the distribution volume (V), $k \times V$ is the clearance (K), which is also constant, since in this overly simplified example we assume that V does not change. Integration of Eq. 3.5 and substituting K/V for k yields:

$$C = C_0 e^{-Kt/V}, \qquad (3.6)$$

C_0 is the initial concentration and C is the concentration at time (t). Logarithmic transformation of Eq. 3.6 yields:

$$Kt/V = \ln\left(C_0 / C\right). \qquad (3.7)$$

The left side of the overly simplified Eq. 3.7 (Kt/V) is the fractional clearance expressed per dialysis and normalized to body size (V). The denominator (V) adds value as a correlate to lean body mass, which is usually more desirable than body weight as a normalizing factor for body size. Equation 3.7 helps to illustrate the strong dependence of the clearance (expressed as Kt/V) on the ratio of solute concentrations in two blood samples, one at the beginning (C_0), and one at the end of the treatment (C). Note that the ratio is used, not the absolute concentrations, and also note that none of the components of the Kt/V expression need to be measured independently, including the treatment time (t).

If urea is the solute, and its generation (G) and volume changes (ΔV) during the dialysis are included, Eq. 3.8 (see below) must be substituted for Eq. 3.7, but the fundamental strong dependence of Kt/V on pre/post-urea concentrations remains.

3.6 Modeling Urea Kinetics

Regardless of what we think is going on within the hollow-fiber membranes during dialysis, it is possible to precisely model solute flux, including the effect of ultrafiltration, using a mass balance approach where input equals output. Figure 3.2 depicts the elements contributing to urea mass balance within the patient during and between dialyses. Equation 3.8 is the solution to the mass balance equations in Fig. 3.2 and provides a practical estimate of fluctuating serum urea concentrations while the patient's urea volume varies usually by several kilograms during and between treatments. Equation 3.8 also incorporates residual native kidney function and urea generation, and is used as the fundamental tool for modeling urea kinetics.

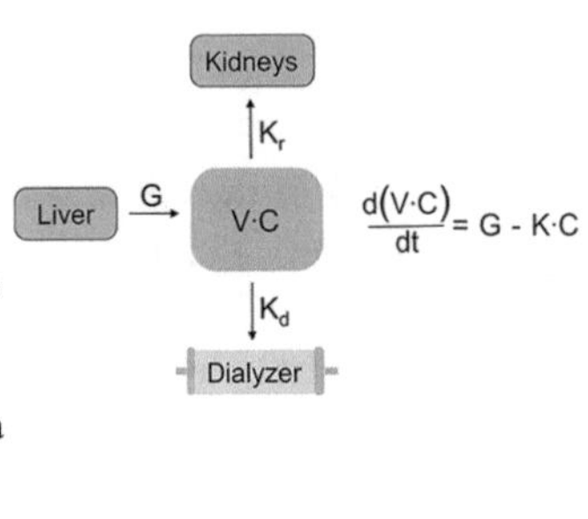

Fig. 3.2 Single-compartment model of urea mass balance. Equation 3.8 is the explicit solution to the differential equation in this figure, which is used to resolve Kt/V and G from a single pre-dialysis BUN and a single post-dialysis BUN. V is the urea distribution volume, C is the urea concentration, K_d is the dialyzer clearance, K_r is the kidney clearance, and G is the urea generation rate. K is the sum of K_d and K_r during dialysis, and is equal to K_r between dialyses

$$C = C_0\left[\frac{V-\Delta V\cdot t}{V}\right]^{\left(\frac{K_r+K_d+\Delta V}{\Delta V}\right)} + \frac{G}{K_r+K_d+\Delta V}\left[1-\left[\frac{V-\Delta V\cdot t}{V}\right]^{\left(\frac{K_r+K_d+\Delta V}{\Delta V}\right)}\right], \quad (3.8)$$

C is the solute concentration at any time (t), C_0 is the initial concentration, V is the solute distribution volume, ΔV is the rate of fluid removal, G is the solute generation rate, K_r is the patient's native kidney solute clearance, and K_d is the dialyzer clearance.

Urea modeling uses Eq. 3.8 in a reverse manner. The modeler measures C and C_0 (analogous to Eq. 3.7) then solves for G and Kt/V using computerized iterations of Eq. 3.8. The modeler must also have knowledge of volume fluxes (ΔV), K_r, and t, although these are less critical. Equation 3.8 yields a profile of the BUN during and between treatments and repeats itself weekly because the interdialysis treatment intervals are asymmetric during the week. Each treatment is assumed to be identical, but the patient begins the treatment differently because of the time asymmetry. For example, if dialysis is performed three times per week, the patient will have accumulated solute for 2 or 3 days depending on the day of the week. Equation 3.8 is solved (by iteration) twice, once during dialysis, and again between dialyses when K_d is zero. Note that the results are expressed in relative terms, as a fraction of the patient's urea volume. For example, to resolve V, knowledge of K_d is necessary and vice versa. Ordinarily, the user provides an estimate of K_d, which is assumed to be constant throughout the treatment as noted above; K_d and KoA can be measured using samples collected simultaneously from the blood inflow and outflow ports or estimated using Eqs. 3.2 and 3.3.

During dialysis, K_d has the major influence; between dialyses G dominates. This means that Kt/V is primarily determined by the pre-dialysis and post-dialysis BUN values (see Eq. 3.7), and G is determined by the post-dialysis and subsequent pre-dialysis BUN values. Because the primary modeling outcome is Kt/V, an independent measure of K_d is not required, and errors in estimates of K_d have little influence on the resulting Kt/V dose measurement. Similar to Eq. 3.7, the ratio of post- to pre-BUN values determines Kt/V; absolute values are not considered. Absolute values, however, can be used to measure G using an iterative method as depicted in Fig. 3.3, eliminating the need to sample blood again at the next dialysis [18]. Since urea is an end product of protein metabolism, G can be converted to a protein equivalent, a net protein catabolic rate normalized to V (PCRn), as shown in Eq. 3.9 [19]. PCRn can be useful as an adjunct to dietary counseling:

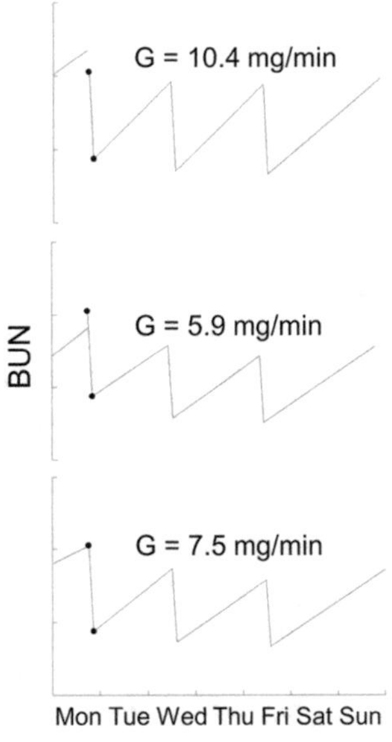

Fig. 3.3 Measuring G with only 2 BUN values. The *upper graph* shows a weekly BUN profile generated by Eq. 3.8 that uses an excessively high value for G. In the *middle graph* the value is too low. By repeated iteration, a value for G is found (*lower graph*) that matches the pre-dialysis BUN with the end-week BUN. [18]

$$PCRn = 5420(G/V) + 0.17. \quad (3.9)$$

3.7 More Refined Modeling

The single-compartment (single V) model diagramed in Fig. 3.2 predicts BUN concentrations during and between dialyses, but the results do not coincide precisely with measured values, especially for short intense dialysis as shown in Fig. 3.4. BUN values are overestimated during dialysis and underestimated between dialyses, especially in the immediate post-dialysis period. The cause of these discrepancies is delayed diffusion among the patient's body compartments, most notably intracellular versus extracellular, which reduces the effective volume of distribution during dialysis and causes a rebound in concentration as the two compartments re-equilibrate post dialysis. Despite the unique and rapid diffusibility of urea across red cell membranes as noted above, urea kinetics in the remainder of the body are better described by a two-compartment model, as shown in Fig. 3.5. This model is similar to the single-compartment model de-

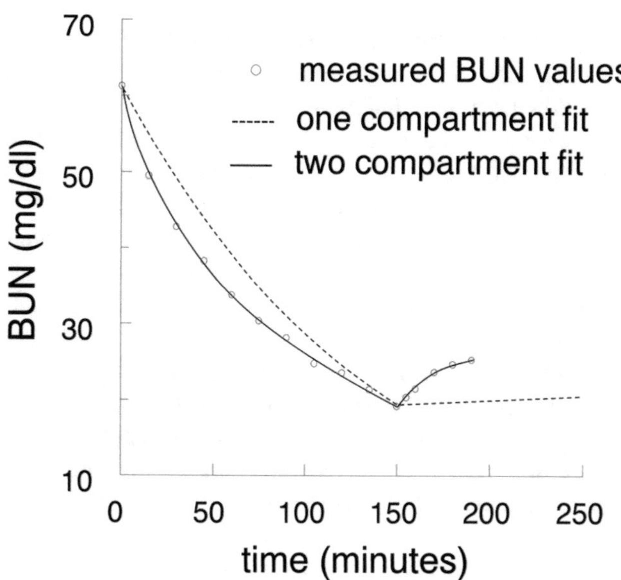

Fig. 3.4 Modeled and measured BUN values compared. The single-compartment prediction of BUN values during and following a short, high-efficiency dialysis is shown as the *dashed line*. Actual values measured every 15 min are shown as *open circles*. The *solid line* shows the prediction of a two-compartment model

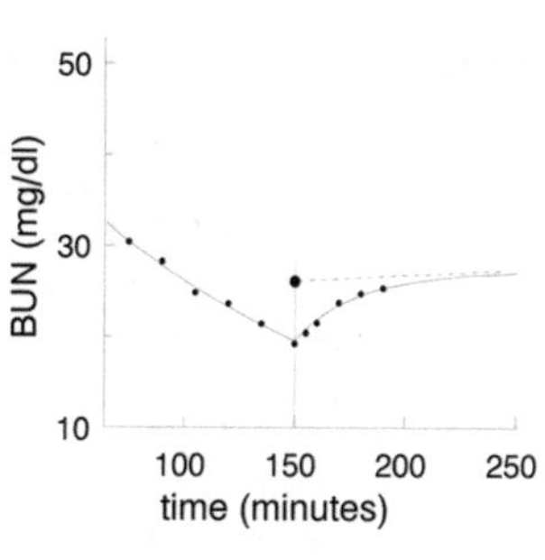

Fig. 3.6 Source of eKt/V. The equilibrated post-dialysis BUN shown here as the *large circle* is obtained by extrapolating measured post-dialysis BUN values. It is always higher than the BUN measured immediately post dialysis (shown just below it). Whole body eKt/V, which is derived from the equilibrated BUN, is always lower than spKt/V, which is derived from the immediate post-dialysis BUN

picted in Fig. 3.2 with an added remote compartment volume (V_2) and concentration (C_2). Unfortunately, the addition of a second compartment complicates the mathematics such that the equations depicted in Fig. 3.5 are not easily resolved explicitly and require more complex mathematical manipulations for a solution [20]. A method using numerical analysis has been implemented and made available on an Internet site devoted to dialysis dosing [21].

The single-compartment assumption causes the errors in predicted concentrations as shown in Fig. 3.4 but when used to calculate the dialysis dose as Kt/V, the two errors during and after the end of dialysis tend to cancel each other; the resulting values for Kt/V (and K_d) calculated by each model

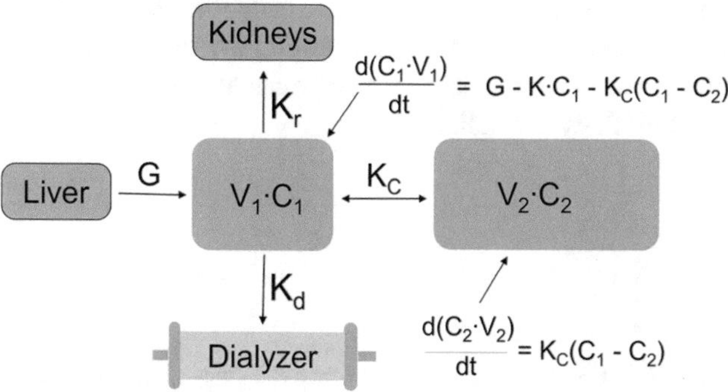

Fig. 3.5 Two-compartment diffusion model. Fast iterative resolution of the two differential equations shown in this figure yield values for V_1, V_2, K_C, and G. V_1 is the dialyzed compartment volume, V_2 is the remote compartment volume, and K_C is the inter-compartment mass transfer coefficient. Other symbols are the same as defined in Fig. 3.2

are similar, justifying clinical use of the simpler model [22]. Despite this minimization of the single-compartment error, some authorities have objected to using the immediate post-dialysis BUN as an indicator of the dialysis dose, since it is falsely low if compared to the equilibrated value shown in Fig. 3.6. The latter is determined by extrapolating the late inter-dialysis concentration curve back to the immediate post-dialysis time, which essentially converts the patient's urea kinetics to a single compartment but with an equilibrated clearance (eK). The resulting eK and eKt/V are always lower than the dialyzer instantaneous clearance and single pool Kt/V (spKt/V). The lowered clearance is an effective whole body clearance defined as the removal rate divided by the average urea concentration in the patient's body compartments at the time the removal rate is measured. eKt/V was used in the HEMO Study (see below) as the target for randomization [23], and by the European Best Practice Guideline Expert Group as a target for HD adequacy in general [24]. Fortunately, a two-compartment model is not needed to calculate eKt/V; approximations based on the intensity of dialysis have been developed [25–27], one of which is shown here [26]:

$$eKt/V = spKt/V(t/(t+30)). \qquad (3.10)$$

To complicate the model further, the immediate rebound in urea concentration post dialysis is not entirely due to delayed diffusion. Disequilibrium within the blood compartment is caused by multiple parallel circuits with markedly different blood flow rates [28]. The most rapidly flowing circuit is the route through the patient's arteriovenous fistula, heart and lungs, and back [29]; this cardiopulmonary (CP) circuit has a round-trip circulation time of 5–15 s depending on the patency of the fistula and the patient's cardiac output. The CP circuit also happens to be the dialyzed circuit, all others feeding into it from venous return. As a result the urea concentration falls to a lower level in the CP circuit during dialysis, as much as 20 mg/dl lower than in the periphery, and it rebounds within about 2 min when the blood pump is stopped [28]. This flow-related disequilibrium differs from

Table 3.2 Flow limited versus diffusion limited clearance; both contribute to rebound

Flow limited	Diffusion limited
Established immediately	Highly dependent on molecular size, diffusibility
Dissipates quickly (within 2 min)	Slow to develop
Not dependent on molecular size, diffusibility	Dissipates slowly (1–4 h)
Multiple flow circuits, no diffusion barrier	Multiple compartments and diffusion barriers

Table 3.3 Blood sampling technique to measure the post-dialysis BUN

Turn off ultrafiltration
Slow the blood pump to 100 ml/min for 10 s then stop the pump
Draw the blood sample from the arterial (dialyzer inflow) port

the diffusion-related disequilibrium (Fig. 3.6) with respect to several factors listed in Table 3.2.

In addition to reducing solute clearance, disequilibrium has a significant impact on the method for drawing the post-dialysis BUN. A method that yields a modeled dialyzer clearance equivalent to the actual cross-dialyzer clearance is shown in Table 3.3. If the sample is drawn too soon, before potential access recirculation has dissipated, the dialysis dose, expressed as a delivered clearance, will be overestimated, putting the patient in jeopardy from under-dialysis. If drawn too late, the dose will be inconsistent from treatment to treatment.

3.8 Intermittent Versus Continuous Dialysis

Solute disequilibrium is a consequence of high clearances applied intermittently. This phenomenon together with the self-limiting nature of intermittent dialysis as described above reduces the treatment efficiency, which means that more dialysis (clearance × time) must be applied to achieve the same concentration-lowering effect as continuous dialysis. When dialysis is applied continuously (e.g., continuous PD) or for native kidney function, constant replenishment of solute on the blood side (G) eliminates this inefficiency, and solute disequilibrium is essentially nonexistent. When minimum standards for PD and HD are compared, it appears that patients maintained with continuous PD require approximately half of the weekly clearance × time required by HD patients. Two theories have been put forth to explain this observation. One is based on peak urea concentrations, claiming that peak concentrations correlate better with overall uremic toxicity than mean levels, and the other is based on solute disequilibrium, claiming that toxic solutes are sequestered in remote compartments that equilibrate more slowly with the dialyzed compartment, essentially preventing the dialyzer from completing its job. Slow continuous treatments eliminate peaks and allow time for equilibration. Both theories have a basis in mathematical modeling and both produce similar solute concentration profiles under a variety of conditions as discussed below under "Dosing Frequent Dialysis" [30].

Although less efficient than continuous treatment, intermittent treatments are much easier to measure. Continuous clearances such as PD or native kidney function require collections of urine and/or dialysate during a defined time period. Intermittent hemodialysis clearances only require measuring the change in blood concentrations from beginning to end of the treatment and applying a model of solute kinetics as described above. Blood sampling alone is required; collection of dialysate is not necessary.

3.9 Practical Differences Between Hemodialysis Kt/V and Native Kidney Glomerular Filtration Rate (GFR)

In comparison with the native kidney, the clearance concept and definition are the same but the methods for measuring and expressing clearance differ, as shown in Table 3.4. For HD, urea is the preferred marker solute instead of creatinine because of the red cell creatinine disequilibrium discussed above, the additional patient-specific information obtained about protein nutrition, and the sensitivity of urea clearances to dialyzer effectiveness. Urea is not favored as a measure of native kidney clearance because tubular urea reabsorption is variable and unpredictable. Most current incenter dialysis treatments are intermittent, so the expression of dose must take into account the time during which the patient is not dialyzed. Expressing the dose as a clearance per dialysis satisfies this requirement as long as the frequency is specified as part of the dose. Instead of body surface area, the denominator for the dialysis dose is the volume of urea distribution, an automatic result of urea kinetic modeling as noted above and a mathematical convenience. Lastly, the fluctuations in urea concentration between and during intermittent dialyses allow measuring the dose by mathematical modeling without need for dialysate collection.

Table 3.4 Hemodialysis Kt/V versus native kidney glomerular filtration rate (GFR)

The marker solute is urea instead of creatinine
The time element is per dialysis instead of per minute
The denominator is V instead of BSA
The measurement doesn't require urine (or dialysate) collection

3.10 Dosing Frequent Dialysis

As noted above, the efficiency of HD depends on the frequency, increasing with more frequent treatments and eventually reaching maximum efficiency with continuous treatment. To include frequency in the dose, the peak concentration hypothesis [31] has been applied, which redefines the clearance as the removal rate divided by the average peak concentration [32]. This newly defined continuous equivalent clearance, called "standard Kt/V" (stdKt/V) is expressed as a fractional clearance similar to spKt/V, but as a weekly clearance similar to PD. The target is slightly higher than the target for continuous PD (2.0 per week) and is independent of dialysis frequency. Figure 3.7 shows the relationship between spKt/V and stdKt/V for different frequencies of dialysis. Of note, the current minimum standard for spKt/V is 1.2 per dialysis 3×/week, which corresponds to a stdKt/V of 2.0/week as shown in Fig. 3.7.

An explicit simplified equation, based on a fixed volume urea kinetic model has been developed for converting eKt/V to stdKt/V [27]:

$$_{\text{std}}\text{Kt}/\text{V} = \frac{10080\dfrac{1-e^{-\text{eKt/V}}}{t}}{\dfrac{1-e^{-\text{eKt/V}}}{\text{eKt}/\text{V}} + \dfrac{10080}{\text{Nt}} - 1}. \qquad (3.11)$$

A recent modification of Eq. 3.11 allows variations in urea volume and K_r [33]:

$$_{\text{std}}\text{Kt}/\text{V} = \frac{\text{S}}{1 - \dfrac{0.74\text{Uf}_\text{W}}{\text{F}\cdot\text{V}}} + \text{Kr}\frac{10080}{\text{V}}, \qquad (3.12)$$

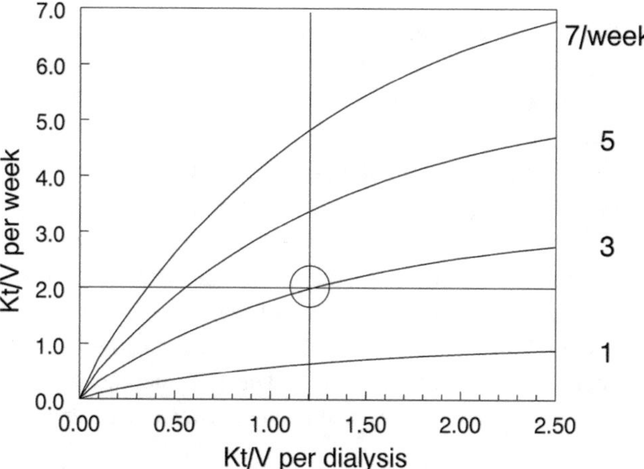

Fig. 3.7 Single pool versus continuous equivalent (standard) Kt/V. The single-pool dose per dialysis on the horizontal axis is compared to the equivalent (standard) weekly dose on the vertical axis. When given three times weekly, the currently accepted minimum dose is 1.2 per dialysis, which closely matches the minimum dose in the USA for continuous PD *(large circle)*

S is the patient's stdKt/V from Eq. 3.11; Uf_w is the patient's weekly fluid removal in ml; F is the dialysis weekly frequency; V is the patient's urea distribution volume in ml; K_r is the patient's native kidney urea clearance in ml/min; 10080 is the number of minutes in a week.

3.11 Adequacy of the Dose

The question of adequacy relates to native kidney function as well as dialysis. We have a vague sense that GFRs >20 ml/min are adequate, but some patients are able to tolerate GFRs as low as 5–10 ml/min for sustained periods of time [34]. The established minimum dose for PD patients is a weekly urea clearance index (Kt/V) of 1.7 [35]. The latter translates, for an average size patient with a urea volume of 30 L, to about 5 ml/min. Recall that GFR overestimates urea clearance because urea is reabsorbed by the native kidney, and it underestimates creatinine clearance because creatinine is secreted. Since the dialyzer has neither reabsorptive nor secretive functions, urea clearance should correspond to native kidney GFR on average. This reasoning leads to a conclusion that the minimum level of dialysis for continuous PD is equivalent to a barely acceptable level of native kidney function; hence the word "minimum" should be emphasized. For HD patients, standard Kt/V (see above) has been introduced to allow comparisons among more frequent and continuous clearances, including native kidney function. Published USA guidelines specify a minimum stdKt/V 2.0/week, which translates to about 7 ml/min for an average size patient. These surprisingly low levels of replacement function are based on outcomes studies such as the HEMO and ADEMEX studies that failed to show improvement in mortality and various secondary outcomes including hospitalization rates when the dose was increased [23, 35].

Reports of improved outcomes in patients dialyzed more frequently led investigators to suggest that intermittent treatments have intrinsic limitations that can only be overcome by increasing the frequency of treatments to 4–6 sessions per week. Solute kinetic analysis also suggested that increasing the treatment time would be more effective when applied more than 3×/week (see Fig. 3.7). In keeping with these theoretical considerations and marked benefits reported from uncontrolled studies, controlled clinical trials showed significant improvements in patient outcomes but somewhat less impressive than anticipated. The US National Institutes of Health-sponsored Frequent Hemodialysis Network study found that short daily incenter dialysis for 1 year improved the primary composite outcome of survival + reduction in left ventricular (LV) mass [36], the latter mainly in patients with ventricular hypertrophy. Quality of life was also improved. A similar improvement in LV mass was noted in a smaller Canadian study that compared frequent nocturnal HD with standard treatments given three times per week [37]. Together with findings of a significant reduction in pre-dialysis blood pressure, the data suggest that accumulation of fluid between dialyses is detrimental, but correctable by an increase in dialysis frequency. Phosphorus control was also improved as evidenced by lower pre-dialysis serum concentrations and a reduced requirement for oral phosphate binders. Whether the predictable increase in removal of other small solutes contributed to the clinical improvements is not possible to dissect from the data. For the present, more frequent dialysis is recommended for patients who prefer it and for patients with poor control of BP, volume, or serum phosphorus.

It is important to distinguish between adequate dialysis and adequate care of the patient. These distinct concepts are sometimes confused. Dialysis is the major focus of the nephrologist, but it is only a subset of the latter. Care certainly would be considered inadequate if it consisted only of dialysis and assessment of the dialysis dose. Measures of the adequacy of care in other spheres are also required. Patients approaching the need for dialysis usually bring with them a legacy of medical problems some of which may have contributed to the decline in kidney function. These problems are not necessarily alleviated or even improved by dialysis, and usually require attention, sometimes more attention than the dialysis itself.

3.12 Influence of Native Kidney Function on the Dose

Considered precious and frequently measured in the months and years prior to starting dialysis, residual native kidney function (K_r) is largely ignored once dialysis has begun. Perhaps use of terminology such as "replacement therapy" gives the impression that it no longer matters. The fallacy of this concept was well shown by the Netherlands Cooperative study where the mortality rate in patients with no K_r exceeded that of patients even with a K_r of 1–3 ml/min by an order of magnitude [38, 39]. For patients managed with PD, K_r is measured with each assessment of dialysis adequacy but the practice of collecting the patient's urine to measure K_r in HD patients is unusual. Several factors may explain this seemingly strange behavior: (1) PD patients are schooled in self-care and tend to be more self-directed. (2) Adequacy of dialysis is more difficult to measure in PD patients so it is done only 3 or 4 times/year instead of monthly in HD patients. (3) Combining K_r with K_d is conceptually easier in PD patients where simple addition suffices (see below).

Once the dialysis dose is reduced, K_r must be monitored carefully to guard against under-dialysis when kidney function deteriorates further. Opponents of K_r measurements point to the negative psychological impact on patients whose treatment time requires an increase when K_r diminishes or is lost. Caregivers must then struggle to convince the patient that a higher dose of dialysis is necessary. Financial providers might also object to equal pay for reduced and full (anuric) doses of dialysis (Table 3.5) [38, 40–48].

Table 3.5 Clinical consequences due to loss of K_r

Lower survival rate [38, 40, 41]
Poorer volume control leading to:
More edema
Less optimal blood pressure control
Left ventricular hypertrophy (LVH)
Reduced clearance of larger molecules (e.g., beta-2 microglobulin) [42, 43]
Reduced clearance of protein-bound molecules (e.g., p-cresol and indoxyl sulfate [44, 45]
Erythropoietin resistance [46]
Lower serum albumin levels [47]
Higher serum phosphorus levels and/or need for more phosphate binders [48]

Table 3.6 To preserve native kidney function

Avoid or reduce exposure to nephrotoxic agents including:
Aminoglycoside antibiotics
Nonsteroidal anti-inflammatory drugs (NSAIDS)
Radiographic contrast agents (take precautions before use)
Use antagonists of the renin–angiotensin system (e.g., ACE inhibitors)
Use diuretics
Manage hypertension
Avoid volume depletion, hypotension

Table 3.7 How to incorporate K_r into Kt/V and stdKt/V

Inflate the native kidney clearance to an intermittent equivalent, then add
Deflate the intermittent dialyzer clearance to a continuous equivalent clearance (e.g., standard Kt/V), then add

Regardless of efforts to measure K_r, efforts to preserve native kidney function in patients prior to initiating dialysis should be continued after dialysis is started. Table 3.6 lists recommended precautions and practices to preserve K_r.

Combining native kidney urea clearance with continuous dialysis clearance is a simple matter of addition, but combining with intermittent (HD) urea clearance requires manipulation of the data to account for their non-simultaneous occurrences. As noted above, intermittent dialysis is less efficient than continuous dialysis, so adjustments for differences in efficiency must be made as well. The first method listed in Table 3.7 was also the first used and continues to be applied:

$$Kt/V = \frac{K_d \times T_d + K_r \times T_r}{V}, \tag{3.13}$$

K_d is the dialyzer clearance, T_d is the treatment time, K_r is the patient's native kidney clearance, T_r is the inter-dialysis

Table 3.8 Inflation of the inter-dialysis interval to account for the greater efficiency of K_r

Treatments per week	Tr (no inflation)	T_r (inflated)
2	5040	9500
3	3360	5500
4	2520	3700
5	2016	2700
6	1680	2100
7	1440	1700

interval, and V is the urea distribution volume. Since K_r has its major impact between dialyses, it is reasonable to use the inter-dialysis time interval (first column in Table 3.8) as a multiplier when calculating $K_r \times T_r$. To account for differences in efficiency, T_r can be inflated, as shown in the second column of Table 3.8.

The second method listed in Table 3.7 involves reducing the dialyzer component to a continuous equivalent clearance (e.g., standard K or stdKt/V as described above), followed by simple addition. Care must be taken to avoid including K_r in the method for downsizing K_d [33].

Alternatives to Urea Modeling

The urea reduction ratio (URR), defined as $(C_0 - C)/C_0$ where C_0 is the pre-dialysis BUN and C is the post-dialysis BUN, is a crude measure of urea extraction during a single dialysis. Its strength is simplicity, and it involves little or no manipulation of the raw data, two advantages that are perhaps the reasons it was chosen by the US Centers for Medicare and Medicaid Services (CMS) for monitoring its constituent dialysis clinics. The URR cannot be used to measure continuous clearances, does not include residual kidney function, and fails to incorporate the additional clearance afforded by ultrafiltration, sometimes as much as 20–30% of the total Kt/V. Urea generation during dialysis is also not accounted for, an especially important factor during prolonged dialysis sessions.

Simplified formulas for estimating Kt/V from formal urea modeling are available as well. The most popular was developed by Daugirdas and recently upgraded to include more frequent dialyses [49, 50]:

$$\frac{K \cdot t}{V} = -\ln(R - 0.03) + (4 - 3.5 \cdot R)\frac{\Delta BW}{BW}, \quad (3.14)$$

R is the ratio of post-dialysis BUN to pre-dialysis BUN. This measure is especially helpful in population studies where the opportunity for modeling individual patients is not available.

Cross-dialyzer solute clearance can be measured as a change in conductivity in response to a pulsed change in the inlet dialysate concentration [51, 52]. Most dialysis delivery systems monitor dilution of a dialysate concentrate using conductivity meters, so the machine is already poised to measure "conductivity clearance," better termed "ionic dialysance."

Since sodium and its accompanying anion are responsible for >90% of the dialysate conductivity, conductivity changes simply reflect sodium dialysance, which is nearly identical to the clearance of urea (and other small solutes). Figure 3.8 shows the pulsed change in conductivity induced on the dialysate inlet side (ΔC_{in}) and the response (ΔC_{out}) on the outlet side recorded by conductivity electrodes placed in the inflow and outflow dialysate lines. The ionic dialysance is calculated as [51, 53]:

$$D_{ionic} = Q_d \left[\frac{\Delta C_{in} - \Delta C_{out}}{\Delta C_{in}}\right]. \quad (3.15)$$

Equation 3.15 provides an instantaneous measure of small solute clearance, equivalent to cross-dialyzer urea clearance. It must be measured several times during the dialysis to obtain an average for the entire treatment to generate a measure equivalent to urea Kt/V. Advantages to this method include real-time monitoring, no blood sampling or analysis, no disposables, and ready use of body surface area as the denominator. Disadvantages include the need for multiple measurements during each dialysis, and need for an independent measure of V to meet current standards, which are measured as Kt/V.

Some authorities have argued that urea is a poor surrogate for uremic toxins, suggesting that Kt/V urea is inappropriate as a measure of dose [54, 55]. This argument fails to consider that absolute levels of urea are not part of Kt/V and that urea is simply a marker for small solute clearance, as noted above. Comparison with PD, however, and the development of standard Kt/V suggest that a sequestered solute might be a better marker [56, 57]. Other solutes too, such as larger (or middle) molecules and protein-bound toxins might be more representative [58–60], especially for the residual syndrome. A comparison among these marker solutes is presented in Table 3.9.

Removal of salt and water has been highlighted as an essential part of the dose or prescription [61]. Fluid accumulation between dialyses must be limited by dietary restriction, and the excess must be removed during dialysis to prevent states of fluid overload and its consequences, including hypertension, pulmonary edema, and death. Rapid removal of

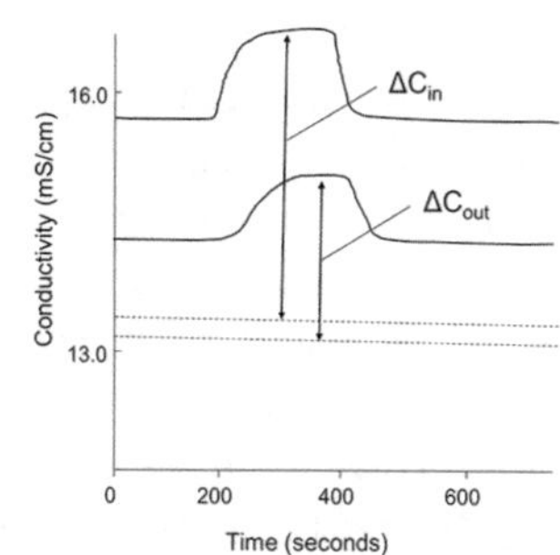

Fig. 3.8 Conductivity profiles illustrate the online clearance method. The *upper graph* shows conductivity in the dialysate inflow line during a 3-min increase in the dialysate concentration. The *lower line* records the conductivity response in the dialysate outflow line

Table 3.9 Solutes cleared less readily than urea

Larger solutes (middle molecules)	Secluded solutes	Protein bound solutes
Low dialyzer clearance rate	High dialyzer clearance rate	High dialyzer clearance of free fraction (clearance of total concentration is low)
Removal depends on membrane porosity (low KoA)	Removal not dependent on membrane porosity (high KoA)	Removal not dependent on membrane porosity
Clearance is significantly enhanced by convection (hemofiltration)	Clearance is minimally enhanced by convection especially because it is already high	Clearance is minimally enhanced by convection
Rebound is variable depending on the distribution volume, ordinarily low or absent	Large rebound due to marked disequilibrium between compartments at the end of dialysis	Minimal rebound as total clearance is low, binding is near-instantaneous
Less shifting of solute into the dialyzed compartment between dialyses	Marked shifting of solutes into the dialyzed compartment between dialyses	Little or no shifting of solute into the dialyzed compartment between dialyses

fluid, however, has been associated with hypotension and adverse cardiac consequences including arrhythmias and myocardial stunning [62]. Uncontrolled studies have shown that these adverse consequences are correlated with the treatment time, leading some to recommend that the patient's treatment time be extended to a minimum of 4 h, regardless of Kt/V, and/or that a maximum rate of fluid removal be set at 10–15 ml/kg body weight [63–65]. These recommendations seem reasonable although they require more of the patient's time, and their validity has not been established in controlled clinical studies.

Although fluid removal by ultrafiltration during dialysis is an essential requirement for most patients, it is not essential for some. In contrast to solute removal, some uremic patients require no fluid removal and conversely, removal of fluid alone will never reverse uremia. Fluid accumulation is therefore not an essential part of the uremic syndrome, and the ultrafiltration component of the dialysis dose must be considered adjunctive therapy.

3.13 The Future of Dosing

In view of continued high morbidity and mortality rates and failed attempts to improve the outcomes of dialysis patients including improved biocompatibility of dialyzer membranes, higher clearances, high-flux dialysis, increases in thrice weekly Kt/V, and more frequent or prolonged treatments, it is reasonable to look elsewhere for an explanation and question current methods for measuring the dialysis dose. Contributions of the native kidney to personal health may be subtle and yet to be discovered, perhaps analogous to erythropoietin support of red cell mass. Patient comorbidities, independent of the kidney failure, may contribute to the high mortality. Poorly dialyzed solutes such as those listed in Table 3.9 may be responsible. However, one must not lose sight of the remarkable ability of dialysis to prolong life that would end within a few days in an anuric patient. The prolongation of life is surely due to removal of small dialyzable (urinary) solutes, reducing their concentrations in the patient to sub-lethal levels. Dialysis does nothing more than remove small solutes by diffusion across a relatively tight semipermeable membrane. There is nothing complex or mysterious about therapeutic dialysis. Therefore, first and foremost in our responsibilities to the patient should be a measure of small solute clearance. After that, the field is open to further exploration and treatment of the residual syndrome, which should be encouraged.

References

1. Abel JJ, Rowntree LG, Turner BB. On the removal of diffusible substances from the circulating blood by means of dialysis. Trans Assoc Am Physicians. 1913;28:51–73.
2. Haas G. Dialysieren des stromenden Blutes am Lebenden: Bemerkung zu der Arbeit von Necheles in dieser Wochenschrift. Klin Wochenschr. 1923;2(Suppl):1888–92.
3. Haas G. Versuche der Blutauswaschung am Lebenden mit Hilfe der Dialyse. Klin Wochenschr. 1925;4:1888–95.
4. Kolff WJ, Berk HTJ, ter Welle M, van der Ley AJW, van Dijk EC, van Noordwijk J. The artificial kidney, a dialyzer with a great area. Acta Med Scand. 1944;117:121–8.
5. Scribner BH, Caner JEZ, Buri R, Hegstrom RM, Burnell JM. The treatment of chronic uremia by means of intermittent dialysis: a preliminary report. Trans Am Soc Artif Intern Organs. 1960;6:114–9.
6. Gotch FA, Sargent JA, Keen ML. Individualized, quantified dialysis therapy of uremia. Proc Clin Dial Transpl Forum. 1974;1:27–37.
7. Graham T. Liquid diffusion applied to analysis. Phil Trans Royal Soc London. 1861;151:183–93.
8. Fick A. Ueber diffusion. Annln Phys. 1855;94:59–74.
9. Michaels AS. Operating parameters and performance criteria for hemodialyzers and other membrane-separation devices. Trans Am Soc Artif Intern Organs. 1966;12:387–92.
10. Cheung AK, Alford MF, Wilson MM, Leypoldt JK, Henderson LW. Urea movement across erythrocyte membrane during artificial kidney treatment. Kidney Int. 1983;23(6):866–9.
11. Sands JM, Timmer RT, Gunn RB. Urea transporters in kidney and erythrocytes. Am J Physiol. 1997;273(3 Pt 2):F321–39.
12. Descombes E, Perriard F, Fellay G. Diffusion kinetics of urea, creatinine and uric acid in blood during hemodialysis. Clinical implications. Clin Nephrol. 1993;40(5):286–95.
13. Schneditz D, Yang Y, Christopoulos G, Kellner J. Rate of creatinine equilibration in whole blood. Hemodial Int. 2009;13(2):215–21.
14. Husted FC, Nolph KD, Vitale FC, Maher JF. Detrimental effects of ultrafiltration on diffusion in coils. J Lab Clin Med. 1976;87:435–42.
15. Baurmeister U, Travers M, Vienken J, Harding G, Million C, Klein E, et al. Dialysate contamination and back filtration may

limit the use of high-flux dialysis membranes. ASAIO Trans. 1989;35(3):519–22.
16. Dellanna F, Wuepper A, Baldamus CA. Internal filtration–advantage in haemodialysis? Nephrol Dial Transplant. 1996;11(Suppl 2):83–6.
17. Santoro A, Conz PA, De Cristofaro V, Acquistapace I, Gaggi R, Ferramosca E, et al. Mid-dilution: the perfect balance between convection and diffusion. Contrib Nephrol. 2005;149:107–14.
18. Depner TA, Cheer A. Modeling urea kinetics with two vs. three BUN measurements. A critical comparison. ASAIO J. 1989;35:499–502.
19. Borah MF, Schoenfeld PY, Gotch FA, Sargent JA, Wolfson M, Humphreys MH. Nitrogen balance during intermittent dialysis therapy of uremia. Kidney Int. 1978;14:491–500.
20. Schneditz D, Daugirdas JT. Formal analytical solution to a regional blood flow and diffusion-based urea kinetic model. ASAIO J. 1994;40:M667–73.
21. Daugirdas JT, Depner TA, Greene T, Silisteanu P. Solute-solver: a web-based tool for modeling urea kinetics for a broad range of hemodialysis schedules in multiple patients. Am J Kidney Dis. 2009;54(5):798–809.
22. Depner TA. Multicompartment models. Prescribing hemodialysis: a guide to urea modeling. Boston: Kluwer Academic Publishers; 1991. pp. 91–126.
23. Eknoyan G, Beck GJ, Cheung AK, Daugirdas JT, Greene T, Kusek JW, et al. Effect of dialysis dose and membrane flux in maintenance hemodialysis. N Engl J Med. 2002;347(25):2010–9.
24. European Best Practice Guidelines Expert Group on Hemodialysis ERA. Section II. Haemodialysis adequacy. Nephrol Dial Transplant. 2002;17(Suppl 7):16–31.
25. Daugirdas JT. Simplified equations for monitoring Kt/V, PCRn, eKt/V, and ePCRn. Adv Ren Replace Ther. 1995;2:295–304.
26. Tattersall JE, DeTakats D, Chamney P, Greenwood RN, Farrington K. The post-hemodialysis rebound: predicting and quantifying its effect on Kt/V. Kidney Int. 1996;50:2094–102.
27. Leypoldt JK, Jaber BL, Zimmerman DL. Predicting treatment dose for novel therapies using urea standard Kt/V. Semin Dial. 2004;17(2):142–5.
28. Depner TA, Rizwan S, Cheer AY, Wagner JM, Eder LA. High venous urea concentrations in the opposite arm. A consequence of hemodialysis-induced compartment disequilibrium. ASAIO J. 1991;37:141–43.
29. Schneditz D, Kaufman AM, Polaschegg HD, Levin NW, Daugirdas JT. Cardiopulmonary recirculation during hemodialysis. Kidney Int. 1992;42:1450–6.
30. Depner TA. Benefits of more frequent dialysis: lower TAC at the same Kt/V. Nephrol Dial Transpl. 1998;13:20–4.
31. Keshaviah PR, Nolph KD, Van Stone JC. The peak concentration hypothesis: a urea kinetic approach to comparing the adequacy of continuous ambulatory peritoneal dialysis (CAPD) and hemodialysis. Peritoneal Dial Int. 1989;9:257–60.
32. Gotch FA. The current place of urea kinetic modelling with respect to different dialysis modalities. Nephrol Dial Transpl. 1998;13(Suppl 6):10–4.
33. Daugirdas JT, Depner TA, Greene T, Levin NW, Chertow GM, Rocco MV. Standard Kt/Vurea: a method of calculation that includes effects of fluid removal and residual kidney clearance. Kidney Int. 2010;77(7):637–44.
34. Cooper BA, Branley P, Bulfone L, Collins JF, Craig JC, Fraenkel MB, et al. A randomized, controlled trial of early versus late initiation of dialysis. N Engl J Med. 2010;363(7):609–19.
35. Paniagua R, Amato D, Vonesh E, Correa-Rotter R, Ramos A, Moran J, et al. Effects of increased peritoneal clearances on mortality rates in peritoneal dialysis: ADEMEX, a prospective, randomized, controlled trial. J Am Soc Nephrol. 2002;13(5):1307–20.
36. Chertow GM, Levin NW, Beck GJ, Depner TA, Eggers PW, Gassman JJ, et al. In-center hemodialysis six times per week versus three times per week. N Engl J Med. 2010;363(24):2287–300.
37. Culleton BF, Walsh M, Klarenbach SW, Mortis G, Scott-Douglas N, Quinn RR, et al. Effect of frequent nocturnal hemodialysis vs conventional hemodialysis on left ventricular mass and quality of life: a randomized controlled trial. JAMA. 2007;298(11):1291–9.
38. Termorshuizen F, Dekker FW, van Manen JG, Korevaar JC, Boeschoten EW, Krediet RT. Relative contribution of residual renal function and different measures of adequacy to survival in hemodialysis patients: an analysis of the Netherlands Cooperative Study on the Adequacy of Dialysis (NECOSAD)-2. J Am Soc Nephrol. 2004;15(4):1061–70.
39. Wang AY, Lai KN. The importance of residual renal function in dialysis patients. Kidney Int. 2006;69(10):1726–32.
40. Maiorca R, Brunori G, Zubani R, Cancarini GC, Manili L, Camerini C, et al. Predictive value of dialysis adequacy and nutritional indices for mortality and morbidity in CAPD and HD patients. A longitudinal study. Nephrol Dial Transplant. 1995;10:2295–305.
41. Bargman JM, Thorpe KE, Churchill DN. Relative contribution of residual renal function and peritoneal clearance to adequacy of dialysis: a reanalysis of the CANUSA study. J Am Soc Nephrol. 2001;12(10):2158–62.
42. Brown PH, Kalra PA, Turney JH, Cooper EH. Serum low-molecular-weight proteins in haemodialysis patients: effect of residual renal function. Nephrol Dial Transplant. 1988;3(2):169–73.
43. Amici G, Virga G, Rin G D, Grandesso S, Vianello A, Gatti P, et al. Serum beta-2-microglobulin level and residual renal function in peritoneal dialysis. Nephron. 1993;65(3):469–71.
44. Bammens B, Evenepoel P, Verbeke K, Vanrenterghem Y. Removal of middle molecules and protein-bound solutes by peritoneal dialysis and relation with uremic symptoms. Kidney Int. 2003;64(6):2238–43.
45. Marquez IO, Tambra S, Luo FY, Li Y, Plummer NS, Hostetter TH, et al. Contribution of residual function to removal of protein-bound solutes in hemodialysis. Clin J Am Soc Nephrol. 2011;6(2):290–6.
46. Wang AY, Wang M, Woo J, Law MC, Chow KM, Li PK, et al. A novel association between residual renal function and left ventricular hypertrophy in peritoneal dialysis patients. Kidney Int. 2002;62(2):639–47.
47. Wang AY, Woo J, Wang M, Sea MM, Sanderson JE, Lui SF, et al. Important differentiation of factors that predict outcome in peritoneal dialysis patients with different degrees of residual renal function. Nephrol Dial Transplant. 2005;20(2):396–403.
48. Wang AY, Woo J, Sea MM, Law MC, Lui SF, Li PK. Hyperphosphatemia in Chinese peritoneal dialysis patients with and without residual kidney function: what are the implications? Am J Kidney Dis. 2004;43(4):712–20.
49. Daugirdas JT. Second generation logarithmic estimates of single-pool variable volume Kt/V: an analysis of error. J Am Soc Nephrol. 1993;4:1205–13.
50. Daugirdas JT, Leypoldt JK, Akonur A, Greene T, Depner TA. Improved equation for estimating single-pool Kt/V at higher dialysis frequencies. Nephrol Dial Transplant. 2013;28(8):2156–60.
51. Petitclerc T, Bene B, Jacobs C, Jaudon MC, Goux N. Non-invasive monitoring of effective dialysis dose delivered to the haemodialysis patient. Nephrol Dial Transplant. 1995;10:212–6.
52. Gotch FA, Panlilio FM, Buyaki RA, Wang EX, Folden TI, Levin NW. Mechanisms determining the ratio of conductivity clearance to urea clearance. Kidney Int Suppl. 2004;89:S3–24.
53. Filippo S D, Manzoni C, Andrulli S, Pontoriero G, Dell'Oro C, La Milia V, et al. How to determine ionic dialysance for the online assessment of delivered dialysis dose. Kidney Int. 2001;59(2):774–82.
54. Vanholder R, DeSmet R, Lesaffer G. Dissociation between dialysis adequacy and Kt/V. Semin Dial. 2002;15(1):3–7.
55. Eloot S, Van Biesen W, Glorieux G, Neirynck N, Dhondt A, Vanholder R. Does the adequacy parameter Kt/V(urea) reflect uremic toxin concentrations in hemodialysis patients? PLoS ONE. 2013;8(11):e76838.

56. Depner TA. Uremic toxicity: urea and beyond. Semin Dial. 2001;14(4):246–51.
57. Ishizaki M, Matsunaga T, Itagaki I. What is a surrogate marker for optimal dialysis? Hemodial Int. 2007;11(4):478–84.
58. Eloot S, Torremans A, De SR, Marescau B, De WD, De Deyn PP, et al. Kinetic behavior of urea is different from that of other water-soluble compounds: the case of the guanidino compounds. Kidney Int. 2005;67(4):1566–75.
59. Meijers BK, Bammens B, De Moor B, Verbeke K, Vanrenterghem Y, Evenepoel P. Free p-cresol is associated with cardiovascular disease in hemodialysis patients. Kidney Int. 2008;73(10):1174–80.
60. Meyer TW, Sirich TL, Hostetter TH. Dialysis cannot be dosed. Semin Dial. 2011;24(5):471–9.
61. Foundation NK. K/DOQI clinical practice guidelines and clinical practice recommendations for 2006 Updates: hemodialysis adequacy, peritoneal dialysis adequacy, and vascular access. Am J Kidney Dis. 2006;48(Suppl 1):S1–322.
62. McIntyre CW, Burton JO, Selby NM, Leccisotti L, Korsheed S, Baker CS, et al. Hemodialysis-induced cardiac dysfunction is associated with an acute reduction in global and segmental myocardial blood flow. Clin J Am Soc Nephrol. 2008;3(1):19–26.
63. Kurella M, Chertow GM. Dialysis session length ("t") as a determinant of the adequacy of dialysis. Semin Nephrol. 2005;25(2):90–5.
64. Flythe JE, Kimmel SE, Brunelli SM. Rapid fluid removal during dialysis is associated with cardiovascular morbidity and mortality. Kidney Int. 2011;79(2):250–7.
65. Flythe JE, Curhan GC, Brunelli SM. Disentangling the ultrafiltration rate-mortality association: the respective roles of session length and weight gain. Clin J Am Soc Nephrol. 2013;8(7):1151–61.

4 Hemodialysis Complications

Nicholas A. Zwang, Sagar U. Nigwekar and David J. R. Steele

4.1 Introduction

Complications related to hemodialysis are frequent. By its nature, the hemodialysis procedure attempts to reproduce the physiological functions of the kidney on a basic level. In doing so, it requires the patient to spend periods of time enduring extracorporeal blood circulation, forced ultrafiltration, and dialysis of solute by way of exposure to large volumes of dialysate. This process is associated with both expected and unexpected complications given the circumstances of the treatment process.

4.2 Access Complications

Vascular access is known as the "Achilles heel" of dialysis. It is the rare dialysis patient who has not undergone access revision, thrombectomy, or insertion of a temporary dialysis catheter. Each of these procedures adds to the burden of care for dialysis patients and the systems of care that serve them. The three main types of long-term dialysis access are tunneled catheters, arteriovenous grafts, and arteriovenous fistulas. Each carries its own special set of risks and complications that merit careful attention.

The most expeditious means to achieve vascular access is with a hemodialysis catheter. Catheters may be situated via a subcutaneous tunnel or may be non-tunneled. The latter are not suitable for outpatient use due to higher rates of infection bleeding and accidental dislodgement. Catheters are the least durable mode of dialysis access. Blood flow and clearance rates are often impaired due to thrombosis and adherence of fibrin, and infectious complications are high, ranging from exit site infections to systemic bacteremia and sepsis. The most common pathogens responsible for catheter-associated infections are skin flora, particularly *Staphylococcus aureus* (including methicillin-resistant *S. aureus* (MRSA)) and coagulase-negative species [1]. Prevention strategies for catheter-associated infections are important. Catheter care with standardized protocols associated with cleansing of the catheter exit site and the surrounding skin [2], application of maximal sterile barriers when accessing catheters, and regular assessment of exit sites by nursing staff are well described, although adherence may not always occur [3, 4]. Intranasal antibacterial applications, such as mupiricon, may reduce catheter infections related to some bacterial species and are a strategy applied in some settings to reduce MRSA-associated infections. Routine catheter exchanges over a guidewire are not recommended to prevent infections. Application of iodine or antibiotic ointments to catheter exit sites is not universally recommended but may help to reduce infections in selected patients [5, 6]. Citrate locks, especially those containing antibiotics, appear superior to heparin for the prevention of catheter-associated bloodstream infection without affecting the risk of poor flow or catheter-associated thrombosis [7]. Clinicians should have a low threshold to draw blood cultures and institute empiric antibiotic therapy in febrile dialysis patients with indwelling dialysis catheters. According to current Infectious Diseases Society of America guidelines, infected catheters can be salvaged with systemic antibiotics and antibiotic locks depending on the associated organ or can be managed with catheter exchanges [8]. Appropriate management, however, depends on the severity of infection. Patients in septic shock with tunneled dialysis catheters are best managed with catheter removal and temporary access placement.

In addition to infection, dialysis catheters frequently fail due to mechanical complications. These failures can be a

D. J. R. Steele (✉)
Department of Medicine, Massachusetts General Hospital, Boston, MA, USA
e-mail: dsteele@partners.org

N. A. Zwang
Department of Nephrology, Massachusetts General Hospital, Boston, MA, USA

S. U. Nigwekar
Department of Internal Medicine/Nephrology, Harvard Medical School, Massachusetts General Hospital, Boston, MA, USA

A. K. Singh et al. (eds.), *Core Concepts in Dialysis and Continuous Therapies*, DOI 10.1007/978-1-4899-7657-4_4

consequence of placement (such as kinking and inadequate length) or thrombotic occlusions (including intraluminal thrombi and external fibrin sheath formation) [9]. Evidence of reduced catheter function includes reduced arterial blood flows (below 300 mL/min), and inadequate dialysis (Kt/V below 1.2), often associated with negative arterial pressures (more negative than 250 mmHg) [10]. First-line strategies to treat intraluminal thrombi include thrombolytic agents and heparin locks at port sites [11]. When external fibrin sheaths form, catheters develop a "valve mechanism" obstructing adequate blood flow [12]. Angiography may be necessary to visualize the presence of a fibrin sheath. Instillation of thrombolytics and catheter exchange over a guidewire with mechanical sheath lysis may be required.

The median patency of a tunneled dialysis catheter is about 200 days, with a nearly 66% failure rate at 6 months and a median time to catheter-associated infection of 163 days [12]. For these reasons, it is preferable to initiate dialysis with more durable access in the form of an arteriovenous fistula or a (bio)prosthetic graft. These forms of dialysis access, however, may be associated with complications of their own. Mechanical complications include maturation failure, stenoses (either within the access or in contiguous native vessels), thrombosis, endovascular infections, aneurysms, and bleeding or rupture. Thrombosis is the most common complication of grafts and fistulas. For functioning fistulas, the 1-year thrombosis rate is about 16%; about half of the fistulas remain patent 2 years after placement [13]. Grafts have higher failure rates and require more interventions. Fistulas have higher rates of non-maturation than grafts, which may make grafts more suitable in patients with a high likelihood of primary access failure or those initiating dialysis with a short life expectancy [13]. More recently, a hybrid central catheter and prosthetic subcutaneously placed graft has become an option to bypass central stenoses in patients with a history of difficult or failed access [14].

The practicing nephrologist should examine a patient's access routinely. The "rule of six" may be used to recognize a mature fistula: access is a minimum of 6 mm in diameter with discernible margins when a tourniquet is in place; is less than 6 mm deep to the skin; blood flow exceeds 600 mL/min; and there is at least a straight 6 cm segment to cannulate [15]. There is strong agreement between abnormalities detected on physical examination of dialysis shunts and those confirmed angiographically [16, 17]. Routine physical examination of a dialysis shunt begins with inspection to assess for signs of infection, skin changes (shiny taut skin may indicate high underlying pressures related to outflow stenosis), and pseudoaneurysms [18]. Evaluation should include auscultation for a continuous bruit and palpation of an adequate thrill without hyperpulsatility. A fistula should normally augment upon distal occlusion, and failure to do so indicates an inflow stenosis; it should collapse upon limb raising, and poor collapsibility indicates an outflow stenosis. Since arteriovenous grafts normally have higher pressures than fistulas, arm raising is not informative for these shunts.

Both fistulas and grafts are susceptible to thrombosis, though grafts tend to have higher rates of thrombotic complications. There are no clearly agreed upon approaches to primary prophylaxis such as active surveillance for preemptive angioplasty or empiric anticoagulation [19]. While access thrombosis is common and increased among patients with underlying thrombophilias, there is no value to screening for inherited thrombophilias [20]. Thrombosis of a fistula, unlike a graft, can be associated with dialytic hypotension and lower pre-dialysis systolic blood pressures [21]. Declotting procedures are often successful in experienced hands. A complication of thrombectomy is thromboembolism [22]. In patients with a patent foramen ovale, paradoxical embolism has been described, although it is rare [23].

When the clinicians suspect dialysis shunt dysfunction, they should assess for recirculation. When venous return to the circulation via a fistula or graft is unimpeded, no recirculation occurs. When there is resistance to venous return, a percentage of blood recirculates to the dialyzer. High rates of recirculation may indicate access stenosis or thrombosis [24]. Urea-based recirculation is calculated as follows: $(\text{BUN}_{\text{serum}} - \text{BUN}_{\text{arterial}})/(\text{BUN}_{\text{serum}} - \text{BUN}_{\text{venous}}) \times 100\%$. A recirculation greater than 10% merits additional investigation [25]. As measurement of recirculation by urea-based methods can be inconsistent, Doppler ultrasound to detect saline bolus dilution may be used [26]. Measurement of saline dilution by online blood volume monitors is another method [27]. Measured by this technology, recirculation greater than 5% is considered abnormal.

Infectious complications of dialysis fistulae and grafts are frequent. Grafts are more prone to infections than fistulae. Protocols for prevention of access infection should be rigidly enforced in the dialysis setting. Accesses should be washed prior to use and sterile procedures should be followed with needle placement. Patient education related to sterility is important. Access infection is associated with hematoma and local tissue injury. Buttonhole access sights are prone to infectious complications due to frequency of use and microtrauma. Local infections of grafts and fistula may present with systemic symptoms (fever, elevated white blood cell count, and failure to thrive symptoms) prior to obvious signs of local infection. Ultrasound imaging may be helpful to define a collection in this setting. Erythema, fluctuation, local tenderness, and pus draining from needle insertions sites are late signs in the process. Indolent infection in a graft or in residual components of resected graft material, as a cause for bacteremia, may represent a particular diagnostic challenge as local signs of infection are often absent in these cases [28].

4.3 Technical Complications

The major technical components of the hemodialysis procedure relate to the water system, including the dialysate delivery system, the hemodialysis machine including its hardware and software, and the interface with the patient, the tubing, and dialysis membrane. All components are multifaceted and failure of any one of the mechanical components can be serious. In the spirit of primary prevention, hemodialysis care delivery is the subject of close regulatory scrutiny, and dialysis relies upon collaboration among physicians and highly trained nurses and technicians.

Beyond leak and rupture, dialysis membranes can precipitate allergic reactions. These reactions are classified as either type A (true hypersensitivity or "first use" syndromes) or type B (nonspecific clinical syndromes associated with incompatibilities between the patient and dialysis membrane) [29]. Type B reactions often present with chest or back pain. An important illustration of type B reactions is the case of polyacrilonitrate (PAN). These PAN dialyzers uniquely promote bradykinin release, which cannot be metabolized in patients taking angiotensin-converting enzyme inhibitors. These reactions tend to resolve quickly with cessation of dialysis and saline reinfusion.

Type A reactions are true hypersensitivity reactions. Ethylene gas, when used to sterilize dialysis membranes, is one of the most common allergens, and skin prick testing can demonstrate preformed IgE antibodies [30]. Gamma radiation sterilization has largely superseded the use of ethylene gas. The use of biocompatible (e.g., polysulfone membranes) as opposed to bio-incompatible membranes (e.g., cellulosic membranes) has resulted in fewer membrane-associated allergic phenomena. Typically, dialysis hypersensitivity provoked by a dialyzer membrane begins with complement activation. Hypocomplementemia and elevated serum tryptase levels may lend support to the diagnosis of a hypersensitivity reaction [30]. Membrane-associated leukopenia in the first 30 min of dialysis, even without an associated hypersensitivity reaction, and platelet activation with thrombocytopenia are associated with polysulfone dialyzers (with various compositions of polyvinylpyrrolidone and particularly those sterilized by electron beam) [31].

A potential approach to managing "first use" dialyzer reactions is to reuse dialyzer membranes for the same patient after appropriate disinfection procedures. While dialyzer reuse decreases costs and may decrease complement-mediated dialyzer reactions, chemicals used for sterilization (bleach, formaldehyde, acetic acid) can be allergenic [32]. Inadequate sterilization can lead infectious complications. Dialyzer reuse has fallen out of favor by many centers.

Hemolysis may occur due to technical complications related to the dialysate preparations, and dialysis tubing may kink and cause mechanical hemolysis in both cases with potentially serious consequences [33]. Post-pump kinks may not trigger either pre-pump or post-pump pressure alarms. Small but simultaneous decreases in both arterial and venous pressures may indicate a post-pump tubing kink [34].

The dialysis circuit itself must be airtight to prevent the introduction of air bubbles that can be the source for embolic events. Venous microbubbles can occur [35]. The air trap along the arterial circulation input is the first defense against large air emboli. Higher rather than lower levels of blood in the air trap can help to reduce microemboli [36]. The consequences of air embolism can be severe. Signs of air embolism include negative venous pressures, bubbles in the venous air trap, chest pain, dyspnea, and hypoxemia [37]. When suspected, one should stop dialysis immediately, apply 100 % oxygen, place the patient in the left lateral decubitus position, and—in severe cases—consider hyperbaric therapy [38].

Dialysate is highly purified water mixed with a liquid or dry concentrate to achieve a desired electrolyte composition. Since water is the basis for dialysate, water treatment to achieve desired component and sterility guidelines is fundamental in terms of patient safety [39, 40]. With a dialysate flow of 800 mL/min, a typical patient can be exposed to almost 200 L of dialysate in a single dialysis session. Therefore, trace contaminants that are inconsequential for the general public take on special significance for the dialysis population. Treatment of water from local sources typically includes softening, reverse osmosis purification, ultra violet (UV) light treatment, ultrafiltration (to remove endotoxin), carbon filtration, and often continuous recirculation to prevent growth of bacterial biofilms [41].

Biofilms typically harboring gram-negative organisms, such as *Pseudomonas, Klebsiella*, and *Enterobacter* species, are very difficult to remove once established, and are the sources of outbreaks [42]. These outbreaks can lead to severe morbidity and mortality from septicemia. Even if bacterial growth in biofilms does not cause overt infections, bacteria—both from biofilms and municipal water supplies—produce endotoxin. Exposure to endotoxin leads to pyogenic reactions ranging from uncomplicated fevers to septic shock. Importantly, pyogenic reactions due to bacterial or endotoxin contamination do not abate with cessation of dialysis [43]. In contrast, most dialyzer reactions or pyogenic reactions due to chemical contaminations can resolve quickly by stopping the dialysis procedure.

The most important chemical contaminants to which end-stage renal disease (ESRD) patients may be exposed are chloramines, derived from chlorine and ammonia used to decontaminate municipal water supplies [44]. Oxidative by-products of chloramine induce acute hemolytic anemia and methemoglobinemia. Low-grade, chronic chloramine exposure can manifest as erythropoietin resistance [45]. Of particular importance, carbon filtration but not reverse osmosis removes waterborne chloramines. Other contaminants that have caused notable outbreaks include lead, copper, aluminum, and sulfates [43].

Whenever an outbreak of infection or pyogenic or hemolytic reactions occur in a dialysis unit, it is essential to review water purification procedures in depth and analyze water and dialysate samples.

The dialysate potassium prescription receives the closest attention from nephrologists and dialysis nurses. Low-potassium dialysate is often needed to treat hyperkalemia. There is conflicting evidence whether low-potassium dialysate causes increased ectopy or QT interval prolongation, a concern in patients who have electrocardiogram (EKG) abnormalities due to acute hyperkalemia [46]. Two well-publicized studies have shown sudden cardiac death during dialysis after the long weekend interval [47, 48]. A proposed explanation for these findings has been an increased potassium gradient at this time, as ESRD patients are often relatively hyperkalemic following the weekend interval. Indeed, there is a correlation between low-potassium dialysate and sudden cardiac death [49]. Some experts, therefore, advise treatment with graded reduction in dialysate potassium for acute hyperkalemia and rarely using low (i.e., below 2 mmol/L) potassium dialysate for outpatients [50]. In cases of life-threatening hyperkalemia, higher-bicarbonate dialysate might help reduce serum potassium via transcellular shift [51]. The benefit of bicarbonate administration to manage acute hyperkalemia, however, is unclear [52]. The drawback to this approach is the potential for potassium rebound post dialysis.

It is also important to focus on dialysate bicarbonate concentrations. The total bicarbonate dose delivered to a patient is the sum of dialysate bicarbonate and the acid anion (e.g., citrate or acetate) added to the pre-infusion dialysate [53]. Addition of these weak acids keeps the dialysate pH below 7.3, thereby preventing salt precipitation. Citrate and acetate, once delivered to the patient, are metabolized to bicarbonate. In this context, epidemiologic studies suggest that higher dialysate bicarbonate concentrations may impact outcomes [54]. While lower dialysate bicarbonate concentrations in acidotic and catabolic patients may predisose to increased mortality [55]. Therefore, clinicians should interpret pre-dialysis serum bicarbonates and dialysate bicarbonate needs, in the context of a patient's general health and nutritional status.

Simplistically, high dialysate sodium leads to salt overload and hypertension, just as sodium retention leads to hypertension in patients with functioning kidneys. A net positive sodium load in dialysis leads to increased serum sodium, thirst, and hypertension. This relationship is the basis for individualized and profiled sodium prescriptions in hemodialysis. The technique of sodium profiling involves a stepwise decrease in dialysate concentration over the course of dialysis. The rationale for this approach is to deliver hypertonic dialysate early in the session, thereby raising the blood pressure to allow for more aggressive ultrafiltration [56]. As the session proceeds, dialysate sodium concentrations decrease in order to decrease the net load of sodium delivered. This approach may allow for increased ultrafiltration volume while decreasing dialytic hypotension [57, 58]. Observational data indeed show a positive, linear correlation between the dialysate and plasma sodium gradient. Many patients managed with sodium profiling finish their dialysis sessions net positive with respect to sodium [59]. This leads to inter-dialytic weight gain due to increased thirst [60, 61]. Sodium profiling is not appropriate for the general dialysis population but may be useful for selected patients with difficult-to-manage dialytic hypotension or inter-dialytic weight gain [62]. An alternative strategy to sodium modeling is to lower or individualize the sodium prescription. Low sodium (135 mEq/L for patients with sodium levels less than 137, 137 mEq/L for patients with sodium levels over 137) has been found to decrease pre-dialysis systolic blood pressures and intradialytic weight gain [63]. Adjusting dialysate sodium concentration for a patient's pre-dialysis sodium concentration may be the most physiologic approach and has been linked to inter-dialytic weight gain and hypotension [64].

Dialysate calcium concentrations require adjustment under certain circumstances, for example, in patients with chronic hypocalcemia (e.g., following parathyroidectomy) or chronic hypercalcemia (e.g., due calciphylaxis or hyperparathyroidism). Dialysate calcium concentrations of 1.25 mM (2.5 mEq/L) yield negative body calcium balance, whereas increased concentrations yield net positive total body calcium balance [65, 66]. Higher calcium dialysate may induce vasoconstriction, and may be an adjunct to manage intradialytic hypotension [67]. Low-calcium dialysate may be associated with an increased risk of sudden cardiac death [68]. Adjusting dialysate calcium concentrations may help manage metabolic bone disease. Decreased dialysate concentrations alongside vitamin D therapy can help to decrease parathyroid hormone (PTH) and even serum phosphate concentrations. Conversely, increased dialysate calcium concentrations might increase PTH and bone turnover in patients with adynamic bone disease [69].

4.4 Complications Related to Dialysis Treatment

Incident dialysis patients are at risk of acute neurologic complications. The "dialysis disequilibrium syndrome" historically has been described in highly uremic patients undergoing hemodialysis initiation [70]. In this context, urea (typically an ineffective osmole) is cleared more rapidly from the plasma than from the cerebrospinal fluid (CSF). As a consequence, CSF is transiently hypertonic to plasma, leading to transient cerebral edema until this gradient dissipates. Patients with dialysis disequilibrium develop symptoms ranging from mild nausea and headache to, in rare circumstances, seizure and coma [71]. Attendant cerebral parenchymal abnormalities are visible on T2-weighted magnetic resonance imaging (MRI) [72]. Rat studies of uremia have shown decreased expression of urea transporters but increased aquaporin expression, which helps to explain the delayed resolution of the CSF–plasma urea gradient with attendant diffusion of water into the CSF [73]. Given the pathophysiology described, most nephrologists introduce patients—particularly highly uremic patients—to dialysis gradually, unless there are life-threatening indications requiring more aggressive dialysis. Many centers also treat incident patients with osmotically active agents, such as mannitol, during their first several hemodialysis sessions in order to reduce the CSF–plasma osmolality gradient. The benefits of this practice, however, have not been proven definitively.

Dialysis-associated cramping is a common symptom and is the most common cause for early sign off from dialysis [74]. Rapid ultrafiltration and osmotic shifts during hemodialysis are often implicated in cramping, but the precise underlying neuromuscular mechanisms that cause cramping in dialysis are not known. While decreasing ultrafiltration or dialysis intensity may improve cramping, these maneuvers may lead to under-dialysis [75]. Of the various remedies offered to treat cramping, a meta-analysis suggests that L-carnitine supplementation does not improve muscle cramping, and the benefits of the antioxidants Vitamin C (which figures into carnitine biosynthesis), E, both, or placebo have not been established [76, 77]. Historically, two small, randomized controlled trials suggested a benefit of quinine, administered pre-dialysis, to prevent cramping [78, 79]. Quinine toxicity including cinchonism, cardiac arrhythmias, thrombocytopenia, hemolytic uremic syndrome, and impaired digoxin and warfarin metabolism, limits the utility of this medication. For these reasons, the Food and Drug Administration (FDA) has warned against this off-label prescribing of quinine to treat hemodialysis-associated muscle cramps [75, 80].

Both dialytic hypotension and hypertension can significantly interrupt dialysis, limiting adequacy and causing significant patient morbidity and even mortality. Dialytic hypotension arises from an imbalance between the rates of ultrafiltration and capillary refill, resulting in a systolic blood pressure drop of more than 20 mmHg or a mean arterial pressure (MAP) drop of more than 10 mmHg [81]. This may result from autonomic dysregulation, inappropriately low dry weight goals, and splanchnic vasodilatation while eating. Prevention of dialytic hypotension begins with careful attention to volume status [82]. In addition to consideration of sodium profiling, as discussed above, bicarbonate (but not acetate) and increased dialysate calcium may prevent dialytic hypotension. Some patients require pre-dialysis administration of α-1 agonists [83]. Although popular, the technique of isolated ultrafiltration followed by hemodialysis appears inferior to standard treatment [84]. Another initially popular preventative treatment—administration of L-carnitine—ultimately was shown to be ineffective in preventing dialytic hypotension [76]. Continued monitoring of noninvasive hematocrits measured by optical transmission may be helpful, but in a randomized controlled trial there was no benefit to preventing dialytic hypotension and increased hospitalization and mortality rates [85]. Techniques to treat acute hypotension include cooling the dialysate and Trendelenburg positioning. Modeling of rates of ultrafiltration is a consideration in certain patients and may be beneficial if individualized. The rates of ultrafiltration have an association with dialysis outcomes and rapid rates for fluid removal have been associated with adverse outcomes. In this context, the risk of all-cause and cardiovascular mortality increases with ultrafiltration rates over 10 ml/h/kg and is associated with a greater risk of all-cause and cardiovascular death [86].

Less common but equally important, and perhaps more difficult to manage, is the problem of dialytic hypertension. Frequently, this is a sign of volume overload, and systolic hypertension improves with increased ultrafiltration and adjustment of the estimated dry weight [87]. Other first-line therapies to manage dialytic hypertension include more aggressive dietary sodium restriction and decreased dialysate sodium, as discussed above [88]. Some patients, however, have underlying neurohormonal dysfunction contributing to their dialytic hypertension. While the renin–angiotensin system is often implicated, it is not clear that this is always the responsible axis [89]. Rather, endothelial dysfunction may be to blame. In terms of treatment options, studies using carvedilol have shown promise [90], and atenolol appears superior to metoprolol to reduce hypertension and morbidity in ESRD patients with intradialytic resistant hypertension [91].

Cardiovascular complications, particularly chest pain and arrhythmias, are common and important occurrences in dialysis patients. The incident rate of atrial fibrillation in dialysis initiates may be up to 10% [92]. Recent data from implantable cardioverter defibrillator (ICD) studies have suggested that the onset of new atrial fibrillation in ESRD patients occurs more frequently on dialysis than on non-dialysis days and, specifically, during dialysis itself [93]. Indeed, older studies have found ECG changes in the first 2 h of dialysis, including decreased T wave amplitude, increased QRS amplitude, and QTc interval changes [94]. When cardiac arrests occur in dialysis units, the underlying arrhythmia is usually ventricular. Survival among these patients tends to be very low: 15% at 1 year [95]. Thus, it is essential for dialysis units to maintain protocols and staff training for evaluation and treatment of cardiac arrhythmias on dialysis.

4.5 Complications Related to Dialysis Adequacy

Chronic uremia leads to generalized failure to thrive in ESRD patients and to the "malnutrition–inflammation complex syndrome" [96]. Such patients are typically hypoalbuminemic, and this may be a contributor to cardiovascular mortality on dialysis [97–99]. Conversely, obese or over-nourished patients enjoy some improved survival outcomes [100]. Identifying at-risk patients requires a multidisciplinary approach to assess biochemical, dietary, and anthropomorphic factors [101]. A surprisingly simple, targeted intervention is to allow dialysis patients to eat during their treatments [102]. This approach is not universally accepted, and risks of eating during dialysis include aspiration, splanchnic vasodilatation causing hypotension, and introduction of microbes into the dialysis treatment environment.

The generalized syndrome of dialysis inadequacy, due to either technical complications or patient characteristics (such as a catabolic, chronically inflamed state), leads to several noteworthy complications, chief among which are cardiac and neurologic diseases.

Incident dialysis patients are at risk of uremic pericarditis, particularly within the first few weeks of initiation [103]. Pericarditis may also develop in prevalent patients and may be a marker of inadequate dialysis. While the pathophysiology of both conditions is similar—chronic inflammation leading to a fibrinous exudate—prevalent dialysis pericarditis is more difficult to treat. Not all pericarditis in dialysis patients is uremic in etiology, and viral and inflammatory etiologies may also occur. Intensive hemodialysis is usually the first step toward managing uremic pericarditis. If hemodynamic compromise due to tamponade is present, pericardiocentesis should be performed [104]. Conservative options for patients whose pericarditis fails to respond to intensive dialysis are limited. Neither nonsteroidal anti-inflammatory medications [105] nor glucocorticoids are recommended for cases that fail to respond to intensive hemodialysis [106]. Rather, pericardiocentesis or pericardial window placement is often required for refractory cases.

There are many neuromuscular sequelae of chronic uremia in dialysis. Peripheral neuropathy related to length-dependent axonal loss and demyelination can occur [107]. Historically, "middle molecules" such as β[beta]$_2$-microglobulin and PTH have been implicated in this pathophysiology [108]. Prior to the widespread use of high-flux dialyzers, accumulation of large molecules such as β[beta]$_2$-microglobulin was an important cause of osteoarthropathy—and constriction neuropathies including spinal stenosis and carpal tunnel syndrome—in long-term hemodialysis patients [109]. The pathogenesis of β[beta]$_2$-microglobulin amyloidosis requires not only deposition of β[beta]$_2$-microglobulin fibrils but also a monocyte-driven inflammatory response. Two rare but clinically important neurologic conditions are important to recognize in hemodialysis patients. First, ischemic optic neuropathy is caused by hypotension in patients with underlying atherosclerotic disease or calcific uremic arteriolopathy [110]. Any hope of treatment requires restoration of optic nerve perfusion. Second, ulnar neuropathy is often subclinical and has a prevalence up to 60% [111]. Many of these cases may be attributable simply to arm positioning during hemodialysis.

4.6 Medical Comorbidities

4.6.1 Cardiovascular Disease

ESRD patients suffer from many underlying systemic diseases, most commonly hypertension, diabetes, and autoimmune conditions. These patients are at high risk of cardiovascular disease. There appears to be a relationship between inadequate dialysis (defined by $Kt/V < 1.2$), short treatment time (<210 min), and sudden cardiac death [112]. Data show increased mortality with dialysis sessions shorter than 240 min [113].

"Uremic cardiomyopathy" is a constellation of left ventricular hypertrophy leading to both systolic and diastolic dysfunction [114]. Uremia itself, independent of hypertension, seems to be associated with a cardiomyopathy and underlying signaling derangements in cardiomyocytes [115–117]. Cardiomyopathy can manifest as left ventricular hypertrophy, left ventricular dilatation, and heart failure—all of which are independently associated with a risk for de novo ischemic heart disease [118]. Cardiac MRI studies suggest that the underlying pathology is a pattern of fibrosis in patients with uremic cardiomyopathy [119]. This cardiomyopathy is frequently progressive, particularly within the first year of starting hemodialysis [120]. Hemodialysis itself induces at least temporary myocardial "stunning." Myocardial blood flow appears to fall during dialysis [121], a finding that correlates with segmental wall motion abnormalities [122]. More frequent dialysis sessions with lower ultrafiltration rates [123] and cooled dialysate [124] may ameliorate this problem.

4.6.2 Gastrointestinal (GI) Bleeding

Dialysis patients are particularly at risk for upper GI bleeding. Their rates of upper GI bleeding exceed those of the general population, and an episode of GI bleeding carries a 30-day mortality rate of nearly 12% [125]. Rates of rebleeding following treatment for peptic ulcer disease are higher in dialysis than in non-dialysis patients [126]. Age and dialysis vintage are independent risk factors for short-term mortality from upper GI bleeding among ESRD patients [127]. Risk factors for incident GI hemorrhage include cardiovascular disease, smoking, and generalized deconditioning in the dialysis population [128]. An especially important source of GI bleeding from any source in dialysis patients is small bowel angiodysplastic lesions, which may be obscure and require capsule endoscopy [129, 130]. In addition, uremia induces platelet dysfunction predisposing ESRD patients toward bleeding [131]. Finally, modality of renal replacement is an important consideration in dialysis patients with GI bleeding. Patients with hemodynamically significant bleeding frequently require ICU-level care and may not be stable enough for hemodialysis. In these cases, sustained low-efficiency dialysis (SLED) or continuous hemofiltration may be indicated.

4.6.3 Malignancy

Malignancy—particularly renal cell carcinoma—is an important consideration in the dialysis population. The incidence of native kidney neoplasms in long-term (10 years or more) dialysis patients approaches 3% [132]. Indeed, older dialysis vintage is associated with renal cell carcinoma arising out of acquired cystic lesions [133, 134]. The logical question, therefore, arises whether screening for renal neoplasms is warranted [135]. Decision analysis studies have suggested that the only population that may benefit from such screening approaches are young patients with long (at least 25 years) life expectancies [136]. These studies call to mind a broader question of whether general population age-appropriate cancer screening is at all warranted in dialysis patients. While age-appropriate cancer screening is appropriate for patients who may undergo renal transplantation, the decision to screen in other ESRD patients must be made on an individualized basis after considering life expectancy and the risks of screening [137]. ESRD patients with failed kidney transplants require special attention to their risks of malignancy, particularly skin cancers in those treated with calcineurin inhibitors [138].

4.6.4 Dermatological Complications

A variety of cutaneous conditions are seen in patients with hemodialysis. Although many of these conditions (e.g., ecchymosis, pruritus) can be seen in non-hemodialysis patients, when these occur in the setting of hemodialysis a few additional considerations apply. These are summarized in Table 4.1.

4.7 Infectious Disease Complications

During dialysis, patients are exposed to pathogens on multiple levels: via the angioaccess, related to community sources, and potentially although rare due to the dialysate or dialysis equipment.

Table 4.1 Special considerations for cutaneous conditions seen in hemodialysis patients

Xerosis	Most common dermopathy in hemodialysis
	Caused due to atrophy of sebaceous follicles and eccrine glands
	Can be a risk factor for ulcerations due to excoriations
	Daily local emollient application can be effective treatment
Pruritus	Although the exact etiology remains unclear, considerations include inadequate dialysis, abnormalities in mineral-bone disorder (e.g., hyperphosphatemia), and xerosis
	Oral antihistamines and low-dose gabapentin are effective treatments in addition to emollients for xerosis
Hyperpigmentation	Etiology unclear
	Sun protection may prevent hyperpigmentation
Ecchymosis	Could be related to platelet dysfunction, trauma, or anticoagulant use
	Optimizing dialysis adequacy and non-anticoagulant-based treatments for preventing access clots can reduce the risk of ecchymosis
	In severe cases, maintaining hemoglobin concentration above 10 g/dL, desmopressin, and estrogen therapy are indicated
Uremic frost	Extremely rare in hemodialysis patients in the modern days
	Indicates inadequate dialysis
Nephrogenic systemic fibrosis	Declining incidence since the use of non-gadolinium-based agents for magnetic resonance imaging studies
	Diagnosis is clinicopathological and requires high index of suspicion and demonstration of dermal fibrocyte proliferation on skin biopsy
	No effective therapy available; renal transplantation offers the best hope
Calciphylaxis	A highly fatal disorder characterized by dermal arteriolar calcification and thrombosis
	Hypercalcemia and warfarin therapy could be risk factors
	No effective therapy available

Hepatitis B infection is historically the best known infectious disease complication of hemodialysis although it is now rare. This in part relates to almost universal screening of all patients at the time of initiation of dialysis and then annually. Patients who are hepatitis B surface antibody seronegative are offered vaccination with a series of three or four exposures over a 6 month period. Seroconversion is not universal in part due to the level of immune suppression engendered for the ESRD chronic disease state.

Non-access-related infection remains a significant problem for patients with ESRD. Rates of chronic viral infections, human immunodeficiency virus (HIV), and hepatitis C are increased, as are rates of common bacterial infections such as pneumonia, urinary tract, and GI infections. Overall, infection accounts for approximately 15 % of deaths in ESRD patients, and in newly started hemodialysis, patient's infection is a frequent cause of readmission following index hospitalization [139]. Rates of pneumonia are five times higher and these rates are increased in smokers [140].

Herpes zoster infection is an important problem related in part to chronic immune suppression and low immunization rates. When treatment is given with antiviral agents, such as valacyclovir, dose adjustment for ESRD clearance rates is needed [141].

Clostridium difficile infection rates are higher and associated with high comorbidity levels and low serum albumin. Drug dosing should also be adjusted due to low intrinsic clearance, and metronidazole dose should be decreased by 50 % and given post dialysis treatment [142].

Urinary tract infections represent a challenge in hemodialysis patients, particularly in those with low urine output and urinary stasis. Pyuria is a common finding and, if associated with bacteriuria and a clinical syndrome of dysuria and fever, should be treated. Pyocystitis is an often overlooked cause of fever in dialysis patients, and when present it requires bladder irrigation in addition to antibiotic therapy. Pyelonephritis likewise should be considered both under the circumstances of a clinical syndrome with back pain and fever and in the asymptomatic patient with fever.

Soft tissue infections related to vascular disease, stasis dermatitis, and chronic pruritus are a frequent cause of emergency room visits and hospitalizations, and in the case of diabetic patients delay in diagnosis may occur due to underlying neuropathy. These cases are associated with the risk of limb loss due to underlying vascular disease. In this light, frequent diabetic foot checks are mandated hoping for early intervention.

Dental infections due to poor oral hygiene and lack of access to appropriate dental care are often overlooked. Chronic gingivitis and dental caries can contribute to impaired nutrition.

4.8 Disorders of Mineral Metabolism

Metabolic bone disease is an important complication of ESRD and encompasses laboratory abnormalities, structural bone abnormalities, and vascular calcification [143]. Laboratory abnormalities include hypocalcemia, hyperphosphatemia, hypovitaminosis D, and hyperparathyroidism. Fibroblast growth factor 23 (FGF 23) is now recognized as one of the earliest detectable abnormalities as the chronic disease progresses; however, routine assaying of FGF 23 is not routinely indicated for clinical purposes since data are insufficient to demonstrate whether targeting a specific level of FGF 23 leads to improved patient outcomes [144]. Serum levels of calcium and phosphorous should be targeted at the normal range, and serum PTH levels should be maintained between two to nine times the upper limit of normal [143]. The optimal 25-hydroxyvitamin D level for hemodialysis patients remains to be defined; however, current expert opinion favors treatment with oral ergocalciferol 50,000 IU (or cholecalciferol 10,000 IU) weekly for 8 weeks, followed by repeated serum 25-hydroxyvitamin D measurement for patients with 25-hydroxyvitamin D levels <30 ng/mL [145]. Bone pathology associated with hemodialysis includes abnormalities in bone turnover, volume, and mineralization. Multiple observational studies have demonstrated that hemodialysis patients are at an increased risk for fractures; however, interventions to reduce this fracture risk have not been investigated in rigorous trials [146–149]. Evaluation of novel risk factors that predict bone health and fracture risk in hemodialysis patients is an area of active investigation [150, 151], and this will inform the future clinical trials.

Recent attention has also focused on the prognostic significance of vascular calcification in hemodialysis patients, and various measures of vascular calcification burden (e.g., coronary calcification score) have been shown to predict the risk of cardiovascular events and mortality in the hemodialysis population [151]. Traditionally, hyperphosphatemia and hypercalcemia have been described as significant contributors to vascular calcification; however, multiple other factors (both stimulatory and inhibitory) control the active calcification process. The current Kidney Disease Improving Global Outcomes (KDIGO) guidelines recommend a lateral abdominal radiograph to screen for vascular calcification, but this recommendation is limited since there is no effective intervention to treat vascular calcification in hemodialysis patients.

Calciphylaxis is a potentially fatal cutaneous complication seen in hemodialysis patients. It is characterized by dermal arteriolar calcification and thrombosis leading to painful skin nodules, livedo, and/or ulcerations [152]. Recent investigations suggest hypercalcemia and warfarin therapy as possible risk factors; however, the studies are limited by small sample size [153, 154]. Calciphylaxis has over 60 %

1-year mortality and significant morbidity associated with nonhealing wounds and pain. A definitive diagnosis requires a skin biopsy with evidence of dermal arteriolar calcification. Sodium thiosulfate is one of the most commonly used treatments; however, evidence to support its efficacy is limited [155, 156].

4.9 Neuropsychiatric Disease and Psychosocial Complications

We have already discussed some of the specific neurologic effects of uremia and dialysis. Dialysis is further associated with both acute neuropsychiatric consequences and chronic conditions owing to mood disturbances, cognitive impairment, and sexual dysfunction.

As with many chronic medical conditions, ESRD is associated with an increased prevalence of depression. In fact, the rate of depression among patients undergoing hemodialysis may be as high as 40% [157]. Even among incident dialysis patients, depression correlates with a 2.7-fold increased risk of mortality at 2 years [158]. An association between dialysis and mortality persists in meta-analysis, even after controlling for other chronic medical comorbidities such as diabetes and cardiovascular disease [159]. Depression and sleep impairment are closely correlated, suggesting a modifiable target for depressed ESRD patients [160]. Thus, it is important to recognize and treat depression in patients treated with hemodialysis.

In addition to mood disturbances, ESRD patients are prone to a decline in cognitive function. Not only does cognitive dysfunction diminish quality of life but it can also interfere with medication and dietary adherence. In one study, 80% of ESRD patients met neuropsychiatric criteria for cognitive dysfunction, compared to 50% of case-matched controls. This risk was independent of vascular disease risk factors [161]. Surprisingly, there is no clear relationship between adequacy and cognitive dysfunction [162]. In fact, some patients manifest impaired cognitive function *after* routine dialysis sessions [163]. Many of these parameters for cognitive dysfunction improve after transplantation [164].

Both men and women with ESRD suffer from sexual dysfunction. Eighty-four percent of women with ESRD reported sexual dysfunction [165]. Reported symptoms were independently associated with—among other variables—age, depression, and diabetes. Nearly half of the men on hemodialysis reported erectile dysfunction, a condition that correlated strongly with depression [166]. Surprisingly, only 4% of men with reported erectile dysfunction actually were receiving pharmacologic treatment.

Finally, it is important for providers to recognize that dialysis is an intensive time commitment for the patient. The time required for transportation, dialysis attendance, and recovery after the dialysis session are associated with a significant financial opportunity cost for the patient. Adherence to a routine dialysis regimen is a job in itself. Often, dialysis patients are unable to hold full-time employment and require additional government assistance. Alternatives forms of renal replacement therapy, such as nocturnal hemodialysis and peritoneal dialysis, can help solve this problem for selected patients. Physicians should be sensitive to these important financial considerations for dialysis patients.

In this final section, we have explored the spectrum of psychosocial complications for patients on hemodialysis, ranging from acute dialysis disequilibrium to depression and financial disadvantages. These findings illustrate the importance of assessing the ESRD patient completely, for whom nearly every aspect of his or her life and health are affected by ESRD.

4.10 Conclusion

The combination of chronically ill patients with high indices of comorbidity and the complexities of the hemodialysis procedure result in risks for many of the complications described in this chapter. To an extent, hemodialysis delivery represents a form of outpatient intensive care. Awareness of the potential for complications and active surveillance as part of the dialysis process is necessary to impact complication rates and optimize the quality of care delivery.

References

1. Dryden MS, Samson A, Ludlam HA, Wing AJ, Phillips I. Infective complications associated with the use of the Quinton 'Permcath' for long-term central vascular access in haemodialysis. J Hosp Infect. 1991;19(4):257–62.
2. Rosenblum A, Wang W, Ball LK, Latham C, Maddux FW, Lacson E Jr. Hemodialysis catheter care strategies: a cluster-randomized quality improvement initiative. Am J Kidney Dis. 2014;63(2):259–67.
3. Rebmann T, Barnes SA, Association for Professionals in Infection Control and Epidemiology. Preventing infections in hemodialysis: an executive summary of the APIC Elimination Guide. Am J Infect Control. 2011;39(1):72–5.
4. O'Grady NP, Alexander M, Burns LA, Dellinger EP, Garland J, Heard SO, et al. Guidelines for the prevention of intravascular catheter-related infections. Clin Infect Dis. 2011;52(9):e162–93.
5. Johnson DW, MacGinley R, Kay TD, Hawley CM, Campbell SB, Isbel NM, Hollett P. A randomized controlled trial of topical exit site mupirocin application in patients with tunneled, cuffed haemodialysis catheters. Nephrol Dial Transplant. 2002;17(10):1802–7.
6. Lok CE, Stanley KE, Hux JE, Richardson R, Tobe SW, Conly J. Hemodialysis infection prevention with polysporin ointment. J Am Soc Nephrol. 2003;14(1):169–79.
7. Zhao Y, Li Z, Zhang L, Yang J, Yang Y, Tang Y, Fu P. Citrate versus heparin lock for hemodialysis catheters: a systematic review and meta-analysis of randomized controlled trials. Am J Kidney Dis. 2014;63(3):479–90.

8. Mermel LA, Allon M, Bouza E, Craven DE, Flynn P, O'Grady NP, et al. Clinical practice guidelines for the diagnosis and management of intravascular catheter-related infection: 2009 update by the Infectious Diseases Society of America. Clin Infect Dis. 2009;49(1):1–45.
9. Rasmussen RL. The catheter-challenged patient and the need to recognize the recurrently dysfunctional tunneled dialysis catheter. Semin Dial. 2010;23(6):648–52.
10. Besarab A, Pandey R. Catheter management in hemodialysis patients: delivering adequate flow. Clin J Am Soc Nephrol. 2011;6(1):227–34.
11. O'Mara NB, Ali S, Bivens K, Sherman RA, Kapoian T. Efficacy of tissue plasminogen activator for thrombolysis in central venous dialysis catheters. Hemodial Int. 2003;7(2):130–4.
12. Shingarev R, Barker-Finkel J, Allon M. Natural history of tunneled dialysis catheters placed for hemodialysis initiation. J Vasc Interv Radiol. 2013;24(9):1289–94.
13. Fokou M, Teyang A, Ashuntantang G, Kaze F, Eyenga VC, Chichom Mefire A, Angwafo F 3rd. Complications of arteriovenous fistula for hemodialysis: an 8-year study. Ann Vasc Surg. 2012;26(5):680–4.
14. Nassar GM, Glickman MH, McLafferty RB, Kevin Croston J, Zarge JI, Katzman HE, et al. A comparison between the HeRO graft and conventional arteriovenous grafts in hemodialysis patients. Semin Dial. 2014;27(3):310–8.
15. Vachharajani TJ. Diagnosis of arteriovenous fistula dysfunction. Semin Dial. 2012;25(4):445–50.
16. Asif A, Leon C, Orozco-Vargas LC, Krishnamurthy G, Choi KL, Mercado C, et al. Accuracy of physical examination in the detection of arteriovenous fistula stenosis. Clin J Am Soc Nephrol. 2007;2(6):1191–4.
17. Tessitore N, Bedogna V, Melilli E, Millardi D, Mansueto G, Lipari G, et al. In search of an optimal bedside screening program for arteriovenous fistula stenosis. Clin J Am Soc Nephrol. 2011;6(4):819–26.
18. Salman L, Beathard G. Interventional nephrology: physical examination as a tool for surveillance for the hemodialysis arteriovenous access. Clin J Am Soc Nephrol. 2013;8(7):1220–7.
19. Allon M. Current management of vascular access. Clin J Am Soc Nephrol. 2007;2(4):786–800.
20. Salmela B, Hartman J, Peltonen S, Albäck A, Lassila R. Thrombophilia and arteriovenous fistula survival in ESRD. Clin J Am Soc Nephrol. 2013;8(6):962–8.
21. Chang TI, Paik J, Greene T, Desai M, Bech F, Cheung AK, Chertow GM. Intradialytic hypotension and vascular access thrombosis. J Am Soc Nephrol. 2011;22(8):1526–33.
22. Smits HF, Van Rijk PP, Van Isselt JW, Mali WP, Koomans HA, Blankestijn PJ. Pulmonary embolism after thrombolysis of hemodialysis grafts. J Am Soc Nephrol. 1997;8(9):1458–61.
23. Wu S, Ahmad I, Qayyum S, Wicky S, Kalva SP. Paradoxical embolism after declotting of hemodialysis fistulae/grafts in patients with patent foramen ovale. Clin J Am Soc Nephrol. 2011;6(6):1333–6.
24. Whittier WL. Surveillance of hemodialysis vascular access. Semin Intervent Radiol. 2009;26(2):130–8.
25. Hemodialysis adequacy work group. Clinical practice guidelines for hemodialysis adequacy, update 2006. Am J Kidney Dis. 2006;48(Suppl 1):S2–90.
26. Depner TA, Krivitski NM. Clinical measurement of blood flow in hemodialysis access fistulae and grafts by ultrasound dilution. ASAIO J. 1995;41(3):M745–9.
27. Yoshida I, Ookawara, S, Ando K, Uchida T, Horiguchi A, Nakajima I, et al. Evaluation of a new method for measuring vascular access recirculation. Ther Apeher Dial. 2011;15(3):319–26.
28. Lok CE, Foley R. Vascular access morbidity and mortality: trends of the last decade. Clin J Am Soc Nephrol. 2013;8(7):1213–9.
29. Daugirdas JT, Ing TS. Classification of first-use reactions. Int J Artif Organs. 1986;9(3):19.
30. Ebo DG, Bosmans JL, Couttenye MM, Stevens WJ. Haemodialysis-associated anaphylactic and anaphylactoid reactions. Allergy. 2006;61(2):211–20.
31. Daugirdas JT, Bernardo AA. Hemodialysis effect on platelet count and function and hemodialysis-associated thrombocytopenia. Kidney Int. 2012;82(2):147–57.
32. Twardowski ZJ. Dialyzer reuse—part II: advantages and disadvantages. Semin Dial. 2006;19(3):217–26.
33. Sweet SJ, McCarthy S, Steingart R, Callahan T. Hemolytic reactions mechanically induced by kinked hemodialysis lines. Am J Kidney Dis. 1996;27(2):262–6.
34. Malinauskas RA. Decreased hemodialysis circuit pressures indicating postpump tubing kinks: a retrospective investigation of hemolysis in five patients. Hemodial Int. 2008;12(3):383–93.
35. Rollé F, Pengloan J, Abazza M, Halimi JM, Laskar M, Pourcelot L, Tranquart F. Identification of microemboli during haemodialysis using Dopper ultrasound. Nephrol Dial Transplant. 2000;15(9):1420–4.
36. Forsberg U, Jonsson P, Stegmayr C, Stegmayr B. High blood level in the air trap reduces microemboli during hemodialysis. Artif Organs. 2012;36(6):525–9.
37. Prince LK, Abbott KC, Green F, Little D, Nee R, Oliver JD 3rd, et al. Expanding the role of objectively structured clinical examinations in nephrology training. Am J Kidney Dis. 2014;63(6):906–12.
38. Baskin SE, Wozniak RF. Hyperbaric oxygenation in the treatment of hemodialysis-associated air embolism. N Engl J Med. 1975;293(4):184–5.
39. HHS, CMS. Conditions for coverage for end stage renal disease facilities. 42 CFR Parts 405, 410, 413, 414, 488, and 494. Baltimore: Department of Human and Health Services, Centers for Medicare and Medicaid Services; 2008
40. ANSI/AAMI/ISO. Guidance for the preparation and quality management of fluids for hemodialysis and related therapies 23500:2011. Arlington: Association for the Advancement of Medical Instrumentation, 2011
41. Lonnemann G. When good water goes bad how it happens, clinical consequences, and possible solutions. Blood Purif. 2004;22(1):124–9.
42. Roth VR, Jarvis WR. Outbreaks of infection and/or pyrogenic reactions in dialysis patients. Semin Dial. 2000;13(2):92–6.
43. Coulliette AD, Arduino MJ. Hemodialysis and water quality. Semin Dial. 2013;26(4):427–38.
44. Pérez García R, Rodríguez-Benítez P. Chloramine, a sneaky contaminant of dialysate. Nephrol Dial Transplant. 1999;14(11):2579–82.
45. Fluck S, McKane W, Cairns T, Fairchild V, Lawrence A, Lee J, et al. Chloramine induced haemolysis presenting as erythropoietin resistance. Nephrol Dial Transplant. 1999;14(7):1687–91.
46. Weisberg LS, Rachoin JS. The safety of low potassium dialysis. Semin Dial. 2010;23(6):556–60.
47. Karnik JA, Young BS, Lew NL, Herget M, Dubinsky C, Lazarus JM, Chertow GM. Cardiac arrest and sudden death in dialysis units. Kidney Int. 2001;60(1):350–7.
48. Bleyer AJ, Hartman J, Brannon PC, Reeves Daniel A, Satko SG, Russell G. Characteristics of sudden death in hemodialysis patients. Kidney Int. 2006;69(12):2268–73.
49. Pun PH, Lehrich RW, Honeycutt EF, Herzog CA, Middleton JP. Modifiable risk factors associated with sudden cardiac arrest within hemodialysis clinics. Kidney Int. 2011;79(2):218–27.
50. Moledina D, Geller D. Is low dialysate potassium ever indicated in outpatient hemodialysis? Semin Dial. 2014;27(3):263–5.
51. Heguilén RM, Sciurano C, Bellusci AD, Fried P, Mittelman G, Rosa Diez G, Bernasconi AR. The faster potassium lowering effect of high dialysate bicarbonate concentrations in chronic haemodialysis patients. Nephrol Dial Transplant. 2005;20(3):591–7.

52. Allon M, Shanklin N. Effect of bicarbonate administration on plasma potassium in dialysis patients interactions with insulin and albuterol. Am J Kidney Dis. 1996;28(4):508–14.
53. Kohn OF, Kjellstrand CM, Ing TS. Dual concentrate bicarbonate-based hemodialysis: know your buffers. Artif Organs. 2012;36(9):765–8.
54. Tentori F, Karaboyas A, Robinson BM, Morgenstern H, Zhang J, Sen A, et al. Association of dialysate bicarbonate concentration with mortality in the Dialysis Outcomes and Practice Patterns Study (DOPPS). Am J Kidney Dis. 2013;62(4):738–46.
55. Bommer J, Locatelli F, Satayathum S, Keen ML, Goodkin DA, Saito A, Akiba T, Port FK, Young EW. Association of predialysis serum bicarbonate levels with risk of mortality and hospitalization in the Dialysis Outcomes and Practice Patterns Study (DOPPS). Am J Kidney Dis. 2004;44(4):661–71.
56. Stewart IJ, Henrich WL. Is there any role for sodium modeling in the prevention of intradialytic hypotension in patients with large interdialytic fluid gains? Semin Dial. 2001;24(4):42–3.
57. Zhou YL, Liu HL, Duan XF, Yao Y, Sun Y, Liu Q. Impact of sodium and ultrafiltration profiling on haemodialysis related hypotension. Nephrol Dial Transplant. 2006;21(11):3231–7.
58. Hilali N A, Al-Humoud HM, Ninan VT, Nampoory MR, Ali JH, Johny KV. Profiled hemodialysis reduces intradialytic symptoms. Transplant Proc. 2004;36(6):1827–8.
59. Song JH, Park GH, Lee SY, Lee SW, Lee SW, Kim MJ. Effect of sodium balance and the combination of ultrafiltration profile during sodium profiling hemodialysis on the maintenance of the quality of dialysis and sodium and fluid balances. J Am Soc Nephrol. 2005;16(1):237–46.
60. Movilli E, Camerini C, Gaggia P, Zubani R, Feller P, Poiatti P, et al. Role of dialysis sodium gradient on intradialytic hypertension an observational study. Am J Nephrol. 2013;38(5):413–9.
61. Santos SF, Peixoto AJ. Revisiting the dialysate sodium prescription as a tool for better blood pressure and interdialytic weight gain management in hemodialysis patients. Clin J Am Soc Nephrol. 2008;3(2):522–30.
62. Stiller S, Bonnie Schorn E, Grassmann A, Uhlenbusch-Körwer I, Mann H. A critical review of sodium profiling for hemodialysis. Semin Dial. 2001;14(5):337–47.
63. Sayarlioglu H, Erkoc R, Tuncer M, Soyoral Y, Esen R, Gumrukcuoglu HA, et al. Effects of low sodium dialysate in chronic hemodialysis patients an echocardiographic study. Ren Fail. 2007;29(2):143–6.
64. De Paula FM, Peixoto AJ, Pinto LV, Dorigo D, Patricio PJ, Santos SF. Clinical consequences of an individualized dialysate sodium prescription in hemodialysis patients. Kidney Int. 2004;66(3):1232–8.
65. Hou SH, Zhao J, Ellman CF, Hu J, Griffin Z, Spiegel DM, Bourdeau JE. Calcium and phosphage fluxes during hemodialysis with low calcium dialysate. Am J Kidney Dis. 1991;18(2):217–24.
66. Argilés A, Kerr PG, Canaud B, Flavier JL, Mion C. Calcium kinetics and the long term effects of lowering dialysate calcium concentration. Kidney Int. 1993;43(3):630–40.
67. McIntyre CW. Calcium balance during hemodialysis. Semin Dial. 2008;21(1):38–42.
68. Pun PH, Horton JR, Middleton JP. Dialysate calcium concentration and the risk of sudden cardiac arrest in hemodialysis patients. Clin J Am Soc Nephol. 2013;8(5):797–803.
69. Hamano T, Oseto S, Fjuii N, Ito T, Katayama M, Horio M, et al. Impact of lowering dialysate calcium concentration on serum bone turnover markers in hemodialysis patients. Bone. 2005;36(5):909–16.
70. Rosen SM, O'Connor K, Shaldon S. Haemodialysis disequilibrium. Br Med J. 1964;2(5410):672–5.
71. Patel N, Dalal P, Panesar M. Dialysis disequilibrium syndrome a narrative review. Semin Dial. 2008;21(5):493–8.
72. Chen CL, Lai PH, ChouKJ, Lee PT, Chung HM, Fang HC. A preliminary report of brain edema in patients with uremia at first hemodialysis evaluation by diffusion-weighted MR imaging. AJNR Am J Neuroradiol. 2007;28(1):68–71.
73. Trinh Trang-Tan MM, Cartron JP, Bankir L. Molecular basis for the dialysis disequilibrium syndrome: altered aquaporin and urea transporter expression in the brain. Nephrol Dial Transplant. 2005;20(9):1984–8.
74. Rocco MV, Burkart JM. Prevalence of missed treatments and early sign offs in hemodialysis patients. J Am Soc Nephrol. 19934(5):1178–83.
75. Kobrin SM, Bens JS. Quinine—a tonic too bitter for hemodialysis associated muscle cramps? Semin Dial. 2007;20(5):396–401.
76. Lynch KE, Feldman HI, Berlin JA, Flory J, Rowan CG, Brunelli SM. Effects of L carnitine on dialysis-related hypotension and muscle cramps: a meta-analysis. Am J Kidney Dis. 200852(5):926–71.
77. Khajehdehi P, Mojerlou M, Behzadi S, Rais Jalali GA. A randomized, double-blind, placebo-controlled trial of supplementary vitamins E, C, and their combination for treatment of haemodialysis cramps. Nephrol Dial Transplant. 2001;16(7):1448–51.
78. Kaji DM, Ackad A, Nottage WG, Stein RM. Prevention of muscle cramps in haemodialysis patients by quinine sulphate. Lancet. 1976;2(7976):66–7.
79. Panader Sandoval J, Pérez García A, martin Abad L, Piqueras A, Garcés L, Chacón JC, Cruz JM. Action of quinine sulphate on the incidence of muscle cramps during hemodialysis. Med Clin (Barc). 1980;76(6):247–9.
80. Derbis J. Serious risks associated with using Quinine to treat nocturnal leg cramps (September 2012) [Internet]. 2012. [updated 2010 Aug 8]. http://www.fda.gov/forhealthprofessionals/articlesofinterest/ucm317811.htm.
81. Reilly RF. Attending rounds a patient with intradialytic hypotension. Clin J Am Soc Nephrol. 2014;9(4):798–803.
82. Kooman J, Basci A, Pizzarelli F, Canaud B, Haage P, Fouque D, et al. EBPG guidelines on haemodynamic instability. Nephrol Dial Transplant. 2007;22(Suppl 2):ii22–44.
83. Cruz DN, Mahnensmith RL, Brickel HM, Perazella MA. Midodrine and cool dialysate are effective therapies for symptomatic intradialytic hypotension. Am J Kidney Dis. 1999;33(5):920–6.
84. Dheenan S, Henrich WL. Preventing dialysis hypotension a comparison of usual protective maneuvers. Kidney Int. 2001;59(3):1175–81.
85. Reddan DN, Szczech LA, Hasselblad V, Lowrie EG, Lindsay RM, Himmelfarb J, et al. Intradialytic blood volume monitoring in ambulatory hemodialysis patients: a randomized trial. J Am Soc Nephrol. 2005;16(7):2162–9.
86. Flythe JE, Kimmel SE, Brunelli SM. Rapid fluid removal during dialysis is associated with cardiovascular morbidity mortality. Kidney Int. 2011;79(2):250–7.
87. Agarwal R, Light RP. Intradialytic hypertension is a marker of volume excess. Nephrol Dial Transplant. 2010;25(10):3355–61.
88. Chazot C, Jean G. Intradialytic hypertension it is time to act. Nephron Clin Pract. 2010;115(3):c182–8.
89. Chou KJ, Lee PT, Chen CL, Chiou CW, Hsu CY, Chung HM, Liu CP, Fang HC. Physiological changes during hemodialysis in patients with intradialysis hypertension. Kidney Int. 2006;69(10):1833–8.
90. Inrig JK, Van Buren P, Kim C, Vongpatanasin W, Povsic TJ, Toto R. Probing the mechanisms of intradialytic hypertension a pilot study targeting endothelial cell dysfunction. Clin J Am Soc Nephrol. 2012;7(8):1300–9.
91. Agarwal R, Sinha AD, Pappas MK, Abraham TN, Tegegne GG. Hypertension in hemodialysis patients treated with atenolol or Lisinopril a randomized controlled trial. Nephrol Dial Transplant. 2014;29(3):627–81.

92. Wetmore JB, Ellerbeck EF, Mahnken JD, Phadnis M, Rigler SK, Mukhopadhyay P, et al. Atrial fibrillation and risk of stroke in dialysis patients. Ann Epidemiol. 2013;23(3):112–8.
93. Buiten MS, de Bie MK, Rotmans JI, Gabreëls BA, van Dorp W, Wolterbeek R, et al. The dialysis procedure as a trigger for atrial fibrillation new insights in the development of atrial fibrillation in dialysis patients. Heart. 2014;100(9):685–90.
94. Shapira OM, Bar Khayim Y. ECG changes and cardiac arrhythmias in chronic renal failure patients on hemodialysis. J Electrocardiol. 1992;25(4):273–9.
95. Davis TR, Young BA, Eisenberg MS, Rea TD, Copass MK, Cobb LA. Outcome of cardiac arrests attended by emergency medical services staff at community outpatient dialysis centers. Kidney Int. 2008;73(8):933–9.
96. Kalantar Zadeh K, Ikizler TA, Block G, Avram MM, Kopple JD. Malnutrition-inflammation complex syndrome in dialysis patients: causes and consequences. Am J Kidney Dis. 2003;42(5):864–81.
97. Kim Y, Molnar MZ, Rattanasompattikul M, Hatamizadeh P, Benner K, Kopple JD, Kovesdy CP, Kalantar-Zadeh K. Relative contributions of inflammation and inadequate protein intake to hypoalbuminemia in patients on maintenance hemodialysis. Int Urol Nephrol. 2013;45(1):215–27. doi:10.1007/s11255-012-0170-8.
98. KaysenGA, DubinJA, Müller HG, Mitch WE, Rosales LM, Levin NW. Relationships among inflammation nutrition and physiologic mechanisms establishing albumin levels in hemodialysis patients. Kidney Int. 2002;61(6):2240–9.
99. Kalantar-Zadeh K, Kilpatrick RD, Kuwae N, McAllister CJ, Alcorhn H, Kopple JD, Greenland S. Revisiting mortality predictability of serum albumin in the dialysis population: time dependency, longitudinal changes and population-attributable fraction. Nephrol Dial Transplant. 2005;20(9):1880–8.
100. Kalantar-Zadeh K, Block G, Humphreys MH, Kopple JD. Reverse epidemiology of cardiovascular risk factors in maintenance dialysis patients. Kidney Int. 2003;63(3):793–808.
101. Kovesdy CP, Kalantar-Zadeh K. Accuracy and limitations of the diagnosis of malnutrition in dialysis patients. Semin Dial. 2012;25(4):423–7.
102. Kalantar-Zadeh K, Ikizler TA. Let them eat during dialysis: an overlooked opportunity to improve outcomes in maintenance hemodialysis. J Ren Nutr. 2013;23(3):157–63.
103. Renfrew R, Buselmeier TJ, Kjellstrand CM. Pericarditis and renal failure. Annu Rev Med. 1980;31:345–60.
104. Wood JE, Mahnensmith RL. Pericarditis associated with renal failure: evolution and management. Semin Dial. 2001;14(1):61–6.
105. Spector D, Alfred H, Siedlecki M, Briefel G. A controlled study of the effect of indomethacin in uremic pericarditis. Kidney Int. 1983;24(5):663–9.
106. Alpert MA, Ravenscraft MD. Pericardial involvement in end-stage renal disease. Am J Med Sci. 2003;325(4):228–36.
107. Krishnan AV, Pussell BA, Kiernan MC. Neuromuscular disease in the dialysis patient: an update for the nephrologist. Semin Dial. 2009;22(3):267–78.
108. Krishanan AV, Phoon RK, Pussell BA, Charlesworth JA, Bostock H, Kiernan MC. Neuropathy, axonal Na+/K+ pump function and activity-dependent excitability changes in end-stage kidney disease. Clin Neurophysiol. 2006;117(5):992–9.
109. Gejyo F, Narita I. Current clinical and pathogenic understanding of beta2-m amyloidosis in long-term hemodialysis patients. Nephrology (Carlton). 2003;8 Suppl:S45–9.
110. Korzets A, Marashek I, Schwartz A, Rosenblatt I, Herman M, Ori Y. Ischemic optic neuropathy in dialyzed patients: a previously unrecognized manifestation of calcific uremic arteriolopathy. Am J Kidney Dis. 2004;44(6):393–7.
111. Nardin R, Chapman KM, Raynor EM. Prevalence of ulnar neuropathy in patients receiving hemodialysis. Arch Neurol. 2005;62(2):271–5.
112. Jadoul M, Thumma J, Fuller DS, Tentori F, Li Y, Morgentstern H, Mendelssohn D, et al. Modifiable practices associated with sudden death among hemodialysis patients in the Dialysis Outcomes and Practice Patterns Study. Clin J Am Soc Nephrol. 2012;7(5):765–74.
113. Flythe JE, Curhan GC, brunelli SM. Shorter length dialysis sessions are associated with increased mortality independent of body weight. Kidney Int. 2014;83(1):104–13.
114. Jardine AG, McLaughlin K. Cardiovascular complications of renal disease. Heart. 2001;86(4):459–66.
115. Alhaj E, Alhaj E, Rahman I, Niazi TO, Berkowitz R, Klapholz M. Uremic cardiomyopathy: an underdiagnosed disease. Congest Heart Fail. 2013;19(4):E40–5.
116. McMahon AC, Greenwald SE, Dodd SM, Hurst MJ, Raine AE. Prolonged calcium transients and myocardial remodeling in early experimental uremia. Nephrol Dial Transplant. 2002;17(5):759–64.
117. Semple D, Smith K, Bhadnari S, Seymour AM. Uremic cardiomyopathy and insulin resistance: a critical role for akt? J Am Soc Nephrol. 2011;22(2):207–15.
118. Parfrey PS, Foley RN, Harnett JD, Kent GM, Murray D, Barre PE. Outcome and risk factors of ischemic heart disease in chronic uremia. Kidney Int. 1996;49(5):1428–34.
119. Mark PB, Johnston N, Groenning BA, Foster JE, Blyth KG, Martin TN, et al. Redefinition of uremic cardiomyopathy by contrast-enhanced cardiac magnetic resonance imaging. Kidney Int. 2006;69(10):1839–45.
120. Foley RN, Parfrey PS, Kent GM, Harnett JD, Murray DC, Barre PE. Long-term evolution of cardiomyopathy in dialysis patients. Kidney Int. 1998;54(5):1720–5.
121. Dasselaar JJ, Slart RH, Knip M, Pruim J, Tio RA, McIntyre CW, de Jong PE, Franssen CF, et al. Haemodialysis is associated with a pronounced fall in myocardial perfusion. Nephrol Dial Transplant. 2009;24(2):604–10.
122. McIntyre CW, Burton JO, Selby NM, Leccisotti L, Korsheed S, Baker CS, Camici PG. Hemodialysis-induced cardiac dysfunction is associated with an acute reduction in global and segmental myocardial blood flow. Clin J Am Soc Nephrol. 2008;3(1):19–26.
123. Jefferies HJ, Virk B, Schiller B, Moran J, McIntyre CW. Frequent hemodialysis schedules are associated with reduced levels of dialysis-induced cardiac injury (myocardial stunning). Clin J Am Soc Nephrol. 2011;6(6):1326–32.
124. Selby NM, Burton JO, Chesterton LJ, McIntyre CW. Dialysis-induced regional left ventricular dysfunction is ameliorated by cooling the dialysate. Clin J Am Soc Nephrol. 2006;1(6):1216–25.
125. Yang JY, Lee TC, Montez-Rath ME, Paik J, Chertow GM, Desai M, Winkelmayer WC. Trends in acute nonvariceal upper gastrointestinal bleeding in dialysis patients. J Am Soc Nephrol. 2012;23(3):495–506.
126. Cheung J, Yu A, LaBossiere J, Zhu Q, Fedorak RN. Peptic ulcer bleeding outcomes adversely affected by end-stage renal disease. Gastrointest Endosc. 2010;71(1):44–9.
127. Yang JY, Lee TC, Montez-Rath ME, Chertow GM. Risk factors of short-term mortality after acute nonvariceal upper gastrointestinal bleeding in patients on dialysis: a population-based study. BMC Nephrol. 2013;14:97.
128. Wasse H, Gillen DL, Ball AM, Kestenbaum BR, Seliger SL, Sherrard D, Stehman-Breen CO. Risk factors for upper gastrointestinal bleeding among end-stage renal disease patients. Kidney Int. 2003;64(4):1455–61.
129. MarcuardSP WJV. Gastrointestinal angiodysplasia in renal failure. J Clin Gastroenterol. 1988;10(5):482–4.
130. Karagiannis S, Goulas S, Kosmadakis G, Galanis P, Arvanitis D, Boletis J, et al. Wireless capsule endoscopy in the investigation of patients with chronic renal failure and obscure gastrointestinal bleeding (preliminary data). World J Gastroenterol. 2006;12(32):5182–5.

131. Kaw D, Malhotra D. Platelet dysfunction and end-stage renal disease. Semin Dial. 2006;19(4):317–22.
132. Stewart JH, Buccianti G, Agodoa L, Gellert R, McCredie MR, Lowenfels AB, et al. Cancers of the kidney and urinary tract in patients on dialysis for end-stage renal disease: analysis of data from the United States, Europe, and Australia and New Zealand. J Am Soc Nephrol. 2003;14(1):197–207.
133. Livio M, gotti E, Marchesi D, Mecca G, Remuzzi G, de Gaetano G. Uraemic bleeding: role of anaemia and beneficial effect of red cell transfusions. Lancet. 1982;2(8306):1013–5.
134. Sassa N, Hattori R, Tsuzuki T, Watarai Y, Fukatsu A, Katsuno S, et al. Renal cell carcinomas in haemodialysis patients: does haemodialysis duration influence pathological cell types and prognosis? Nephrol Dial Transplant. 2011;26(5):1677–82.
135. Singanamala S, Brewster UC. Should screening for acquired cystic disease and renal malignancy be undertaken in dialysis patients? Semin Dial. 2011;24(4):365–6.
136. Sarasin FP, Wong JB, Levey AS, Meyer KB. Screening for acquired cystic kidney disease: a decision analytic perspective. Kidney Int. 1995;48(1):207–19.
137. Holley JL. Screening, diagnosis, and treatment of cancer in long-term dialysis patients. Clin J Am Soc Nephrol. 2007;2(3):604–10.
138. Alberú J. Clinical insights for cancer outcomes in renal transplant patients. Transplant Proc. 2010;42(9 Suppl):S36–40.
139. USRDS Annual Data Report. 2013 [Internet]. 2013. www.usrds.org/adr.
140. Naqvi SB, Collins AJ. Infectious complications of chronic kidney disease. Adv Chronic Kidney Dis. 2006;13(3):199.
141. Kuo C, Lee CT, Lee IM, Ho SC, Yang CY. Risk of herpes zoster in patients with long-term hemodialysis: a matched cohort study. Am J Kidney Dis. 2012;59(3):428–33.
142. Sheth H, Bernardini J, Burr R, Lee S, Miller RG, Shields M, Vergis EN, Piraino B. Clostridium difficile infections in outpatient dialysis cohort. Infect Control Hosp Epidemiol. 2010;31(1):89–9.
143. Kidney D. Improving Global Outcomes CKDMBDWG. KDIGO clinical practice guideline for the diagnosis, evaluation, prevention, and treatment of Chronic Kidney Disease-Mineral and Bone Disorder (CKD-MBD). Kidney Int Suppl. 2009;113:S1–130.
144. Wolf M. Forging forward with 10 burning questions on FGF23 in kidney disease. J Am Soc Nephrol. 2010;21(9):1427–35.
145. Nigwekar SU, Bhan I, Thadhani R. Ergocalciferol and cholecalciferol in CKD. Am J Kidney Dis. 2012;60(1):139–56.
146. Lin ZZ, Wang JJ, Chung CR, Huang PC, Su BA, Cheng KC, et al. Epidemiology and mortality of hip fracture among patients on dialysis: Taiwan National Cohort Study. Bone. 2014;64:235–9.
147. Beaubrun AC, Kilpatrick RD, Freburger JK, Bradbury BD, Wang L, Brookhart MA. Temporal trends in fracture rates and postdischarge outcomes among hemodialysis patients. J Am Soc Nephrol. 2013;24(9):1461–9.
148. Chen YJ, Kung PT, Wang YH, Huang CC, Hsu SC, Tsai WC, et al. Greater risk of hip fracture in hemodialysis than in peritoneal dialysis. Osteoporos Int. 2014;25(5):1513–8.
149. Miller PD. Bone disease in CKD: a focus on osteoporosis diagnosis and management. Am J Kidney Dis. 2014;64(2):290–304.
150. Nigwekar SU, Wenger J, Thadhani R, Bhan I. Hyponatremia, mineral metabolism, and mortality in incident maintenance hemodialysis patients: a cohort study. Am J Kidney Dis. 2013;62(4):755–62.
151. Barreto DV, Barreto FC, Carvalho AB, Cuppari L, Cendoroglo M, Draibe SA, et al. Coronary calcification in hemodialysis patients: the contribution of traditional and uremia-related risk factors. Kidney Int. 2005;67(4):1576–82.
152. Hayashi M. Calciphylaxis: diagnosis and clinical features. Clin Exp Nephrol. 2013;17(4):498–50.
153. Nigwekar SU, Bhan I, Turchin A, Skentzos SC, Hajhosseiny R, Steele D, et al. Statin use and calcific uremic arteriolopathy: a matched case-control study. Am J Nephrol. 2013;37(4):325–32.
154. Hayashi M, Takamatsu I, Kanno Y, Yoshida T, Abe T, Sato Y, et al. A case-control study of calciphylaxis in Japanese end-stage renal disease patients. Nephrol Dial Transplant. 2012;27(4):1580–4.
155. Nigwekar SU, Brunelli SM, Meade D, Wang W, Hymes J, Lacson E Jr. Sodium thiosulfate therapy for calcific uremic arteriolopathy. Clinical J Am Soc Nephrol. 2013;8(7):1162–70.
156. O'Neill WC. Sodium thiosulfate: mythical treatment for a mysterious disease? Clinical J Am Soc Nephrol. 2013;8(7):1068–9.
157. Su SF, Ng HY, Huang TL, Chi PJ, Lee YT, Lai CR, et al. Survey of depression by Beck Depression Inventory in uremic patients undergoing hemodialysis and hemodiafiltration. Ther Apher Dial. 2012;16(6):573–9.
158. Chilcot J, Davenport A, Wellsted D, Firth J, Farrington K. An association between depressive symptoms and survival in incident dialysis patients. Nephrol Dial Transplant. 2011;26(5):1627–34.
159. Farrokhi F, Abedi N, Beyene J, Kurdyak P, Jassal SV. Association between depression and mortality in patients receiving long-term dialysis: a systematic review and meta-analysis. Am J Kidney Dis. 2014;63(4):623–35.
160. Rodriguez L, Tighiouart H, Scott T, Lou K, Giang L, Sorensen E, et al. Association of sleep disturbances with cognitive impairment and depression in maintenance hemodialysis patients. J Nephrol. 2013;26(1):101–10.
161. Post JB, Morin KG, Sano M, Jegede AB, Langhoff E, Spungen AM. Increased prevalence of cognitive impairment in hemodialysis patients in the absence of neurological events. Am J Nephrol. 2012;35(2):120–6.
162. Giang LM, Weiner DE, Agganis BT, Scott T, Sorensen EP, Tighiouart H, Sarnak MJ. Cognitive function and dialysis adequacy: no clear relationship. Am J Nephrol. 2011;33(1):33–8.
163. Costa AS, Tiffin-Richards FE, Holschbach B, Frank RD, Vassiliadou A, Krüger T, et al. Clinical predictors of individual cognitive fluctuations in patients undergoing hemodialysis. Am J Kidney Dis. 2014;pii: S0272–6386(14):00592–7.
164. Radić J, Ljutić D, Radić M, Kovačić V, Dodig-Ćurković K, Šain M. Kidney transplantation improves cognitive and psychomotor functions in adult hemodialysis patients. Am J Nephrol. 2011;34(5):399–406.
165. Strippoli GF, Vecchio M, Palmer S, De Berardis G, Craig J, Lucisano G, et al. Sexual dysfunction in women with ESRD requiring hemodialysis. Clin J Am Soc Nephrol. 2012;7(6):974–81.
166. Vecchio M, Palmer S, De Berardis G, Craig J, Johnson D, Pellegrini F, et al. Prevalence and correlates of erectile dysfunction in men on chronic haemodialysis: a multinational cross-sectional study. Nephrol Dial Transplant. 2012;27(6):2479–88.

5 Nutrition Management in Hemodialysis

Katrina Campbell, Megan Rossi and Juan Jesus Carrero

5.1 Introduction

Dietary intervention is a cornerstone strategy in the management of end-stage kidney disease (ESKD). In fact, during the 1960s, before dialysis was accepted as a regular form of renal replacement therapy, many patients were treated with diet alone. The role of the kidneys includes the elimination of metabolic waste products as well as maintenance of fluid, electrolyte, and hormone homeostasis. Thereby, ESKD requiring renal replacement therapy is associated with a range of metabolic and nutritional issues. Undergoing hemodialysis treatment, where only partial replacement of renal function is possible, the resulting metabolic and nutritional consequences require a range of management approaches.

Potentially significant dietary changes are necessary for patients undergoing hemodialysis treatment. The overarching goals for the nutritional management in hemodialysis include:

1. Optimizing nutritional status, including prevention and treatment of protein-energy wasting (PEW) and correction of nutrient deficiency
2. Management of electrolyte and fluid balance

This chapter will briefly address the range of factors that affect nutritional status in ESKD, including the prevalence, methods of assessment, and management of the following issues:

- PEW
- Electrolyte disturbance
- Fluid balance
- Vitamin and mineral deficiencies

5.2 Protein-Energy Wasting in Hemodialysis

Protein Energy Wasting (PEW) refers to nutritional problems related to altered protein and energy metabolism. This is influenced by two major factors. The first factor is an imbalance between protein and energy intake and requirements, attributed to inadequate intake. The second factor is the catabolic processes associated with dialysis and metabolic consequences of end-stage disease (including inflammation and oxidative stress) resulting in accelerated breakdown of protein stores. In clinical practice, it may be difficult to separate these two processes, which work synergistically while exacerbating one another (Fig. 5.1).

The following section will address the prevalence, etiology, and methods of assessment and management of PEW in hemodialysis.

5.2.1 Prevalence of PEW and Effect of PEW on Outcome in Hemodialysis

PEW remains a common issue even in the modern day dialysis patient. As illustrated in Fig. 5.1, approximately 20–60 % of patients undergoing hemodialysis around the world may have PEW [1–9]. Importantly, we should bear in mind that the actual prevalence may be higher, as these data are from observational studies that include only those patients who are clinically stable.

Nutrients are the substrates for energy, tissue synthesis, and metabolism, and are necessary for life. Undernutrition and/or micro/macronutrient deficiencies specifically are contributors to the metabolic complications and poor outcomes of hemodialysis patients. Most markers of PEW have been

M. Rossi (✉)
School of Medicine, University of Queensland, Brisbane, QLD, Australia
e-mail: megan.rossi@uq.net.au

K. Campbell
Department of Nutrition & Dietetics, Princess Alexandra Hospital, Woolloongabba, QLD, Australia

J. J. Carrero
Department of Renal Medicine, Karolinska Institute, Huddinge, Sweden

A. K. Singh et al. (eds.), *Core Concepts in Dialysis and Continuous Therapies,* DOI 10.1007/978-1-4899-7657-4_5

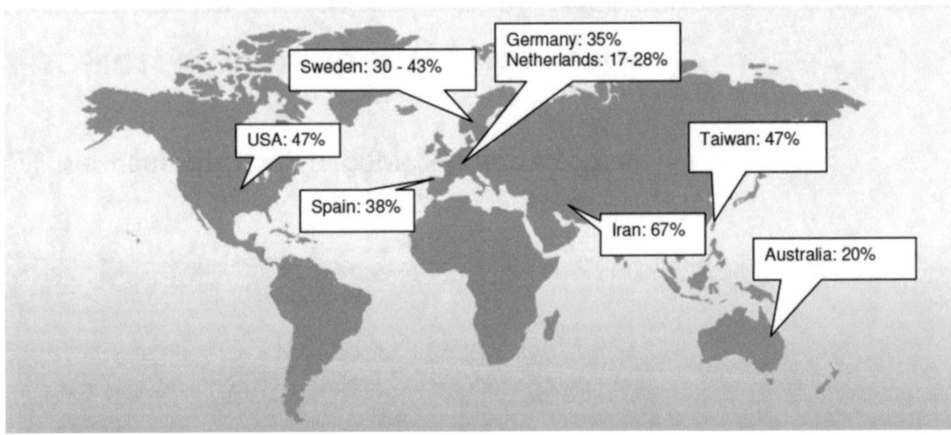

Fig. 5.1 Prevalence of protein-energy wasting in hemodialysis populations throughout the world

associated with poor quality of life, infections, atherosclerosis, cardiovascular events, graft rejection, and mortality [1, 2, 10–12]. Simple markers of nutritional status, such as serum albumin, serum prealbumin, and poor appetite, are strongly associated with the incidence of hospitalizations [13, 14], which impacts health-care costs. Health-care costs for PEW hemodialysis patients have been suggested up to threefold as compared with non-PEW individuals [13]. Although we currently lack of randomized controlled trials targeting PEW to reduce hard outcomes in hemodialysis patients, three large epidemiological analyses have explored this issue based on the potential of providing oral nutritional support to hypoalbuminemic patients. In one study, hypoalbuminemic individuals receiving nutritional support had a 34% reduction in 1-year mortality risk as compared to those who did not receive it [15]. Nutritional support in persistently hypoalbuminemic hemodialysis patients reduced hospitalizations rates during the subsequent year by approximately 20% [16] versus those who did not receive it. Implementation of a protocol to provide nutritional support during hemodialysis upon diagnosis of hypoalbuminemia and to maintain albumin within normal range associated with 20–30% reduced mortality as compared to similar patients not receiving nutritional support. Despite these reports being observational in nature, they provide solid background regarding the importance of ensuring good nutritional status in hemodialysis patients.

PEW has short-term impact on mortality, and its consequences are so rapid and devastating that in epidemiological studies things that are normally risk factors appear as protective. A clear example is the association between cholesterol and mortality. In hemodialysis patients, a high- rather than a low-level of cholesterol associates with improved survival [17], which is opposite to the effect observed in the general population. When chronic kidney disease (CKD) patients are stratified according to the presence/absence of PEW, it is observed that this mortality paradox is seen only in people with signs of PEW [17]. The explanation is likely that patients undergoing hemodialysis die of the short-term consequences of PEW and do not live long enough to die of cardiovascular disease associated with high cholesterol. In this case, high cholesterol may actually be a sign of higher fat stores that allows the patient to survive the wasting process longer. A similar paradox has been reported repeatedly for obesity [18]; dialysis patients are at such high risk of PEW that obesity may provide a measure of protection by excess energy store to stand the PEW catabolic process. Hyperhomocysteinemia, an important cardiovascular risk factor in the general population, has also been associated with improved survival in hemodialysis patients [19]. Again, homocysteine levels in this setting may be a reflection of overall better amino acid stores.

5.2.2 Etiology of PEW Is Multifactorial in ESKD

There are a wide range of drivers that affect the nutritional and metabolic state in CKD (Fig. 5.2). Understanding the features that contribute to the etiology of PEW is critical to inform appropriate assessment and treatment strategies. Not all of these alterations are directly or fully tackled by adequate nutritional support and will not be discussed in this chapter. These include, for instance, inflammation-induced hypercatabolism, increased energy expenditure, hormonal disorders (such as insulin resistance or growth hormone alterations), and poor physical activity and/or frailty. A multifaceted therapeutic approach for this complex syndrome is therefore necessary.

5.2.2.1 Appetite

Reduced appetite in ESKD is an independent predictor of poor outcome [10, 20] and important contributor of PEW, as a result of driving an inadequate dietary intake. Appetite disturbance present in ESKD is generally reported between 35 and 50% of hemodialysis patients from samples in Europe and the USA [10, 12, 20–22]. Appetite is typically driven by the endocrine system; however, in hemodialysis patients, factors related to the dialysis procedure, alterations in the gastrointestinal system, as well as hedonic and social implications are also important to consider.

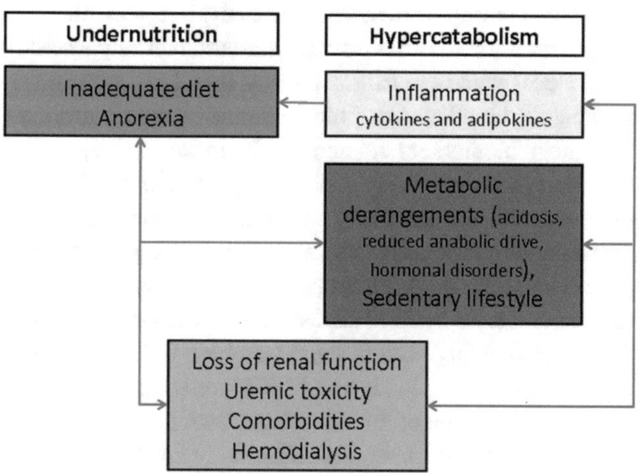

Fig. 5.2 A simple overview of etiology of protein-energy wasting in dialysis

Appetite hormones and neuropeptides serve to regulate hunger to respond with adequate energy intake; however, their actions are altered in ESKD. Studies indicate that patients undergoing dialysis treatment who exhibit appetite disturbance show signs of slower eating and report higher ratings of fullness prior to meals compared with controls [23]. This response has been associated with high circulating levels of anorectic hormones (cholecystokinin (CCK), leptin and peptide-YY (PYY)) [24, 25] and stimulation of serotonin [26]. To add to this picture of dysregulation, ghrelin, an appetite-stimulating hormone, appears to have reduced function in ESKD [27]. These appetite hormones, which are typically cleared by dialysis, peak prior to a dialysis session, resulting in reduced appetite leading up to dialysis [28]. Therefore, we see a typical cycling of appetite along dialysis days with reduced appetite being common before dialysis session [29].

5.2.2.2 Effect of Hedonic Drivers of Food Intake

The food and drink "experience" or hedonic factors driving appetite and food intake may be negatively influenced by a range of disturbances that manifest in ESKD, both physiological and psychological. CKD changes both smell and taste functions, thereby reducing the ability to detect basic tastes for salt and bitter, as well as reducing taste sensitivity compared with healthy controls [30–32]. Taste is thought to be affected in CKD patients by a range of factors, including reduced saliva volume and altered composition, as well as reduced neural function resulting in impaired activity of taste receptors [33]. Other oral manifestations including a high prevalence of oral disease, increased uremic by-products, buffering, and reduced salivary flow rate increase erosion and malocclusion [34]. Such dental problems may create chewing or biting problems, interfering with the ability to consume a variety of nutrient-dense foods [35]. Hedonic experience can also be influenced in the setting of hemodialysis by a range of psychological factors, including anxiety due to past (or present) food restrictions or coping with the disease, and presence of depression, which has been demonstrated to be a strong driver of appetite in hemodialysis patients [21]. These together with a range of social issues, including food security [36] and social isolation [37], dialysis patients experience a range of factors that influence their food experience and therefore it is important to consider them in the context of nutritional management.

5.2.2.3 Gastrointestinal Disturbance

Gastrointestinal symptoms are also potential contributors to PEW observed in ESKD. Prevalent conditions in dialysis patients include constipation, impaired gastric emptying, and motility disorders [38–41]. The pathogenesis of these disorders is largely unknown; however, it may be related to bacterial overgrowth in the small [42] and large [43] intestines. This state of "dysbiosis" has been hypothesized in ESRD as a driver of increased inflammation and anorexia [43]. In relation to this, comorbid diabetes may also increase the risk of diabetic gastroparesis, resulting in delayed gastric emptying, nausea, and prolonged satiety [44]. Nonetheless, the prevalence of gastrointestinal symptoms in ESKD patients with diabetes does not appear to be any different to the remaining ESKD population, although the studies are few [39, 40].

5.2.2.4 Inflammation

Inflammation is a major contributor to PEW and cardiovascular disease in dialysis [45, 46]. ESKD is characterized by persistent low-grade, inflammatory state [47]. Increased concentration of inflammatory cytokines and adipokines are due to both reduced renal clearance and stimulation of increased production [48]. Furthermore, factors that have been hypothesized to promote a state of chronic inflammation in dialysis patients include membrane bio-incompatibility, comorbid conditions, persistent infection, diet, and genetic factors [48].

Inflammation contributes to PEW as a driver for appetite dysregulation and protein catabolism. Key inflammatory cytokines trigger both central and peripheral mechanisms to drive appetite regulation [49]. High concentrations of each of these cytokines have been reported in the dialysis population and are associated with uremic anorexia [10, 50, 51]. Furthermore, muscle wasting is a significant consequence of chronic inflammation [52, 53]. The action of IL-6 as a result of muscle proteolysis appears to stimulate further protein catabolism [54]. Therefore, the synergistic action of poor appetite and increased muscle wasting resulting from the inflammatory cascade represents a key mechanistic driver of PEW. Treatment targeting the source of inflammation (i.e., optimizing dialysis therapy, including access and prescription, appropriate fluid management, etc.) is critical with nutrition interventions having limited success in isolation.

5.2.2.5 Dialysis Procedure

The hemodialysis procedure in itself is a catabolic stimulus: Interaction between the blood flowing through the dialysis membrane gives rise to an inflammatory cascade, which appears to be dependent on the dialysis membrane used [55]. Furthermore, inflammatory stimuli include limited clearance of uremic toxins, particularly protein-bound uremic toxins, along with increased gut ischemia leading to increased endotoxemia. Amino acid and protein losses during the dialysis session, together with low nutrient intake, promote low nutrient availability for muscle synthesis and acute-phase reactant synthesis [56–58]. The consequence is breakdown of muscle protein to compensate for these losses [59, 60]. Concurrent amino acid supplementation during the dialysis session can prevent or reverse these adverse effects [61, 62]. Furthermore, optimizing dialysis provision and/or increasing the frequency of the dialysis procedure has been associated with improvements in nutritional markers [63, 64]; however, this has not been confirmed in a subsequent randomized trial [65]. Finally, hemodialysis results in a more rapid loss of residual renal function, which has been shown to relate to rates of malnutrition [66]. Proposed mechanisms for this include reduced regulation of amino acid metabolism, particularly conversion of essential amino acids (phenylalanine to tyrosine and glycine to serine), thereby limiting the amino acid profile available for protein synthesis [67] .

5.2.2.6 Metabolic Acidosis

Metabolic acidosis is a common consequence of the reduced buffering capacity of the kidney in ESKD and an important contributor to net protein catabolism and uremic anorexia. Correction of acidosis has shown to improve nutritional status [68], likely through decreased protein turnover, improved appetite, and total protein intake. The mechanism of action through decreased protein degradation has been demonstrated in both hemodialysis [69] and peritoneal dialysis [70].

5.2.3 Assessment of Protein-Energy Wasting in Hemodialysis

Systematic screening and assessment of nutritional status is essential in the management of hemodialysis patients. The key goal of this process is to identify potential nutrition risk early (screening) and undertake thorough assessment in order to form a diagnosis of PEW and indicate targets for intervention, evaluation, and monitoring [71]. An ideal nutrition assessment tool should not only predict outcome, but also respond to nutritional therapy, without being affected by nonnutritional factors. In addition, nutrition assessment in hemodialysis must be easily applied in practice, preferably achievable during or soon after the dialysis treatment.

However, there is not a single measure that can provide a valid assessment of nutritional status; therefore, nutrition assessment is based on a combination of measures. Nutritional laboratory biomarkers are and can be influenced by uremic retention (and conversely residual renal function), fluid status, inflammation (as many nutritional markers also function as acute-phase reactants), and renal replacement therapy (losses into dialysate). Anthropometry and body composition tools are affected by fluid status. Careful consideration of all these confounding factors must be given before making a diagnosis. Given that drivers of PEW are complex and multifactorial, parameters for assessment therefore need to capture a range of measures, including body composition, biochemical parameters, and dietary intake [72]. An overview of nutrition assessment parameters is provided in Table 5.1.

5.2.3.1 Anthropometry and Body Composition for PEW Assessment

Monitoring of weight and body composition is useful to identify depleted fat and/or muscle stores; however, the precision is dependent on the tool used [73]. In general, the most clinically applicable tools are the least precise. For example, assessment of weight and weight change is a standard routine practice in the dialysis setting. Weight gain or loss is influenced by fluctuations in body water related to breaks in dialysis therapy; however, long-term trends of adjustments to "dry" or target weight may provide insights into actual weight change. Even when the weight change is established, it is not known the degree of weight loss from muscle wasting, compared with fat mass. Anthropometric measures including skinfold thickness (in particular, triceps and biceps) and circumferences (typically mid-arm) are also applicable to routine care and may be used together with weight to identify where weight changes may be coming from. Handgrip strength is another clinically applicable tool that can be used to assess change in muscle function over time and has been shown to be a good predictor of outcome [74, 75].

More advanced methods, including body composition instruments, are more likely to be applied in a research situation rather than in daily practice in the hemodialysis setting. Dual X-ray absorptiometry, total body potassium, and total body nitrogen are generally isolated from the research setting due to their high cost and limited application to the clinical practice setting. Bioimpedance analysis (BIA) tools are becoming more common in the routine assessment of nutrition status in hemodialysis. BIA relies on several assumptions; it is important to use equipment validated for dialysis patients and to also account for consistent hydration status. As this is constantly variable in the hemodialysis patients, it is important to perform this measurement at a consistent timeframe, for example, 30 min after dialysis. Longitudinal

Table 5.1 Overview of parameters used in hemodialysis for assessing protein-energy wasting

Assessment tool	Ease of measurement	Clinical applicability	Considerations
Anthropometry and body composition			
Weight and weight change, including BMI	High	Moderate	Does not distinguish body compartments. Dry weight change of 5 % or more clinically applicable
Lean muscle mass (and/or fat mass) using body composition instruments	Low	High	Tools to assess directly are expensive and not clinically applicable (e.g., total body potassium, total body nitrogen); or open to error due to indirect measure and body water fluctuations (bioimpedance, DEXA)
Anthropometrics including skinfold thickness and mid-arm muscle circumference	Moderate	Moderate	Require training to optimize validity and reproducibility, low-cost and to be undertaken after dialysis session
Handgrip strength	High	Moderate	Measure of muscle function, non-invasive. Evaluation of longitudinal change required
Biochemistry			
Serum proteins	High	Low	Inverse relationship with inflammation and hydration status
Inflammation markers	Moderate	Moderate	Indicator of stress response, may decrease protein synthesis and raise energy expenditure
Nutrition assessment tools			
Subjective global assessment	High	High	Draw on a range of data from medical histories and physical examination to evaluate overall nutritional status
Malnutrition inflammation score			
Dietary intake			
Adequacy of protein and energy intake (diet history)	Moderate	High	For reliable data from detailed diet histories require skills and training, however, important to evaluate, given the high protein and energy requirements in hemodialysis
Adequacy of protein intake (PNA)	High	Moderate	PNA can be calculated by estimating the generation of urea nitrogen in blood. Assumes patient is metabolically stable

BMI body mass index, *DEXA* dual-energy X-ray absorptiometry, *PNA* protein of nitrogen appearance

changes from BIA have been used to predict body cell mass in dialysis patients [76] and were associated with morbidity and mortality [77].

5.2.3.2 Biochemistry for PEW Assessment

Biochemical parameters are commonly used to estimate dietary needs and to monitor nutritional status [78]. However, this assessment method requires caution in interpretation. In clinically stable hemodialysis patients, protein of nitrogen appearance (PNA) can be used to estimate protein intake. The total nitrogen appearance of the body should be equal to or slightly smaller than the nitrogen intake. Because urea nitrogen appearance is highly correlated with total nitrogen appearance and measurement of total nitrogen losses in urine, dialysate, and stool is inconvenient and laborious, regression equations to estimate PNA have been developed. In hemodialysis patients, PNA can be calculated by estimating the generation of urea nitrogen in blood [79], usually followed by normalization (nPNA) by body weight or body weight derived from the urea distribution space. nPNA assessment is recommended with a monthly frequency [79]. nPNA would not be a valid indicator of protein intake in cases of catabolism, growth/anabolism (children, pregnant women, recovering from an intercurrent illness), or day-to-day changes in dietary protein intake. PNA should not be used to evaluate nutritional status in isolation, but rather as one of several independent measures when evaluating nutritional status.

Synthesis of serum proteins commonly used to assess nutritional status (albumin, prealbumin, etc.) is directly impacted by inflammation. Therefore, there is a direct inverse correlation between serum proteins and serum inflammatory markers in dialysis patients [80], rendering the assessment of nutrition status using serum proteins problematic. A low serum albumin concentration is highly prognostic; however, it may not only reflect an acute-phase response, but also be the result of fluid overload and dialysate loss. This is also reflective of other serum proteins, including pre-albumin, transferrin, and retinol-binding protein. Inadequate dietary protein intake can affect serum protein in the short term, as it decreases the rate of serum protein synthesis [81]. However, longer term, compensatory shifts in serum protein from extravascular to intravascular space occur, thereby limiting the value of serum proteins for evaluating nutritional status. To overcome some of these limitations, it can be useful to evaluate inflammatory markers, such as C-reactive protein (CRP), and interdialytic fluid gains to assess the validity of these markers for predicting PEW.

Pre-dialysis serum bicarbonate can provide an indication of the etiology for PEW. Metabolic acidosis may lead to stimulation of protein breakdown and subsequent muscle wasting, indicated by low serum bicarbonate. However, in the event of both low and high pre-dialysis, bicarbonate may be indicative of PEW risk. When low, this may indicate severe malnutrition due to the lack of endogenous protein [82, 83].

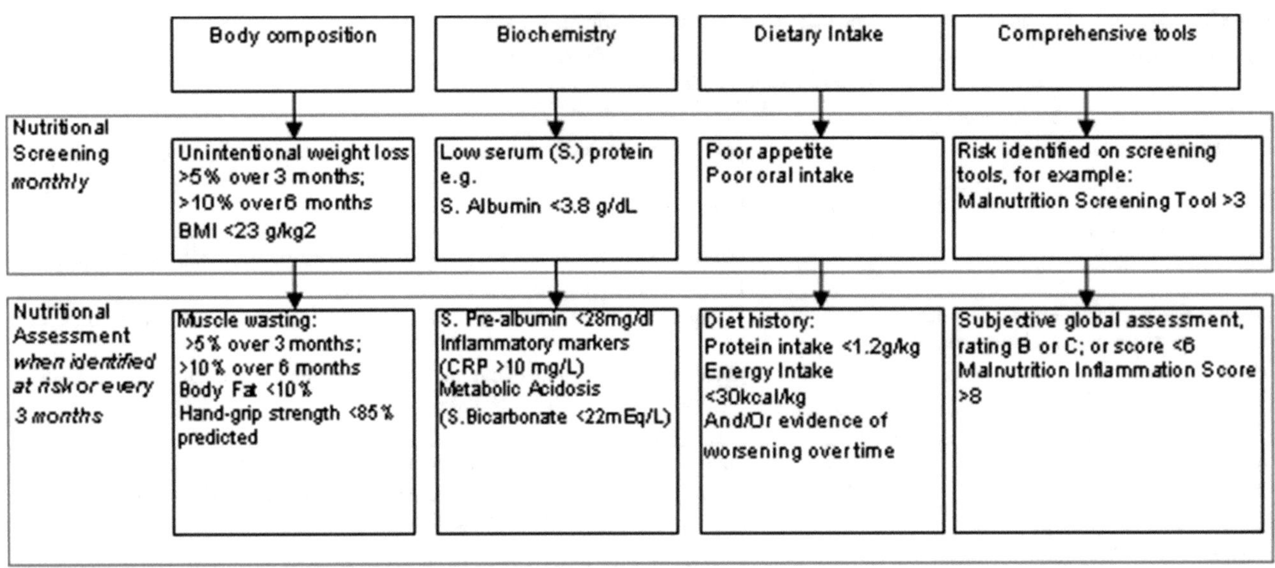

Fig. 5.3 Suggested nutrition screening and assessment parameters for use in hemodialysis

5.2.3.3 Nutrition Assessment Tools for PEW Assessment

The most comprehensive nutrition assessment tools to evaluate PEW in the hemodialysis setting include the subjective global assessment (SGA) and the malnutrition inflammation score (MIS) [84]. These tools combine features of a medical history (e.g., weight change, gastrointestinal symptoms, dietary intake change, functional capacity, and in the case of MIS, biochemistry) as well as a physical examination (accounting for fat and muscle wasting). SGA differs from MIS, by not requiring biochemistry, and is also based on a global rating rather than a summative score. Both tools have been shown to be prognostic indicators of clinical outcome, although may not be sensitive to detect small changes over time [85] .

5.2.4 Treatment of Protein-Energy Wasting

Once a nutrition screening and assessment process is in place (as detailed in Fig. 5.3), it is critical to be followed up by an appropriate management plan to treat PEW, or indeed prevent the exacerbated nutrition risk [71]. The recommended energy and protein requirements in hemodialysis are 35 kcal/kg/day (over 30 kcal/kg/day for >60 years old) and over 1 g protein/kg/day [72, 86]. Most studies demonstrate that these targets are rarely met, particularly for protein. In the event of PEW, nutrition support is required. There are a number of different forms of nutrition support as outlined in Fig. 5.4.

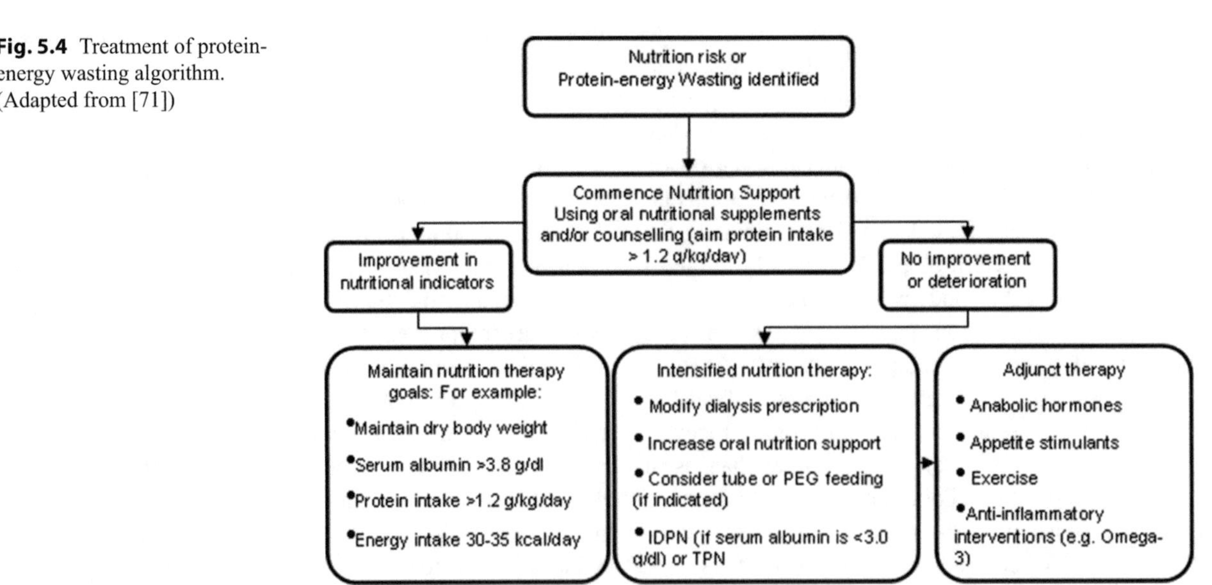

Fig. 5.4 Treatment of protein-energy wasting algorithm. (Adapted from [71])

5.2.4.1 Oral and Enteral Nutritional Supplements

Oral nutritional supplements (ONS) are considered a first-line treatment for PEW in hemodialysis. In addition to dietary counseling to optimize nutritional intake from food, ONS can provide an added 7–10 kcal/day and 0.3–0.4 g/kg protein/day [87]. Provision of ONS to dialysis patients has shown improvements in serum albumin, in the order of 0.23 g/dL [88]. Additional benefits observed have included increased body weight [89], lean body mass [90], global nutrition status, and quality of life (QOL) [91]. Recent large observational studies have demonstrated reduced hospitalizations [15] and improved survival [16] in hemodialysis patients in those who received ONS, compared with patients who did not.

ONS are best incorporated into routine intake away from main meals and/or provided during a dialysis session. Meals and ONS provided on dialysis have several benefits including improved protein turnover [61] and compliance, and should therefore be considered in all patients at risk of PEW [92].

Enteral nutrition, in the form of tube feeding, is an option for patients who are unable to tolerate sufficient oral intake. This involves nasogastric tubes (through nose to stomach), percutaneous endoscopic gastroscopy (PEG, direct to stomach), or jejunostomy tubes (through to the jejunum) [93]. Generally, tube feeding would be utilized in the situation of comorbid conditions impacting the nutritional status and/or functional oral intake, including dysphagia or severe anorexia.

5.2.4.2 Intradialytic Parenteral Nutrition

Intradialytic parenteral nutrition (IDPN) provides nutrition support during the hemodialysis procedure directly via the venous access. IDPN is considered when ONS have been tried and intake remains considerably inadequate (e.g., <20 kcal/kg/day) [89]. Formations of IDPN come in the form of multi- or single macronutrients (dextrose, amino acids, and/or lipids) and, therefore, may be somewhat individualized for the patients needs [71]. The effectiveness of this treatment over any other nutrition support option has yet to be demonstrated; however, it is a safe and convenient option for patients who cannot meet their needs orally.

5.2.4.3 Other Treatments

There are a range of other treatments that warrant consideration, including optimization of dialysis, use of appetite stimulants, and growth hormone. Appetite stimulants such as megestrol acetate have been evaluated in pilot randomized-controlled trials in maintenance hemodialysis patients [94, 95]. Although this agent has been shown to improve appetite and food intake, it has been associated with increase in body fat, not muscle mass, notwithstanding considerable side effects [96]. However, a pilot study in malnourished dialysis patients demonstrated improved energy balance with subcutaneous ghrelin administration [97]. Finally, small, short-term metabolic studies investigating the use of growth hormone in maintenance hemodialysis have demonstrated an indication for achieving positive nitrogen balance (reviewed in [71]). However, important consideration into side effects of growth hormone, including hyperglycemia and acromegaly, has prevented its approval for treatment of PEW in the maintenance hemodialysis population. This is an area which is likely to receive increasing attention, in addition to agents targeting inflammation and gut microbiota in the prevention and treatment of PEW in hemodialysis.

5.3 Electrolyte Disturbance

5.3.1 Hyperkalemia

Disturbance in potassium balance is a management challenge in kidney disease, in particular, for anuric patients receiving hemodialysis treatment. While a small percentage is chronically hypokalemic, hyperkalemia is by far the more common disturbance of potassium homeostasis. Hyperkalemia is potentially life threatening with muscular cells highly sensitive to changes in intracellular concentrations of potassium, precipitating muscle weakening, paralysis, and potentially fatal arrhythmias[98]. Hyperkalemia is a risk factor for sudden cardiac death, the leading cause of mortality in hemodialysis patients [99], and is associated with a twofold risk of all-cause and cardiovascular mortality [100].

There are a number of different causes of elevated serum potassium, many of which are not diet related. Common causes in the dialysis population include acute infection, medications such as angiotensin-converting-enzyme inhibitors and non-steroidal anti-inflammatory agents, and factors that may indirectly be related to suboptimal nutrition, including metabolic acidosis, increased catabolism, poor glycemic control, and constipation.

5.3.1.1 Assessment of Hyperkalemia

Hyperkalemia, categorized as mild or moderate (serum potassium 5.5–6.5 mEq/L) to severe (>6.5 mEq/L), is often asymptomatic and detection generally relies on biochemical tests, or electrocardiography, in the acute setting. An understanding of the underlying cause of hyperkalemia is needed when considering treatment options to avoid any unnecessary dietary restrictions in this population already at high risk of malnutrition. For instance, hyperkalemia can also occur in situations of underdialysis or alterations in the gastrointestinal (GI) tract (site of potassium elimination). Steroids, ACEIs, and potassium-sparing diuretics may raise potassium levels. Acidosis and hyperglycemia promote loss of intracellular potassium and raise potassium levels.

Table 5.2 Example of a simple potassium food guide

High (>5 mmol/serve[a])	Medium (3–5 mmol/serve[a])	Low (≤2 mmol/serve[a])
Fruit		
Banana	Pear	Canned fruit (drained)
Fruit mixes (fresh juice/dried)	Melon	Berries
Peach	Plum	Rhubarb
Vegetables		
Starchy vegetables	Broccoli	Asparagus
Tomato	Carrot	Peas
Avocado	Silver beet	Lettuce
Dairy		
Cow, butter and soy milk	Ice cream	Cheese
Yogurt	Creamed rice	Rice milk
Extra foods		
Iced coffee	Liquorice	Oatmeal/plain biscuits
Worcestershire sauce	Chocolate	Plain muesli bars

Unit conversion: 1 mmol potassium=39 mg potassium
[a] Based on standard portion size

A diet history targeting sources of potassium is a method for determining whether diet may be the primary or a contributory cause of hyperkalemia. Identification of total potassium intake as well as the sources of high potassium foods is needed for targeted intervention. Food frequency questionnaires using a checklist of high potassium foods, as exemplified in Table 5.2, may also add to the dietary assessment. This technique may assist patient recall of high potassium foods consumed less frequently although potentially in high quantities, contributing to the unexplained occasional hyperkalemia.

Twenty-four-hour urine tests are another method of assessing potassium intake, although logistics including timeliness and patient burden limits its clinical applicability.

5.3.1.2 Management of Hyperkalemia

In the case of hyperkalemia where diet has been identified as a contributing factor, limiting intake of high potassium foods is recommended as the first-line intervention. This generally precedes medical treatments such as potassium exchange resins and changes to the concentration of the dialysis bath. As a guide, limiting potassium intake to 1 mmol/kg of ideal body weight through education on potassium sources and individualizing meal plans may help in the treatment or prevention of hyperkalemia.

Depending on the resources available, however, intervention can be as basic as providing patients with lists of high, medium, and low foods from each food group with the recommendation of avoiding foods from the "high" category. Only reputable food lists obtained from government agencies should be used, many of which are freely accessible and reviewed by qualified dieticians [101]. It is important that dialysis patients do not exclude any food groups from their diet (including fruit and vegetables), instead select the lower potassium options within each food group. Following this method limits the risk of malnutrition, nutrient deficiencies, and enhances patient satisfaction.

Individualized counseling with a qualified dietitian is the gold standard diet intervention for hyperkalemia. This management strategy allows recommendations to be tailored to patients' normal diet intakes, enhancing patient knowledge and compliance. In specific dialysis populations, generally younger patients, up-skilling using a potassium point system may be an effective strategy. Patients are given a daily potassium allowance (calculated based on 1 mmol/kg) and are educated on individual foods' potassium contents. This technique promotes patient autonomy, allowing patients to select how they use their daily allowance of potassium. Nonetheless, the lack of mandatory labeling for potassium on nutrition information panels is a major barrier for many patients.

Food preparation techniques including soaking and boiling have been shown to decrease the potassium content by up to 70% in some foods [102]. However, it is important to consider the loss of other water-soluble nutrients when recommending this technique.

5.3.1.3 Key Management Strategies

1. Dietary counseling
   a. Limiting foods from the high potassium category (see Table 5.2)
   b. Potassium point system (higher level knowledge)
2. Food preparation techniques
3. Potassium exchange resins
4. Adjusting concentration of dialysis bath

5.3.2 Hyperphosphatemia

The kidneys play a vital role in mineral metabolism, maintaining homeostasis between serum and tissue stores of essential minerals including phosphorus. The kidney's ability to excrete phosphorous is progressively compromised with deterioration in kidney function leading to hypophosphatemia and hormonal disturbances. This presents as CKD-mineral and bone disorder (CKD-MBD), which encompasses mineral, bone, and extra skeletal (vascular) abnormalities. Despite a lack of intervention studies linking phosphorous manipulation to clinical outcomes, the strength of observational and experimental data has warranted the development of guidelines for phosphorous control [103].

Table 5.3 Guideline recommendations for dietary intake on hemodialysis

Nutrient	Guideline recommendation
Energy [86]	35 kcal/kg 30–35 kcal/kg > 60 years
Protein [86]	For clinically and weight stable patients aim for at least 1.2 g/kg of ideal body weight/day protein
Sodium [86]	Less than 2.3 g/day (or < 100 mmol/day)
Fluid [86]	Target range: 500 mL plus previous day urine output
Phosphate [103]	Target range: < 1.6 mEq/L Phosphorus intake of 800–1000 mg/day and aiming for 10–12 mg/g
Potassium [86]	Target range: Potassium 3.5–5.5 mEq/L Low potassium diet: individualized, approximately 40 mg/kg IBW or adjusted weight [141]

5.3.2.1 Assessment of Hyperphosphatemia

Routine blood tests are used to measure phosphorous, with KDIGO guidelines recommending a target below 1.6 mmol/L (see Table 5.3). Test results should be based on trends rather than single laboratory values when determining the need for intervention. In the short term, significant elevation of phosphorous may present as severe itchiness, while long-term elevation can manifest in visible calcification deposits in bones and joints of extremities.

There are two main forms of dietary phosphorous, organic and inorganic phosphorous, which need to be targeted in diet history assessments (whether diet history records or food frequency questionnaires are employed). Sources of organic phosphorus include animal products such as dairy, meat, fish, and eggs, as well as plant foods such as whole grains, legumes, and nuts. Inorganic phosphorus is found primarily in processed foods in the form of food additives for a range of properties including anticaking, leavening, emulsification, flavor enhancement, and color and moisture retention. The phosphorus content of foods is determined not only by the total amount but also by the bioavailability of the phosphorous. Organic phosphorus from plant and animal sources is absorbed at a rate of 20–40 and 40–60 %, respectively, while inorganic forms of phosphorus are thought to be absorbed between 90 and 100 % [104] (see Table 5.4 for a list of common phosphorous-based food additives).

5.3.2.2 Management of Hyperphosphatemia

The National Kidney Foundation-Kidney Disease Outcomes Quality Initiative (NKF-KDOQI) guidelines and the European Best Practice Guidelines recommend daily phosphorus intake of 800–1000 mg/day for patients on maintenance hemodialysis therapy. However, intakes adjusted to dietary protein requirements (10–12 mg/g protein) may be more appropriate for patients with higher protein needs [105].

Dietary restrictions must be carefully recommended and followed up because limiting naturally rich phosphorus foods can increase the risk of undernutrition and low protein intake [106]. Restriction should be directed toward processed foods with phosphorous-based additives. This should be the first-line intervention because of the high bioavailability of the phosphorous additives in addition to the low nutrient density of most processed foods. Educating patients to identify phosphorous-based additives on the food ingredient lists is an effective strategy shown to lower serum phosphorous levels [107]. This strategy is becoming more important with the increasing use of phosphorus-based additives in the food supply [107]. A barrier to this strategy, however, is that phosphorus listing on the nutrition panel is not mandated. In addition, the ingredient list commonly reports additives as E-numbers instead of names in much of Europe and other non-US countries. This makes it difficult to determine which foods contain phosphorus additives. The name and E-number for each of the 18 commonly used additives are provided in Table 5.4 [108].

Often a simplified message of promoting home-cooked meals from fresh ingredients and limiting processed and takeaway foods is a more practical approach to achieve restriction of phosphorous additives. Food preparation techniques including boiling have been shown to decrease the phosphorus content considerably [109]. However, again, it is important to consider the loss of other water-soluble nutrients when recommending this technique.

The next line strategy is to ensure that a low phosphorus to protein ratio is adopted and/or dietary protein is not excessive (e.g., < 1.5 g/kg, see dietary protein guidelines in Table 5.5). One strategy to balance the phosphorous intake without compromising on protein is to limit high phosphorus to protein ratio foods. Ideally, foods with ratios of 12–16 mg

Table 5.4 Common phosphorous-based food additives

E-number	Additive name	E-number	Additive name
101	Riboflavin	452	Polyphosphates
322	Lecithins	541	Sodium aluminum phosphate acidic
338	Phosphoric acid	627	Disodium guanylate
339	Sodium phosphates	631	Disodium inosinate
340	Potassium phosphates	635	Disodium 5′-ribonucleotides
341	Calcium phosphates	1410	Monostarch phosphate
343	Magnesium phosphates	1412	Distarch phosphate
442	Ammonium phosphatides	1413	Phosphated distarch phosphate
450	Diphosphates	1414	Acetylated distarch phosphate
451	Triphosphates	1442	Hydroxy propyl distarch phosphate

Table 5.5 Phosphorous-to-protein ratio of selected food items [2]

Food	Phosphorous-to-protein ratio
Seafood	
Orange roughy fish	4.5
Tuna, canned in water	6.4
Lobster	9.0
Salmon, sockeye	10.0
Crab, blue	10.2
Rainbow trout	11.0
Chicken egg	
Egg white	1.4
Egg substitute	10.1
Whole egg	13.3
Egg yolk	24.7
Meat	
Lamb	6.3
Beef (excludes organ meats)	7.0
Chicken breast	7.5
Pork (excludes organ meats)	9.3
Frankfurter, beef	14.1
Chicken liver	16.5
Dairy	
Cream cheese	16.7
Soymilk	17.4
Cheddar cheese	20.4
Milk, low fat (2%)	28.3

of phosphorous to 1 g of protein are recommended [110]. It is important to note, however, that more restrictive prescription of dietary phosphate is associated with poorer indices of nutritional status and, therefore, it is paramount that patients are given clear messages not to overrestrict protein intakes to achieve phosphate targets [111]. Phosphorous from plant sources, such as whole grains, is not essential to restrict due to the importance of their dietary fiber, vitamin and mineral content, and the low bioavailability of plant-based phosphorus. Suggestions of typically ingested foods according to phosphorus/protein content are listed in Table 5.5.

Despite optimal dietary management, phosphate binders remain a common adjunct therapy. There are different types of phosphate binders on the market, which vary in cost, although the data to date do not support superiority of the more expensive novel non-calcium binding agents [112]. To enhance the effectiveness of this medication, educating patients on matching their binder medication to the phosphorous load of their meals can improve serum levels [113]. Although this self-adjusting binder technique promotes autonomy, limits dietary restrictions, and enhances patient satisfaction, it is time intensive to implement and is restricted by patients' cognitive capacity. Another important, but often overlooked, point is to ensure that patients are taken binders appropriately, such as timing at the start of meals.

5.3.2.3 Key Management Strategies

1. Restrict phosphorous-based additives
   a. Promotion of fresh food is best
   b. Check ingredient lists for phosphorous-based additives (higher level knowledge)
2. Ensure dietary protein is not excessive (see protein guidelines)
3. Limit foods with high phosphorus: protein ratios
4. Phosphate binder prescription
   a. Ensure appropriate use and compliance to binders
   b. Self-adjusting binder education (higher level knowledge)

5.3.3 Fluid Balance

Fluid overload is highly prevalent in dialysis patients. In fact, acute fluid overload is a common cause for not only emergency dialysis but also hospital admissions manifesting as heart failure and pulmonary edema. This contributes a significant cost burden on the health-care system [114]. Chronic hypervolemia is thought to be the cause of at least 80% of all hypertension in dialysis patients [115]. Furthermore, fluid overload is closely linked to markers of cardiovascular disease and stroke, the leading cause of morbidity and mortality in this population. In addition, removal of excessive fluid during dialysis requires high ultrafiltration rates, leading to an increased risk of hypotensive episodes and cramps.

5.3.3.1 Assessment

There is a lack of consensus on the definition for excessive fluid gains, termed interdialytic weight gain (IDWG). Excessive IDWG may be defined using an absolute amount (i.e., 2–5 kg) or a percentage of the individual's body weight (usually 4%). Due to the lack of consensus surrounding the recommended cutoffs, it is important to develop and communicate local policies and standards based on the dialysis unit, or individual patient, accounting to comorbidities. Furthermore, despite the existence of many assessment tools, no single method has emerged as a gold standard.

The average IDWG from six consecutive sessions (over a 2-week period) is generally used to determine compliance to fluid restrictions. Peripheral edema, hypertension, and visible distension of jugular veins are commonly used in the clinical setting to determine fluid overload.

Biochemical assessment of sodium is a poor indicator of hydration due to the body's tight control of this parameter. There are a series of serum natriuretic peptides that hold promise as prognostic biomarkers of fluid status, although to date their lack of specificity limits utilization in practice [115].

Bioimpedance analysis is another method that has shown to be useful for determining fluid status, although most of the validation studies have been undertaken in the nonuremic population. Nonetheless, recent studies have demonstrated that clinical decision-making based on hydration management from bioimpedance resulted in improved management and reduced cardiovascular markers such as arterial stiffness and all-cause mortality [116].

More invasive measures of chronic fluid overload that offer good prognosis for cardiovascular risk include left ventricular dysfunction and hypertrophy from echocardiogram or cardiac magnetic resonance imaging.

5.3.3.2 Management

Most patients' fluid intakes are limited to 0.5 L fluid/day (plus a quantity equal to any residual urine output). However, prescribing a fluid allowance without a sodium restriction is futile, with thirst strongly linked to sodium intake. In fact, for every 8 g of salt, 1 L of fluid is required to meet the associated thirst [117]. Therefore, compliance to sodium guidelines of less than 6 g of salt/day (equivalent of 2 g sodium) is fundamental for achieving fluid control.

Patients often fear salt restricted diets due to their association with bland, un-pleasurable food. Identified barriers to adherence to a salt restrictive diet are (a) perceived taste/palatability of low-sodium foods, (b) convenience/difficulty (e.g., time, availability of low-sodium foods, interference with socialization, and cost) or, (c) lack of knowledge or understanding (e.g., lack of perceived benefit and inability to identify low-sodium foods). For this reason, it is important to begin any sodium dietary education with reassuring patients of sodium's acquired taste and, thus, slow decreases over time lead to increased salt sensitivity. With this in mind, it is important that realistic goals are set and sodium reduction occurs gradually over several months.

Bread, baked products, pre-cooked foods, and sausages are the most common sources of sodium in a Western diet besides the salt added to meals. Most of the sodium (75 %) comes from processed foods and, therefore, advocating for fresh, unprocessed food should underpin all sodium education. Other principles such as not adding salt to cooking, but instead utilizing other salt-free flavors and spices such as garlic, freshly ground pepper, and dry mustard powder, can enhance compliance without compromising flavor. Caution should also be given against using salt substitutes due to their high potassium content. Fortunately, there is mandatory labeling of sodium on nutrition information panels, enhancing the transparency for patients. As a general rule, foods with more than 120 mg of sodium per 100 g should be limited, and the importance of checking-specific brands is also apparent, with some brands containing several fold more sodium for equivalent food products [118]. Individualized counseling with a qualified dietitian remains the gold standard. This allows for patient-specific recommendations of food alternatives based on the patient's reported diet history. This method maybe perceived as less overwhelming for patients who struggle with adjusting their dietary habits.

Clearing up myths is another important strategy to increase patient awareness. Common myths include the need for extra salt in hotter months as well as for preventing dialysis-associated cramps.

Once patients have a grasp on sodium restrictions, education on what constitutes a fluid becomes more relevant. Anything that forms a liquid at mouth temperature or even foods with high fluid contents, such as rice and melon fruits, should be considered in fluid allowances. There are a number of government approved resources available which offer practical tips including the use of peppermints or slices of lemon to stimulate saliva flow, as well as freezing some of the fluid allowance to extend its thirst-quenching capacity [101].

5.3.3.3 Key Management Strategies

1. Limiting processed foods
2. Replacing salt in cooking with other flavors and spices
3. Reading food labels (higher level knowledge)
4. Choosing lower salt food options within each food group
5. Dispelling sodium myths
6. Educating on what constitutes a fluid
7. Practical tips for fluid management
   a. Stimulating saliva
   b. Extending fluid allowance

5.3.4 Vitamins and Trace Elements

There are a range of factors that contribute to vitamin and mineral disturbances common in the hemodialysis population, which manifest as both primary and secondary deficiencies. Primary causes, defined by low nutrient intakes, may result from symptoms of anorexia, taste changes, as well as the burden of potassium and oxalate dietary restrictions. Secondary causes include medication interactions, particularly with phosphate binders; enhanced gastrointestinal malabsorption, possibly relating to gut edema; altered kidney and cellular synthesis and metabolism, specifically with vitamin D; and the significant loss of water-soluble vitamins in dialysate. Toxicity from vitamin and trace elementals is also a concern in this population due to their limited clearance, particularly in anuric patients.

Studies have reported that more than 90 % of maintenance hemodialysis patients exhibit some level of vitamin abnormality [119] and similar prevalences have been observed with trace elements, particularly in anemic patients [120].

The literature linking vitamin and elemental supplementation with clinically relevant outcomes is sparse. One prominent observation study, which has led to a significant uptake in routine supplementation, demonstrated that patients who consumed water-soluble vitamins had better nutrition status, in addition to a 16% decrease in mortality, compared to those who did not [121]. Importantly, the benefit of vitamin supplementation persisted even after adjusting for traditional risk factors such as age, gender, race, body mass index, and other potential confounders.

Nonetheless, the importance of undertaking prospective intervention studies to confirm this association is clear. This has been highlighted by the disappointing results of a number of intervention studies demonstrating a lack of efficacy for homocysteine lowering therapy (through vitamin B supplementation) on clinical outcomes, despite initial promise suggested in observation studies [122].

5.3.4.1 Assessment

The hemodialysis population's complex biochemistry and nutrient metabolism limit the application of the recommended dietary intake (RDI) reference values which are targeted at the general population [123]. This shortcoming makes assessment of nutritional adequacy an ongoing challenge for dialysis patients. In addition, the lack of consensus on optimal methods to assess nutritional status for many vitamins and minerals further compounds the issue.

Nonetheless, the European Renal Association in conjunction with the European Dietitian and Transplant Nurses Association (ERA-EDTNA) has published recommendations for nutrient adequacy in the dialysis population [124]. The ERA-EDTNA make clear the distinction, however, between their recommendations based on expert opinion and clinical guidelines, which have been hampered by the lack of research in this area.

There are large differences in the distribution and size of body stores between nutrients and, therefore, assessment of adequacy requires a range of techniques. Common methods include (1) dietary intake, (2) serum or plasma concentration, (3) urine concentration, and (4) enzymatic activity. In addition, clinical manifestations of deficiency or toxicity, particularly where early signs are well defined, may offer better insight into overall body adequacy. In fact, the ERA-EDTNA have suggested that zinc supplementation should be given in the case of chronic inadequate protein/energy intakes with physical symptoms evoking signs of zinc deficiency (such as impaired taste or smell, skin fragility, and peripheral neuropathy), rather than relying solely on serum measures.

There are a number of robust, non-invasive techniques for measuring vitamins including erythrocyte transketolase activity coefficients (ETK-AC) (thiamine adequacy) and erythrocyte glutamic pyruvic transaminase (EGPT) activity (pyridoxine adequacy) [125]. Unfortunately, the complexity and cost associated with these biochemical measures limits the translation into routine clinical care in many dialysis units.

5.3.4.2 Management

Following a balanced diet is the preferred method to achieve recommended nutrient intakes as it limits not only the risk of toxicity that presents with taking commercial supplements but also the interaction between nutrients. For example, iron supplements have been shown to promote zinc deficiencies through inhibiting absorption [124].

The significant impact of dietary intake on nutrient adequacy in hemodialysis patients was demonstrated in a study that compared the vitamin intake of patients reliant on processed foods with those relied on traditional meals, and found the former group were significantly lower, particularly in B6 and folic acid [126].

Nonetheless, dietary intakes are often insufficient to meet the increased needs of many vitamins and trace elements in this population, as outlined in Table 5.6.

5.3.4.3 Vitamin Supplementation

The ERA-EDTNA working group is the only body to provide recommendations on a compressive list of vitamin and mineral supplementations, with many other groups opting against due to the lack of evidence in this area [127]. Since the inception of these recommendations in 2007, there has only been one significant change. The ERA-EDTNA's recommendation for vitamin E supplementation (400–800 IU/day) was based on the findings of a high-impact study which demonstrated that α-tocopherol supplementation in maintenance hemodialysis prevented vascular events [128]. Unfortunately, subsequent studies, including Heart Outcomes Prevention Evaluation (HOPE) [129] and HOPE-The Ongoing Outcomes (HOPE-TOO), have not only showed no benefit but also a possible risk for heart failure with vitamin E supplementation [130]. For this reason, prudence dictates that recommendations for supplementation of vitamin E should be withdrawn until further research is undertaken.

Vitamin D is unique to the other fat-soluble vitamins in that its metabolism, bioactivity, and supplementation requirements are dependent on phosphocalcic metabolism and bone status. For this reason, clinical guidelines recommend vitamin D supplementation should be individualized [131].

Due to the limited clearance of fat-soluble vitamins, toxicity from this group poses a significant risk. Irrespective of that, caution in supplementing water-soluble vitamins, such as vitamin C, can also be detrimental, with levels well below what is considered toxic in the general population, proving to be harmful [132].

5.3.4.4 Trace—Element Supplementation

Like vitamin D, the need for iron supplementation is variable and depends on a number factors including hemoglobin levels and the use of erythropoiesis-stimulating agents. Therefore, guidelines recommend routine evaluation and individualized management of iron stores should be followed, with supplementation in the form of intravenous iron if needed.

Table 5.6 Vitamin and trace element requirements [138–140]

	RDA/AI[a] 19–50 years	Recommended supplementation on hemodialysis	RDI/AI recommended (%)	Food sources	Toxicity[b]
Water-soluble vitamins					
Thiamine (B1)	1.2 mg (male); 1.1 mg (female)	1.1–1.2 mg	100	Enriched, fortified, or whole-grain products, including ready-to-eat cereals	No
Riboflavin (B2)	1.3 mg (male); 1.1 mg (female)	1.1–1.3 mg	100	Organ meats, milk, bread products and fortified cereals	No
Pyridoxine (B6)	1.3 mg $\geq$50 years: 1.7 mg (male) 1.5 mg (female)	10 mg	>700	Fortified cereals, organ meats, fortified soy-based meat substitutes	Yes
Ascorbic acid (C)	90 mg (male); 75 mg (female)	75–90 mg	100	Citrus fruits, tomatoes, potatoes, Brussel sprouts, cauliflower, broccoli, strawberries	Yes
Folic acid (B9)	400 μg	1 mg	250	Enriched cereal grains and breads, dark leafy vegetables, fortified ready-to-eat cereals	Yes
Cobalamin (B12)	2.4 μg	2.4 μg	100	Fortified cereals, organ meats, fortified soy-based meat substitutes	No
Niacin (B3, nicotinamide, nicotinic acid)	16 mg (males); 14 mg (females)	14–16 mg	100	Meat, fish, poultry, enriched and wholegrain breads and bread products, fortified ready-to-eat cereals	Yes
Biotin (B8)	30 μg[a]	30 mg	100	Liver and smaller amounts in fruits and meats	No
Pantothenic acid (B5)	5 mg[a]	5 mg	100	Chicken, beef, potatoes, oats, cereals, tomato products, liver, kidney, egg yolk, broccoli, whole grains	No
Fat-soluble vitamins					
Retinol (A)	900 μg (males); 700 μg (females)	Nil	n/a	Liver, dairy products, fish, darkly colored fruits, leafy vegetables	Yes
Alpha-tocopherol (E)	15 mg	Up to RDA if deficiency exists	n/a	Vegetable oils, unprocessed cereal grains, nuts, fruits, vegetables, meats	Yes
Vitamin K	120 μg[a] (male); 90 μg (female)	Unknown	n/a	Green vegetables (collards, spinach, salad greens, broccoli), brussel sprouts, cabbage, plant oils and margarine	No
Calciferol (D)	15 μg 20 μg (>70 years)	Individualized approach	n/a	Fish liver oils, flesh of fatty fish, egg yolk, fortified dairy products and fortified cereals	Yes
Trace elements					
Iron	8 mg (men; women post-menopause); 18 mg (women pre-menopause)	IV iron dose case specific[c]	n/a	Fruits, vegetables and fortified bread and grain products such as cereal (nonheme iron sources), meat and poultry (heme iron sources)	Yes
Zinc	11 mg (men); 8 mg (women)	Nil	n/a	Fortified cereals, red meats, certain seafood	Yes
Selenium	55 μg	Nil	n/a	Organ meats, seafood, plants (depending on soil selenium content)	Yes

[a] *RDAs* recommended dietary allowances, *AIs* adequate intakes
[b] For normal individuals defined by the presence of an upper limit
[c] [131]

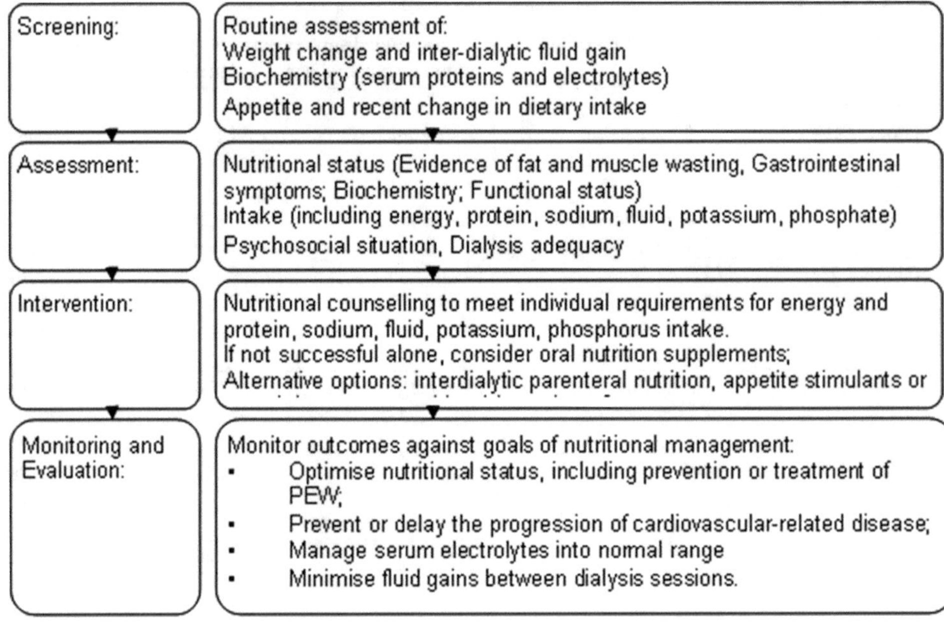

Fig. 5.5 Overview of the process for providing medical nutrition therapy for hemodialysis patients

Despite the lack of routine recommendation for both zinc and selenium, studies have shown symptom improvement with supplementation [133, 134]. Therefore, supplementation for 3–6 months may be considered where symptoms evoking signs of deficiency are suspected.

The high prevalence of commercial dietary supplements in the general population, which was reported to be 50% in a large cohort of older Americans [135], highlights the importance of reviewing patients' supplement use. Purchase of regular vitamin and mineral supplements should be strongly discouraged, where supplements such as B-100 or multivitamins can contain dangerously high amounts of B vitamins as well as containing hazardous minerals (phosphorous and potassium) and vitamins (A and K). There are a number of renal-specific formulations available, which comply with the recommended dose defined in Table 5.6.

5.4 Summary of Nutritional Management in Hemodialysis

The goal of nutritional management in hemodialysis is to (1) optimize the nutritional status, including prevention or treatment of PEW, (2) prevent or delay the progression of cardiovascular-related disease, (3) manage bone mineral metabolism through optimizing phosphate management, and (4) manage serum electrolytes and fluid. Dietary requirements for dialysis patients span both macronutrients (protein and energy) and micronutrients (vitamins and trace minerals) and essential nutrients in the form of amino acids and fatty acids. Optimizing nutritional status requires adherence to minimum requirements. Guideline recommendations for intake in maintenance dialysis patients are summarized in Table 5.3 [71, 79, 86, 105, 136].

Figure 5.5 outlines the process that should be undertaken for the nutritional management of hemodialysis patients. Providing routine review of dialysis patients results in improved outcomes, including reduced rates of malnutrition, improvements in control of serum phosphate and potassium [137].

References

1. de Mutsert R, Grootendorst DC, Boeschoten EW, Brandts H, van Manen JG, Krediet RT, Dekker FW, Group ftNCSotAoD-S. Subjective global assessment of nutritional status is strongly associated with mortality in chronic dialysis patients. Am J Clin Nutr. 2009;89:787–93.
2. Rambod M, Bross R, Zitterkoph J, Benner D, Pithia J, Colman S, Kovesdy CP, Kopple JD, Kalantar-Zadeh K. Association of Malnutrition-Inflammation Score with quality of life and mortality in hemodialysis patients: a 5-year prospective cohort study. Am J Kidney Dis. 2009;53:298–309.
3. Cordeiro AC, Qureshi AR, Stenvinkel P, Heimburger O, Axelsson J, Barany P, Lindholm B, Carrero JJ. Abdominal fat deposition is associated with increased inflammation, protein-energy wasting and worse outcome in patients undergoing haemodialysis. Nephrol Dial Transpl. 2010;25:562–8.
4. Miyamoto T, Carrero JJ, Qureshi AR, Anderstam B, Heimburger O, Barany P, Lindholm B, Stenvinkel P. Circulating follistatin in patients with chronic kidney disease: implications for muscle strength, bone mineral density, inflammation, and survival. Clin J Am Soc Nephrol. 2011;6:1001–8.
5. Tabibi H, As'habi A, Heshmati BN, Mahdavi-Mazdeh M, Hedayati M. Prevalence of protein-energy wasting and its various types in Iranian hemodialysis patients: a new classification. Ren Fail. 2012;34:1200–5.

6. Tsai HB, Chen PC, Liu CH, Hung PH, Chen MT, Chiang CK, Kao JH, Hung KY. Association of hepatitis C virus infection and malnutrition-inflammation complex syndrome in maintenance hemodialysis patients. Nephrol Dial Transpl. 2012;27:1176–83.
7. Fiedler R, Dorligjav O, Seibert E, Ulrich C, Markau S, Girndt M. Vitamin D deficiency, mortality, and hospitalization in hemodialysis patients with or without protein-energy wasting. Nephron Clin Pract. 2011;119:220–6.
8. Leal VO, Moraes C, Stockler-Pinto MB, Lobo JC, Farage NE, Velarde LG, Fouque D, Mafra D. Is a body mass index of 23 kg/m^2 a reliable marker of protein–energy wasting in hemodialysis patients? Nutrition. 2012;28:973–7.
9. Steiber A, Leon JB, Secker D, McCarthy M, McCann L, Serra M, Sehgal AR, Kalantar-Zadeh K. Multicenter study of the validity and reliability of subjective global assessment in the hemodialysis population. J Ren Nutr. 2007;17:336–42.
10. Kalantar-Zadeh K, Block G, McAllister CJ, Humphreys MH, Kopple JD. Appetite and inflammation, nutrition, anemia, and clinical outcome in hemodialysis patients. Am J Clin Nutr. 2004;80:299–307.
11. Kalantar-Zadeh K, Kopple JD, Block G, Humphreys MH. A malnutrition-Inflammation Score is correlated with morbidity and mortality in maintenance hemodialysis patients. Am J Kidney Dis. 2001;38:1251–63.
12. Burrowes JD, Larive B, Chertow GM, Cockram DB, Dwyer JT, Greene T, Kusek JW, Leung J, Rocco MV. Self-reported appetite, hospitalization and death in haemodialysis patients: findings from the hemodialysis (HEMO) study. Nephrol Dial Transpl. 2005;20:2765–74.
13. Kaysen GA, Muller HG, Young BS, Leng X, Chertow GM. The influence of patient- and facility-specific factors on nutritional status and survival in hemodialysis. J Ren Nutr. 2004;14:72–81.
14. Dalrymple LS, Johansen KL, Chertow GM, Cheng S-C, Grimes B, Gold EB, Kaysen GA. Infection-related hospitalizations in older patients with ESRD. Am J Kidney Dis. 56:522–30.
15. Cheu C, Pearson J, Dahlerus C, Lantz B, Chowdhury T, Sauer PF, Farrell RE, Port FK, Ramirez SPB. Association between oral nutritional supplementation and clinical outcomes among patients with ESRD. Clin J Am Soc Nephrol. 2012;8(1):100–7.
16. Lacson E Jr, Wang W, Zebrowski B, Wingard R, Hakim RM. Outcomes associated with intradialytic oral nutritional supplements in patients undergoing maintenance hemodialysis: a quality improvement report. Am J Kidney Dis. 2012;60:591–600.
17. Liu Y, Coresh J, Eustace JA, Longenecker JC, Jaar B, Fink NE, Tracy RP, Powe NR, Klag MJ. Association between cholesterol level and mortality in dialysis patients: role of inflammation and malnutrition. JAMA. 2004;291:451–9.
18. Kalantar-Zadeh K, Block G, Humphreys MH, Kopple JD. Reverse epidemiology of cardiovascular risk factors in maintenance dialysis patients. Kidney Int. 2003;63:793–808.
19. Suliman ME, Stenvinkel P, Qureshi AR, Barany P, Heimburger O, Anderstam B, Alvestrand A, Lindholm B. Hyperhomocysteinemia in relation to plasma free amino acids, biomarkers of inflammation and mortality in patients with chronic kidney disease starting dialysis therapy. Am J Kidney Dis. 2004;44:455–65.
20. Carrero JJ, Qureshi AR, Axelsson J, Avesani CM, Suliman ME, Kato S, Bárány P, Snaedal-Jonsdottir S, Alvestrand A, Heimbürger O, Lindholm B, Stenvinkel P. Comparison of nutritional and inflammatory markers in dialysis patients with reduced appetite. Am J Clin Nutr. 2007;85:695–701.
21. Lopes AA, Elder SJ, Ginsberg N, Andreucci VE, Cruz JM, Fukuhara S, Mapes DL, Saito A, Pisoni RL, Saran R, Port FK. Lack of appetite in haemodialysis patients–associations with patient characteristics, indicators of nutritional status and outcomes in the international DOPPS. Nephrol Dial Transpl. 2007;22:3538–46.
22. Curtin RB, Bultman DC, Thomas-Hawkins C, Walters BA, Schatell D. Hemodialysis patients' symptom experiences: effects on physical and mental functioning. Nephrol Nurs J. 2002;29:562, 567–74. discussion 575, 598.
23. Wright M, Woodrow G, O'Brien S, King N, Dye L, Blundell J, Brownjohn A, Turney J. Disturbed appetite patterns and nutrient intake in peritoneal dialysis patients. Perit Dial Int. 2003;23:550–6.
24. Chung SH, Carrero JJ, Lindholm B. Causes of Poor Appetite in Patients on Peritoneal Dialysis. J Ren Nutr. 2011;21:12–5.
25. Suneja M, Murry DJ, Stokes JB, Lim VS. Hormonal regulation of energy-protein homeostasis in hemodialysis patients: an anorexigenic profile that may predispose to adverse cardiovascular outcomes. Am J Physiol Endocrinol Metab. 2011. 300:55–64.
26. Aguilera A, Codoceo R, Bajo MA, Iglesias P, Diéz JJ, Barril G, Cigarrán S, Álvarez V, Celadilla O, Fernández-Perpén A, Montero A, Selgas R. Eating behavior disorders in uremia: a question of balance in appetite regulation. Semin Dial. 2004;17:44–52.
27. Cheung WW, Mak RH. Ghrelin and its analogues as therapeutic agents for anorexia and cachexia in end-stage renal disease. Kidney Int. 2009;76:135–7.
28. Bossola M, Tazza L, Giungi S, Luciani G. Anorexia in hemodialysis patients: an update. Kidney Int. 2006;70:417–22.
29. Burrowes JD, Larive B, Cockram DB, Dwyer J, Kusek JW, McLeroy S, Poole D, Rocco MV. Effects of dietary intake, appetite, and eating habits on dialysis and non-dialysis treatment days in hemodialysis patients: cross-sectional results from the HEMO study. J Ren Nutr. 2003;13:191–8.
30. Manley K, Haryono RY, Keast RSJ. Taste changes and saliva composition in chronic kidney disease. Ren Soc Australas J. 2012;8:56–60.
31. Middleton RA, Allman-Farinelli MA. Taste sensitivity is altered in patients with chronic renal failure receiving continuous ambulatory peritoneal dialysis. J Nutr. 1999;129:122–5.
32. Raff AC, Lieu S, Melamed ML, Quan Z, Ponda M, Meyer TW, Hostetter TH. Relationship of impaired olfactory function in ESRD to malnutrition and retained uremic molecules. Am J Kidney Dis. 2008;52:102–10.
33. Boltong A, Campbell K. 'Taste' changes: a problem for patients and their dietitians. Nutr Diet. 2013;70:262–9.
34. Akar H, Akar GC, Carrero JJ, Stenvinkel P, Lindholm B. Systemic consequences of poor oral health in chronic kidney disease patients. Clin J Am Soc Nephrol. 2011;6:218–26.
35. Carrero JJ. Identification of patients with eating disorders: clinical and biochemical signs of appetite loss in dialysis patients. J Ren Nutr. 2009;19:10–5.
36. Crews DC, Kuczmarski MF, Grubbs V, Hedgeman E, Shahinian VB, Evans MK, Zonderman AB, Burrows NR, Williams DE, Saran R, Powe NR. Effect of food insecurity on chronic kidney disease in lower-income Americans. Am J Nephrol. 2014;39:27–35.
37. Untas A, Thumma J, Rascle N, Rayner H, Mapes D, Lopes AA, Fukuhara S, Akizawa T, Morgenstern H, Robinson BM, Pisoni RL, Combe C. The associations of social support and other psychosocial factors with mortality and quality of life in the dialysis outcomes and practice patterns study. Clin J Am Soc Nephrol. 2011;6:142–52.
38. Bossola M, Luciani G, Rosa F, Tazza L. Appetite and gastrointestinal symptoms in chronic hemodialysis patients. J Ren Nutr. 2011;21:448–54.
39. Strid H, Simrén M, Johansson AC, Svedlund J, Samuelsson O, Björnsson ES. The prevalence of gastrointestinal symptoms in patients with chronic renal failure is increased and associated with impaired psychological general well-being. Nephrol Dial Transpl. 2002;17:1434–9.
40. Shirazian S, Radhakrishnan J. Gastrointestinal disorders and renal failure: exploring the connection. Nat Rev Nephrol. 2010;6:480–92.
41. Cano AE, Neil AK, Kang J-Y, Barnabas A, Eastwood JB, Nelson SR, Hartley I, Maxwell D. Gastrointestinal symptoms in patients

with end-stage renal disease undergoing treatment by hemodialysis or peritoneal dialysis. Am J Gastroenterol. 2007;102:1990–7.
42. Strid H, Simrén M, Stotzer PO, Ringström G, Abrahamsson H, Björnsson ES. Patients with chronic renal failure have abnormal small intestinal motility and a high prevalence of small intestinal bacterial overgrowth. Digestion. 2003;67:129–37.
43. Aguilera A, Gonzalez-Espinoza L, Codoceo R, Jara Mdel C, Pavone M, Bajo MA, Del Peso G, Celadilla O, Martinez MV, Lopez-Cabrera M, Selgas R. Bowel bacterial overgrowth as another cause of malnutrition, inflammation, and atherosclerosis syndrome in peritoneal dialysis patients. Adv Perit Dial. 2010;26:130–6.
44. Strid H, Simren M, Stotzer PO, Abrahamsson H, Bjornsson ES. Delay in gastric emptying in patients with chronic renal failure. Scand J Gastroenterol. 2004;39:516–20.
45. Stenvinkel P, Heimburger O, Paultre F, Diczfalusy U, Wang T, Berglund L, Jogestrand T. Strong association between malnutrition, inflammation, and atherosclerosis in chronic renal failure. Kidney Int. 1999;55:1899–911.
46. Kalantar-Zadeh K, Ikizler TA, Block G, Avram MM, Kopple JD. Malnutrition-inflammation complex syndrome in dialysis patients: causes and consequences. Am J Kidney Dis. 2003;42:864–81.
47. Carrero JJ, Stenvinkel P. Persistent inflammation as a catalyst for other risk factors in chronic kidney disease: a hypothesis proposal. Clin J Am Soc Nephrol. 2009;4:S49–S55.
48. Carrero JJ, Yilmaz MI, Lindholm B, Stenvinkel P. Cytokine dysregulation in chronic kidney disease: how can we treat it? Blood Purif. 2008;26:291–9.
49. Plata-Salaman CR. Cytokines and feeding. Int J Obes Relat Metab Disord. 2001;25(Suppl 5):48–52.
50. Aguilera A, Codoceo R, Selgas R, Garcia P, Picornell M, Diaz C, Sanchez C, Bajo MA. Anorexigen (TNF-alpha, cholecystokinin) and orexigen (neuropeptide Y) plasma levels in peritoneal dialysis (PD) patients: their relationship with nutritional parameters. Nephrol Dial Transpl. 1998;13:1476–83.
51. Bossola M, Luciani G, Giungi S, Tazza L. Anorexia, fatigue and plasma interleukin-6 levels in chronic hemodialysis patients. Ren Fail. 2010;32:1049–54.
52. Carrero JJ, Chmielewski M, Axelsson J, Snaedal S, Heimbürger O, Bárány P, Suliman ME, Lindholm B, Stenvinkel P, Qureshi AR. Muscle atrophy, inflammation and clinical outcome in incident and prevalent dialysis patients. Clin Nutr. 2008;27:557–64.
53. Kaizu Y, Ohkawa S, Odamaki M, Ikegaya N, Hibi I, Miyaji K, Kumagai H. Association between inflammatory mediators and muscle mass in long-term hemodialysis patients. Am J Kidney Dis. 2003;42:295–302.
54. Raj DSC, Moseley P, Dominic EA, Onime A, Tzamaloukas AH, Boyd A, Shah VO, Glew R, Wolfe R, Ferrando A. Interleukin-6 modulates hepatic and muscle protein synthesis during hemodialysis. Kidney Int. 2008;73:1054–61.
55. Cheung AK. Biocompatibility of hemodialysis membranes. J Am Soc Nephrol. 1990;1:150–61.
56. Mokrzycki MH, Kaplan AA. Protein losses in continuous renal replacement therapies. J Am Soc Nephrol. 1996;7:2259–63.
57. Davies SP, Reaveley DA, Brown EA, Kox WJ. Amino acid clearances and daily losses in patients with acute renal failure treated by continuous arteriovenous hemodialysis. Crit Care Med. 1991;19:1510–5.
58. Schepky AG, Bensch KW, Schulz-Knappe P, Forssmann WG. Human hemofiltrate as a source of circulating bioactive peptides: determination of amino acids, peptides and proteins. Biomed Chromatogr. 1994;8:90–4.
59. Raj DS, Zager P, Shah VO, Dominic EA, Adeniyi O, Blandon P, Wolfe R, Ferrando A. Protein turnover and amino acid transport kinetics in end-stage renal disease. Am J Physiol Endocrinol Metab. 2004;286:136–43.
60. Ikizler TA, Pupim LB, Brouillette JR, Levenhagen DK, Farmer K, Hakim RM, Flakoll PJ. Hemodialysis stimulates muscle and whole body protein loss and alters substrate oxidation. Am J Physiol Endocrinol Metab. 2002;282:107–16.
61. Pupim LB, Majchrzak KM, Flakoll PJ, Ikizler TA. Intradialytic oral nutrition improves protein homeostasis in chronic hemodialysis patients with deranged nutritional status. J Am Soc Nephrol. 2006;17:3149–57.
62. Veeneman JM, Kingma HA, Boer TS, Stellaard F, De Jong PE, Reijngoud DJ, Huisman RM. Protein intake during hemodialysis maintains a positive whole body protein balance in chronic hemodialysis patients. Am J Physiol Endocrinol Metab. 2003;284:954–65.
63. Azar AT, Wahba K, Mohamed AS, Massoud WA. Association between dialysis dose improvement and nutritional status among hemodialysis patients. Am J Nephrol. 2007;27:113–9.
64. Galland R, Traeger J, Arkouche W, Cleaud C, Delawari E, Fouque D. Short daily hemodialysis rapidly improves nutritional status in hemodialysis patients. Kidney Int. 2001;60:1555–60.
65. Chertow GM, Levin NW, Beck GJ, Depner TA, Eggers PW, Gassman JJ, Gorodetskaya I, Greene T, James S, Larive B, Lindsay RM, Mehta RL, Miller B, Ornt DB, Rajagopalan S, Rastogi A, Rocco MV, Schiller B, Sergeyeva O, Schulman G, Ting GO, Unruh ML, Star RA, Kliger AS. In-center hemodialysis six times per week versus three times per week. N Engl J Med. 2010;363:2287–300.
66. Wang AYM, Lai KN. The importance of residual renal function in dialysis patients. Kidney Int. 2006;69:1726–32.
67. Carrero JJ, Heimburger O, Chan M, Axelsson J, Stenvinkel P, Lindholm B. Protein-energy malnutrition/wasting during peritoneal dialysis. In Khanna R, RTK, editor. Nolph and Gokal's textbook of peritoneal dialysis. New York: Springer; 2009.
68. de Brito-Ashurst I, Varagunam M, Raftery MJ, Yaqoob MM. Bicarbonate supplementation slows progression of CKD and improves nutritional status. J Am Soc Nephrol. 2009;20:2075–84.
69. Graham KA, Reaich D, Channon SM, Downie S, Goodship TH. Correction of acidosis in hemodialysis decreases whole-body protein degradation. J Am Soc Nephrol. 1997;8:632–7.
70. Graham KA, Reaich D, Channon SM, Downie S, Gilmour E, Passlick-Deetjen J, Goodship TH. Correction of acidosis in CAPD decreases whole body protein degradation. Kidney Int. 1996;49:1396–400.
71. Ikizler TA, Cano NJ, Franch H, Fouque D, Himmelfarb J, Kalantar-Zadeh K, Kuhlmann MK, Stenvinkel P, TerWee P, Teta D, Wang AY-M, Wanner C. Prevention and treatment of protein energy wasting in chronic kidney disease patients: a consensus statement by the International Society of Renal Nutrition and Metabolism. Kidney Int. 2013;84:1096–107.
72. Fouque D, Kalantar-Zadeh K, Kopple J, Cano N, Chauveau P, Cuppari L, Franch H, Guarnieri G, Ikizler TA, Kaysen G, Lindholm B, Massy Z, Mitch W, Pineda E, Stenvinkel P, Trevinho-Becerra A, Wanner C. A proposed nomenclature and diagnostic criteria for protein-energy wasting in acute and chronic kidney disease. Kidney Int. 2007;73:391–8.
73. Chumlea WC. Anthropometric and body composition assessment in dialysis patients. Semin Dial. 2004;17:466–70.
74. Heimburger O, Qureshi AR, Blaner WS, Berglund L, Stenvinkel P. Hand-grip muscle strength, lean body mass, and plasma proteins as markers of nutritional status in patients with chronic renal failure close to start of dialysis therapy. Am J Kidney Dis. 2000;36:1213–25.
75. Wang AY, Sea MM, Ho ZS, Lui SF, Li PK, Woo J. Evaluation of handgrip strength as a nutritional marker and prognostic indicator in peritoneal dialysis patients. Am J Clin Nutr. 2005;81:79–86.
76. Barbosa-Silva MCG, Barros AJ, Wang J, Heymsfield SB, Pierson RN. Bioelectrical impedance analysis: population reference val-

ues for phase angle by age and sex. Am J Clin Nutr. 2005;82:49–52.
77. Beberashvili I, Azar A, Sinuani I, Shapiro G, Feldman L, Stav K, Sandbank J, Averbukh Z. Bioimpedance phase angle predicts muscle function, quality of life and clinical outcome in maintenance hemodialysis patients. Eur J Clin Nutr. 2014;68:683–9.
78. Carrero JJ, Chen J, Kovesdy CP, Kalantar-Zadeh K. Critical appraisal of biomarkers of dietary intake and nutritional status in patients undergoing dialysis. Semin Dial. 2014;27(6):586–9.
79. National Kidney Foundation. Clinical practice guidelines for nutrition in chronic renal failure. K/DOQI, National Kidney Foundation. Am J Kidney Dis. 2000;35:1–140.
80. Suliman ME, Qureshi AR, Stenvinkel P, Pecoits-Filho R, Bárány P, Heimbürger O, Anderstam B, Rodríguez Ayala E, Divino Filho JC, Alvestrand A, Lindholm B. Inflammation contributes to low plasma amino acid concentrations in patients with chronic kidney disease. Am J Clin Nutr. 2005;82:342–9.
81. Kaysen GA, Dubin JA, Muller H-G, Rosales L, Levin NW, Mitch WE. Inflammation and reduced albumin synthesis associated with stable decline in serum albumin in hemodialysis patients. Kidney Int. 2004;65:1408–15.
82. Bommer J, Locatelli F, Satayathum S, Keen ML, Goodkin DA, Saito A, Akiba T, Port FK, Young EW. Association of predialysis serum bicarbonate levels with risk of mortality and hospitalization in the Dialysis outcomes and practice patterns study (DOPPS). Am J Kidney Dis. 2004;44:661–71.
83. Lisawat P, Gennari FJ. Approach to the hemodialysis patient with an abnormal serum bicarbonate concentration. Am J Kidney Dis. 2014;64:151–5.
84. Steiber AL, Kalantar-Zadeh K, Secker D, McCarthy M, Sehgal A, McCann L. Subjective global assessment in chronic kidney disease: a review. J Ren Nutr. 2004;14:191–200.
85. Campbell KL, Ash S, Bauer J, Davies PSW. Critical review of nutrition assessment tools to measure malnutrition in chronic kidney disease. Nutr Diet. 2007;64:23–30.
86. Ash S, Campbell KL, Bogard J, Millichamp A. Nutrition prescription to achieve positive outcomes in chronic kidney disease: a systematic review. Nutrients. 2014;6:416–51.
87. Kalantar-Zadeh K, Cano NJ, Budde K, Chazot C, Kovesdy CP, Mak RH, Mehrotra R, Raj DS, Sehgal AR, Stenvinkel P, Ikizler TA. Diets and enteral supplements for improving outcomes in chronic kidney disease. Nat Rev Nephrol. 2011;7:369–84.
88. Stratton RJ, Bircher G, Fouque D, Stenvinkel P, de Mutsert R, Engfer M, Elia M. Multinutrient oral supplements and tube feeding in maintenance dialysis: a systematic review and meta-analysis. Am J Kidney Dis. 2005;46:387–405.
89. Cano NJM, Fouque D, Roth H, Aparicio M, Azar R, Canaud B, Chauveau P, Combe C, Laville M, Leverve XM, tFSGfNiD. Intradialytic parenteral nutrition does not improve survival in malnourished hemodialysis patients: a 2-year multicenter, prospective, randomized study. J Am Soc Nephrol. 2007;18:2583–91.
90. Hiroshige K, Sonta T, Suda T, Kanegae K, Ohtani A. Oral supplementation of branched-chain amino acid improves nutritional status in elderly patients on chronic haemodialysis. Nephrol Dial Transpl. 2001;16:1856–62.
91. Fouque D, McKenzie J, de Mutsert R, Azar R, Teta D, Plauth M, Cano N. Use of a renal-specific oral supplement by haemodialysis patients with low protein intake does not increase the need for phosphate binders and may prevent a decline in nutritional status and quality of life. Nephrol Dial Transpl. 2008;23:2902–10.
92. Kalantar-Zadeh K, Ikizler TA. Let them eat during dialysis: an overlooked opportunity to improve outcomes in maintenance hemodialysis patients. J Ren Nutr. 2013;23:157–63.
93. Cano N, Fiaccadori E, Tesinsky P, Toigo G, Druml W, Kuhlmann M, Mann H, Hörl WH. ESPEN Guidelines on enteral nutrition: adult renal failure. Clin Nutr. 2006;25:295–310.
94. Yeh S, Wu SY, Levine DM, Parker TS, Olson JS, Stevens MR, Schuster MW. Quality of life and stimulation of weight gain after treatment with megestrol acetate: correlation between cytokine levels and nutritional status, appetite in geriatric patients with wasting syndrome. J Nutr Health Aging. 2000;4:246–51.
95. Monfared A, Heidarzadeh A, Ghaffari M, Akbarpour M. Effect of megestrol acetate on serum albumin level in malnourished dialysis patients. J Ren Nutr. 2009;19:167–71.
96. Ruiz Garcia V, Lopez-Briz E, Carbonell Sanchis R, Gonzalvez Perales JL, Bort-Marti S. Megestrol acetate for treatment of anorexia-cachexia syndrome. Cochrane Database Syst Rev. 2013;3:CD004310.
97. Ashby DR, Ford HE, Wynne KJ, Wren AM, Murphy KG, Busbridge M, Brown EA, Taube DH, Ghatei MA, Tam FW, Bloom SR, Choi P. Sustained appetite improvement in malnourished dialysis patients by daily ghrelin treatment. Kidney Int. 2009;76:199–206.
98. Sanghavi S, Whiting S, Uribarri J. Potassium balance in dialysis patients. Semin Dial. 2013;26:597–603.
99. Glassock RJ, Pecoits-Filho R, Barberato SH. Left ventricular mass in chronic kidney disease and ESRD. Clin J Am Soc Nephrol. 2009;4(Suppl 1):79–91.
100. Kovesdy CP, Regidor DL, Mehrotra R, Jing J, McAllister CJ, Greenland S, Kopple JD, Kalantar-Zadeh K. Serum and dialysate potassium concentrations and survival in hemodialysis patients. Clin J Am Soc Nephrol. 2007;2:999–1007.
101. Queensland Government QH, Nutrition Education Materials Online (NEMO). Renal resources. Australia: Queensland Government QH; 2014.
102. Picq C, Asplanato M, Bernillon N, Fabre C, Roubeix M, Ricort JM. Effects of water soaking and/or sodium polystyrene sulfonate addition on potassium content of foods. Int J Food Sci Nutr. 2014;65(6):673–7.
103. KDIGO. Kidney disease: improving global outcomes (KDIGO) clinical practice guideline for the diagnosis, evaluation, prevention, and treatment of chronic kidney disease-mineral and bone disorder (CKD-MBD). Kidney Int Suppl. 2009;113:1–130.
104. Williams C, Ronco C, Kotanko P. Whole grains in the renal diet–is it time to reevaluate their role? Blood Purif. 2013;36:210–4.
105. American Dietetic Association. Chronic kidney disease evidence-based nutrition practice guideline. Chicago: American Dietetic Association; 2010.
106. Shinaberger CS, Kilpatrick RD, Regidor DL, McAllister CJ, Greenland S, Kopple JD, Kalantar-Zadeh K. Longitudinal associations between dietary protein intake and survival in hemodialysis patients. Am J Kidney Dis. 2006;48:37–49.
107. Sullivan C, Sayre SS, Leon JB, Machekano R, Love TE, Porter D, Marbury M, Sehgal AR. Effect of food additives on hyperphosphatemia among patients with end-stage renal disease: a randomized controlled trial. JAMA. 2009;301:629–35.
108. The European Parliament and Council. Amending Annex II to Regulation (EC) No 1333/2008: Union list of food additives. Off J Eur Union. 2011;1–177. http://eur-lex.europa.eu/legal-content/EN/ALL/?uri=CELEX%3A32011R1129
109. Cupisti A, Comar F, Benini O, Lupetti S, D'Alessandro C, Barsotti G, Gianfaldoni D. Effect of boiling on dietary phosphate and nitrogen intake. J Ren Nutr. 2006;16:36–40.
110. National Kidney Foundation. K/DOQI clinical practice guidelines for bone metabolism and disease in chronic kidney disease. Am J Kidney Dis. 2003;42:S1–201.
111. Lynch KE, Lynch R, Curhan GC, Brunelli SM. Prescribed dietary phosphate restriction and survival among hemodialysis patients. Clin J Am Soc Nephrol. 2011;6:620–9.
112. Navaneethan SD, Palmer SC, Vecchio M, Craig JC, Elder GJ, Strippoli GF. Phosphate binders for preventing and treating bone disease in chronic kidney disease patients. Cochrane Database Syst Rev. 2011;2:CD006023.

113. Ahlenstiel T, Pape L, Ehrich JH, Kuhlmann MK. Self-adjustment of phosphate binder dose to meal phosphorus content improves management of hyperphosphataemia in children with chronic kidney disease. Nephrol Dial Transplant. 2010;25:3241–9.
114. Arneson TJ, Liu J, Qiu Y, Gilbertson DT, Foley RN, Collins AJ. Hospital treatment for fluid overload in the Medicare hemodialysis population. Clin J Am Soc Nephrol. 2010;5:1054–63.
115. Jaeger JQ, Mehta RL. Assessment of dry weight in hemodialysis: an overview. J Am Soc Nephrol. 1999;10:392–403.
116. Onofriescu M, Hogas S, Voroneanu L, Apetrii M, Nistor I, Kanbay M, Covic AC. Bioimpedance-guided fluid management in maintenance hemodialysis: a pilot randomized controlled trial. Am J Kidney Dis. 2014;64:111–8.
117. Lindley EJ. Reducing sodium intake in hemodialysis patients. Semin Dial. 2009;22:260–3.
118. Sullivan CM, Leon JB, Sehgal AR. Phosphorus-containing food additives and the accuracy of nutrient databases: implications for renal patients. J Ren Nutr. 2007;17:350–4.
119. Allman MA, Truswell AS, Tiller DJ, Stewart PM, Yau DF, Horvath JS, Duggin GG. Vitamin supplementation of patients receiving haemodialysis. Med J Aust. 1989;150:130–3.
120. Fukushima T, Horike H, Fujiki S, Kitada S, Sasaki T, Kashihara N. Zinc deficiency anemia and effects of zinc therapy in maintenance hemodialysis patients. Ther Apher Dial. 2009;13:213–9.
121. Fissell RB, Bragg-Gresham JL, Gillespie BW, Goodkin DA, Bommer J, Saito A, Akiba T, Port FK, Young EW. International variation in vitamin prescription and association with mortality in the dialysis outcomes and practice patterns study (DOPPS). Am J Kidney Dis. 2004;44:293–9.
122. Jardine MJ, Kang A, Zoungas S, Navaneethan SD, Ninomiya T, Nigwekar SU, Gallagher MP, Cass A, Strippoli G, Perkovic V. The effect of folic acid based homocysteine lowering on cardiovascular events in people with kidney disease: systematic review and meta-analysis. BMJ. 2012;344:e3533.
123. Institute of Medicine. DRI dietary reference intakes: applications in dietary assessment. Washington, DC: National Academies Press; 2000.
124. Fouque D, Vennegoor M, ter Wee P, Wanner C, Basci A, Canaud B, Haage P, Konner K, Kooman J, Martin-Malo A, Pedrini L, Pizzarelli F, Tattersall J, Tordoir J, Vanholder R. EBPG guideline on nutrition. Nephrol Dial Transpl. 2007;22(Suppl 2):ii45–i87.
125. Steiber AL, Kopple JD. Vitamin status and needs for people with stages 3–5 chronic kidney disease. J Ren Nutr. 2011;21:355–68.
126. Ribeiro MM, Araujo ML, Netto MP, Cunha LM. Effects of customary dinner on dietetical profile of patients undergoing hemodialysis. J Bras Nefrol. 2011;33:69–77.
127. K/DOQI. Clinical practice guidelines for nutrition in chronic renal failure. National Kidney Foundation. Am J Kidney Dis. 2000; 35:1–140.
128. Boaz M, Smetana S, Weinstein T, Matas Z, Gafter U, Iaina A, Knecht A, Weissgarten Y, Brunner D, Fainaru M, Green MS. Secondary prevention with antioxidants of cardiovascular disease in endstage renal disease (SPACE): randomised placebo-controlled trial. Lancet. 2000;356:1213–8.
129. Mann JF, Lonn EM, Yi Q, Gerstein HC, Hoogwerf BJ, Pogue J, Bosch J, Dagenais GR, Yusuf S. Effects of vitamin E on cardiovascular outcomes in people with mild-to-moderate renal insufficiency: results of the HOPE study. Kidney Int. 2004;65:1375–80.
130. Lonn E, Bosch J, Yusuf S, Sheridan P, Pogue J, Arnold JM, Ross C, Arnold A, Sleight P, Probstfield J, Dagenais GR. Effects of long-term vitamin E supplementation on cardiovascular events and cancer: a randomized controlled trial. JAMA. 2005;293:1338–47.
131. KDIGO. KDIGO 2012 Clinial practice guidelines for the evaluation and management of chronic kidney disease. Kidney Int. 2013;3:1–150.
132. Pru C, Eaton J, Kjellstrand C. Vitamin C intoxication and hyperoxalemia in chronic hemodialysis patients. Nephron. 1985;39:112–6.
133. Sprenger KB, Bundschu D, Lewis K, Spohn B, Schmitz J, Franz HE. Improvement of uremic neuropathy and hypogeusia by dialysate zinc supplementation: a double-blind study. Kidney Int Suppl. 1983;16:S315–8.
134. Napolitano G, Bonomini M, Bomba G, Bucci I, Todisco V, Albertazzi A, Monaco F. Thyroid function and plasma selenium in chronic uremic patients on hemodialysis treatment. Biol Trace Elem Res. 1996;55:221–30.
135. Qato DM, Alexander GC, Conti RM, Johnson M, Schumm P, Lindau ST. Use of prescription and over-the-counter medications and dietary supplements among older adults in the United States. JAMA. 2008;300:2867–78.
136. Naylor HL, Jackson H, Walker GH, Macafee S, Magee K, Hooper L, Stewart L, MacLaughlin HL. British dietetic association evidence-based guidelines for the protein requirements of adults undergoing maintenance haemodialysis or peritoneal dialysis. J Hum Nutr Diet. 2013;26:315–28.
137. Campbell KL, Ash S, Zabel R, McFarlane C, Juffs P, Bauer JD. Implementation of standardized nutrition guidelines by renal dietitians is associated with improved nutrition status. J Ren Nutr. 2009;19:136–44.
138. Institute of Medicine. Dietary reference intakes for vitamin C, vitamin E, selenium, and carotenoids. Washington, DC: National Academies Press; 2000.
139. Institute of Medicine. Dietary reference intakes for thiamin, riboflavin, niacin, vitamin B6, folate, vitamin B12, pantothenic acid, biotin, and choline. Washington, DC: National Academies Press; 1998.
140. Institute of Medicine. Dietary reference intakes for vitamin A, vitamin K, arsenic, boron, chromium, copper, iodine, iron, manganese, molybdenum, nickel, silicon, vanadium, and zinc. Washington, DC: National Academies Press; 2001.
141. Wiggins K. Guidelines for nutritional care of renal patients. 3rd ed. (Renal Dietitians Dietetic Practice Group, ADA). Chicago: American Dietetic Association; 2002.

Vascular Access in Hemodialysis

6

Timmy Lee and Roman Shingarev

6.1 Introduction

The vascular access remains the "lifeline" for the hemodialysis patient [1, 2]. The vascular access provides the conduit to the patient's bloodstream for the dialysis machine to receive and return blood. The recommended and most preferred type of vascular access is the native arteriovenous fistula (AVF), followed by the arteriovenous graft (AVG) and tunneled dialysis catheter (TDC) [3]. In recent years, vascular access has been described as the "Achilles heel" of the hemodialysis procedure because of high rates of AVF maturation failure, recurrent AVG stenosis requiring frequent interventions to maintain patency, and frequent TDC infections leading to hospitalizations [1, 2]. Achieving adequate vascular access for the hemodialysis patient requires balancing process of care challenges related to early nephrology referral, surgical referral for vascular access evaluation and placement, and successful cannulation and biological factors that play a role in vascular access dysfunction after vascular access creation.

This chapter seeks to provide a comprehensive overview of vascular access for hemodialysis by reviewing the epidemiology of vascular access use, primary advantages and disadvantages of each vascular access type, current and future therapies for vascular access dysfunction, the role of the interventional nephrologist to improve vascular issues, and future areas of investigation to improve comprehensive vascular access care.

T. Lee (✉)
Department of Medicine, University of Alabama, Birmingham, AL, USA
e-mail: txlee@uab.edu

R. Shingarev
Department of Nephrology, Memorial Sloan Kettering Center, Birmingham, AL, USA

6.2 Epidemiologic Trends in Vascular Access Use

6.2.1 Practice Patterns and Vascular Access Utilization

The landscape of vascular access use has evolved over the past several decades. In the 1980s, there were relatively few issues related to vascular access dysfunction and few complications. During that era, patient selection for hemodialysis initiation was generally reserved for patients who were young, without diabetes, and had few comorbidities such as cardiovascular or peripheral vascular disease [4–6]. This patient population had vessels that were ideal and adequate quality and size for construction of a native AVF that would mature and be durable for long-term use [6]. Furthermore, patients during this era could frequently be adequately dialyzed at low blood flow rates such as 250 ml/min due to lower rates of obesity, which permitted use of AVFs that were of smaller diameters [7]. During this period, the large majority of hemodialysis patients utilized AVFs and the maturation failure rates were very low at approximately 10% [6].

Beginning in the 1990s the demographic landscape of the hemodialysis population dramatically shifted. The criteria for patient selection for dialysis became significantly less stringent, as more diabetic, elderly, and female patients (who have smaller vessels sizes compared to males) with more cardiovascular and peripheral vascular comorbidities were allowed to enter the United States End stage Renal Disease (ESRD) program [4–6]. Consequently, these patients had poorer quality vasculature to create native AVFs. Moreover, during this same period there was also a greater emphasis on increasing dialysis adequacy (Kt/V), which could be achieved with high blood flows in AVGs in addition to AVFs [6, 7]. These two factors played an important role in leading to increased utilization of AVGs and reduction of AVFs in the 1990s [6]. By the mid-1990s, only 20% of US patients were utilizing AVFs for hemodialysis [6]. As their use became more prominent and widespread, it became clearly evident that AVGs developed stenoses and thromboses more frequently (compared to AVFs),

A. K. Singh et al. (eds.), *Core Concepts in Dialysis and Continuous Therapies*, DOI 10.1007/978-1-4899-7657-4_6

requiring recurrent interventions to maintain and restore patency [6, 8–12]. Furthermore, the costs of treating vascular access complications during this time period was estimated to be greater than US$1 billion annually [13].

In part due to the high number of interventions and costs required to maintain AVG patency, a paradigm shift occurred in the mid-1990s emphasizing increased placement and use of native AVFs once again. In 1997, the first National Kidney Foundation Kidney Disease Outcomes Quality Initiative (KDOQI) Guidelines for Vascular Access was published [14], which emphasized increased placement of native AVFs. The Centers for Medicare and Medicaid Services (CMS) later embraced these recommendations with implementation of the Fistula First Breakthrough Initiative (FFBI). FFBI in collaboration with subsequent KDOQI Guidelines (2001 and 2006) endorsed AVF rates of 50 % or greater for incident patients and at least 40 % for prevalent patients undergoing hemodialysis [3, 15, 16]. These initiatives and guidelines have resulted in a substantial growth in AVF prevalence (Fig. 6.1) [15]. In 2009, the FFBI reset the goal for prevalent AVF use to 66 % [15]. Currently, in 2014, the prevalent AVF rate in the USA is 61 % [15]. However, one of the unintended consequences of increased AVF placement has been a prevalent TDC rate greater than 20 % [15], likely due to the high proportion of AVF maturation failure.

6.2.2 Processes of Care to Increase AVF Use

While the prevalent AVF rates have dramatically improved in recent years, incident AVFs have remained remarkably low at 20 % with almost 80 % of hemodialysis patients initiating dialysis with a TDC [15, 17]. In the incident patient population, multiple care providers are responsible for the vascular access care of the pre-ESRD patient. These individuals include nephrologists, vascular access surgeons, interventional nephrologists, nurse practitioners, and social workers. Central to the coordination and communication of these individuals with the future dialysis patient is a dedicated vascular access coordinator. The primary goal of this centralized coordinated care is to achieve a functional AVF in eligible patients by the time the patient initiates dialysis. The major steps and hurdles in achieving a functional AVF at dialysis initiation include (Fig. 6.2) [18]: (1) early nephrology referral and evaluation, (2) adequate predialysis nephrology care, (3) timely surgical evaluation for preemptive vascular access prior to reaching ESRD and placement of AVF before dialysis initiation, (4) nephrology and surgical follow-up post AVF creation, and (5) successful AVF cannulation at dialysis initiation. Due to the many steps required to overcome these hurdles, a multidisciplinary approach has been shown to successfully improve AVF placement in pre-ESRD patients [19, 20].

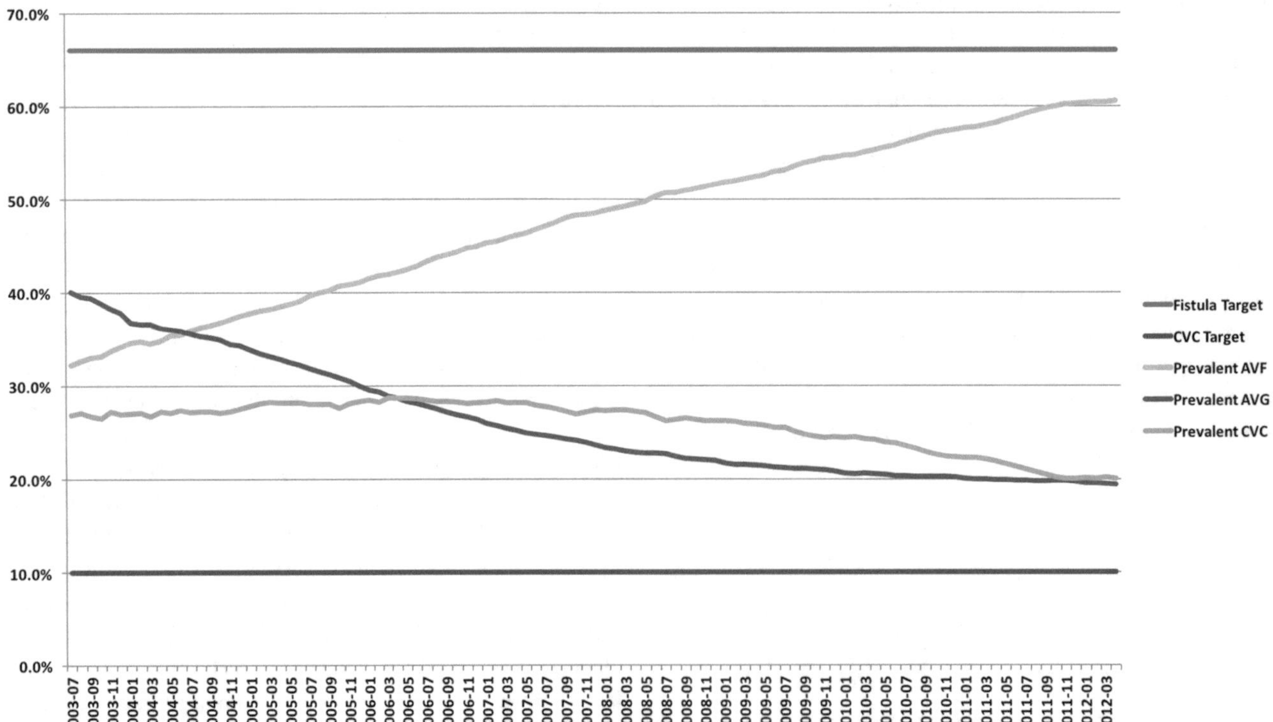

Fig. 6.1 Epidemiologic trends in prevalent vascular access utilization in the USA. Trends in arteriovenous fistula *(AVF)*, arteriovenous graft *(AVG)*, and tunneled dialysis catheter *(TDC)* use in the USA. Since 2003, there has been a steady increase in prevalent AVF use with a concurrent decrease in AVG utilization. TDC has modestly decreased and remains at approximately 20 %. The goal for AVF use set by the Fistula First Initiative is 66 % and prevalent catheter target is 10 %. *CVC* central venous catheter. (Data from the Fistula First Initiative dashboard, www.fistulafirst.org)

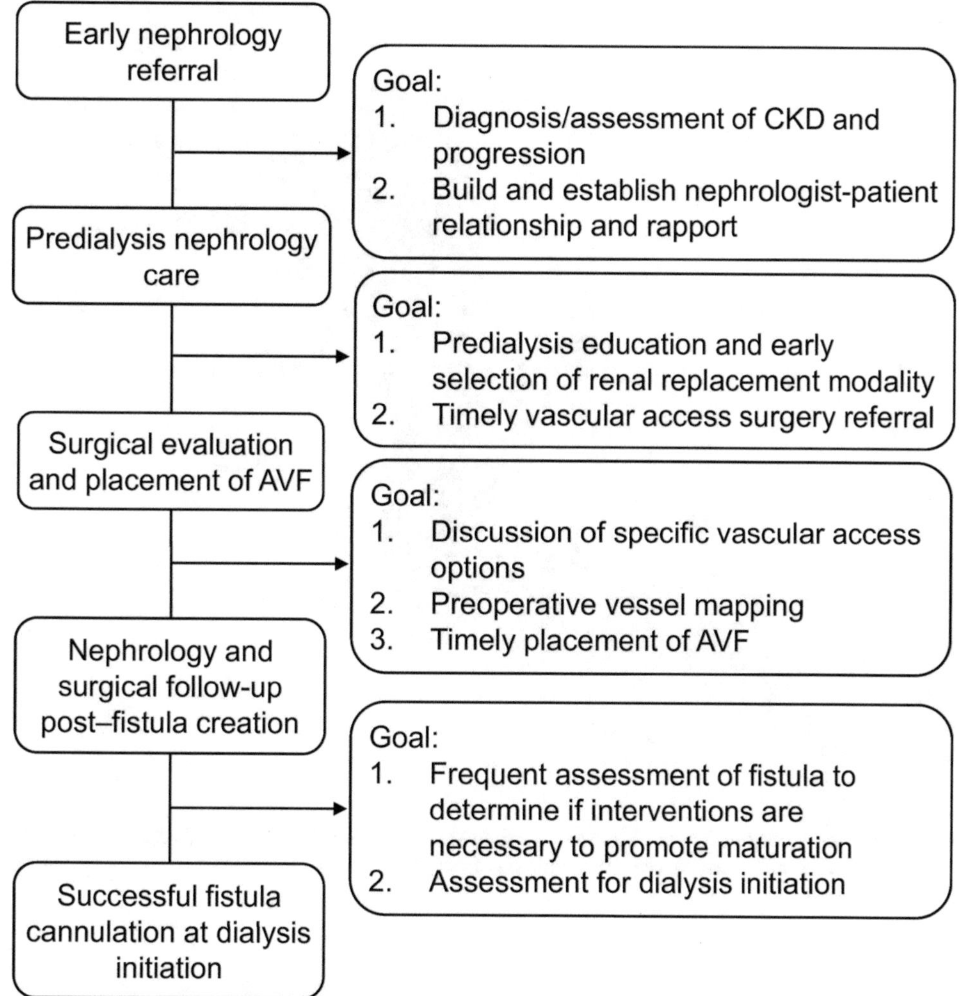

Fig. 6.2 Model for achieving successful arteriovenous fistula *(AVF)* for incident hemodialysis patients. *CDK* chronic kidney disease (Reprinted from [18] with permission from Elsevier Inc.)

6.3 Types of Vascular Access

6.3.1 Arteriovenous Fistulas

AVFs are the preferred type of vascular access for most hemodialysis patients. The major advantage of AVFs compared to AVGs are that AVFs require fewer interventions to maintain patency, if they mature successfully for dialysis [6]. Published studies have reported that AVGs require 2.4–7.1 more interventions to maintain patency compared to AVFs [6]. Furthermore, infectious complications occur more frequently in AVGs compared to AVFs [6]. However, the major disadvantages of AVFs compared to AVGs are the longer maturation time (ranging from 6 weeks to 6 months) and higher rates of maturation failures [21]. In recent years, AVF maturation failure rates have been reported to range anywhere between 20–50 % in the literature [22–35]. In fact, a recent multicenter randomized controlled trial reported AVF maturation failure to be 60 % in a US population [21].

6.3.1.1 Arteriovenous Fistula Configurations

There are several anatomical options and sites for vascular access placement in a hemodialysis patient. The main vessels used for vascular creation (AVF and AVG) include the radial and brachial artery and the cephalic and basilic veins (Fig. 6.3) [36]. The first AVF initially described in 1966 was the radiocephalic AVF [36, 37]. The radiocephalic AVF is an anastomotic connection between the radial artery and cephalic vein at the level of the wrist (Fig. 6.4) [36]. The cephalic veins are usually of very poor quality in the antecubital region because of frequent cannulation for phlebotomy. Thus, these AVFs have high maturation failure rates [38, 39]. For those patients without suitable vasculature to create radiocephalic AVFs in the forearm, brachiocephalic AVFs in the upper arm are the next alternative. The brachiocephalic AVF is an anastomotic connection between the radial artery and cephalic vein in the upper arm and provides good blood flow (Fig. 6.5). Usually considered the last resort, transposed brachiobasilic AVFs can be created if the cephalic vein is unavailable in its entirety. Transposed brachiobasilic AVFs are more

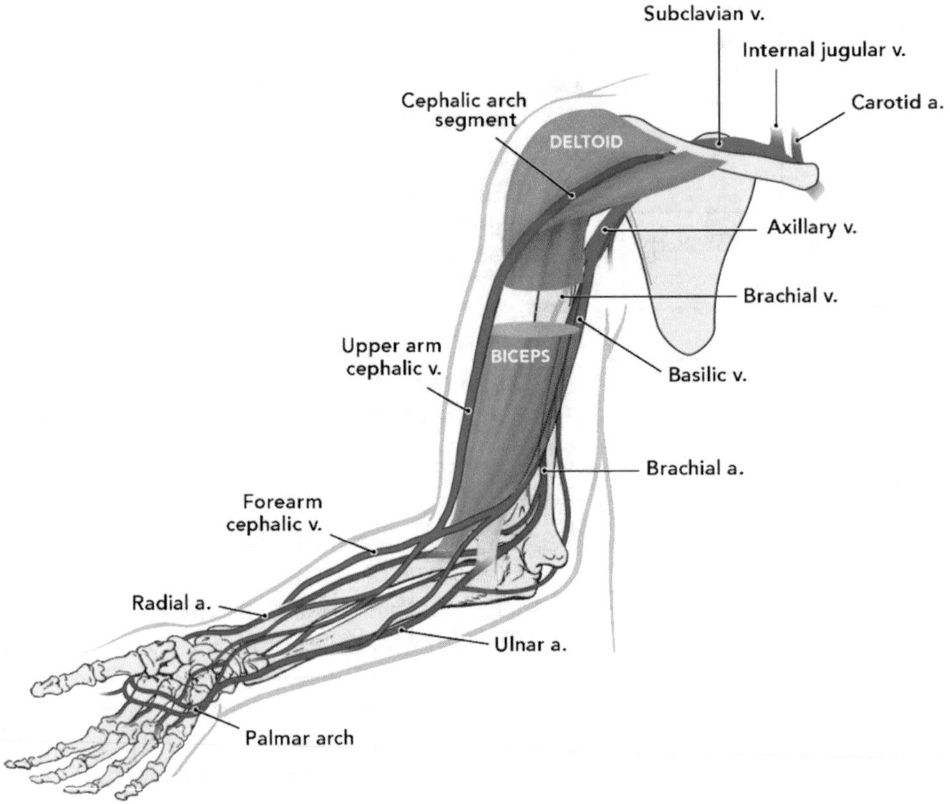

Fig. 6.3 Anatomy of upper extremity vessels for vascular access creation. This figure displays the potential upper extremity anatomic vessels used to create arteriovenous fistulas and grafts. (Reproduced with permission from [36])

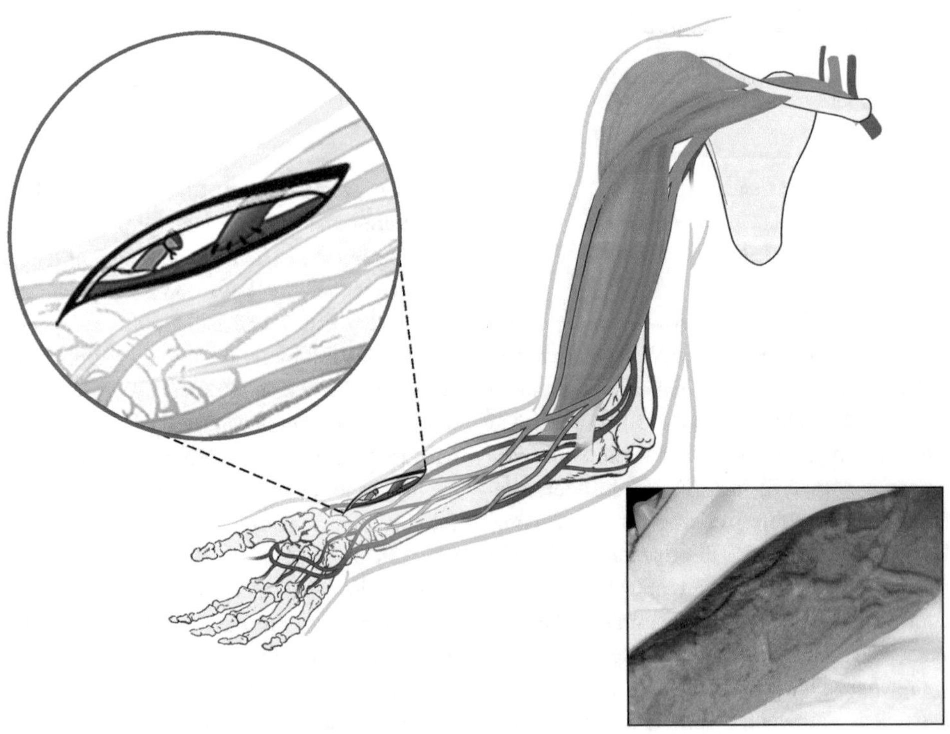

Fig. 6.4 Radiocephalic arteriovenous fistula. In the radiocephalic arteriovenous fistula, the anastomotic connection occurs between the radial artery and cephalic vein. (Reproduced with permission from [36])

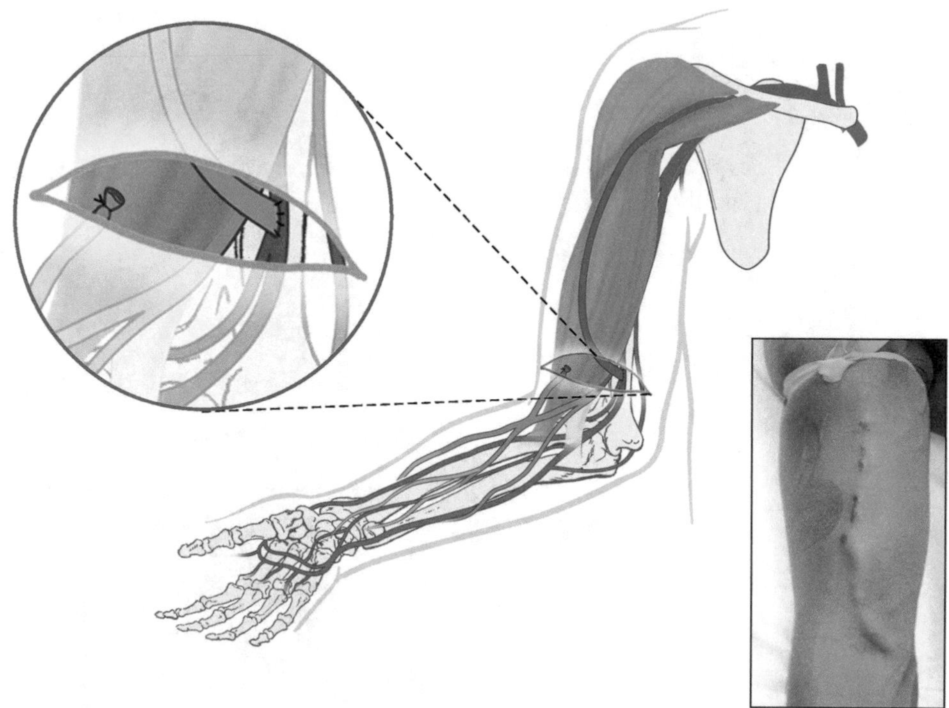

Fig. 6.5 Brachiocephalic arteriovenous fistula. In the brachiocephalic arteriovenous fistula, the anastomotic connection occurs between the brachial artery and cephalic vein. (Reproduced with permission from [36])

challenging and time consuming to create and require greater surgical experience (Fig. 6.6). However, the basilic vein is an important vessel for AVF creation because it runs deeper and is typically spared from phlebotomy injury and has a large enough diameter for the creation of AVF. However, because of the depth of the basilic vein from the skin, it frequently needs to be transposed or it can be very difficult to cannulate. The transposed brachiobasilic AVF can be created either using a one-stage or two-stage procedure [40–42]. Basilic vein AVFs have equal if not better outcomes compared to cephalic vein AVFs [43, 44], and should be considered in patients who exhaust distal extremity vasculature sites.

6.3.1.2 Preoperative Vascular Studies to Assess AVF Suitability

Preoperative vascular access mapping has been the standard of care in the USA to assess both artery and vein diameters prior to AVF creation. Ultrasound has been the predominant modality used to assess preoperative vessel diameter. Studies evaluating preoperative vessel mapping have demonstrated its utility in increasing overall placement of AVF and improving prevalent use of AVF in their dialysis programs [28, 29, 32, 45]. KDOQI guidelines recommend preoperative vessel mapping in all patients being considered for new permanent vascular access placement, which can include ultrasound; and suggest AVF creation in patients with arterial diameter greater than 2.0 mm and vein diameter greater than 2.5 mm [3]. Another common imaging modality used for preoperative vessel mapping is angiography. It allows for a more detailed assessment of the central venous system. The procedure requires administration of intravenous contrast, but has been demonstrated to be safe with very low rates of contrast-induced acute kidney injury complications in pre-ESRD patients [46].

6.3.1.3 Biology of AVF Failure

While the AVFs are the preferred vascular access for hemodialysis patients, the emerging scientific problem is related to the high proportion of AVFs that fail to mature successfully for use on dialysis after creation. A recent multicenter randomized clinical trial reported that 60 % of AVFs created failed to mature for dialysis [21]. Venous neointimal hyperplasia is the main histologic lesion seen in AVF maturation failure and primarily occurs at the vein–artery anastomosis [47–50] (Fig. 6.7). A number of biological factors play a role in AVF maturation failure. These factors are often divided into upstream events and downstream events. Upstream events are related to the initial vascular injury to the vessels prior to and at the time of AVF creation [1, 2, 51]. Downstream events refer to the biological response to the initial upstream vascular injury [1, 2, 51]. The major upstream events include [1, 2, 51] (Fig. 6.8): (1) surgical injury to the vessel at the time of AVF creation, (2) hemodynamic changes related to sheer stress and turbulent flow at the arteriovenous (AV) anastomosis, (3) surgical injury to the vessel at the time of AVF creation, and (4) uremic and inflammatory damage to the vessels from complications of progressive and advanced CKD. These upstream events lead to injury to the vascular endothelium and

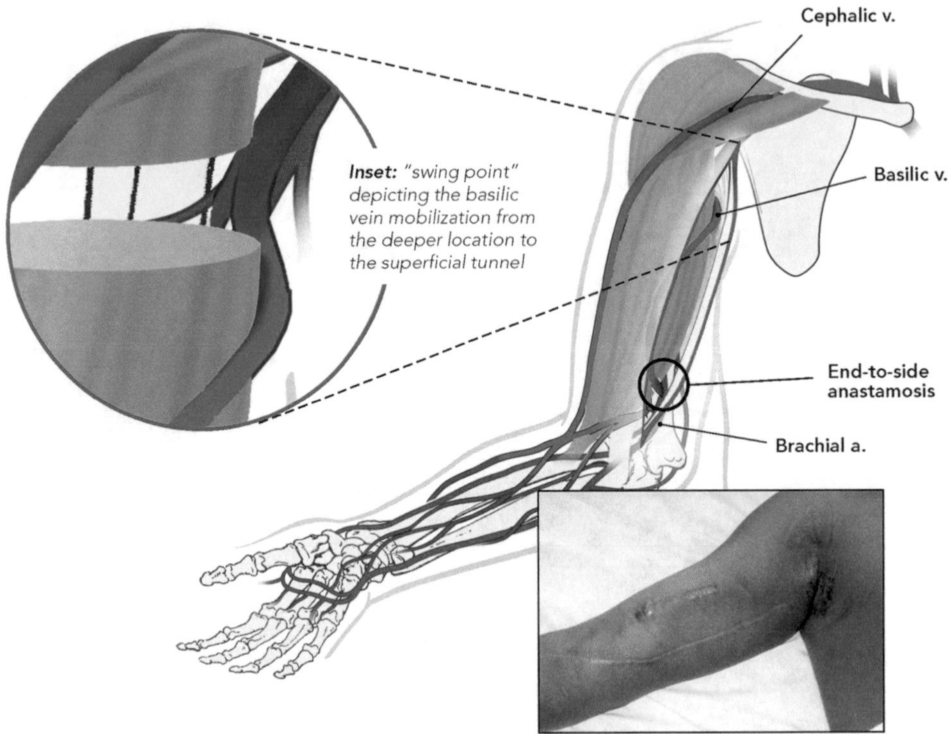

Fig. 6.6 Transposed basilic vein arteriovenous fistula. In the transposed basilic vein arteriovenous fistula, the anastomotic connection occurs between the basilic vein and brachial artery. It can be created in one or two stages. (Reproduced with permission from [36])

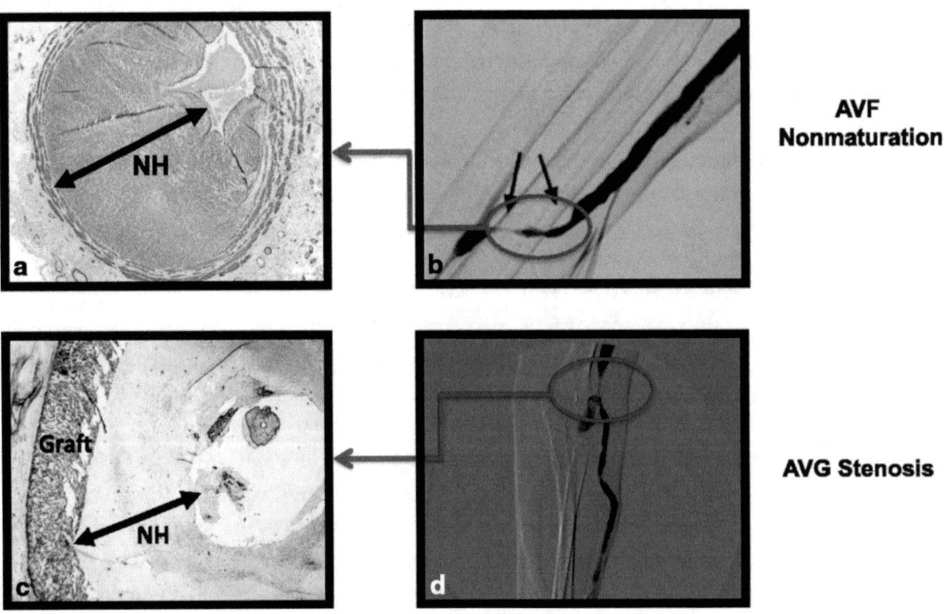

Fig. 6.7 Histology and angiography of venous stenosis in arteriovenous fistula and arteriovenous graft. **a** and **b** represent angiography and histology of arteriovenous fistula maturation failure. Note aggressive venous neointimal hyperplasia. **c** and **d** represent angiography and histology of arteriovenous graft stenosis. Note aggressive neointimal hyperplasia at graft–vein anastomosis. *AVF* arteriovenous fistula, *AVG* arteriovenous graft, *NH* Neointimal hyperplasia. (Reprinted from [1] with permission from the American Society of Nephrology)

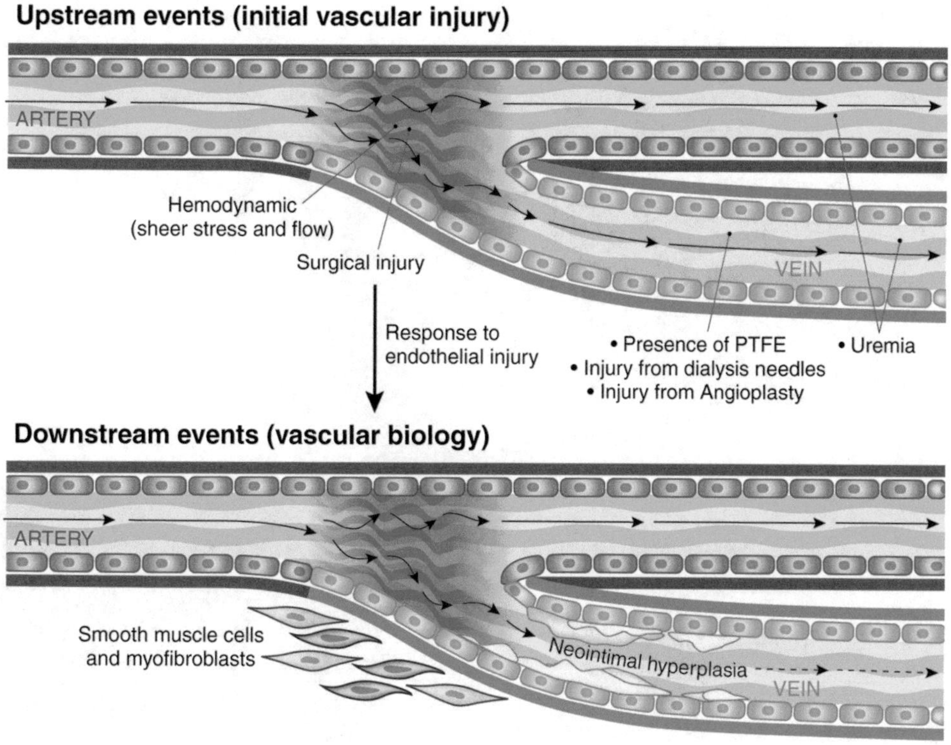

Fig. 6.8 Upstream and downstream events in hemodialysis vascular access dysfunction. Upstream events result in initial vascular injury. Downstream events are the vascular biologic response to upstream injury. Downstream biology involves mediators of oxidative stress and inflammation that regulate activation, proliferation, and migration of fibroblasts, smooth muscle cells, and myofibroblasts. *PTFE* polytetrafluoroethylene. (Reprinted from [1] with permission from the American Society of Nephrology)

a subsequent cascade of downstream events. The downstream events are the biological response to these upstream vascular injuries. The biological response to upstream vascular injuries remains poorly understood at this time, but fibroblast, smooth muscle cell, and myofibroblast activation, proliferation, and migration from the adventitial layer of the vessel to the media and intima are believed to play major roles in the process of neointimal hyperplasia development [1, 2, 51]. Furthermore, mediators of inflammation and oxidative stress have been shown to modulate the fibroblast, smooth muscle cell, and myofibroblast response [52–54]. Improving the understanding of the biological factors that impact AVF maturation and stenosis will ultimately allow for better therapies and devices that target upstream and downstream AVF events.

6.3.1.4 Interventions to Treat AVF Dysfunction

Balloon angioplasties are most commonly performed in AVFs for maturation failure. Stenoses of AVFs typically occur at the vein–artery anastomosis (juxta-anastomosis) and are most commonly treated with serial balloon angioplasty dilations. Six-month primary patency following angioplasty in AVFs ranges from 34 to 67 %. When AVFs are thrombosed, thrombectomy procedures in addition to angioplasty are required to salvage AVFs. The primary patency following thrombectomy of AVFs has ranged from 27 to 81 % at 6 months and 18–70 % at 1 year [55–60]. In many circumstances surgical revision of AVF can be performed to salvage stenotic or thrombotic AVFs by proximalization of the anastomosis. Several studies have reported better long-term AVF outcomes in patients receiving surgical revision to treat AVF stenosis compared to angioplasty [61–64].

6.3.2 Arteriovenous Grafts

Arteriovenous grafts are created using a synthetic conduit in place of a native vein. The most common synthetic materials used for AVGs are polytetrafluoroethylene (PTFE) and polyurethane. AVGs are usually placed when the vein diameters are not of suitable size to place a native AVF. AVGs can be placed at several different anatomic locations, such as the forearm and upper arm, and with a straight, curved, or looped configuration (Fig. 6.9). The main advantage of AVG placement is that the maturation period is usually short. AVGs can typically be used 2–3 weeks after surgical placement, thus, sparing the patient from prolonged TDC use. Furthermore, some AVGs can be used immediately after placement [65]. However, the main disadvantage of AVGs, compared to AVFs, is the high rate of thrombosis and stenosis requiring frequent procedures to reestablish patency [66]. A second major disadvantage is a higher frequency of infectious complications in AVG compared to AVF [67].

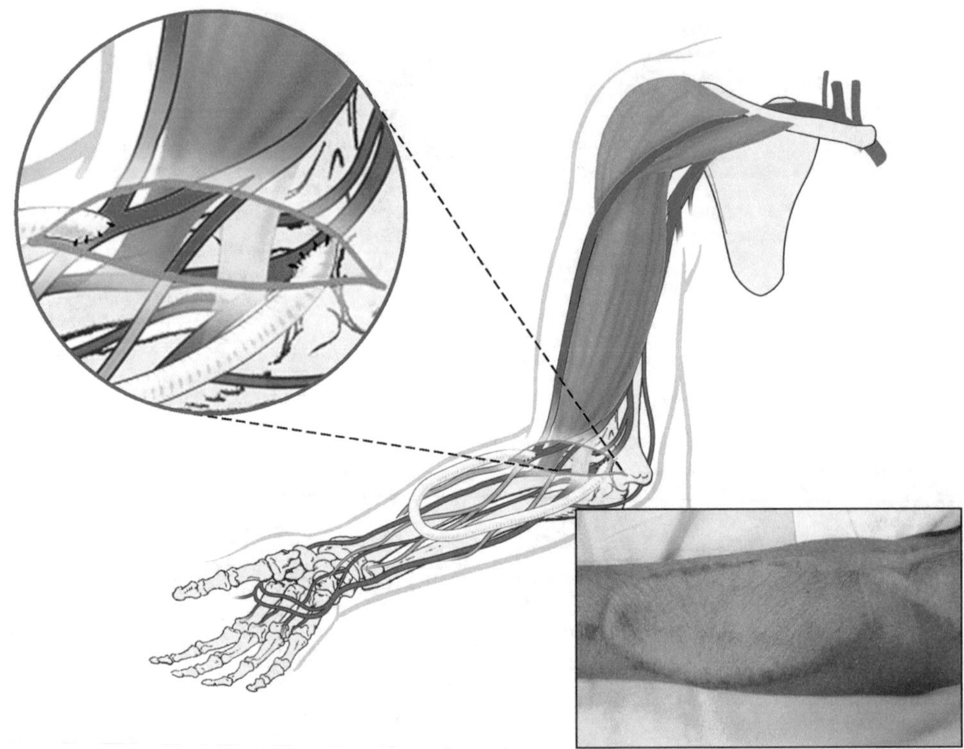

Fig. 6.9 Forearm loop arteriovenous graft. (Reproduced with permission from [36])

6.3.2.1 Complications of AVGs

Thrombosis is the main complication that results from AVG use and it accounts for nearly 80% of all AVG failures [66, 68, 69]. The most common location of AVG stenosis and thrombosis is at the vein–graft anastomosis [70–74]. Salvage of thrombosed AVFs usually requires both thrombectomy and angioplasty procedures. However, the primary patency following interventions to salvage AVGs are very poor with outcomes worse after salvage of clotted AVGs compared to preemptively treating stenosis with angioplasty. In clotted AVGs, after thrombectomy and angioplasty, the primary patency ranges from 33 to 63% at 3 months and 11 to 39% at 6 months [56, 66, 73, 75–81]. In sharp contrast, the primary patency is significantly better after elective angioplasty for stenosis and without clotted AVG, ranging from 70 to 85% at 3 months and 47 to 63% at 6 months [11, 66, 70, 73, 74, 82].

6.3.2.2 Surveillance and Clinical Monitoring of AVGs

Recognizing the possibility that both preventing and intervening prior to AVG thrombosis occurring may impact AVG patency, a number of observational studies have compared outcomes of monitoring versus surveillance and clinical trials have been performed using surveillance technology for early detection of thrombosis compared to routine clinical monitoring. Clinical monitoring consists of a physical examination of the AVG examining for absent thrill, abnormal bruit, or edema, abnormalities during dialysis treatments such as prolonged bleeding from needle sites or difficulty with cannulation, and unexpected decreases in dialysis adequacy as measured by Kt/V [66, 83]. Surveillance of AVG typically utilizes specialized technology to identify and document increases in intra-access pressure or decreased access flows as a result of a developing stenosis. Observational studies have shown that implementation of AVG surveillance or clinical monitoring programs decrease AVG thrombosis from 41 to 77% compared to historical controls [9, 11, 12, 19, 84, 85]. However, in randomized controlled trials comparing surveillance to routine clinical monitoring, the benefit of surveillance programs has been less convincing. To date, there have been six published randomized controlled trials directly studying the clinical impact of AVG graft surveillance versus clinical monitoring to detect stenosis [86–91]. The surveillance techniques used in these six studies have included either Doppler ultrasound, monitoring of access flow, or dynamic venous pressure [86–91]. All of these studies have reported that patients in the surveillance programs have higher frequencies of angioplasty procedures, suggesting that surveillance does increase the detection of stenosis. However, only one of these six randomized controlled trials showed improved cumulative AVG survival in patients receiving access surveillance [90], with none of them showing surveillance programs decreasing thrombosis rates. One explanation why the surveillance programs may in general not improve AVG outcomes is because the vascular injury from angioplasty may accelerate stenosis faster than de novo stenosis itself occurs [66, 92]. Currently, there are few therapies available to enhance the short- and long-term survival of AVG following angioplasty, potentially minimizing the benefits of surveillance at the present time.

6.3.2.3 Biology of AVG Failure

Venous stenosis in AVG results from aggressive venous neointimal hyperplasia (Fig. 6.7) [48, 93, 94]. The venous neointimal hyperplasia in AVGs is characterized by smooth muscle cells, myofibroblasts, and fibroblasts, and by macrophages that line the perivascular region of the AVG [48, 93, 94]. Similar to AVFs, the pathophysiology of AVG dysfunction remains poorly understood, but similar upstream and downstream events play an important role in development of venous stenosis and neointimal hyperplasia (Fig. 6.8) [51]. However, one major difference in AVGs is that the AVG material itself elicits a foreign body reaction by recruiting macrophages and producing an abundance of cytokines [93]. Furthermore, repeated injury needle cannulation may also impact development of stenosis [51]. Currently, there are very few if any effective therapies available to treat and prevent AVG stenosis, in part due to the limited understanding of the pathobiology of neointimal hyperplasia development in AVGs.

6.3.2.4 Interventions to Treat AVG Failure

The major therapy to treat AVG stenosis remains the percutaneous AVG angioplasty. It is preceded by an angiogram to visualize the venous limb of the AVG and the draining vein and central veins. Stenotic lesions are assessed in different locations, such as the arterial anastomosis, intragraft region, venous anastomosis, draining vein, and central veins. When lesions of greater than 50 % are identified, they typically undergo balloon angioplasty. In cases of AVG thrombosis, thrombectomy is also performed in addition to angioplasty. The primary patency following interventions to AVGs is extremely poor, ranging from 50 to 60 % at 6 months and 30 to 40 % at 1 year following elective angioplasty [11, 56, 70, 73, 74, 82]. Clinical outcomes following thrombectomy and angioplasty of AVGs are considerably worse with primary patency at 3 and 6 months ranging from 30 to 63 % and 11 to 39 %, respectively [56, 73, 75–81, 95]. Clinical outcomes following these procedures are poor because of injury to the endothelium from the angioplasty and development of recurrent and often more aggressive neointimal hyperplasia [92]. Due to the poor primary patency following angioplasty, endovascular stents have been evaluated as a potential therapy to prolong patency. The function of stents is to form a rigid scaffold to prevent elastic recoil and assist in maintaining lumen patency. There are no randomized controlled trials comparing stents versus angioplasty alone. However, a nonrandomized study comparing outcomes of clotted AVGs treated with thrombectomy and stent placement at the venous anastomosis with matched control patients treated with only thrombectomy and angioplasty showed a significantly longer primary patency in AVGs treated with a stent compared to angioplasty treatment alone [96]. Stent grafts are a type of stent consisting of a metallic stent covered with graft material. In a recent multicenter randomized controlled trial comparing treatment of AVG stenosis (> 50 %) at the venous anastomosis with either stent graft or angioplasty, primary patency at 2 and 6 months was significantly better in the stent graft group compared to angioplasty alone [97].

6.3.3 Tunneled Dialysis Catheters

TDCs are most commonly placed in the central venous system, but can also be placed in the lower extremity venous system. TDCs are the most common type of vascular access used when patients initiate hemodialysis. Currently, in the USA, approximately 80 % of patients initiate hemodialysis with a TDC. There are several advantages of TDCs. TDC provides immediate access to the circulation, can be placed with relative ease and in an outpatient setting, and there is no pain because it does not require cannulation of the arm with needles. However, TDCs have significant disadvantages and complications, which limit their successful long-term use. These disadvantages and complications include frequent thrombosis, stenosis, and infection. Furthermore, numerous studies have shown a significant mortality and hospitalization risk in patients utilizing catheters compared to AVF or AVG [98–102].

6.3.3.1 Etiologies of TDC Dysfunction

TDC dysfunction is defined by KDOQI as "failure to attain and maintain an extracorporeal blood flow sufficient to perform hemodialysis without significantly lengthening treatment" [3]. Early impairment in TDC function is usually associated with poor TDC position and placement techniques [103–106]. Late TDC dysfunction, which is generally more common than early dysfunction, is typically associated with thrombus formation (intraluminal or extraluminal) or fibrin sheath development [104, 107]. Thrombosis is a major cause of TDC dysfunction. Extraluminal thrombus formation is related to either central vein thrombosis or right arterial thrombosis. The frequency of central vein thrombosis has been reported to range from 2 to 64 % [108, 109]. The majority of TDC dysfunction related to flow impairment is the result of intrinsic thrombi, which is intraluminal, at the tip of the catheter, or surrounding the TDC in a sheath-like configuration [104, 110]. Upon insertion of the TDC, the vascular endothelium is injured leading to the initiation of inflammatory and coagulation cascades which activate leukocytes and platelets and results in thrombi formation [106]. Prevention of thrombosis includes TDC lock solutions. The most common catheter lock solution is heparin administered in concentrations ranging from 1000 to 10,000 U within the lumen. The incidence of TDC thrombosis ranges from 4.0 to 5.5 episodes/1000 catheter days [106, 111, 112]. Trisodium citrate lock has been evaluated as an alternative to heparin and reported to be equivalent if not superior to heparin to prevent thrombosis [111, 113]. Finally, results from a recent randomized clinical trial reported that tissue plasminogen activator (tPA), once weekly instead of heparin, reduces TDC thrombosis [114].

Development of a fibrin sheath is another common cause of TDC dysfunction and may also contribute to thrombi formation. Fibrin sheaths develop within 24 h dialysis catheter placement at the point of TDC contact with the vessel wall and can frequently encase the entire vessel wall [106, 107]. The pathophysiology of fibrin sheath development remains poorly understood but is thought to involve an inflammatory reaction that occurs at the time the catheter contacts the vessel wall and is exacerbated with constant movement of the catheter and irritation of the foreign body against the vessel wall [106, 115]. Histologically, the fibrin sheath layer is primarily composed of a collagenous layer with smooth muscle cells and overlying endothelial cell layer [115]. One treatment for TDC dysfunction from fibrin sheaths is stripping or disruption of the fibrin sheath with a snare catheter under fluoroscopy [116–118]. An alternative approach is exchanging the catheter over a guidewire and disrupting the fibrin sheath at the time of catheter exchange [119, 120].

6.3.3.2 Infectious Complications of TDC Use

Complications from infection are another major reason for TDC loss. These infections can involve the exit site, tunneled track, or blood stream. TDC-related bacteremia is a frequent complication in dialysis patients who utilize TDCs for a prolonged period of time. An exit-site infection is a soft tissue infection localized primarily in the region from the catheter cuff to the exit site. Common features of exit-site infections include erythema, site tenderness, and purulent drainage. Exit-site infections can also spread down the tunnel track if timely treatment is not initiated. The large majority of exit-site infections result from *Staphylococcus aureus* infections [3, 121].

A tunnel infection is suspected when the catheter tunnel superior to the cuff develops erythema, tenderness, or develops drainage through the exit site that is culture positive [3]. The infection often can spread more centrally resulting in TDC-related bacteremia. Unfortunately, there is no standard uniform definition for TDC-related bacteremia, which is critical for diagnostic and treatment purposes. KDOQI has established three definitions for diagnosis of TDC-related bacteremia (possible, probable, and definite catheter-related bacteremia) based on Center for Disease Control definitions [3]. KDOQI [3] considers a: (1) possible TDC-related infection as "defervescence of symptoms after antibiotic treatment or after removal of catheter in the absence of laboratory confirmation of bloodstream infection in a symptomatic patient with no other apparent source of infection," (2) probable TDC-related infection as "defervescence of symptoms after antibiotic therapy with or without removal of catheter, in the setting in which blood cultures confirm infection, but catheter tip does not (or catheter tip does, but blood cultures do not) in a symptomatic patient with no other apparent source of infection," and (3) a "definite bloodstream infection as the same organism from a semiquantitative culture of the catheter tip (>15 colony-forming units per catheter segment) and from a peripheral or catheter blood sample in a symptomatic patient with no other apparent source of infection." However, there are many limitations to clinical application of these definitions, such as availability of the patients' dialysis units resources to make the diagnosis and exclude other etiologies of infection, the patients' peripheral veins are often unavailable to obtain blood, and the catheter not being removed prior to initiation of antibiotic therapy and drawing blood cultures. Thus, a more practical definition may be the presence of positive blood cultures in a patient who is catheter-dependent, where there is no clear source or etiology of infection [66, 122].

6.3.3.3 Pathogenesis of TDC-Bacteremia

The pathogenesis of TDC-related bacteremia begins from the attachment of the microorganism to the catheter, which leads to development of a biofilm. A biofilm is a self-sustaining colony of microorganisms protected by an exopolysaccharide matrix that is stimulated and secreted by the bacteria [123–125]. The polysaccharides form the matrix that connects the microorganism to one another and to the surface of the catheter (Fig. 6.10). The exopolysaccharide layer of the biofilm may be 100-fold greater than the microorganisms it protects, making it very challenging to penetrate and eradicate with antibiotic therapy [125, 126]. The most common organisms present within the biofilm layer include *Staphylococcus, Candida*, and *Pseudomonas* [123–125]. Determinants of biofilm development include the type of microorganism, type of material of the dialysis catheter, and the type of fluid and fluid hemodynamics within the catheter. Thus, it appears a critical component of management of TDC-related bacteremia is to prevent biofilm development on the catheter.

6.3.3.4 Prevention and Treatment of TDC Infections

Since 80 % of patients initiate hemodialysis in the USA with a TDC [17], both prevention and treatment of TDC-related bacteremia is critical in the overall care of patients utilizing catheters for dialysis. Routine sterile technique from dialysis nurses should be performed during each dialysis session. KDOQI recommends that dialysis staff should adhere to uniform sterile precautions and hygienic measures and wear masks and sterile gloves while manipulating the catheter [3, 125]. The site should be cleaned with either 2 % chlorhexidine, 70 % alcohol, or 10 % povidone-iodine solution every treatment [3, 125, 127]. However, several randomized studies have shown that chlorhexidine is the preferred and superior antiseptic agent for cleansing of the exit site [125, 128–133]. Multiple studies have shown that administration of topical antibiotic ointment at the exit site reduces TDC-related bacteremia by 75–93 % [125, 134–137]. The major antibiotic topical ointments evaluated to date include mupirocin, povidine-iodine, and polysporin [138]. However, use of topical antibiotics may promote development of resis-

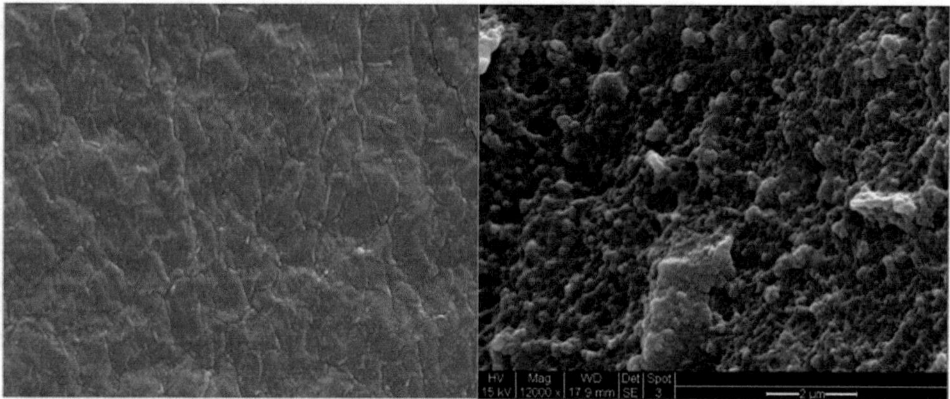

Fig. 6.10 Biofilm development in tunneled dialysis catheter. Panel on the left shows the scanning electron microscopy (SEM) of lumen of new catheter showing no biofilm. On the right panel is SEM of the lumen of a 6-week old tunneled catheter removed after arteriovenous fistula maturation. The 6-week old tunneled dialysis catheter demonstrates substantial biofilm development

tant microorganisms. *Staphylococcus aureus* nasal colonization has also been shown to be a major risk factor for development of infections in dialysis patients [139]. Both rifampin and mupirocin have been shown to reduce nasal carriage of *Staphylococcus aureus* nasal carriage and bacteremia [139, 140], but may also lead to emergence of resistant strains [139]. Recently, prophylactic TDC lock solutions have emerged as a promising strategy to prevent TDC-related bacteremia. Prophylactic TDC lock solutions compared to standard heparin locks have been reported to reduce TDC-related infections in the range of 51–99% (Table 6.1) [141–157]. While prophylactic TDC lock therapies have demonstrated excellent ability to reduce TDC-related bacteremia, the main concern regarding their long-term use is the emerging reports of antibiotic-resistant gram-positive organisms [158, 159].

While the ideal goal is to prevent TDC-related bacteremia from occurring, TDC-bacteremia will, nevertheless, remain a frequent complication of the dialysis treatment. The frequency of catheter-related bacteremia ranges from 2.0 to 5.5 episodes/1000-catheter-days [66, 134, 145, 160–167]. Serious complications associated with TDC-related bacteremia include endocarditis, osteomyelitis, septic arthritis, epidural abscess, or death [66, 122]. Thus, immediate treatment is imperative for suspected TDC-related infection. The initial treatment of TDC-related bacteremia consists of broad-spectrum antibiotics to empirically cover both gram-positive and gram-negative organisms. Due to the high prevalence of methicillin-resistant *Staphylococcus aureus* in the dialysis population, vancomycin should be included as an initial choice of antibiotics. Antibiotic therapy needs to be modified once specific culture and sensitivity results are obtained. The most common strategies to manage TDC-related bacteremia include: (1) catheter salvage without antibiotic locking, (2) catheter salvage with antibiotic locking, (3) catheter removal with delayed placement, and (4) catheter exchange over guidewire. Intravenous antibiotics alone rarely treat TDC-related infections successfully. The majority of clini-

Table 6.1 Summary of clinical trials of catheter lock solutions for prophylaxis for catheter-related bacteremia

Study	Type of lock solution	Rate of catheter-related bacteremia per 1000 catheter-days		*P* value
		Control	Intervention	
Dogra et al. [145]	Gentamicin	4.2	0.3	0.003
Allon [146]	Taurolidine	5.6	0.6	<0.001
McIntyre et al. [147]	Gentamicin	4.0	0.3	0.02
Betjes et al. [148]	Taurolidine	2.1	0	0.047
Weijmer et al. [149]	30% citrate	4.1	1.1	<0.0001
Kim et al. [150]	Gentamicin/cefazolin	3.1	0.4	0.031
Saxena et al. [151]	Cefotaxime	3.2	1.4	<0.001
Al-Hwiesh et al. [152]	Vancomycin/gentamicin	13.1	4.54	0.05
Winnett et al. [153]	46.7% citrate	2.1	0.81	<0.001
Power et al. [154]	46.7% citrate	0.7	0.7	0.9
Venditto et al. [155]	Gentamicin	2.9	0.4	0.06
Solomon et al. [157]	Taurolidine/citrate	2.4	1.4	0.1
Moran et al. [156]	Gentamicin/citrate	0.9	0.28	0.003

cal studies have reported >75 % recurrence of bacteremia in attempting to salvage infected TDC with intravenous antibiotics alone [163, 166, 168–172]. Studies evaluating exchange of the TDC over a guidewire with antibiotics for TDC-related bacteremia have demonstrated high cure rates [166, 173–175]. In fact, a nonrandomized controlled study has shown that the infection free survival time among patients with guidewire exchange is equivalent to those patients with TDC removal and delayed placement of a new catheter [176]. Successful treatment with intravenous antibiotics and antibiotic locking solution varies depending on the type of organism present. Cure rates have been reported to be between 87–100 % for gram-negative infections, 75–84 % for *Staphylococcus epidermidis* infections, but only 55 % for *Staphylococcus aureus* infections [165, 177, 178]. Finally, in these subset of patients the TDC should always be immediately removed with delayed placement of TDC [125]: (1) patients who are clinically unstable, (2) patients with persistent fever for 48 h despite intravenous antibiotic therapy, (3) presence of a tunnel infection, (4) metastatic infectious complications, (5) recurrence of TDC-related bacteremia after exchange, (6) and TDC-related infection with fungemia.

6.4 Interventional Nephrology

As prevalence of ESRD patients grows, medical care for this population is burdened to a significant extent by its fragmented care. There are many responsibilities that are shared by nephrologists, radiologists, and surgeons in the vascular access care of patients, sometimes without a recognizable leader. Interventional nephrology was born out of necessity to streamline care for vascular access by capitalizing on nephrologists' familiarity with vascular access complications in the settings of dialysis clinics, longitudinal nature of ESRD care and close relationship with other specialists involved in the process.

As a very young field, interventional nephrology has relied on and borrowed from other, more traditional specialties, such as radiology and cardiology. Even today there are very few tools and equipment designed specifically for vascular access interventions. However, application of well-known interventional tools and techniques to treat dialysis access complications was pioneered by nephrologists in the private practice sector driven in part by their desire to improve patient satisfaction and reign in growing costs. As a great example of such an approach, Gerald Beathard was able to demonstrate in the early 1990s that percutaneous angioplasty can be used to treat venous stenosis—a common problem plaguing AVFs and AVGs [70, 72, 75, 179]. The procedure proved to be safe and effective and the ability to perform it in outpatient settings helped minimize disruption of ESRD care and drove down the costs. At present, percutaneous angioplasty is performed using an angioplasty balloon catheter (Fig. 6.11) inflated at the stenotic segment of an AVF or an AVG (Fig. 6.12a, b). In cases of elastic or rapidly recurrent stenosis, where success cannot be achieved with angioplasty alone, a bare metal stent can be deployed to provide support to the vessel wall (Fig. 6.13). In cases of iatrogenic venous dissection, large aneurysms or refractory stenoses, a graft (covered) stent can be placed to seal off a vascular defect (Fig. 6.14). Gradually, interventional nephrologists acquired progressively more complex procedures in their armamentarium and many now perform AVG stenting for elastic venous stenoses, coil deployment for accessory venous tributaries, banding of large caliber AVFs in cases of steal syndrome and many others [180, 181].

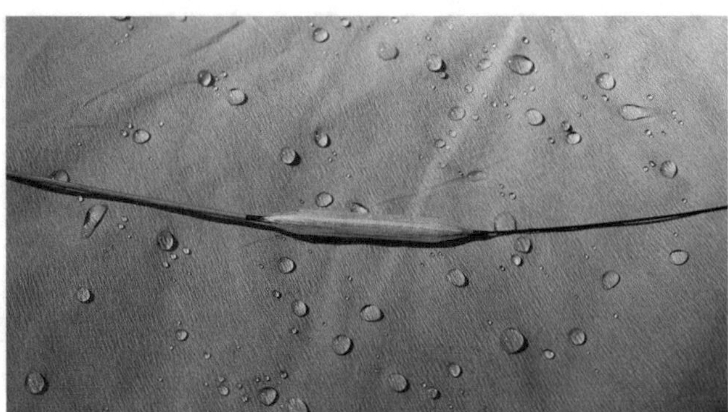

Fig. 6.11 Inflated angioplasty balloon over guidewire. This figure depicts a representative angioplasty balloon utilized for arteriovenous fistula and graft interventions

Early success of interventional nephrology pioneers captivated audiences of their colleagues translating into rapid initial growth of this field with multiple interventional nephrology centers emerging across the USA [182–186]. Interventional nephrologists are now estimated to perform at least a quarter of all vascular access procedures in this country [185–187]. However, further growth of the specialty has been limited by scarce opportunities to disseminate proper knowledge and skills to those nephrologists interested in performing vascular access interventions. Traditionally, a single interventionalist would share his or her expertise with members of a particular private practice group leading to the establishment of a vascular access center able to provide care for hemodialysis patients followed by this group. Resultant divergence of practice standards across the country and difficulty in assessing their relative success emphasized the need for establishing a governing body. In 2000, the American Society of Diagnostic and Interventional Nephrology (ASDIN) was founded with the mission "to promote the proper application of new and existing procedures in the practice of nephrology with the goal of improving the care on nephrology patients" [188, 189]. With nephrologists in leadership positions, the ASDIN has been gaining weight in medical community by accrediting training programs in interventional nephrology, certifying physicians in specific procedures, and establishing practice standards. ASDIN was successful in promoting its goals by incorporating post-graduate courses in interventional nephrology within the American Society of Nephrology (ASN) meetings and maintaining a vibrant section in its official journal,

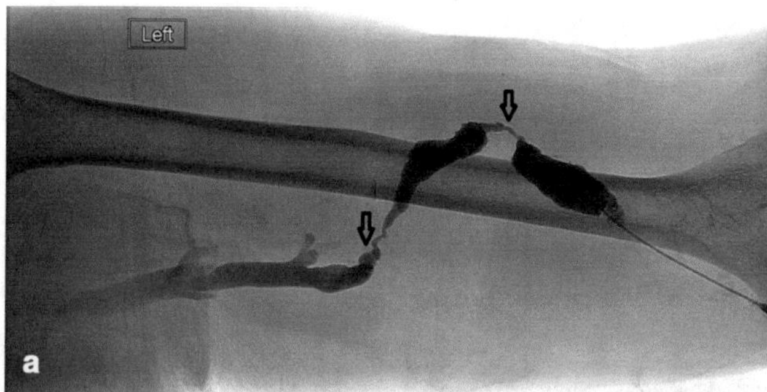

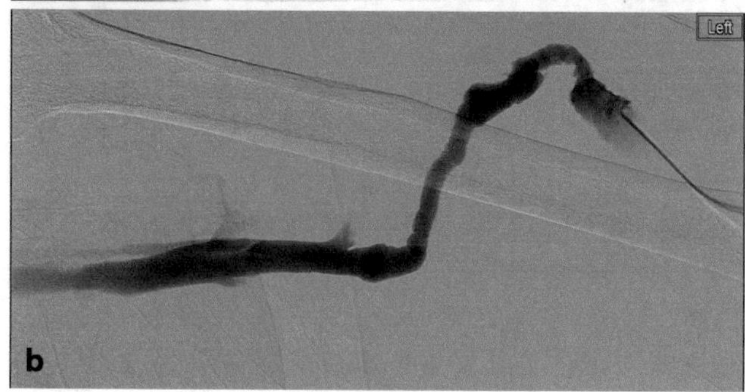

Fig. 6.12 Arteriovenous fistula stenosis before and after angioplasty. Two segments of near-occlusive stenosis *(arrows)* affecting transposed brachiobasilic fistula before (**a**) and after (**b**) percutaneous angioplasty

Seminars in Dialysis. ASDIN's own annual scientific meeting serves as an annual platform for evaluating the specialty's progress, launching new initiatives, and exchange of ideas among attendees from wide spectrum of medical specialties, nurses, technologists, and industry representatives.

Evolving into a full-fledged discipline interventional nephrology faces challenges in its goal to further dialysis patient care. Clinical and translational research plays a quintessential role in enabling physicians to improve patients' life expectancy and well-being. Many nephrologists have embraced this belief generating vast amounts of new and unique information through clinical trials that have dramatically changed the landscape of interventional nephrology in the past decade [2, 51, 66, 190]. Unfortunately, interventional nephrology trials constitute a very trivial proportion of all nephrology trials in a recent review of ClinicalTrials.gov database [191]. Moreover, nephrology as a whole is known to be woefully lagging behind other medical specialties in quality and sheer number of clinical trials [192–194]. While many factors have been identified adversely affecting the quality of published studies (e.g., high rates of loss to follow-up and heterogeneous methods for handling missing data), the conclusions that are usually drawn highlight the importance of standardization of trial protocols, establishing common clinical endpoints for research community, and collaboration between different medical centers. Interventional nephrologists are uniquely positioned to promote such endeavors in the field of dialysis access. In fact, ASDIN and Interventional Nephrology Advisory Group (INAG) for ASN have recently spearheaded efforts directed at defining meaningful clinical outcomes in the framework of vascular access clinical studies [195].

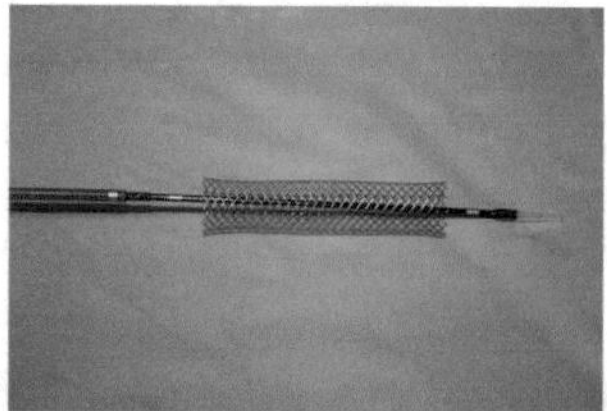

Fig. 6.13 Bare metal stent for dialysis access. This figure depicts a representative bare metal stent used to treat recurrent venous stenosis and vascular recoil

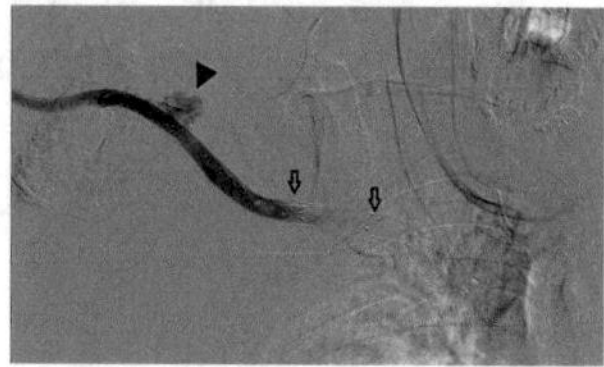

Fig. 6.14 Complication during angioplasty procedure in arteriovenous fistula. Contrast extravasation *(arrowhead)* due to fistula dissection, partially covered by graft-stents *(arrows)*

While clinical trials can produce data valuable for day-to-day clinical care of dialysis patients, there is a growing recognition of limitations of such studies, as our understanding of clinical problems deepens. Identification of neointimal hyperplasia as a culprit in the process of stenosis formation in arteriovenous fistulas and grafts led to the rapid expansion of our knowledge of its pathophysiology drawing from the expertise of vascular biologists, pathologists, and cardiologists. However, most publications on this subject are generated by a handful of scientists in this country [1, 2, 47, 50, 51, 93, 196–198]. Further understanding of this important issue necessitates greater involvement by interventional nephrologists nationwide and major advances in therapeutics designed to control neointimal hyperplasia will require a bench-to-bedside approach using in vitro experimentation and animal models. Interventional nephrologists are ideal candidates for leadership roles in these research efforts, but with most of them practicing in private sector (similarly to other medical subspecialties), procurement of translational research skills and collaboration with basic scientists will be challenging.

6.5 Therapies for Hemodialysis Vascular Access Dysfunction

At present there are few, if any, effective therapies to treat hemodialysis vascular access dysfunction. The standard therapy to date to treat vascular access dysfunction in AVF and AVG has been balloon angioplasty with stent therapy when warranted. This section will discuss clinical trials from systemic therapies in AVF and AVG and current studies evaluating novel therapies and delivery systems in AVF and AVG.

Table 6.2 Randomized studies of pharmacologic therapies to prevent graft stenosis and thrombosis

Reference	Pharmacologic agent	Total number of subjects	Primary outcome	Results	*P*-value
Sreedhara et al. [198]	Dipyridamole, aspirin, or dipyridamole + aspirin	84	Cumulative thrombosis rate	21 % dipyridamole alone, 42 % dipyridamole and aspirin, and 80 % aspirin alone	0.02
Schmitz et al. [199]	Fish oil	24	Primary patency at 1 year	14.9 % in placebo and 75.6 % in fish oil group	<0.03
Crowther et al. [202]	Warfarin	107	Time to AVG failure	83 days in placebo and 199 days in warfarin	0.74
Kaufman et al. [203]	Clopidogrel + aspirin	200	Cumulative incidence on time to first episode of thrombosis	HR 0.81 in favor of aspirin and clopidogrel group versus placebo	0.45
Dixon et al. [200]	Dipyridamole + aspirin	649	Loss of primary unassisted patency at 1 year	Loss of unassisted primary patency at 1 year 23 % in aspirin + dipyridamole group and 28 % in placebo group	0.03
Lok et al. [201]	Fish oil	196	Loss of native patency within 12 months	43 % in fish oil group and 62 % in placebo group	0.064

6.5.1 Pharmacologic Therapies for AVGs

There have been several randomized controlled studies evaluating pharmacologic therapies in AVGs (Table 6.2). Two of these smaller studies have shown that both dipyridamole [199] and fish oil [200] decrease graft thrombosis. Recently, two larger clinical trials evaluating the dipyridamole and aspirin combination and fish oil have recently been published [201, 202]. The first study was a multicenter randomized controlled trial, sponsored by the National Institutes of Health Dialysis Access Consortium, which evaluated dipyridamole and aspirin compared to placebo [201]. To date this study is the largest randomized controlled trial in AVGs. The primary outcome from this study was 1-year primary unassisted patency. In the treatment group which received dipyridamole and aspirin ($n=321$) the 1-year primary unassisted patency was 28 % compared to 23 % in the placebo group ($n=328$, $p=0.03$). While the patients in the dipyridamole and aspirin group showed a significant but modest benefit in improvement of primary unassisted patency, 72 % of patients still lost AVG patency within 1 year of AVG placement [201]. Whether dipyridamole and aspirin is a cost-effective therapy to prevent AVG failure remains debatable. The second study was a Canadian multicenter randomized controlled trial evaluating the impact oral fish oil therapy ($n=99$) compared to placebo ($n=97$) [202]. The primary outcome was to evaluate 12 month loss of native AVG patency. There was no significant difference in loss of native patency within 12 months between the fish oil group compared to placebo (48 vs. 62 %; $p=0.06$) [202]. This was in part likely due to the investigators not reaching target recruitment goals and the study being slightly underpowered, as there was a trend toward benefit in the fish oil group. However, among the clinical meaningful secondary outcomes, fish oil showed significant benefit when compared to placebo when evaluating rates of thrombosis, frequency of AVG interventions, and cardiovascular events [202]. One randomized study has evaluated warfarin and showed no decrease in AVG patency, but increased in major bleeds in the warfarin group [203].

6.5.2 Pharmacologic Therapies for AVFs

The major hurdle that remains to improve incident and prevalent AVF rates is addressing the problem of AVF maturation failure. Small randomized studies focused on antiplatelet agents to prevent early AVF thrombosis have showed that they may reduce the risk for early thrombosis after AVF creation [204]. Recently, the largest multicenter randomized controlled trial to date in AVFs, sponsored by the National Institutes of Health Dialysis Access Consortium, was completed and evaluated clopidogrel therapy compared to placebo in newly created AVFs [21]. The primary outcome of this study was to determine whether clopidogrel therapy for 6 weeks after creation of AVF reduces AVF thrombosis at 6 weeks. In patients who received clopidogrel ($n=441$), AVF thrombosis was significantly reduced at 6 weeks compared to placebo ($n=436$), 12.2 versus 19.5 %, respectively ($p=0.18$) [21]. However, the most pertinent outcome from this study was the more clinically relevant outcome, AVF suitability, which the investigators defined as use of the AVF on the dialysis machine at a minimum pump rate of 300 ml/min during 8 out of 12 dialysis sessions during 1 month [21]. In the clopidogrel group, 61 % of patients and in the placebo group 60 % patients had suitability failure [21]. This study has lead to a renewed interest in understanding the pathobiology of AVF maturation and neointimal hyperplasia development [205].

6.5.3 Novel Therapies to Treat Dialysis Access Dysfunction

In recent years, a number of novel therapies have been developed and tested to both prevent and treat vascular access stenosis. The main rationale of local delivery therapies is to deliver a target drug directly at the site of the AV anastomosis in AVF and AVG because this is the area where neointimal hyperplasia and vascular stenosis most commonly develops. There have been several early phase randomized controlled trials evaluating local delivery therapies. These include perivascular-delivered: (1) endothelial cell implants [206, 207], (2) recombinant elastase [208–210], (3) and sirolimus [211]. These studies have all demonstrated appropriate safety and feasibility for these novel drugs. Endothelial cell implant and recombinant elastase therapies are currently being evaluated in phase III studies. Recently, a novel arteriovenous anastomotic conduit device was tested in early phase studies and showed good safety and feasibility as well as promising efficacy when assessing maturation and assisted patency [212]. This device is also currently being tested in phase III clinical trials. Far-infrared therapy is a novel and local therapy that has demonstrated to prolong AVF patency after dialysis initiation and angioplasty and promote AVF maturation in several randomized controlled studies [213–215]. To date far-infrared therapy is the only therapy shown to be consistently effective in treating AVF dysfunction.

The primary therapy to treat vascular access dysfunction in AVF and AVG remains balloon angioplasty with or without stent therapy. As described in previous sections, these therapies unfortunately have very poor patency outcomes due to frequent restenosis. However, there are currently randomized controlled trials underway to evaluate drug-coated balloons and drug-eluting stents to reduce frequent restenosis after balloon angioplasty [216].

6.6 Future Perspectives to Improve Hemodialysis Vascular Access Outcomes

The current epidemiologic landscape from the United States Renal Data System (USRDS) data projects a continued increase in both the incident and prevalent hemodialysis population for the foreseeable future [17]. Thus, the current hemodialysis vascular access challenges, such as improving AVF utilization and maturation failure, decreasing overall dialysis catheter use, reducing stenosis and thromboses in AVG, etc. will likely be magnified in future years. In order to successfully address these current and future issues in dialysis access, a balanced approach needs to be taken to improve the processes of care issues and biological issues related to hemodialysis vascular access dysfunction.

6.6.1 Improving Processes of Care Issues for Vascular Access Care

The most common process of care issues related to improving vascular access care include early referral to nephrologist, referral to a dedicated vascular surgeon, and timely placement of a permanent access prior to initiation of hemodialysis. Continued improvement of each of these benchmarks will impact vascular access utilization at dialysis initiation and will require coordinated multidisciplinary care. However, new and emerging issues related to process of care, which need more clinical research, include access selection, individualization of care, and end of life care in the elderly. The elderly population is the one of the fastest growing ESRD populations. In this population, both quality life (pain, number of vascular access interventions to promote maturation, life expectancy, etc.) and patient preferences need to be balanced with both guidelines and quality initiatives, which do not acknowledge the trade-offs involved in managing the elderly patients with multiple chronic conditions and limited life expectancy or the value that patients place on achieving these outcomes [217, 218]. Approximately 30% of AVF placed in elderly patients are never utilized for dialysis because they die prior to initiating dialysis [219, 220]. Furthermore, among elderly patients, the initial choice of vascular access (AVF or AVG) does not significantly affect survival after initiating dialysis [102, 221]. Thus, the goals in this population may need to be aligned to a more patient-centered approach that focuses and addresses the extent to which the process of decision-making of vascular access selection support the goals and preferences of the individual patient [221, 222].

6.6.2 Advancing the Understanding of the Pathobiology of Vascular Access Dysfunction

Currently, there are few, if any, effective therapies to prevent or treat vascular access dysfunction. A better fundamental understanding of the biology of vascular stenosis and neointimal hyperplasia development, utilizing a "bench-to-bedside" approach, will be necessary to improve therapeutic targets. This will require utilizing animal models, imaging technology, and human biological samples from veins, arteries, and AVFs. Currently, the National Institutes of Health has invested in a multicenter consortium (Hemodialysis Fistula Maturation Consortium) to study both clinical, anatomical, and biological predictors of AVF maturation utilizing a prospective observational study [205] in 600 patients. There must be further and continued investment from government and industry resources to develop and translate therapies from the "bench to the bedside."

Another major hurdle in development of novel vascular access therapies is the paucity of randomized controlled trials in vascular access [193]. However, recently the ASN has founded a collaborative partnership with the Federal Drug Administration (FDA), the Kidney Health Initiative, where the kidney community can interact more efficiently to enhance the process of optimizing the evaluation of drugs, biologics, devices, and food products [223]. The goal of this initiative is to foster an environment and partnerships (academic institutions, industry, and FDA) that will facilitate development and delivery of innovative therapies in a timely fashion to patients with kidney disease, including those requiring novel therapies for dialysis access [223].

6.7 Conclusions

The vascular access remains the lifeline to achieving successful hemodialysis therapy for ESRD patients. Achieving optimal vascular access outcomes will require improving our processes and delivery of care, as well as incorporating a more patient-centered approach when considering vascular access selection. Moreover, there is currently an unmet need to better understand the biological mechanisms of vascular access dysfunction in AVF, AVG, and TDC, so that this knowledge can be successfully translated and developed into new innovations and technologies to treat vascular access dysfunction in hemodialysis patients.

References

1. Lee T. Novel paradigms for dialysis vascular access: downstream vascular biology-is there a final common pathway? Clin J Am Soc Nephrol. 2013;8:2194–2201.
2. Lee T, Roy-Chaudhury P. Advances and new frontiers in the pathophysiology of venous neointimal hyperplasia and dialysis access stenosis. Adv Chronic Kidney Dis. 2009;16(5):329–38.
3. Clinical practice guidelines for vascular access. Am J Kidney Dis. 2006;48:S176–273.
4. Levinsky NG. The organization of medical care. Lessons from the medicare end stage renal disease program. N Engl J Med. 1993;329(19):1395–9.
5. Rostand SG, Gretes JC, Kirk KA, Rutsky EA, Andreoli TE. Ischemic heart disease in patients with uremia undergoing maintenance hemodialysis. Kidney Int. 1979;16(5):600–11.
6. Allon M, Robbin ML. Increasing arteriovenous fistulas in hemodialysis patients: problems and solutions. Kidney Int. 2002;62(4):1109–24.
7. Port FK. Morbidity and mortality in dialysis patients. Kidney Int. 1994;46(6):1728–37.
8. Schwab SJ, Harrington JT, Singh A, Roher R, Shohaib SA, Perrone RD, et al. Vascular access for hemodialysis. Kidney Int. 1999;55(5):2078–90.
9. Schwab SJ, Raymond JR, Saeed M, Newman GE, Dennis PA, Bollinger RR. Prevention of hemodialysis fistula thrombosis. Early detection of venous stenoses. Kidney Int. 1989;36(4):707–11.
10. Besarab A, Sullivan KL, Ross RP, Moritz MJ. Utility of intra-access pressure monitoring in detecting and correcting venous outlet stenoses prior to thrombosis. Kidney Int. 1995;47(5):1364–73.
11. Safa AA, Valji K, Roberts AC, Ziegler TW, Hye RJ, Oglevie SB. Detection and treatment of dysfunctional hemodialysis access grafts: effect of a surveillance program on graft patency and the incidence of thrombosis. Radiology. 1996;199(3):653–7.
12. McCarley P, Wingard RL, Shyr Y, Pettus W, Hakim RM, Ikizler TA. Vascular access blood flow monitoring reduces access morbidity and costs. Kidney Int. 2001;60(3):1164–72.
13. Feldman HI, Kobrin S, Wasserstein A. Hemodialysis vascular access morbidity. J Am Soc Nephrol. 1996;7(4):523–35.
14. NKF-DOQI clinical practice guidelines for vascular access. National Kidney Foundation-dialysis outcomes quality initiative. Am J Kidney Dis. 1997;30(4 Suppl 3):S150–91.
15. Fistula First National Access Improvements Initiative. 2014. http://www.fistulafirst.org/. Accessed 3 June 2014.
16. National Kidney Foundation. DOQI clinical practice guidelines for vascular access: update 2000. Am J Kidney Dis. 2001;37(1):137–S81.
17. Collins AJ, Foley RN, Herzog C, Chavers B, Gilbertson D, Herzog C, et al. US Renal Data System 2012 annual data report. Am J Kidney Dis. 2013;61(1 Suppl 1):A7, e1–476.
18. Lee T, Roy-Chaudhury P, Thakar CV. Improving incident fistula rates: a process of care issue. Am J Kidney Dis. 2011;57(6):814–7.
19. Allon M, Bailey R, Ballard R, Deierhoi MH, Hamrick K, Oser R, et al. A multidisciplinary approach to hemodialysis access: prospective evaluation. Kidney Int. 1998;53(2):473–9.
20. Lok CE, Oliver MJ. Overcoming barriers to arteriovenous fistula creation and use. Semin Dial. 2003;16(3):189–96.
21. Dember LM, Beck GJ, Allon M, Delmez JA, Dixon BS, Greenberg A, et al. Effect of clopidogrel on early failure of arteriovenous fistulas for hemodialysis: a randomized controlled trial. JAMA. 2008;299(18):2164–71.
22. Hodges TC, Fillinger MF, Zwolak RM, Walsh DB, Bech F, Cronenwett JL. Longitudinal comparison of dialysis access methods: risk factors for failure. J Vasc Surg. 1997;26(6):1009–19.
23. Silva MB Jr, Hobson RW 2nd, Pappas PJ, Jamil Z, Araki CT, Goldberg MC, et al. A strategy for increasing use of autogenous hemodialysis access procedures: impact of preoperative noninvasive evaluation. J Vasc Surg. 1998;27(2):302–7. discussion 7–8.
24. Miller PE, Tolwani A, Luscy CP, Deierhoi MH, Bailey R, Redden DT, et al. Predictors of adequacy of arteriovenous fistulas in hemodialysis patients. Kidney Int. 1999;56(1):275–80.
25. Murphy GJ, White SA, Knight AJ, Doughman T, Nicholson ML. Long-term results of arteriovenous fistulas using transposed autologous basilic vein. Br J Surg. 2000;87(6):819–23.
26. Revanur VK, Jardine AG, Hamilton DH, Jindal RM. Outcome for arterio-venous fistula at the elbow for haemodialysis. Clin Transpl. 2000;14(4 Pt 1):318–22.
27. Wolowczyk L, Williams AJ, Donovan KL, Gibbons CP. The snuffbox arteriovenous fistula for vascular access. Eur J Vasc Endovasc Surg. 2000;19(1):70–6.
28. Gibson KD, Caps MT, Kohler TR, Hatsukami TS, Gillen DL, Aldassy M, et al. Assessment of a policy to reduce placement of prosthetic hemodialysis access. Kidney Int. 2001;59(6):2335–45.
29. Allon M, Lockhart ME, Lilly RZ, Gallichio MH, Young CJ, Barker J, et al. Effect of preoperative sonographic mapping on vascular access outcomes in hemodialysis patients. Kidney Int. 2001;60(5):2013–20.
30. Oliver MJ, McCann RL, Indridason OS, Butterly DW, Schwab SJ. Comparison of transposed brachiobasilic fistulas to upper arm grafts and brachiocephalic fistulas. Kidney Int. 2001;60(4):1532–9.
31. Sedlacek M, Teodorescu V, Falk A, Vassalotti JA, Uribarri J. Hemodialysis access placement with preoperative noninvasive vascular mapping: comparison between patients with and without diabetes. Am J Kidney Dis. 2001;38(3):560–4.
32. Dixon BS, Novak L, Fangman J. Hemodialysis vascular access survival: upper-arm native arteriovenous fistula. Am J Kidney Dis. 2002;39(1):92–101.
33. Lee T, Ullah A, Allon M, Succop P, El-Khatib M, Munda R, et al. Decreased cumulative access survival in arteriovenous fistulas

requiring interventions to promote maturation. Clin J Am Soc Nephrol. 2011;6(3):575–81.
34. Lee T, Barker J, Allon M. Comparison of survival of upper arm arteriovenous fistulas and grafts after failed forearm fistula. J Am Soc Nephrol. 2007;18(6):1936–41.
35. Kats M, Hawxby AM, Barker J, Allon M. Impact of obesity on arteriovenous fistula outcomes in dialysis patients. Kidney Int. 2007;71(1):39–43.
36. Vachharajani TJ. Atlas of vascular access. 2014. http://www.fistulafirst.org. Accessed 1 June 2014.
37. Brescia MJ, Cimino JE, Appel K, Hurwich BJ. Chronic hemodialysis using venipuncture and a surgically created arteriovenous fistula. N Engl J Med. 1966;275(20):1089–92.
38. Lauvao LS, Ihnat DM, Goshima KR, Chavez L, Gruessner AC, Mills JL Sr. Vein diameter is the major predictor of fistula maturation. J Vasc Surg. 2009;49(6):1499–504.
39. Tordoir JH, Rooyens P, Dammers R, van der Sande FM, de Haan M, Yo TI. Prospective evaluation of failure modes in autogenous radiocephalic wrist access for haemodialysis. Nephrol Dial Transpl. 2003;18(2):378–83.
40. Rao RK, Azin GD, Hood DB, Rowe VL, Kohl RD, Katz SG, et al. Basilic vein transposition fistula: a good option for maintaining hemodialysis access site options? J Vasc Surg. 2004;39(5):1043–7.
41. Paulson KA, Gordon V, Flynn L, Lorelli D. Modified two-stage basilic vein transposition for hemodialysis access. Am J Surg. 2011;202(2):184–7.
42. Jennings WC, Sideman MJ, Taubman KE, Broughan TA. Brachial vein transposition arteriovenous fistulas for hemodialysis access. J Vasc Surg. 2009;50(5):1121–5. discussion 5–6.
43. Ramanathan AK, Nader ND, Dryjski ML, Dosluoglu HH, Cherr GS, Curl GR, et al. A retrospective review of basilic and cephalic vein-based fistulas. Vascular. 2011;19(2):97–104.
44. Maya ID, O'Neal JC, Young CJ, Barker-Finkel J, Allon M. Outcomes of brachiocephalic fistulas, transposed brachiobasilic fistulas, and upper arm grafts. Clin J Am Soc Nephrol. 2009;4(1):86–92.
45. Miller A, Holzenbein TJ, Gottlieb MN, Sacks BA, Lavin PT, Goodman WS, et al. Strategies to increase the use of autogenous arteriovenous fistula in end-stage renal disease. Ann Vasc Surg. 1997;11(4):397–405.
46. Asif A, Cherla G, Merrill D, Cipleu CD, Tawakol JB, Epstein DL, et al. Venous mapping using venography and the risk of radiocontrast-induced nephropathy. Semin Dial. 2005;18(3):239–42.
47. Roy-Chaudhury P, Arend L, Zhang J, Krishnamoorthy M, Wang Y, Banerjee R, et al. Neointimal hyperplasia in early arteriovenous fistula failure. Am J Kidney Dis. 2007;50(5):782–90.
48. Roy-Chaudhury P, Wang Y, Krishnamoorthy M, Zhang J, Banerjee R, Munda R, et al. Cellular phenotypes in human stenotic lesions from haemodialysis vascular access. Nephrol Dial Transpl. 2009;24(9):2786–91.
49. Lee T, Wang Y, Arend L, Cornea V, Campos B, Munda R, et al. Comparative analysis of cellular phenotypes within the neointima from vein segments collected prior to vascular access surgery and stenotic arteriovenous dialysis accesses. Semin Dial. 2014;27(3):303–9.
50. Lee T, Somarathna M, Hura A, Wang Y, Campos B, Arend L, et al. Natural history of venous morphologic changes in dialysis access stenosis. J Vasc Access. 2014;0(0):0.
51. Roy-Chaudhury P, Sukhatme VP, Cheung AK. Hemodialysis vascular access dysfunction: a cellular and molecular viewpoint. J Am Soc Nephrol. 2006;17(4):1112–27.
52. Juncos JP, Grande JP, Kang L, Ackerman AW, Croatt AJ, Katusic ZS, et al. MCP-1 contributes to arteriovenous fistula failure. J Am Soc Nephrol. 2011;22(1):43–8.
53. Juncos JP, Tracz MJ, Croatt AJ, Grande JP, Ackerman AW, Katusic ZS, et al. Genetic deficiency of heme oxygenase-1 impairs functionality and form of an arteriovenous fistula in the mouse. Kidney Int. 2008;74(1):47–51.
54. Misra S, Fu AA, Anderson JL, Sethi S, Glockner JF, McKusick MA, et al. The rat femoral arteriovenous fistula model: increased expression of matrix metalloproteinase-2 and -9 at the venous stenosis. J Vasc Interv Radiol. 2008;19(4):587–94.
55. Haage P, Vorwerk D, Wildberger JE, Piroth W, Schurmann K, Gunther RW. Percutaneous treatment of thrombosed primary arteriovenous hemodialysis access fistulae. Kidney Int. 2000;57(3):1169–75.
56. Turmel-Rodrigues L, Pengloan J, Baudin S, Testou D, Abaza M, Dahdah G, et al. Treatment of stenosis and thrombosis in haemodialysis fistulas and grafts by interventional radiology. Nephrol Dial Transpl. 2000;15(12):2029–36.
57. Rajan DK, Clark TW, Simons ME, Kachura JR, Sniderman K. Procedural success and patency after percutaneous treatment of thrombosed autogenous arteriovenous dialysis fistulas. J Vasc Interv Radiol. 2002;13(12):1211–8.
58. Liang HL, Pan HB, Chung HM, Ger LP, Fang HC, Wu TH, et al. Restoration of thrombosed brescia-cimino dialysis fistulas by using percutaneous transluminal angioplasty. Radiology. 2002;223(2):339–44.
59. Shatsky JB, Berns JS, Clark TW, Kwak A, Tuite CM, Shlansky-Goldberg RD, et al. Single-center experience with the Arrow-Trerotola Percutaneous Thrombectomy Device in the management of thrombosed native dialysis fistulas. J Vasc Interv Radiol. 2005;16(12):1605–11.
60. Jain G, Maya ID, Allon M. Outcomes of percutaneous mechanical thrombectomy of arteriovenous fistulas in hemodialysis patients. Semin Dial. 2008;21(6):581–3.
61. Lee T, Tindni A, Roy-Chaudhury P. Improved cumulative survival in fistulas requiring surgical interventions to promote fistula maturation compared with endovascular interventions. Semin Dial. 2013;26(1):85–9.
62. Long B, Brichart N, Lermusiaux P, Turmel-Rodrigues L, Artru B, Boutin JM, et al. Management of perianastomotic stenosis of direct wrist autogenous radial-cephalic arteriovenous accesses for dialysis. J Vasc Surg. 2011;53(1):108–14.
63. Ito Y, Sato T, Okada R, Nakamura N, Kimura K, Takahashi R, et al. Comparison of clinical effectiveness between surgical and endovascular treatment for thrombotic obstruction in hemodialysis access. J Vasc Access. 2011;12(1):63–6.
64. Tessitore N, Mansueto G, Lipari G, Bedogna V, Tardivo S, Baggio E, et al. Endovascular versus surgical preemptive repair of forearm arteriovenous fistula juxta-anastomotic stenosis: analysis of data collected prospectively from 1999 to 2004. Clin J Am Soc Nephrol. 2006;1(3):448–54.
65. Kakkos SK, Andrzejewski T, Haddad JA, Haddad GK, Reddy DJ, Nypaver TJ, et al. Equivalent secondary patency rates of upper extremity vectra vascular access grafts and transposed brachial-basilic fistulas with aggressive access surveillance and endovascular treatment. J Vasc Surg. 2008;47(2):407–14.
66. Allon M. Current management of vascular access. Clin J Am Soc Nephrol. 2007;2(4):786–800.
67. Minga TE, Flanagan KH, Allon M. Clinical consequences of infected arteriovenous grafts in hemodialysis patients. Am J Kidney Dis. 2001;38(5):975–8.
68. Miller PE, Carlton D, Deierhoi MH, Redden DT, Allon M. Natural history of arteriovenous grafts in hemodialysis patients. Am J Kidney Dis. 2000;36(1):68–74.
69. Miller CD, Robbin ML, Barker J, Allon M. Comparison of arteriovenous grafts in the thigh and upper extremities in hemodialysis patients. J Am Soc Nephrol. 2003;14(11):2942–7.
70. Beathard GA. Percutaneous transvenous angioplasty in the treatment of vascular access stenosis. Kidney Int. 1992;42(6):1390–7.
71. Beathard GA, Marston WA. Endovascular management of thrombosed dialysis access grafts. Am J Kidney Dis. 1998;32(1):172–5.
72. Beathard GA. Angioplasty for arteriovenous grafts and fistulae. Semin Nephrol. 2002;22(3):202–10.

73. Lilly RZ, Carlton D, Barker J, Saddekni S, Hamrick K, Oser R, et al. Predictors of arteriovenous graft patency after radiologic intervention in hemodialysis patients. Am J Kidney Dis. 2001;37(5):945–53.
74. Maya ID, Oser R, Saddekni S, Barker J, Allon M. Vascular access stenosis: comparison of arteriovenous grafts and fistulas. Am J Kidney Dis. 2004;44(5):859–65.
75. Beathard GA. Mechanical versus pharmacomechanical thrombolysis for the treatment of thrombosed dialysis access grafts. Kidney Int. 1994;45(5):1401–6.
76. Beathard GA. Thrombolysis versus surgery for the treatment of thrombosed dialysis access grafts. J Am Soc Nephrol. 1995;6(6):1619–24.
77. Beathard GA, Welch BR, Maidment HJ. Mechanical thrombolysis for the treatment of thrombosed hemodialysis access grafts. Radiology. 1996;200(3):711–6.
78. Cohen MA, Kumpe DA, Durham JD, Zwerdlinger SC. Improved treatment of thrombosed hemodialysis access sites with thrombolysis and angioplasty. Kidney Int. 1994;46(5):1375–80.
79. Trerotola SO, Vesely TM, Lund GB, Soulen MC, Ehrman KO, Cardella JF. Treatment of thrombosed hemodialysis access grafts: Arrow-Trerotola Percutaneous Thrombolytic Device versus pulse-spray thrombolysis. Arrow-Trerotola Percutaneous Thrombolytic Device clinical trial. Radiology. 1998;206(2):403–14.
80. Trerotola SO, Lund GB, Scheel PJ Jr, Savader SJ, Venbrux AC, Osterman FA. Jr Thrombosed dialysis access grafts: percutaneous mechanical declotting without urokinase. Radiology. 1994;191(3):721–6.
81. Valji K, Bookstein JJ, Roberts AC, Davis GB. Pharmacomechanical thrombolysis and angioplasty in the management of clotted hemodialysis grafts: early and late clinical results. Radiology. 1991;178(1):243–7.
82. Kanterman RY, Vesely TM, Pilgram TK, Guy BW, Windus DW, Picus D. Dialysis access grafts: anatomic location of venous stenosis and results of angioplasty. Radiology. 1995;195(1):135–9.
83. Asif A, Leon C, Orozco-Vargas LC, Krishnamurthy G, Choi KL, Mercado C, et al. Accuracy of physical examination in the detection of arteriovenous fistula stenosis. Clin J Am Soc Nephrol. 2007;2(6):1191–4.
84. Cayco AV, Abu-Alfa AK, Mahnensmith RL, Perazella MA. Reduction in arteriovenous graft impairment: results of a vascular access surveillance protocol. Am J Kidney Dis. 1998;32(2):302–8.
85. Besarab A, Frinak S, Sherman RA, Goldman J, Dumler F, Devita MV, et al. Simplified measurement of intra-access pressure. J Am Soc Nephrol. 1998;9(2):284–9.
86. Lumsden AB, MacDonald MJ, Kikeri D, Cotsonis GA, Harker LA, Martin LG. Prophylactic balloon angioplasty fails to prolong the patency of expanded polytetrafluoroethylene arteriovenous grafts: results of a prospective randomized study. J Vasc Surg. 1997;26(3):382–90. discussion 90–2.
87. Ram SJ, Work J, Caldito GC, Eason JM, Pervez A, Paulson WD. A randomized controlled trial of blood flow and stenosis surveillance of hemodialysis grafts. Kidney Int. 2003;64(1):272–80.
88. Moist LM, Churchill DN, House AA, Millward SF, Elliott JE, Kribs SW, et al. Regular monitoring of access flow compared with monitoring of venous pressure fails to improve graft survival. J Am Soc Nephrol. 2003;14(10):2645–53.
89. Dember LM, Holmberg EF, Kaufman JS. Randomized controlled trial of prophylactic repair of hemodialysis arteriovenous graft stenosis. Kidney Int. 2004;66(1):390–8.
90. Malik J, Slavikova M, Svobodova J, Tuka V. Regular ultrasonographic screening significantly prolongs patency of PTFE grafts. Kidney Int. 2005;67(4):1554–8.
91. Robbin ML, Oser RF, Lee JY, Heudebert GR, Mennemeyer ST, Allon M. Randomized comparison of ultrasound surveillance and clinical monitoring on arteriovenous graft outcomes. Kidney Int. 2006;69(4):730–5.
92. Chang CJ, Ko PJ, Hsu LA, Ko YS, Ko YL, Chen CF, et al. Highly increased cell proliferation activity in the restenotic hemodialysis vascular access after percutaneous transluminal angioplasty: implication in prevention of restenosis. Am J Kidney Dis. 2004;43(1):74–84.
93. Roy-Chaudhury P, Kelly BS, Miller MA, Reaves A, Armstrong J, Nanayakkara N, et al. Venous neointimal hyperplasia in polytetrafluoroethylene dialysis grafts. Kidney Int. 2001;59(6):2325–34.
94. Swedberg SH, Brown BG, Sigley R, Wight TN, Gordon D, Nicholls SC. Intimal fibromuscular hyperplasia at the venous anastomosis of PTFE grafts in hemodialysis patients. Clinical, immunocytochemical, light and electron microscopic assessment. Circulation. 1989;80(6):1726–36.
95. Sands JJ, Patel S, Plaviak DJ, Miranda CL. Pharmacomechanical thrombolysis with urokinase for treatment of thrombosed hemodialysis access grafts. A comparison with surgical thrombectomy. Asaio J. 1994;40(3):M886–8.
96. Maya ID, Allon M. Outcomes of thrombosed arteriovenous grafts: comparison of stents vs angioplasty. Kidney Int. 2006;69(5):934–7.
97. Haskal ZJ, Trerotola S, Dolmatch B, Schuman E, Altman S, Mietling S, et al. Stent graft versus balloon angioplasty for failing dialysis-access grafts. N Engl J Med. 2010;362(6):494–503.
98. Lacson E Jr, Wang W, Lazarus JM, Hakim RM. Change in vascular access and hospitalization risk in long-term hemodialysis patients. Clin J Am Soc Nephrol. 2010;5(11):1996–2003.
99. Lacson E Jr, Wang W, Hakim RM, Teng M, Lazarus JM. Associates of mortality and hospitalization in hemodialysis: potentially actionable laboratory variables and vascular access. Am J Kidney Dis. 2009;53(1):79–90.
100. Allon M, Daugirdas J, Depner TA, Greene T, Ornt D, Schwab SJ. Effect of change in vascular access on patient mortality in hemodialysis patients. Am J Kidney Dis. 2006;47(3):469–77.
101. Lacson E Jr, Wang W, Lazarus JM, Hakim RM. Change in vascular access and mortality in maintenance hemodialysis patients. Am J Kidney Dis. 2009.
102. Desilva RN, Patibandla BK, Vin Y, Narra A, Chawla V, Brown RS, et al. Fistula first is not always the best strategy for the elderly. J Am Soc Nephrol. 2013;24(8):1297–304.
103. Wong JK, Sadler DJ, McCarthy M, Saliken JC, So CB, Gray RR. Analysis of early failure of tunneled hemodialysis catheters. AJR Am J Roentgenol. 2002;179(2):357–63.
104. Liangos O, Gul A, Madias NE, Jaber BL. Long-term management of the tunneled venous catheter. Semin Dial. 2006;19(2):158–64.
105. Schwab SJ, Beathard G. The hemodialysis catheter conundrum: hate living with them, but can't live without them. Kidney Int. 1999;56(1):1–17.
106. Mokrzycki MH, Lok CE. Traditional and non-traditional strategies to optimize catheter function: go with more flow. Kidney Int. 2010;78(12):1218–31.
107. Hoshal VL Jr, Ause RG, Hoskins PA. Fibrin sleeve formation on indwelling subclavian central venous catheters. Arch Surg. 1971;102(4):353–8.
108. Agraharkar M, Isaacson S, Mendelssohn D, Muralidharan J, Mustata S, Zevallos G, et al. Percutaneously inserted silastic jugular hemodialysis catheters seldom cause jugular vein thrombosis. ASAIO J. 1995;41(2):169–72.
109. Karnik R, Valentin A, Winkler WB, Donath P, Slany J. Duplex sonographic detection of internal jugular venous thrombosis after removal of central venous catheters. Clin Cardiol. 1993;16(1):26–9.
110. Beathard GA. Catheter thrombosis. Semin Dial. 2001;14(6):441–5.
111. Lok CE, Appleton D, Bhola C, Khoo B, Richardson RM. Trisodium citrate 4%—an alternative to heparin capping of haemodialysis catheters. Nephrol Dial Transp. 2007;22(2):477–83.
112. Negulescu O, Coco M, Croll J, Mokrzycki MH. Large atrial thrombus formation associated with tunneled cuffed hemodialysis catheters. Clin Nephrol. 2003;59(1):40–6.

113. Buturovic J, Ponikvar R, Kandus A, Boh M, Klinkmann J, Ivanovich P. Filling hemodialysis catheters in the interdialytic period: heparin versus citrate versus polygeline: a prospective randomized study. Artif Organs. 1998;22(11):945–7.
114. Hemmelgarn BR, Moist LM, Lok CE, Tonelli M, Manns BJ, Holden RM, et al. Prevention of dialysis catheter malfunction with recombinant tissue plasminogen activator. N Engl J Med. 2011;364(4):303–12.
115. Forauer AR, Theoharis CG, Dasika NL. Jugular vein catheter placement: histologic features and development of catheter-related (fibrin) sheaths in a swine model. Radiology. 2006;240(2):427–34.
116. Crain MR, Mewissen MW, Ostrowski GJ, Paz-Fumagalli R, Beres RA, Wertz RA. Fibrin sleeve stripping for salvage of failing hemodialysis catheters: technique and initial results. Radiology. 1996;198(1):41–4.
117. Brady PS, Spence LD, Levitin A, Mickolich CT, Dolmatch BL. Efficacy of percutaneous fibrin sheath stripping in restoring patency of tunneled hemodialysis catheters. AJR Am J Roentgenol. 1999;173(4):1023–7.
118. Gray RJ, Levitin A, Buck D, Brown LC, Sparling YH, Jablonski KA, et al. Percutaneous fibrin sheath stripping versus transcatheter urokinase infusion for malfunctioning well-positioned tunneled central venous dialysis catheters: a prospective, randomized trial. J Vasc Interv Radiol. 2000;11(9):1121–9.
119. Janne d'Othee B, Tham JC, Sheiman RG. Restoration of patency in failing tunneled hemodialysis catheters: a comparison of catheter exchange, exchange and balloon disruption of the fibrin sheath, and femoral stripping. J Vasc Interv Radiol. 2006;17(6):1011–5.
120. Alomari AI, Falk A. The natural history of tunneled hemodialysis catheters removed or exchanged: a single-institution experience. J Vasc Interv Radiol. 2007;18(2):227–35.
121. Onder AM, Chandar J, Coakley S, Francoeur D, Abitbol C, Zilleruelo G. Controlling exit site infections: does it decrease the incidence of catheter-related bacteremia in children on chronic hemodialysis? Hemodial Int. 2009;13(1):11–8.
122. Allon M. Dialysis catheter-related bacteremia: treatment and prophylaxis. Am J Kidney Dis. 2004;44(5):779–91.
123. Costerton JW, Stewart PS, Greenberg EP. Bacterial biofilms: a common cause of persistent infections. Science. 1999;284(5418):1318–22.
124. Donlan RM. Biofilms and device-associated infections. Emerg Infect Dis. 2001;7(2):277–81.
125. Lok CE, Mokrzycki MH. Prevention and management of catheter-related infection in hemodialysis patients. Kidney Int. 2011;79(6):587–98.
126. Tapia G, Yee J. Biofilm: its relevance in kidney disease. Adv Chronic Kidney Dis. 2006;13(3):215–24.
127. Ishizuka M, Nagata H, Takagi K, Kubota K. Comparison of 0.05 % chlorhexidine and 10 % povidone-iodine as cutaneous disinfectant for prevention of central venous catheter-related bloodstream infection: a comparative study. Eur Surg Res (Europaische chirurgische Forschung Recherches chirurgicales europeennes). 2009;43(3):286–90.
128. Onder AM, Chandar J, Billings A, Diaz R, Francoeur D, Abitbol C, et al. Chlorhexidine-based antiseptic solutions effectively reduce catheter-related bacteremia. Pediatr Nephrol. 2009;24(9):1741–7.
129. Darouiche RO, Wall MJ Jr, Itani KM, Otterson MF, Webb AL, Carrick MM, et al. Chlorhexidine-alcohol versus povidone-iodine for surgical-site antisepsis. N Engl J Med. 2010;362(1):18–26.
130. Paocharoen V, Mingmalairak C, Apisarnthanarak A. Comparison of surgical wound infection after preoperative skin preparation with 4 % chlorhexidine [correction of chlohexidine] and povidone iodine: a prospective randomized trial. J Med Assoc Thai. 2009;92(7):898–902.
131. Valles J, Fernandez I, Alcaraz D, Chacon E, Cazorla A, Canals M, et al. Prospective randomized trial of 3 antiseptic solutions for prevention of catheter colonization in an intensive care unit for adult patients. Infect Control Hosp Epidemiol. 2008;29(9):847–53.
132. Mimoz O, Villeminey S, Ragot S, Dahyot-Fizelier C, Laksiri L, Petitpas F, et al. Chlorhexidine-based antiseptic solution vs alcohol-based povidone-iodine for central venous catheter care. Arch Intern Med. 2007;167(19):2066–72.
133. Chaiyakunapruk N, Veenstra DL, Lipsky BA, Saint S. Chlorhexidine compared with povidone-iodine solution for vascular catheter-site care: a meta-analysis. Ann Intern Med. 2002;136(11):792–801.
134. Lok CE, Stanley KE, Hux JE, Richardson R, Tobe SW, Conly J. Hemodialysis infection prevention with polysporin ointment. J Am Soc Nephrol. 2003;14(1):169–79.
135. Levin A, Mason AJ, Jindal KK, Fong IW, Goldstein MB. Prevention of hemodialysis subclavian vein catheter infections by topical povidone-iodine. Kidney Int. 1991;40(5):934–8.
136. Sesso R, Barbosa D, Leme IL, Sader H, Canziani ME, Manfredi S, et al. *Staphylococcus aureus* prophylaxis in hemodialysis patients using central venous catheter: effect of mupirocin ointment. J Am Soc Nephrol. 1998;9(6):1085–92.
137. Johnson LB, Jose J, Yousif F, Pawlak J, Saravolatz LD. Prevalence of colonization with community-associated methicillin-resistant *Staphylococcus aureus* among end-stage renal disease patients and healthcare workers. Infect Control Hosp Epidemiol. 2009;30(1):4–8.
138. Battistella M, Bhola C, Lok CE. Long-term follow-up of the hemodialysis infection prevention with polysporin ointment (HIPPO) study: a quality improvement report. Am J Kidney Dis. 2011;57(3):432–41.
139. Yu VL, Goetz A, Wagener M, Smith PB, Rihs JD, Hanchett J, et al. *Staphylococcus aureus* nasal carriage and infection in patients on hemodialysis. Efficacy of antibiotic prophylaxis. N Engl J Med. 1986;315(2):91–6.
140. Boelaert JR, De Smedt RA, De Baere YA, Godard CA, Matthys EG, Schurgers ML, et al. The influence of calcium mupirocin nasal ointment on the incidence of *Staphylococcus aureus* infections in haemodialysis patients. Nephrol Dial Transpl. 1989;4(4):278–81.
141. James MT, Conley J, Tonelli M, Manns BJ, MacRae J, Hemmelgarn BR. Meta-analysis: antibiotics for prophylaxis against hemodialysis catheter-related infections. Ann Intern Med. 2008;148(8):596–605.
142. Yahav D, Rozen-Zvi B, Gafter-Gvili A, Leibovici L, Gafter U, Paul M. Antimicrobial lock solutions for the prevention of infections associated with intravascular catheters in patients undergoing hemodialysis: systematic review and meta-analysis of randomized, controlled trials. Clin Infect Dis. 2008;47(1):83–93.
143. Jaffer Y, Selby NM, Taal MW, Fluck RJ, McIntyre CW. A meta-analysis of hemodialysis catheter locking solutions in the prevention of catheter-related infection. Am J Kidney Dis. 2008;51(2):233–41.
144. Snaterse M, Ruger W, Scholte O, Reimer WJ, Lucas C. Antibiotic-based catheter lock solutions for prevention of catheter-related bloodstream infection: a systematic review of randomised controlled trials. J Hosp Infect. 2010;75(1):1–11.
145. Dogra GK, Herson H, Hutchison B, Irish AB, Heath CH, Golledge C, et al. Prevention of tunneled hemodialysis catheter-related infections using catheter-restricted filling with gentamicin and citrate: a randomized controlled study. J Am Soc Nephrol. 2002;13(8):2133–9.
146. Allon M. Prophylaxis against dialysis catheter-related bacteremia with a novel antimicrobial lock solution. Clin Infect Dis. 2003;36(12):1539–44.
147. McIntyre CW, Hulme LJ, Taal M, Fluck RJ. Locking of tunneled hemodialysis catheters with gentamicin and heparin. Kidney Int. 2004;66(2):801–5.
148. Betjes MG, van Agteren M. Prevention of dialysis catheter-related sepsis with a citrate-taurolidine-containing lock solution. Nephrol Dial Transpl. 2004;19(6):1546–51.

149. Weijmer MC, van den Dorpel MA, Van de Ven PJ, ter Wee PM, van Geelen JA, Groeneveld JO, et al. Randomized, clinical trial comparison of trisodium citrate 30% and heparin as catheter-locking solution in hemodialysis patients. J Am Soc Nephrol. 2005;16(9):2769–77.
150. Kim SH, Song KI, Chang JW, Kim SB, Sung SA, Jo SK, et al. Prevention of uncuffed hemodialysis catheter-related bacteremia using an antibiotic lock technique: a prospective, randomized clinical trial. Kidney Int. 2006;69(1):161–4.
151. Saxena AK, Panhotra BR, Sundaram DS, Morsy MN, Al-Ghamdi AM. Enhancing the survival of tunneled haemodialysis catheters using an antibiotic lock in the elderly: a randomised, double-blind clinical trial. Nephrology (Carlton). 2006;11(4):299–305.
152. Al-Hwiesh AK, Abdul-Rahman IS. Successful prevention of tunneled, central catheter infection by antibiotic lock therapy using vancomycin and gentamycin. Saudi J Kidney Dis Transpl. 2007;18(2):239–47.
153. Winnett G, Nolan J, Miller M, Ashman N. Trisodium citrate 46.7% selectively and safely reduces staphylococcal catheter-related bacteraemia. Nephrol Dial Transpl. 2008;23(11):3592–8.
154. Power A, Duncan N, Singh SK, Brown W, Dalby E, Edwards C, et al. Sodium citrate versus heparin catheter locks for cuffed central venous catheters: a single-center randomized controlled trial. Am J Kidney Dis. 2009;53(6):1034–41.
155. Venditto M, du Montcel ST, Robert J, Trystam D, Dighiero J, Hue D, et al. Effect of catheter-lock solutions on catheter-related infection and inflammatory syndrome in hemodialysis patients: heparin versus citrate 46% versus heparin/gentamicin. Blood Purif. 2010;29(3):268–73.
156. Moran J, Sun S, Khababa I, Pedan A, Doss S, Schiller B. A randomized trial comparing gentamicin/citrate and heparin locks for central venous catheters in maintenance hemodialysis patients. Am J Kidney Dis. 2012;59(1):102–7.
157. Solomon LR, Cheesbrough JS, Ebah L, Al-Sayed T, Heap M, Millband N, et al. A randomized double-blind controlled trial of taurolidine-citrate catheter locks for the prevention of bacteremia in patients treated with hemodialysis. Am J Kidney Dis. 2010;55(6):1060–8.
158. Pervez A, Ahmed M, Ram S, Torres C, Work J, Zaman F, et al. Antibiotic lock technique for prevention of cuffed tunnel catheter associated bacteremia. J Vasc Access. 2002;3(3):108–13.
159. Landry DL, Braden GL, Gobeille SL, Haessler SD, Vaidya CK, Sweet SJ. Emergence of gentamicin-resistant bacteremia in hemodialysis patients receiving gentamicin lock catheter prophylaxis. Clin J Am Soc Nephrol. 2010;5(10):1799–804.
160. Stevenson KB, Hannah EL, Lowder CA, Adcox MJ, Davidson RL, Mallea MC, et al. Epidemiology of hemodialysis vascular access infections from longitudinal infection surveillance data: predicting the impact of NKF-DOQI clinical practice guidelines for vascular access. Am J Kidney Dis. 2002;39(3):549–55.
161. Beathard GA. Management of bacteremia associated with tunneled-cuffed hemodialysis catheters. J Am Soc Nephrol. 1999;10(5):1045–9.
162. Krishnasami Z, Carlton D, Bimbo L, Taylor ME, Balkovetz DF, Barker J, et al. Management of hemodialysis catheter-related bacteremia with an adjunctive antibiotic lock solution. Kidney Int. 2002;61(3):1136–42.
163. Marr KA, Sexton DJ, Conlon PJ, Corey GR, Schwab SJ, Kirkland KB. Catheter-related bacteremia and outcome of attempted catheter salvage in patients undergoing hemodialysis. Ann Intern Med. 1997;127(4):275–80.
164. Mokrzycki MH, Schroppel B, von Gersdorff G, Rush H, Zdunek MP, Feingold R. Tunneled-cuffed catheter associated infections in hemodialysis patients who are seropositive for the human immunodeficiency virus. J Am Soc Nephrol. 2000;11(11):2122–7.
165. Poole CV, Carlton D, Bimbo L, Allon M. Treatment of catheter-related bacteraemia with an antibiotic lock protocol: effect of bacterial pathogen. Nephrol Dial Transpl. 2004;19(5):1237–44.
166. Saad TF. Bacteremia associated with tunneled, cuffed hemodialysis catheters. Am J Kidney Dis. 1999;34(6):1114–24.
167. Schwab SJ, Weiss MA, Rushton F, Ross JP, Jackson J, Kapoian T, et al. Multicenter clinical trial results with the LifeSite hemodialysis access system. Kidney Int. 2002;62(3):1026–33.
168. Kovalik EC, Raymond JR, Albers FJ, Berkoben M, Butterly DW, Montella B, et al. A clustering of epidural abscesses in chronic hemodialysis patients: risks of salvaging access catheters in cases of infection. J Am Soc Nephrol. 1996;7(10):2264–7.
169. Ashby DR, Power A, Singh S, Choi P, Taube DH, Duncan ND, et al. Bacteremia associated with tunneled hemodialysis catheters: outcome after attempted salvage. Clin J Am Soc Nephrol. 2009;4(10):1601–5.
170. Capdevila JA, Segarra A, Planes AM, Ramirez-Arellano M, Pahissa A, Piera L, et al. Successful treatment of haemodialysis catheter-related sepsis without catheter removal. Nephrol Dial Transpl. 1993;8(3):231–4.
171. Lund GB, Trerotola SO, Scheel PF Jr, Savader SJ, Mitchell SE, Venbrux AC, et al. Outcome of tunneled hemodialysis catheters placed by radiologists. Radiology. 1996;198(2):467–72.
172. Swartz RD, Messana JM, Boyer CJ, Lunde NM, Weitzel WF, Hartman TL. Successful use of cuffed central venous hemodialysis catheters inserted percutaneously. J Am Soc Nephrol. 1994;4(9):1719–25.
173. Beathard GA, Settle SM, Shields MW. Salvage of the nonfunctioning arteriovenous fistula. Am J Kidney Dis. 1999;33(5):910–6.
174. Robinson D, Suhocki P, Schwab SJ. Treatment of infected tunneled venous access hemodialysis catheters with guidewire exchange. Kidney Int. 1998;53(6):1792–4.
175. Shaffer D. Catheter-related sepsis complicating long-term, tunnelled central venous dialysis catheters: management by guidewire exchange. Am J Kidney Dis. 1995;25(4):593–6.
176. Tanriover B, Carlton D, Saddekni S, Hamrick K, Oser R, Westfall AO, et al. Bacteremia associated with tunneled dialysis catheters: comparison of two treatment strategies. Kidney Int. 2000;57(5):2151–5.
177. Fernandez-Hidalgo N, Almirante B, Calleja R, Ruiz I, Planes AM, Rodriguez D, et al. Antibiotic-lock therapy for long-term intravascular catheter-related bacteraemia: results of an open, non-comparative study. J Antimicrob Chemother. 2006;57(6):1172–80.
178. Vardhan A, Davies J, Daryanani I, Crowe A, McClelland P. Treatment of haemodialysis catheter-related infections. Nephrol Dial Transpl. 2002;17(6):1149–50.
179. Beathard GA, Litchfield T, Physician Operators Forum of RMS Lifeline Inc. Effectiveness and safety of dialysis vascular access procedures performed by interventional nephrologists. Kidney Int. 2004;66(4):1622–32.
180. Beathard GA. Gianturco self-expanding stent in the treatment of stenosis in dialysis access grafts. Kidney Int. 1993;43(4):872–7.
181. Leon C, Asif A. Arteriovenous access and hand pain: the distal hypoperfusion ischemic syndrome. Clin J Am Soc Nephrol. 2007;2(1):175–83.
182. Jackson JW, Lewis JL, Brouillette JR, Brantley RR Jr. Initial experience of a nephrologist-operated vascular access center. Semin Dial. 2000;13(6):354–8.
183. Jackson J, Litchfield TF. How a dedicated vascular access center can promote increased use of fistulas. Nephrol Nurs J. 2006;33(2):189–96.
184. Asif A, Besarab A, Roy-Chaudhury P, Spergel LM, Ravani P. Interventional nephrology: from episodic to coordinated vascular access care. J Nephrol. 2007;20(4):399–405.
185. Vachharajani TJ, Moossavi S, Salman L, Wu S, Dwyer AC, Ross J, et al. Dialysis vascular access management by interventional

nephrology programs at University Medical Centers in the United States. Semin Dial. 2011;24(5):564–9.
186. Vachharajani TJ, Moossavi S, Salman L, Wu S, Maya ID, Yevzlin AS, et al. Successful models of interventional nephrology at academic medical centers. Clin J Am Soc Nephrol. 2010;5(11):2130–6.
187. Beathard GA, Schon D. ASDIN news and update. Semin Dial. 2009;22(3):312–7.
188. American Society of Diagnostic and Interventional Nephrology (ASDIN). http://www.asdin.org. Accessed 7 July 2014.
189. Sachdeva B, Abreo K. The history of interventional nephrology. Adv Chronic Kidney Dis. 2009;16(5):302–8.
190. Yevzlin A, Asif A. Stent placement in hemodialysis access: historical lessons, the state of the art and future directions. Clin J Am Soc Nephrol. 2009;4(5):996–1008.
191. Inrig JK. Intradialytic hypertension: a less-recognized cardiovascular complication of hemodialysis. Am J Kidney Dis. 2010;55(3):580–9.
192. Strippoli GF, Craig JC, Schena FP. The number, quality, and coverage of randomized controlled trials in nephrology. J Am Soc Nephrol. 2004;15(2):411–9.
193. Kian K, Asif A. Status of research in vascular access for dialysis. Nephrol Dial Transpl. 2010;25(11):3682–6.
194. Palmer SC, Sciancalepore M, Strippoli GF. Trial quality in nephrology: how are we measuring up? Am J Kidney Dis. 2011;58(3):335–7.
195. American Society of Nephrology. http://www.asn-online.org/about/committees/committee.aspx?panel=INAG. Accessed 7 July 2014.
196. Roy-Chaudhury P, Lee TC. Vascular stenosis: biology and interventions. Curr Opin Nephrol Hypertens. 2007;16(6):516–22.
197. Roy-Chaudhury P, Spergel LM, Besarab A, Asif A, Ravani P. Biology of arteriovenous fistula failure. J Nephrol. 2007;20(2):150–63.
198. Lee T, Chauhan V, Krishnamoorthy M, Wang Y, Arend L, Mistry MJ, et al. Severe venous neointimal hyperplasia prior to dialysis access surgery. Nephrol Dial Transpl. 2011;26(7):2264–70.
199. Sreedhara R, Himmelfarb J, Lazarus JM, Hakim RM. Anti-platelet therapy in graft thrombosis: results of a prospective, randomized, double-blind study. Kidney Int. 1994;45(5):1477–83.
200. Schmitz PG, McCloud LK, Reikes ST, Leonard CL, Gellens ME. Prophylaxis of hemodialysis graft thrombosis with fish oil: double-blind, randomized, prospective trial. J Am Soc Nephrol. 2002;13(1):184–90.
201. Dixon BS, Beck GJ, Vazquez MA, Greenberg A, Delmez JA, Allon M, et al. Effect of dipyridamole plus aspirin on hemodialysis graft patency. N Engl J Med. 2009;360(21):2191–201.
202. Lok CE, Moist L, Hemmelgarn BR, Tonelli M, Vazquez MA, Dorval M, et al. Effect of fish oil supplementation on graft patency and cardiovascular events among patients with new synthetic arteriovenous hemodialysis grafts: a randomized controlled trial. JAMA. 2012;307(17):1809–16.
203. Crowther MA, Clase CM, Margetts PJ, Julian J, Lambert K, Sneath D, et al. Low-intensity warfarin is ineffective for the prevention of PTFE graft failure in patients on hemodialysis: a randomized controlled trial. J Am Soc Nephrol. 2002;13(9):2331–7.
204. Kaufman JS. Antithrombotic agents and the prevention of access thrombosis. Semin Dial. 2000;13(1):40–6.
205. Dember LM, Imrey PB, Beck GJ, Cheung AK, Himmelfarb J, Huber TS, et al. Objectives and design of the hemodialysis fistula maturation study. Am J Kidney Dis. 2013;63:104–12.
206. Conte MS, Nugent HM, Gaccione P, Guleria I, Roy-Chaudhury P, Lawson JH. Multicenter phase I/II trial of the safety of allogeneic endothelial cell implants after the creation of arteriovenous access for hemodialysis use: the V-HEALTH study. J Vasc Surg. 2009;50(6):1359–68 e1.
207. Conte MS, Nugent HM, Gaccione P, Roy-Chaudhury P, Lawson JH. Influence of diabetes and perivascular allogeneic endothelial cell implants on arteriovenous fistula remodeling. J Vasc Surg. 2011;54(5):1383–9.
208. Dwivedi AJ, Roy-Chaudhury P, Peden EK, Browne BJ, Ladenheim ED, Scavo VA, et al. Application of human type I pancreatic elastase (PRT-201) to the venous anastomosis of arteriovenous grafts in patients with chronic kidney disease. J Vasc Access. 2014;15(5):376–84.
209. Peden EK, Leeser DB, Dixon BS, El-Khatib MT, Roy-Chaudhury P, Lawson JH, et al. A multi-center, dose-escalation study of human type I pancreatic elastase (PRT-201) administered after arteriovenous fistula creation. J Vasc Access. 2013;14(2):143–51.
210. Hye RJ, Peden EK, O'Connor TP, Browne BJ, Dixon BS, Schanzer AS, et al. Human type I pancreatic elastase treatment of arteriovenous fistulas in patients with chronic kidney disease. J Vasc Surg. 2014;60(2):454–61.
211. Paulson WD, Kipshidze N, Kipiani K, Beridze N, DeVita MV, Shenoy S, et al. Safety and efficacy of local periadventitial delivery of sirolimus for improving hemodialysis graft patency: first human experience with a sirolimus-eluting collagen membrane (Coll-R). Nephrol Dial Transpl. 2012;27(3):1219–24.
212. Chemla E, Tavakoli A, Nikam M, Mitra S, Malete T, Evans J, et al. Arteriovenous fistula creation using the optiflow vascular anastomotic connector: the OPEN (Optiflow PatEncy and MaturatioN) study. J Vasc Access. 2014;15(1):38–44.
213. Lai CC, Fang HC, Mar GY, Liou JC, Tseng CJ, Liu CP. Post-angioplasty far infrared radiation therapy improves 1-year angioplasty-free hemodialysis access patency of recurrent obstructive lesions. Eur J Vasc Endovasc Surg. 2013;46(6):726–32.
214. Lin CC, Chang CF, Lai MY, Chen TW, Lee PC, Yang WC. Far-infrared therapy: a novel treatment to improve access blood flow and unassisted patency of arteriovenous fistula in hemodialysis patients. J Am Soc Nephrol. 2007;18(3):985–92.
215. Lin CC, Yang WC, Chen MC, Liu WS, Yang CY, Lee PC. Effect of far infrared therapy on arteriovenous fistula maturation: an open-label randomized controlled trial. Am J Kidney Dis. 2013;62(2)304–11.
216. Katsanos K, Karnabatidis D, Kitrou P, Spiliopoulos S, Christeas N, Siablis D. Paclitaxel-coated balloon angioplasty vs. plain balloon dilation for the treatment of failing dialysis access: 6-month interim results from a prospective randomized controlled trial. J Endovasc Ther. 2012;19(2):263–72.
217. Moist LM, Lok CE, Vachharajani TJ, Xi W, AlJaishi A, Polkinghorne KR, et al. Optimal hemodialysis vascular access in the elderly patient. Semin Dial. 2012;25(6):640–8.
218. Vachharajani TJ, Moist LM, Glickman MH, Vazquez MA, Polkinghorne KR, Lok CE, et al. Elderly patients with CKD—dilemmas in dialysis therapy and vascular access. Nat Rev Nephrol. 2014;10(2):116–22.
219. O'Hare AM, Choi AI, Bertenthal D, Bacchetti P, Garg AX, Kaufman JS, et al. Age affects outcomes in chronic kidney disease. J Am Soc Nephrol. 2007;18(10):2758–65.
220. O'Donohoe MK, Schwartz LB, Radic ZS, Mikat EM, McCann RL, Hagen PO. Chronic ACE inhibition reduces intimal hyperplasia in experimental vein grafts. Ann Surg. 1991;214(6):727–32.
221. O'Hare AM. Vascular access for hemodialysis in older adults: a "patient first" approach. J Am Soc Nephrol. 2013;24(8):1187–90.
222. Reuben DB, Tinetti ME. Goal-oriented patient care—an alternative health outcomes paradigm. N Engl J Med. 2012;366(9):777–9.
223. Archdeacon P, Shaffer RN, Winkelmayer WC, Falk RJ, Roy-Chaudhury P. Fostering innovation, advancing patient safety: the kidney health initiative. Clin J Am Soc Nephrol. 2013;8(9):1609–17.

7 Managing Anemia and Metabolic Bone Disease in Dialysis Patients

Ajay K. Singh and Jameela Kari

7.1 Anemia

Anemia occurs over 95% of patients with end-stage renal disease requiring dialysis [1]. The three most important causes of anemia in dialysis patients are: erythropoietin deficiency, because the kidney is the exclusive producer of erythropoietin; iron deficiency, because patients on dialysis have both reduced intestinal absorption of iron and some degree of blood loss during dialysis from frequent blood draws and loss of blood in the dialysis tubing and filter; and inflammation, which is almost ubiquitous among dialysis patients [1].

In most patients on dialysis, the assumption should be that erythropoietin deficiency, iron deficiency, and inflammation combine to varying degrees in determining the degree of anemia [1–3]. Understanding this balance is key to effectively managing anemia in dialysis patients. Figure 7.1a provides a practical alogrithm for managing patients. At various points, iron deficiency may be a dominant issue—for example, early in the initiation of erythropoiesis-stimulating agent (ESA) where a burst of erythropoiesis may consume available iron and exacerbate iron deficiency, which if uncorrected leads to a state of iron-restricted erythropoiesis. At other times, with a smoldering infection or a rejected allograft in place, an inflammatory mileau may induce a profound state of erythropoietin resistance where the anemia persists despite large doses of both ESA and intravenous iron [1].

Understanding the differential contribution of each of the three major causes of anemia requires work-up of patients for anemia, with a particular focus on excluding the possibility of iron deficiency, and for inflammation. Kidney Disease—Improving Global Outcomes (KDIGO) recommendations on how frequently to measure hemoglobin (Hb) and iron parameters are listed in Tables 7.1 and 7.2, respectively [1]. Although assessment of iron by a bone marrow biopsy may represent the gold standard in assessing iron stores, it is clinically impractical and measurement of serum ferritin and transferrin saturation provides the best indicators of iron stores [4, 5]. The serum ferritin is an "acute phase reactant" and is affected by inflammation. Thus, ferritin values are of greatest predictive value when low (<100 ng/mL), but of limited value when elevated. In this setting, a transferrin saturation (TSAT; serum iron × 100 divided by total iron-binding capacity) measures circulating iron that is available for erythropoiesis, and may provide actionable information on body iron stores.

The observation that there is sluggish or suboptimal correction of anemia despite treating with ESA and iron should prompt a search for an inflammatory source [6]. There are more precise definitions of ESA resistance [1]. One definition that remains in use is from the National Kidney Foundation, which defines ESA resistance as the failure to achieve the target Hb in the presence of adequate iron stores with epoetin at doses of 450 IU/kg/week intravenously or 300 IU/kg/week subcutaneously within 4–6 months of treatment initiation, or a failure to maintain the target Hb subsequently at these doses [7]. The most common laboratory indicators of ESA resistance are two acute phase reactants—ferritin and albumin—the ferritin is usually markedly elevated with a normal or low transferrin saturation, and the albumin is low despite an absence of weight loss. A CRP can also be measured and is markedly elevated in the context of inflammation.

7.1.1 The Target Hb in Patients with CKD Anemia

Four large randomized control trials (RCTs) have explored the effect of anemia correction on clinical outcomes [8–11]. These studies have examined both non-dialysis and dialysis patients.

A. K. Singh (✉)
Global and Continuing Education
Harvard Medical School, Boston, MA 02115, USA
e-mail: Ajay_Singh@hms.harvard.edu

J. Kari
Department of Pediatrics, King Abdulaziz University, Jeddah 21943, Saudi Arabia

A. K. Singh et al. (eds.), *Core Concepts in Dialysis and Continuous Therapies*, DOI 10.1007/978-1-4899-7657-4_7

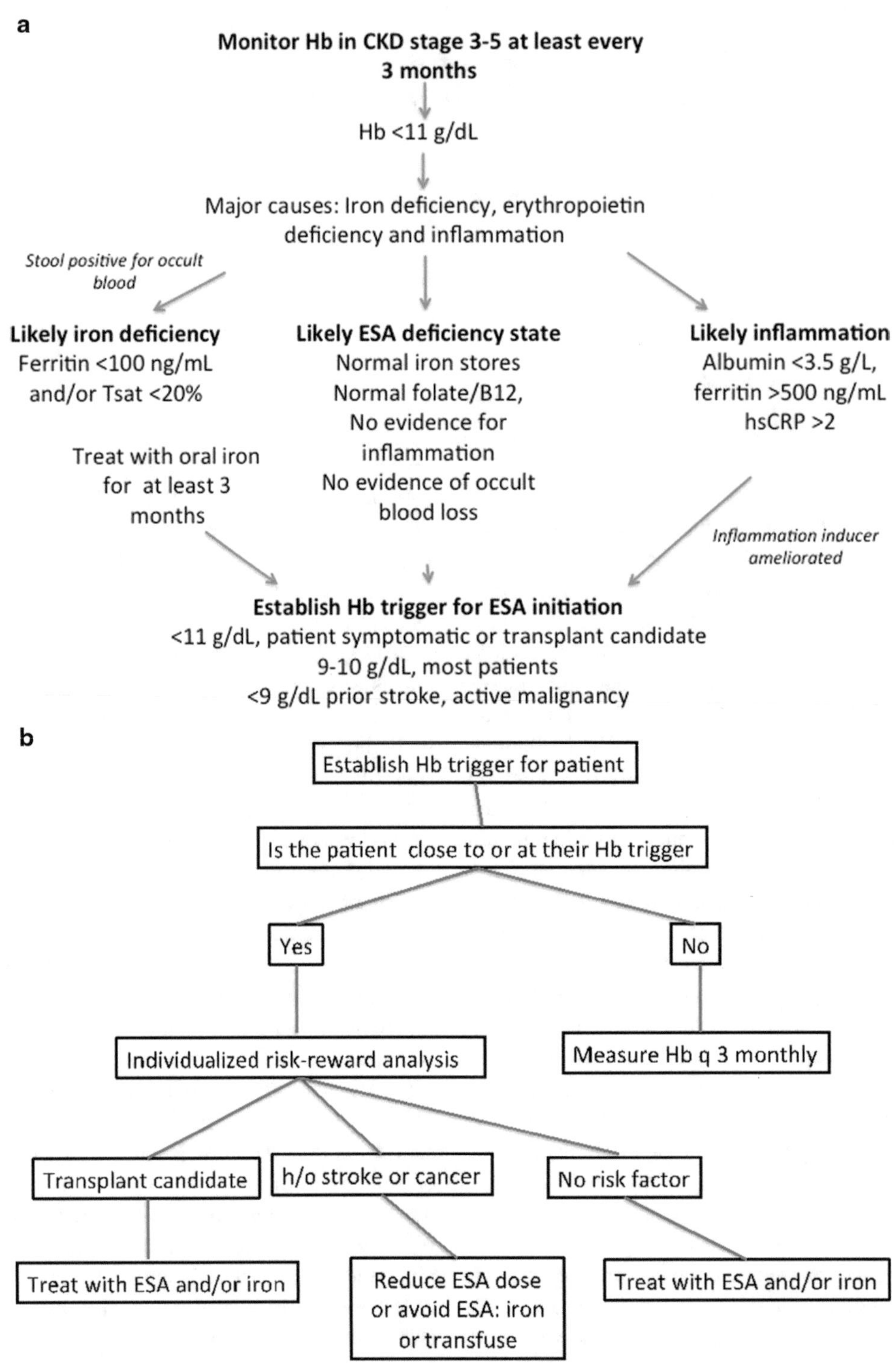

Fig. 7.1 **a** Algorithm for managing anemia in dialysis patients. **b** An alternative approach for identifying an individualized hemoglobin (Hb) concentration

The Normal Hematocrit study evaluated symptomatic dialysis patients and tested the hypothesis that the correction of anemia with epogen in hemodialysis patients with clinical evidence of congestive heart failure or ischemic heart disease would result in improved outcomes (Fig. 7.2). The primary endpoint was the length of time to death or a first nonfatal myocardial infarction. Patients were randomized to either a higher Hb concentration of 13–15 g/dL or a lower Hb arm of

Table 7.1 Testing for anemia and investigation of anemia

For CKD patients without anemia, measure Hb concentration when clinically indicated and
At least annually in patients with CKD 3
At least twice per year in patients with CKD 4–5 ND
At least every 3 months in patients with CKD 5HD and 5PD
For CKD patients with anemia not being treated with an ESA, measure Hb concentration when clinically indicated and
At least every 3 months in patients with CKD 3–5 ND and 5PD
At least monthly in patients with CKD 5HD

CKD chronic kidney disease, *Hb* hemoglobin, *ND* not on dialysis, *HD* on hemodialysis, *PD* on peritoneal dialysis, *ESA* erythropoiesis-stimulating agent

Table 7.2 Use of iron to treat anemia in chronic kidney disease (CKD)

Evaluate iron status (TSAT and ferritin) at least every 3 months during ESA therapy, including the decision to start or continue iron therapy
Test iron status (TSAT and ferritin) more frequently when initiating or increasing ESA dose, when there is blood loss, when monitoring response after a course of IV iron, and in other circumstances where iron stores may become depleted

TSAT transferrin saturation, *ESA* erythropoiesis-stimulating agent

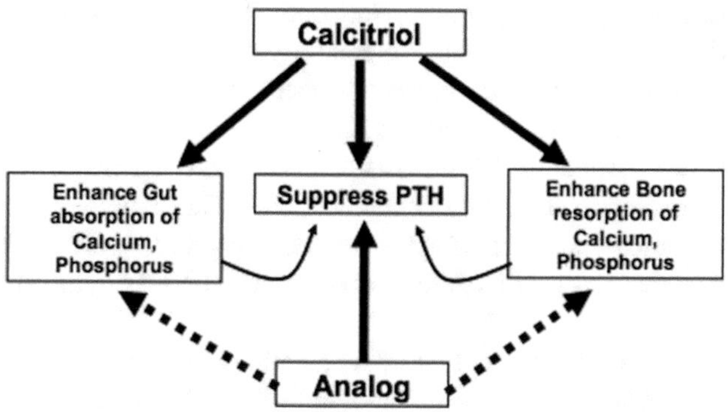

Fig. 7.2 Vitamin D action

9–11 g/dL. Patients were treated with a mean epoetin dosage of 460 U/kg/week in the high Hb arm and 160 U/kg/week in the low Hb arm. The study was halted at the third interim analysis on the recommendation of the Data Safety Monitoring Board. At 29 months, there were 183 deaths and 19 first nonfatal myocardial infarctions in the group with a normal hematocrit and 150 deaths and 14 nonfatal myocardial infarctions in the low hematocrit group (risk ratio (RR), 1.3; 95% confidence interval (CI), 0.9–1.9). There was also a higher rate of vascular thrombosis and strokes in patients in the higher Hb arm as compared to patients randomized to the lower Hb arm [8].

Three RCTs have evaluated non-dialysis chronic kidney disease (CKD) patients—Cardiovascular Reduction Early Anemia Treatment Epoetin beta (CREATE), Correction of Hemoglobin and Outcomes in Renal Insufficiency (CHOIR), Trial to Reduce Cardiovascular Events with Aranesp Therapy (TREAT) [9–11]. In all three studies, no improvement with anemia correction but instead harm with respect to a composite mortality and cardiovascular endpoint or components of the composite endpoint was observed. Taken collectively, the Normal Hematocrit, CREATE, CHOIR, and TREAT demonstrate that there is increased risk for either death or cardiovascular disease (CVD) outcomes or renal outcomes with targeting a higher Hb with higher doses of ESA. Recent meta-analyses have also reached similar conclusions. In the meta-analysis by Phrommintikul et al. [12] nine RCTs were selected on the basis of quality, sample size, and follow-up, and lumped together for a total sample of 5143 patients. Both dialysis and non-dialysis CKD trials were included. There was a higher risk of all-cause mortality (RR, 1.17; 95% CI, 1.01–1.35; p=0.031) and arteriovenous access thrombosis (RR, 1.34; 95% CI, 1.16–1.54; p=0.0001) in the higher Hb target group compared to the lower Hb target group. However, it remains uncertain whether normalization of anemia versus treatment with an ESA explains the higher risk of CVD. Synthesizing secondary analyses of the randomized trials and taking the results of the observational studies into account, the preponderance of evidence suggests that a relationship between ESA exposure and adverse outcomes is plausible—a conclusion that is also supported by evidence of adverse outcomes in non-renal populations. The US Food and Drug Administration (FDA) now recommends more conservative dosing guidelines for ESAs commensurate with these concerns.

The US FDA has also provided guidelines on the target Hb level when treating dialysis (and non-dialysis) patients with an ESA [13] (Table 7.3). While emphasizing the importance of individualizing therapy, the FDA recommends a narrow Hb "window" for treatment: initiating ESA therapy when the Hb level is <10 g/dL and interrupting or reducing ESA dose when the Hb level approaches or exceeds 11 g/dL.

The Hb targets recommended by the FDA are reasonable in a stable chronic dialysis patient, although these recommendations have generated much controversy [1, 13, 14]. However, when a dialysis patient has an acute illness and becomes more severely anemic, it becomes very challenging to manage anemia. In these circumstances, an alternative approach should be considered for identifying an individualized Hb concentration at which to intervene—identifying, if you will, the patient's "Hb trigger" (Fig. 7.1b).

The Hb trigger is the Hb level at which the patient becomes symptomatic and an intervention should be considered. For

Table 7.3 FDA recommendations for anemia treatment with an erythropoiesis-stimulating agent

Individualize therapy using the lowest ESA dose possible to reduce the need for red blood cell transfusions, and weighing the possible benefits of using ESAs to decrease the need for red blood cell transfusions against the increased risks for serious adverse cardiovascular events
For patients with CKD who have anemia and are receiving dialysis, ESA should be started when the hemoglobin level is less than 10 g/dL, and the dose should be reduced or interrupted if the hemoglobin level approaches or exceeds 11 g/dL

ESA erythropoiesis-stimulating agent, *CDK* chronic kidney disease each patient this may be different. Generally, increasing the ESA dose or treating the patient with iron is not required because the patient is already on an optimal ESA dose or already iron replete. Here, the acute illness has created a state of heightened inflammation, and either treatment of the underlying acute problem is necessary or a blood transfusion is indicated because of patient-related factors. For a young dialysis patient, an Hb of 8 g/dL may necessitate treatment for symptoms of fatigue. In contrast, for a frail patient with underlying CVD, the Hb trigger might be 10 or 11 g/dL. How high or low one lets the Hb drift has generated much controversy [15, 16], but in general needs to be individualized. Transfusing blood might be a reasonable strategy to maintain the patient above his or her individualized Hb trigger [17, 18].

Another scenario in which individualization may be necessary is when there is a need to use ESAs sparingly. For example, the KDIGO guidelines recommend caution in using ESAs in patients with a history of a stroke or in patients actively being treated with chemotherapy for a curable cancer [1]. Here, especially in a patient with cancer, a dialysis patient may be managed on a low dose or even no ESA, and decisions around transfusion will depend on the patient's individualized Hb trigger [19] .

7.1.2 Erythropoiesis-Stimulating Agents

In the era prior to the discovery of epoetin alfa (Epo), that is, before 1989, the treatment of CKD anemia consisted largely of blood transfusion and anabolic steroids. With the introduction of Epo, a transformation occurred in the management of anemia. By the 1990s, almost all patients on dialysis were receiving Epo therapy. At least initially, normalization of the Hb level in dialysis patients was recommended because observational studies, dating back to the 1990s, suggested an association between better outcomes and higher levels of Hb—lower rate of cardiovascular complications, lower mortality risk, and higher health-related quality of life. However, in 1998 with the publication of the Normal Hematocrit trial in hemodialysis patients, and in 2006 and 2009 with the publication of the CHOIR and TREAT studies in non-dialysis patients, respectively, it became clear that treatment of mild anemia with normalization of the Hb was not associated with clinically meaningful benefits. Rather, there was an increased risk of cardiovascular complications and kidney disease progression without clinically meaningful improvement in quality of life in patients assigned to a higher Hb target level. Based on these studies, the US FDA has recommended that end-stage renal disease (ESRD) patients should be treated to Hb target less than 11 g/dL.

The 2012 KDIGO Anemia guidelines backed this up by recommending against normalization of the Hb concentration and advocated for a target Hb of 9.0–11.5 g/dL [1]. The guidelines emphasized that ESAs should be used "cautiously, if at all, in patients with a prior history of a stroke or a history of cancer." The KDIGO guidelines recommend that anemia treatment in dialysis patients should be individualized based on the rate of fall of Hb concentration, prior response to iron therapy, the risk of needing a transfusion, and the risks attributable to anemia as well as those related to ESA therapy.

7.1.3 ESA Therapeutic Options

There are many ESAs currently in the market, but only two currently in the USA (Table 7.4) [19–24]. Available ESAs can be broadly divided into short- and long-acting agents. The very first ESA was Epo, marketed in the USA as Epogen and approved in 1989 by the US FDA, which is short-acting (half-life ($t_{1/2}$) of approximately 8.5 h). Epo can be administered subcutaneously or intravenously. Epo is the only short-acting ESA available currently in the USA. There are three other short-acting ESAs available in non-US markets: epoetin-beta, epoetin-omega (Repotin®, South Africa), epoetin-theta (Biopoin®, Eporatio®, Ratioepo®, Europe). Differences exist in potency, safety, tolerability, and immunogenicity among these various forms of epoetin. In addition, to different classes of short-acting Epos, Epo biosimilars are also widely available. Biosimilars are "copy-cat" agents to the innovator or originally developed ESA. Currently, no Epo biosimilar has received approval from the US FDA, although the emergence of biosimilar agents in the USA is imminent [25].

The most commonly used long-acting Epo is darbepoetin alfa (Aranesp®, Amgen, Thousand Oaks, CA, USA). Darbepoetin alfa is a hyperglycosylated Epo analogue designed for prolonged survival in the circulation and with consequent greater bioavailability than the shorter-acting epoetins (darbepoietin has a three-fold longer $t_{1/2}$ than Epo: 25.3 vs. 8.5 h) [26]. Although darbepoietin alfa was approved by the US FDA and the European Medicines Agency (EMA) in 2001, it is currently used mostly in non-dialysis CKD patients, even though it has a much longer half-life than epoetin and can

Table 7.4 Types of ESAs currently available

Available in the USA	
Type of ESA	*Duration of action*
Epoetin alfa (Epogen®/Procrit®)	Short acting
Darbepoetin-alfa (Aranesp®)	Longer acting
Not available in the USA	
Epoetin omega (Epomax)	Short acting
Epoetin delta (Dynepo)	Short acting
Epoetin beta (NeoRecormon®)	Short acting
CERA (Mircera®)	Longer acting

ESA erythropoiesis-stimulating agent

therefore be dosed less frequently ($t_{1/2}$ of darbepoetin-alfa compared with Epo is 54 vs. 16–24 h in dialysis patients).

The other long-acting epoetin that is approved worldwide is "Continuous Erythropoietin Receptor Activator (CERA)" [27]. Notably, CERA is approved in the USA but not marketed because of patent infringement issues. CERA is a molecule that has a water-soluble polyethylene glycol (PEG) moiety added to the epoetin beta molecule. The $t_{1/2}$ after intravenous administration is approximately 134 and 139 h after subcutaneous administration, and the dose is the same by either route. Peginesatide, introduced with much excitement a few years ago [28, 29], has now been withdrawn because of a series of unexpected adverse effects, including over 50 deaths among dialysis patients.

7.1.4 Iron Supplementation to Treat Anemia in Dialysis Patients

Iron deficiency is a common finding in patients in dialysis patients. Absolute iron deficiency reflects no stores of iron, and occurs when both transferrin saturation and ferritin levels are low (<20% and 100 ng/mL, respectively; reviewed extensively in reference [1] and references [30–34]). Functional iron deficiency is the inadequate release of iron to support erythropoiesis, despite the presence of adequate stores of iron. ESA therapy can be associated with functional iron deficiency when patients are inflamed (e.g., with a coexisting smoldering infection or a failed kidney allograft still in place. Functional iron deficiency should be suspected when the serum ferritin is high but transferrin saturation is low. Iron deficiency can lead to decreased effectiveness of ESA therapy, and iron therapy without ESA therapy is usually unsuccessful in patients with CKD. Untreated iron deficiency is a major cause of hyporesponsiveness to ESA treatment.

Iron deficiency is treated with iron administered either by the oral or intravenous route. Oral iron therapy is the preferred method of treating non-dialysis CKD patients. Various oral iron agents are available (Table 7.5).

Oral iron may be tried initially, but is generally not effective in hemodialysis patients because of concerns about lack of absorption due to a hepcidin-mediated functional block in absorption of iron at the level of the enterocyte iron channel. Recently, ferric citrate was approved for the control of serum phosphorus levels in ESRD patients. In addition, ferric citrate repletes iron in dialysis patients. In the ferric citrate phase 3 trials, dialysis patients treated with ferric citrate attained a higher Hb and required less intravenous iron and ESA than control patients [35, 36].

Table 7.5 Oral iron agents and elemental iron content

Iron preparations	Number of pills required to provide ~200 mg of iron	Tablet size (mg)	Amount of elemental iron (mg)/pill
Ferrous sulfate	3	325	65
Ferrous gluconate	6	325	35
Ferrous fumarate	2	325	108
Iron polysaccharide	2	150	150

Table 7.6 Intravenous iron preparations commonly used in treating iron deficiency in dialysis patients*

Product	Indication	Warnings	Total dose infusion	Relative cost
Ferric gluconate (Ferrlecit)	HD pts receiving ESA	General	No	$$$
Iron sucrose (Venofer)	HD, PD, CKD pts	General	No	$$$
LMW iron dextran (INFeD)	Iron-deficiency anemia	Black box	Yes	$$
HMW iron dextran (DexFerrum)	Iron-deficiency anemia	Black box	Yes	$

ESA erythropoiesis-stimulating agent, *CDK* chronic kidney disease, *LMW* low molecular weight, *HMW* high molecular weight
*Ferumoxytol is approved but not commonly used

Four intravenous agents are currently used the USA: iron dextran, ferrous gluconate, and iron sucrose. These agents have low molecular weight and are safer than high molecular weight iron dextran that preceded them and was associated with a high risk of anaphylaxis (Table 7.6).

The 2012 KDIGO Anemia Clinical Practice Guidelines make several recommendations about the use of iron [1]. Most of these recommendations are based on opinion rather than evidence derived from randomized trials. The KDIGO guidelines recommend that decision-making around the route of iron therapy should be governed by the severity of iron deficiency, availability of venous access, response to prior oral or intravenous iron therapy and tolerance of side effects, patient compliance, and cost. Furthermore, KDIGO suggests that decisions to continue iron therapy may be based on recent patient responses to iron therapy, TSAT and ferritin, Hb concentration, ESA responsiveness, ESA dose, ongoing blood losses, and patient's clinical status. There is much debate about when to administer intravenous iron, particularly in relation to the TSAT and ferritin levels [37]. Table 7.7 summarizes one approach that is consistent with KDIGO.

When oral iron is being considered in correcting iron deficiency in a dialysis patient, it is important to dose iron adequately. In general, 200 mg of elemental iron is necessary (ferrous sulfate 325 mg three times daily). If iron supplementation with oral iron after a 1–3-month trial is ineffective (measured by no rise in Hb level and/or no fall in ESA requirement) then it is appropriate to consider intravenous iron. Intravenous iron can be administered as a single large

Table 7.7 Practical approach to repleting iron in end stage renal disease (ESRD) patients

Hb at target	Hb<target	Hb<target	Hb<target
TSAT >20% Ferritin 200–500	TSAT >20% Ferritin 200–500	TSAT >20% Ferritin 500–800	TSAT > 20% Ferritin >800
No iron	Iron	Individualize iron	Hold iron

TSAT transferrin saturation

dose or repeated smaller doses depending on the specific intravenous iron preparation used. The initial course of intravenous iron is approximately 1000 mg in divided doses, which may be repeated if there is no effect on Hb level and/or decreased ESA dose.

Iron status should be monitored every 3 months with TSAT and ferritin while on ESA therapy [1]. When initiating or increasing ESA dose, in the setting of ongoing blood loss, or in circumstances where iron store may become depleted, it is also appropriate to monitor TSAT and ferritin more frequently. A common setting in which to monitor iron status more frequently is infection or inflammation.

7.2 Metabolic Bone Disease

Disturbances in calcium and phosphorus metabolism are common in CKD patients [38–40]. The spectrum of disorders observed in CKD patients has been defined by the KDIGO guideline group (Fig. 7.3).

As glomerular filtration rate (GFR) declines, the kidney's ability to excrete phosphorus decreases as a result of lower nephron mass and the serum phosphate level rises. In order to maintain normophosphatemia there is increased secretion of fibroblast growth factor 23 (FGF23) [41, 42], the main hormonal regulator of phosphorus homeostatis. In patients with early CKD, FGF23 stimulates increased phosphate excretion in order to maintain phosphorus homeostasis. However, in more advanced CKD, FGF23 is unable to enhance renal phosphate excretion, and hyperphosphatemia results. In addition to its effects on phosphate excretion, FGF23 stimulates parathyroid hormone (PTH) production by the parathyroid glands and reduces $1,25(OH)_2D_3$ levels through inhibition of 1-alfa hydroxylase, an enzyme produced in the kidney. Advanced kidney failure independently contributes to reduced activity of 1 alfa hydroxylase [43, 44]. Reduced $1,25(OH)_2D_3$ levels result in reduced gastrointestinal (GI) calcium absorption and hypocalcemia [45].

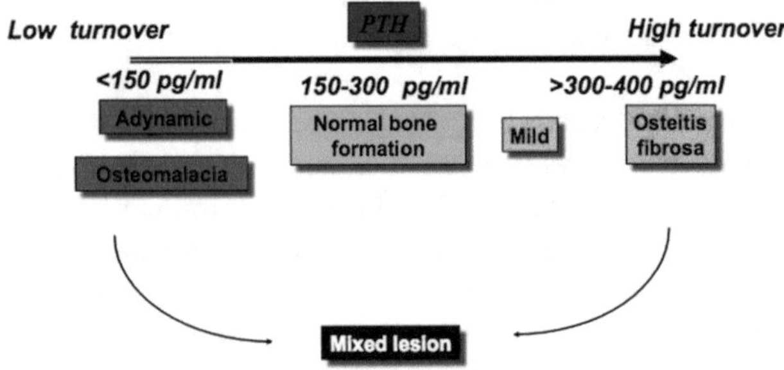

Fig. 7.3 Spectrum of mineral bone density (MBD)

The parathyroid gland is highly sensitive to even very small changes in ionized extracellular calcium and rapidly releases PTH in response to a decrease in calcium concentration. This response is mediated by the calcium-sensing receptor (CaR), the primary regulator of PTH secretion.

Calcitriol inhibits gene transcription of precursors of PTH, and therefore a decline in calcitriol leads to increased PTH production (Fig. 7.2). Decreased calcitriol has also been linked to decreased expression of vitamin D receptors (VDR) and of CaR in parathyroid tissue, which also contributes to increases in serum PTH levels.

High PTH results in osteoclast-mediated bone demineralization and in the long-term renal bone disease or osteodystrophy [43, 44].

Elevated PTH is known to contribute to pathogenesis of renal osteodystrophy and has also been implicated in damage to other systems, including cardiac, cutaneous, endocrine, immunologic, and nervous systems [45–47]. Associated imbalances in mineral homeostasis probably also contribute to organ system damage.

7.2.1 Hyperphosphatemia

In dialysis patients, the focus of management is to prevent metabolic bone disease by aiming for a serum phosphorus level within normal limits [48–51]. The normal ranges are listed in Table 7.8.

This is accomplished by controlling the serum phosphorus and PTH to normal or near-normal levels. In patients with stage 5 CKD, the target serum level of phosphorus is between 3.5 and 5.5 mg/dL [1]. To achieve these levels, a phosphate-restricted diet (800–1000 mg/day) and treatment with a phosphate binder to decrease dietary absorption of phosphate is necessary.

In patients on dialysis, it is necessary to use both a calcium-containing and non-calcium-containing phosphate binder because use of only a calcium-containing binder frequently results in a positive calcium balance and a higher risk of arterial calcification. On the other hand, managing hyperphosphatemia with only non-calcium-containing binders requires large doses of the binders leading to higher risk

Table 7.8 Normal ranges for mineral bone density (MBD) biochemical parameters

Normal phosphorus	2.5–4.5 mg/dL
Normal calcium	8.5–10 mg/dL
Normal iPTH	15–65 pg/mL (varies with the assay used)

of side-effects from these agents (e.g., bloating and GI discomfort with the use of sevelemar) and greater expense.

7.2.1.1 Calcium-Containing Binders

Calcium-containing phosphate binders are available as the calcium salts of carbonate, acetate, and citrate [52]. Calcium citrate increases aluminum absorption and should be avoided. Calcium acetate is the most potent phosphate binder in this class. Although calcium-containing binders provide an effective means of controlling phosphorus, their use may not be without risk. Calcium excess induced by the prescription of large doses of calcium-containing phosphate binders has been associated with calcifications of the aorta and the carotid and coronary arteries; calcium-containing phosphate binders have been implicated in the acceleration of vascular disease that accompanies advancing CKD. Widespread use of these drugs may also play a contributory role in the development of calciphylaxis.

Calcium-containing binders should not be used if the patient has hypercalcemia (>10.2 mg/dL), a PTH <150 pg/mL, or evidence of severe extraskeletal calcification. The total intake of elemental calcium should not exceed 2000 mg/day, and the total dose of elemental calcium provided by calcium-based binders should not exceed 1500 mg/day.

7.2.1.2 Non-Calcium-Containing Binders

There are 4 types of non-calcium-containing phosphorus binders: Sevelamer, lanthanum, aluminum hydroxide, and ferric citrate [53–55].

Sevelamer is available as sevelemar hydrochloride (RenaGel) or sevelamer carbonate (Renvela). Both are calcium- and aluminum-free phosphate binders that control serum phosphorus and reduce PTH levels without inducing hypercalcemia. In addition, both lower serum cholesterol levels. Sevelamer hydrochloride is an exchange resin that releases chloride in exchange for phosphate. The subsequent formation of hydrochloric acid creates an acid load and may cause metabolic acidosis; sevelamer carbonate is less likely to cause acidosis.

Lanthanum carbonate (Fosrenol) is also a calcium- and aluminum-free binder that is approved for the treatment of hyperphosphatemia in patients with ESRD. The initial clinical experience has shown the drug to be both effective and well tolerated. Oral bioavailability of lanthanum is very low, and the drug is excreted largely unabsorbed in the feces. There has been concern about the long-term safety of lanthanum because of reports of tissue deposition of lanthanum in the liver, lung, and kidney in animal models exposed to lanthanum. However, no long-term toxicity has been reported in humans.

Aluminum is a powerful phosphate binder because it forms a very strong ionic bond with phosphorus. However, because of concerns about long-term toxicity, including dementia and aluminum bone disease, aluminum-containing binders have largely fallen from favor. In patients with severe hyperphosphatemia refractory to treatment, aluminum-containing compounds such as aluminum hydroxide and aluminum carbonate may be used as a short-term therapy (for up to 1 month); thereafter, they should be replaced with either lanthanum or sevelamer.

Ferric citrate is a newly approved phosphate binder, effective in both reducing hyperphosphatemia and correcting iron deficiency [56]. Ferric citrate works as well as sevelemar or calcium carbonate as a phosphate binder. Ferric citrate also effectively reduces both intravenous iron and ESA utilization and thus could become the default therapeutic agent in dialysis patients, both for phosphate control and iron repletion. A maximum of 12 tablets of ferric citrate may be given with meals. It is likely, however, that 12 tablets each day (doses as much as 12 g of ferric citrate) are unlikely to be well tolerated by patients—the most common adverse effects being GI (nausea, vomiting, diarrhea, and constipation). Each tablet of ferric citrate (1 g ferric citrate) is 210 mg of ferric iron.

7.3 Metabolic Bone Disease

There are a spectrum of metabolic bone disease abnormalities in ESRD patients [57] (Fig. 7.3). On one end of the spectrum is low turnover "adynamic bone disease" (ABD), which occurs in a minority of patients. On the other side of the spectrum is secondary and tertiary hyperparathyroidism—high-turnover bone disease osteitis fibrosa.

7.3.1 Low Turnover Adynamic Bone Disease

ABD is characterized by extremely low bone turnover with reduced synthesis of bone matrix owing to decreased osteoblastic and osteoclastic activity [58]. In association with reduced bone formation rates (BFR), there is a lack of osteoid accumulation differentiating this abnormality from osteomalacia. Whether ABD is a benign, asymptomatic condition of ESRD has been a matter of debate since its first description. The two major concerns with ABD are the frequent episodes of hypercalcemia with possible soft tissue calcification, and increased risk for fractures due to the impaired remodeling process. The most likely mechanism for the occurrence of ABD is the relative hypoparathyroidism seen in these patients. As the serum-ionized calcium level is one of the most powerful factors affecting PTH secretion, a continuously positive calcium balance associated with oral calcium carbonate ($CaCO_3$) treatment, vitamin D administration, and supraphysiological dialysate calcium may lead to oversuppression of parathyroid gland activity.

7.3.2 High Turnover Bone Disease

When PTH levels remain persistently elevated, secondary hyperparathyroidism develops. Left untreated, secondary hyperparathyroidism can progress to refractory hyperparathyroidism, a condition in which the parathyroid glands become autonomous and release high amounts of PTH out of proportion to a patient's hypocalcemia or hyperphosphatemia; this may occur in late-stage CKD or in ESRD. Secondary hyperparathyroidism is associated with effects on bone—ostitis fibrosis cystica, where osteoclasts stimulated by chronically elevated concentrations of PTH cause severe bone loss and predispose patients to fractures and bone cysts.

Monitoring and treatment of an elevated PTH level may help prevent the development of secondary hyperparathyroidism. The KDIGO guidelines recommend a PTH target in dialysis patients of 2–9 times the upper limit of the normal PTH range (the Kidney Disease Outcomes Quality Initiative (KDOQI) target is 150–300 pg/mL). The target values for PTH in patients with dialysis patients is higher than normal because higher levels are thought to be required for normal bone remodeling, and suppression of PTH to normal nonuremic values may be associated with a higher prevalence of adynamic bone disease. Monthly monitoring of PTH is necessary in order to calibrate the use of active vitamin D therapy. Monthly monitoring of serum calcium and phosphorus levels is also recommended.

In addition to vitamin D and its analogues, cinacalcet (Sensipar) is now widely used [59–61]. Cinacalcet was approved in 2004 and is a calcimimetic that binds to the calcium-sensing receptor in the parathyroid gland and leads to reductions in PTH release. However, to date, there is no definitive proof that cinacalcet improves hard outcomes in patients with CVD or bone disease. In this regard, EValuation Of Cinacalcet Hydrochloride Therapy to Lower CardioVascular Events (EVOLVE) [62–64], a double-blind randomized trial of 3883 hemodialysis patients with moderate to severe hyperparathyroidism (cinacalcet versus placebo) was null with respect to the primary composite endpoint of time to death, myocardial infarction (MI), hospitalization for unstable angina, heart failure, or a peripheral vascular event [62]. The fracture rate between the two arms of the study was not different. However, patients randomized to cinacalcet had a 50 % lower rate of parathyroidectomy, but hypocalcemia was common in the active treatment arm. Importantly, however, the trial has been criticized for the high rate of cross-overs between the two arms of the study and for imbalances in baseline characteristics [63, 64].

As with active vitamin D therapy, cinacalcet effectively lowers the circulating levels of PTH; however, it does not cause the increased GI absorption of calcium and phosphorus associated with vitamin D therapy. Hypocalcemia can occur in a small percentage of patients. In patients with ESRD, combination therapy with cinacalcet and active vitamin D is advantageous, but the optimal mix has not yet been determined.

7.3.3 Parathroidectomy in Dialysis Patients

While most dialysis patients are now managed successfully with cinacalcet, active vitamin D, and management of hyperphosphatemia, some patients become refactory to medical management. These patients are usually characterized by severe clinical, biochemical, and radiological hyperparathyroidism. The PTH levels are usually very high (8–20-fold higher than the upper limit of normal (ULN) for PTH) and resistant to high-dose vitamin D and cinacalcet therapy. The serum calcium is either normal or more commonly elevated. Morphologically, there is evidence of nodular hyperplasia in very enlarged parathyroid glands. There is also evidence of monoclonality (monoclonal proliferation) in the nodules.

While ethanol injection into the largest parathyroid glands is sometimes used to treat refractory hyperparathyroidism, the mainstay is surgical parathyroidectomy [65, 66]. There are three surgical options: subtotal parathyroidectomy, total parathyroidectomy with parathyroid autotransplantation, and total parathyroidectomy without autografting. The main disadvantage of the first two options is recurrence of hyperparathyroidism, whereas the main disadvantage of the latter approach, that is, total parathyroidectomy without autografting is the risk of adynamic bone disease and vascular calcification. Even with this approach, however, detectable PTH levels have been reported because residual tissue is left behind following surgery.

References

1. Kidney Disease. Improving global outcomes (KDIGO) Anemia Work Group. KDIGO clinical practice guideline for anemia in chronic kidney disease. Kidney Int Suppl. 2012;2:279–335.
2. Hsu CY. Epidemiology of anemia associated with chronic renal insufficiency. Curr Opin Nephrol Hypertens. 2002;11:337.
3. Babitt JL, Lin HY. Mechanisms of anemia in CKD. J Am Soc Nephrol. 2012;23(10):1631–4.
4. Lipschitz DA, Cook JD, Finch CA. A clinical evaluation of serum ferritin as an index of iron stores. N Engl J Med. 1974;290(22):1213–6.
5. Fishbane S, Kowalski EA, Imbriano LJ, Maesaka JK. The evaluation of iron status in hemodialysis patients. J Am Soc Nephrol. 1996;7(12):2654–7.
6. Singh AK, Coyne DW, Shapiro W, Rizkala AR, DRIVE Study Group. Predictors of the response to treatment in anemic hemodialysis patients with high serum ferritin and low transferrin saturation. Kidney Int. 2007;71(11):1163–71. Epub 2007 Mar 28.
7. National Kidney Foundation/Kidney disease outcomes quality initiative NKF/KDOQI clinical practice guidelines and clinical practice recommendations for anemia in chronic kidney disease; http://www2.kidney.org/professionals/KDOQI/guidelines_anemiaUP/
8. Besarab A, Bolton WK, Browne JK, Egrie JC, Nissenson AR, Okamoto DM, Schwab SJ, Goodkin DA. The effects of normal as compared with low hematocrit values in patients with cardiac disease who are receiving hemodialysis and epoetin. N Engl J Med. 1998;339(9):584–90.

9. Drueke TB, Locatelli F, Clyne N, Eckardt KU, Macdougall IC, Tsakiris D, Burger HU, Scherhag A, CREATE Investigators. Normalization of hemoglobin level in patients with chronic kidney disease and anemia. N Engl J Med. 2006;355(20):2071–84.
10. Singh AK, Szczech L, Tang KL, Barnhart H, Sapp S, Wolfson M, Reddan D, CHOIR Investigators. Correction of anemia with epoetin alfa in chronic kidney disease. N Engl J Med. 2006;355(20):2085–98.
11. Pfeffer MA, Burdmann EA, Chen CY, Cooper ME, de Zeeuw D, Eckardt KU, Feyzi JM, Ivanovich P, Kewalramani R, Levey AS, Lewis EF, McGill JB, McMurray JJ, Parfrey P, Parving HH, Remuzzi G, Singh AK, Solomon SD, Toto R, the TREAT Investigators. A trial of darbepoetin alfa in type 2 diabetes and chronic kidney disease. N Engl J Med. 2009;361(21):2019–32. [Epub ahead of print].
12. Phrommintikul A, Haas SJ, Elsik M, et al. Mortality and target haemoglobin concentrations in anaemic patients with chronic kidney disease treated with erythropoietin: a meta-analysis. Lancet. 2007;369:381.
13. http://www.fda.gov/Drugs/DrugSafety/ucm259639.htm. Accessed 24 June 2011.
14. Singh AK. ESAs in dialysis patients: are you a hedgehog or a fox? J Am Soc Nephrol. 2010;21(4):543–6. [Epub ahead of print].
15. Rosner MH, Bolton WK. The mortality risk associated with higher hemoglobin: is the therapy to blame? Kidney Int. 2008;74(6):695–7.
16. Fishbane S, Masani NN, Hazzan AD. Should target hemoglobin levels in dialysis patients be lowered to 9–10 g/dl? Semin Dial. 2014;27(3):282–4. doi:10.1111/sdi.12211. Epub 2014 Mar 25. Review. PubMed PMID: 24666175.
17. Macdougall IC, Obrador GT. How important is transfusion avoidance in 2013? Nephrol Dial Transpl. 2013;28(5):1092–9. doi:10.1093/ndt/gfs575. Epub 2013 Mar 13. Review. PubMed PMID: 23486660.
18. Carless PA, Henry DA, Carson JL, Hebert PP, McClelland B, Ker K. Transfusion thresholds and other strategies for guiding allogeneic red blood cell transfusion. Cochrane Database Syst Rev. 2010;10:CD002042.
19. Hazzan AD, Shah HH, Hong S, Sakhiya V, Wanchoo R, Fishbane S. Treatment with erythropoiesis-stimulating agents in chronic kidney disease patients with cancer. Kidney Int. 2014;86(1):34–9. doi:10.1038/ki.2013.528. Epub 2014 Jan 8. PubMed PMID: 24402094.
20. Palmer SC, Navaneethan SD, Craig JC, et al. Erythropoiesis-stimulating agents in patients with chronic kidney disease. Ann Intern Med. 2010;153:23.
21. Del Vecchio L, Locatelli F. Anemia in chronic kidney disease patients: treatment recommendations and emerging therapies. Expert Rev Hematol. 2014;7(4):495–506. doi:10.1586/17474086.2014.941349. Review. PubMed PMID: 25025373.
22. Malyszko J. New renal anemia drugs: is there really anything new on the horizon? Expert Opin Emerg Drugs. 2014;19(1):1–4. doi:10.1517/14728214.2014.872239. Epub 2013 Dec 18. Review. PubMed PMID: 24344917.
23. Fishbane S, Shah HH. Choice of erythropoiesis stimulating agent in ESRD. Nephrol News Issues. 2013;27(7):10–2. PubMed PMID: 23855143.
24. Macdougall IC. New anemia therapies: translating novel strategies from bench to bedside. Am J Kidney Dis. 2012;59(3):444–51. doi:10.1053/j.ajkd.2011.11.013. Epub 2011 Dec 21. Review. PubMed PMID: 22192713.
25. Fishbane S, Shah HH. The emerging role of biosimilar epoetins in nephrology in the United States. Am J Kidney Dis. 2015;65(4):537–42. doi:10.1053/j.ajkd.2014.11.018. Epub 2015 Jan 10. PubMed PMID: 25582283.
26. Macdougall IC. An overview of the efficacy and safety of novel erythropoiesis stimulating protein (NESP). Nephrol Dial Transpl. 2001;16(Suppl 3):14–21. Review. PubMed PMID: 11402086.
27. Macdougall IC. CERA (Continuous Erythropoietin Receptor Activator): a new erythropoiesis-stimulating agent for the treatment of anemia. Curr Hematol Rep. 2005;4(6):436–40. Review. PubMed PMID: 16232379.
28. Macdougall IC, Provenzano R, Sharma A, Spinowitz BS, Schmidt RJ, Pergola PE, Zabaneh RI, Tong-Starksen S, Mayo MR, Tang H, Polu KR, Duliege AM, Fishbane S, PEARL Study Groups. Peginesatide for anemia in patients with chronic kidney disease not receiving dialysis. N Engl J Med. 2013;368(4):320–32. doi:10.1056/NEJMoa1203166. PubMed PMID: 23343062.
29. Fishbane S, Schiller B, Locatelli F, Covic AC, Provenzano R, Wiecek A, Levin NW, Kaplan M, Macdougall IC, Francisco C, Mayo MR, Polu KR, Duliege AM, Besarab A, EMERALD Study Groups. Peginesatide in patients with anemia undergoing hemodialysis. N Engl J Med. 2013;368(4):307–19. doi:10.1056/NEJMoa1203165. PubMed PMID: 23343061.
30. Auerbach M. Intravenous iron and chronic kidney disease. Am J Hematol. 2014;89(11):1083. doi:10.1002/ajh.23849. Epub 2014 Sep 26. PubMed PMID: 25219516.
31. Charytan DM, Pai AB, Chan CT, Coyne DW, Hung AM, Kovesdy CP, Fishbane S, Dialysis Advisory Group of the American Society of Nephrology. Considerations and challenges in defining optimal iron utilization in hemodialysis. J Am Soc Nephrol. 2015;26(6):1238–47. doi:10.1681/ASN.2014090922. Epub 2014 Dec 26. PubMed PMID: 25542967; PubMed Central PMCID: PMC4446883.
32. Malyszko J, Koc-Zorawska E, Levin-Iaina N, Slotki I, Matuszkiewicz-Rowinska J, Glowinska I, Malyszko JS. Iron metabolism in hemodialyzed patients—a story half told? Arch. Med Sci. 2014;10(6):1117–22. doi:10.5114/aoms.2014.47823. PubMed PMID: 25624847; PubMed Central PMCID: PMC4296069.
33. Goodkin DA, Bailie GR. Intravenous iron, inflammation, and ventricular dysfunction during hemodialysis. Am J Kidney Dis. 2015;65(3):518. doi:10.1053/j.ajkd.2014.09.030. PubMed PMID: 25704045.
34. Coyne DW. It's time to compare anemia management strategies in hemodialysis. Clin J Am Soc Nephrol. 2010;5(4):740–2. doi:10.2215/CJN.02490409. Epub 2010 Mar 18. PubMed PMID: 20299363.
35. Umanath K, Jalal DI, Greco BA, Umeukeje EM, Reisin E, Manley J, Zeig S, Negoi DG, Hiremath AN, Blumenthal SS, Sika M, Niecestro R, Koury MJ, Ma KN, Greene T, Lewis JB, Dwyer JP; for the Collaborative Study Group. Ferric citrate reduces intravenous iron and erythropoiesis-stimulating agent use in ESRD. J Am Soc Nephrol. 2015;26(10):2578–87. pii: ASN.2014080842. [Epub ahead of print] PubMed PMID: 25736045.
36. Block GA, Fishbane S, Rodriguez M, Smits G, Shemesh S, Pergola PE, Wolf M, Chertow GM. A 12-week, double-blind placebo-controlled trial of ferric citrate for the treatment of iron deficiency anemia and reduction of serum phosphate in patients with CKD Stages 3–5. Am J Kidney Dis. 2015;65(5):728–36. doi:10.1053/j.ajkd.2014.10.014. Epub 2014 Nov 4. PubMed PMID: 25468387.
37. Sharma A, Vanderhalt K, Ryan KJ, Sclafani J. Refining the approach to IV iron use in hemodialysis patients: a post-DRIVE analysis. Nephrol News Issues. 2010;24(4):22–6, 29–35. PubMed PMID: 20458992.
38. Kidney Disease. Improving global outcomes (KDIGO) CKD-MBD Work Group. KDIGO clinical practice guide- line for the diagnosis, evaluation, prevention, and treatment of Chronic Kidney Disease-Mineral and Bone Disorder (CKD-MBD). Kidney Int Suppl. 2009;113:S1–S130.
39. Moe S, Drueke T, Cunningham J, et al. Definition, evaluation, and classification of renal osteodystrophy: a position statement from kidney disease: improving global outcomes (KDIGO). Kidney Int. 2006;69(11):1945–53.

40. National Kidney Foundation. K/DOQI clinical practice guidelines for bone metabolism and disease in chronic kidney disease. Am J Kidney Dis. 2003;42(Suppl 3):1–202.
41. Zoccali C, Yilmaz MI, Mallamaci F. FGF23: a mature renal and cardiovascular risk factor? Blood Purif. 2013;36(1):52–7. doi:10.1159/000351001. Epub 2013 May 25. Review. PubMed PMID: 23735695.
42. Wolf M. Update on fibroblast growth factor 23 in chronic kidney disease. Kidney Int. 2012;82(7):737–47. doi:10.1038/ki.2012.176. Epub 2012 May 23. Review. PubMed PMID: 22622492; PubMed Central PMCID: PMC3434320.
43. Isakova T. Fibroblast growth factor 23 and adverse clinical outcomes in chronic kidney disease. Curr Opin Nephrol Hypertens. 2012;21(3):334–40. doi:10.1097/MNH.0b013e328351a391. Review. PubMed PMID: 22487610; PubMed Central PMCID: PMC3353875.
44. Li YC. Vitamin D in chronic kidney disease. Contrib Nephrol. 2013;180:98–109. doi:10.1159/000346789. Epub 2013 May 3. Review. PubMed PMID: 23652553.
45. Duranton F, Rodriguez-Ortiz ME, Duny Y, Rodriguez M, Daurès JP, Argilés A. Vitamin D treatment and mortality in chronic kidney disease: a systematic review and meta-analysis. Am J Nephrol. 2013;37(3):239–48. doi:10.1159/000346846. Epub 2013 Mar 5. Review. PubMed PMID: 23467111.
46. Danese MD, Halperin M, Lowe KA, Bradbury BD, Do TP, Block GA. Refining the definition of clinically important mineral and bone disorder in hemodialysis patients. Nephrol Dial Transpl. 2015;30(8):1336–44. pii:gfv034. [Epub ahead of print] PubMed PMID: 25817224.
47. Block GA, Kilpatrick RD, Lowe KA, Wang W, Danese MD. CKD-mineral and bone disorder and risk of death and cardiovascular hospitalization in patients on hemodialysis. Clin J Am Soc Nephrol. 2013;8(12):2132–40. doi:10.2215/CJN.04260413. Epub 2013 Sep 19. PubMed PMID: 24052218; PubMed Central PMCID: PMC3848404.
48. Block GA, Hulbert-Shearon TE, Levin NW, et al. Association of serum phosphorus and calcium x phosphate product with mortality risk in chronic hemodialysis patients: a national study. Am J Kidney Dis. 1998;31(4):607–17.
49. Block GA, Ix JH, Ketteler M, Martin KJ, Thadhani RI, Tonelli M, Wolf M, Jüppner H, Hruska K, Wheeler DC. Phosphate homeostasis in CKD: report of a scientific symposium sponsored by the National Kidney Foundation. Am J Kidney Dis. 2013;62(3):457–73. doi:10.1053/j.ajkd.2013.03.042. Epub 2013 Jun 12. Review. PubMed PMID: 23763855.
50. Cannata-Andía JB, Martin KJ. The challenge of controlling phosphorus in chronic kidney disease. Nephrol Dial Transpl. 2015;pii:gfv055. [Epub ahead of print] Review. PubMed PMID: 25770169.
51. Centre for Clinical Practice at NICE (UK). Hyperphosphataemia in chronic kidney disease: management of hyperphosphataemia in patients with stage 4 or 5 chronic kidney disease. Manchester: National Institute for Health and Clinical Excellence (UK); 2013. PubMed PMID: 25340244.
52. Finn WF. Phosphorus management in end-stage renal disease. Semin Dial. 2005;18:8.
53. Slatopolsky EA, Burke SK, Dillon MA. RenaGel, a nonabsorbed calcium- and aluminum-free phosphate binder, lowers serum phosphorus and parathyroid hormone. The RenaGel Study Group. Kidney Int. 1999;55:299.
54. Pai AB, Shepler BM. Comparison of sevelamer hydrochloride and sevelamer carbonate: risk of metabolic acidosis and clinical applications. Pharmacotherapy. 2009;29(5):554–61.
55. Joy MS, Kshirsagar A, Candiani C. Lanthanum carbonate. Ann Pharmacother. 2006;40:234.
56. Yokoyama K, Hirakata H, Akiba T, Fukagawa M, Nakayama M, Sawada K, Kumagai Y, Block GA. Ferric citrate hydrate for the treatment of hyperphosphatemia in nondialysis-dependent CKD. Clin J Am Soc Nephrol. 2014;9(3):543–52. doi:10.2215/CJN.05170513. Epub 2014 Jan 9. PubMed PMID: 24408120; PMCID: PMC3944759.
57. Al-Badr W, Martin KJ. Vitamin D and kidney disease. Clin J Am Soc Nephrol. 2008;3(5):1555–60.
58. Frazão JM, Martins P. Adynamic bone disease: clinical and therapeutic implications. Curr Opin Nephrol Hypertens. 2009;18(4):303–7. doi:10.1097/MNH.0b013e32832c4df0. Review. PubMed PMID: 19424062.
59. Ballinger AE, Palmer SC, Nistor I, Craig JC, Strippoli GF. Calcimimetics for secondary hyperparathyroidism in chronic kidney disease patients. Cochrane Database Syst Rev. 2014;12:CD006254. doi:10.1002/14651858.CD006254.pub2. Epub 2014 Dec 9. Review. PubMed PMID: 25490118.
60. Drüeke TB. Calcimimetics and outcomes in CKD. Kidney Int Suppl (2011). 2013;3(5):431–5. Review. PubMed PMID: 25028644; PubMed Central PMCID: PMC4089624.
61. Plosker GL. Cinacalcet: a pharmacoeconomic review of its use in secondary hyperparathyroidism in end-stage renal disease. Pharmacoeconomics. 2011;29(9):807–21. doi:10.2165/11207220-000000000-00000. Review. PubMed PMID:21838333.
62. EVOLVE Trial Investigators, Chertow GM, Block GA, Correa-Rotter R, Drüeke TB, Floege J, Goodman WG, Herzog CA, Kubo Y, London GM, Mahaffey KW, Mix TC, Moe SM, Trotman ML, Wheeler DC, Parfrey PS. Effect of cinacalcet on cardiovascular disease in patients undergoing dialysis. N Engl J Med. 2012;367(26):2482–94. doi:10.1056/NEJMoa1205624. Epub 2012 Nov 3. PubMed PMID:23121374.
63. Perkovic V, Neal B. Trials in kidney disease—time to EVOLVE. N Engl J Med. 2012;367(26):2541–2. doi:10.1056/NEJMe1212368. Epub 2012 Nov 3. PubMed PMID: 23121375.
64. Moe SM, Thadhani R. What have we learned about chronic kidney disease-mineral bone disorder from the EVOLVE and PRIMO trials? Curr Opin Nephrol Hypertens. 2013;22(6):651–5. doi:10.1097/MNH.0b013e328365b3a3. Review. PubMed PMID: 24100218; PubMed Central PMCID: PMC3983668.
65. Kuo LE, Wachtel H, Karakousis G, Fraker D, Kelz R. Parathyroidectomy in dialysis patients. J Surg Res. 2014;190(2):554–8. doi:10.1016/j.jss.2014.05.027. Epub 2014 May 20. PubMed PMID: 24950795.
66. Ishani A, Liu J, Wetmore JB, Lowe KA, Do T, Bradbury BD, Block GA, Collins AJ. Clinical outcomes after parathyroidectomy in a nationwide cohort of patients on hemodialysis. Clin J Am Soc Nephrol. 2015;10(1):90–7. doi:10.2215/CJN.03520414. Epub 2014 Dec 16. PubMed PMID: 25516915; PubMed Central PMCID: PMC4284409.

Part II

Home Therapies

8 Technology of Peritoneal Dialysis

Seth B. Furgeson and Isaac Teitelbaum

8.1 Introduction

Peritoneal dialysis (PD) is a home dialysis modality that provides patients with flexibility and control over their dialysis treatments and often the freedom to continue employment. In addition, for reasons that are incompletely understood—perhaps related to greater hemodynamic stability—peritoneal dialysis is associated with a slower decline in residual renal function. On the other hand, patients performing home dialysis must assume the responsibility for administering and monitoring the therapy. In contrast to home hemodialysis , PD can be performed as a continuous therapy without the need for vascular access. However, in order for PD to be successful, numerous technical details of the therapy need to be optimized. This chapter will describe the best practices regarding peritoneal catheter placement, PD solutions, and efforts to maintain a healthy peritoneal membrane.

8.2 Peritoneal Dialysis Catheter

A well-functioning PD catheter is crucial for the long-term success of PD. Catheters that have migrated or have been trapped in omentum may not drain appropriately leading to fluid retention and inadequate solute clearance. Dialysate leaks at the catheter exit site can impair ultrafiltration and adversely affect patients' quality of life. Finally, since peritonitis and catheter infections are leading causes of PD technique failure, catheter designs and implantation practices that minimize infection risk may also improve technique survival.

S. B. Furgeson (✉)
University of Colorado-Anschutz Medical Campus, Aurora, CO, USA
e-mail: seth.furgeson@ucdenver.edu

I. Teitelbaum
Department of Medicine, University of Colorado Hospital, Aurora, CO, USA

Table 8.1 Modifiable components of peritoneal dialysis (PD) catheters

Silicone or polyurethane composition
Coiled or straight intraperitoneal segment
Single or double cuffed catheter
Curved (swan-neck) or straight catheter
Abdominal exit site or extender for presternal exit site

8.2.1 Catheter Characteristics

PD catheters have many potential modifications (Table 8.1). Catheters are made from polyurethane or silicone rubber. The intra-abdominal portion of the catheter can be coiled or straight and the portion within the anterior abdominal wall can have one or two cuffs. Furthermore, there are many modifications that can be made in the subcutaneous portion of the catheter to guide the catheter exit from the abdominal wall. Since the catheter possesses "memory," they tend to revert to their initial conformation. Swan-neck catheters possess a preformed bend that promotes a downward-directed exit from the abdominal wall exit site as well as a downward direction of the intraperitoneal portion of the catheter thereby preventing catheter migration. Other catheters have a straight segment between two cuffs to promote a lateral exit. Some of the above modifications have been compared in randomized trials; however, many of the trials have significant methodological limitations that limit the conclusions.

As compared to catheters made of silicone rubber, polyurethane catheters have greater tensile strength with a thinner wall and larger internal diameter. Those characteristics are desirable as they will positively influence dialysate flow rate. However, polyurethane is prone to damage with numerous antimicrobial solutions. Mupirocin ointment (containing polyethylene glycol) and alcohol have both been reported to cause damage to the catheter wall. Spontaneous rupture of the PD catheter has been reported with mupirocin ointment [1]. Therefore, most catheters used today are made of silicone rubber.

A. K. Singh et al. (eds.), *Core Concepts in Dialysis and Continuous Therapies*, DOI 10.1007/978-1-4899-7657-4_8

Catheters with a coiled intraperitoneal segment offer some potential advantages over straight catheters. Coiled catheters were designed to create better separation between loops of bowel and contain numerous side ports. Since a smaller amount of dialysate moves through each side port, coiled catheters may reduce infusion pain. However, clear benefits of coiled catheters have not been seen in most studies. Comparisons between coiled and straight catheters have been the subject of numerous trials [2]. Most of the early randomized trials were small (fewer than 50 total patients) and reached different conclusions regarding the superiority of either catheter. Furthermore, some of the earlier studies had very high rates of catheter dysfunction raising questions about the generalizability of the results. The two most recent randomized studies of straight versus coiled catheters have also been the largest, enrolling 80 and 132 patients, respectively. The smaller study found that catheter migration occurred more commonly with coiled catheters [3]. The study by Johnson et al. demonstrated better catheter survival with straight catheters, an effect thought to be related to improved small solute clearance [4]. Given small sample sizes from all studies, firm recommendations from the trials are not possible. It should also be noted that the surgical implantation techniques and exit site management may differ significantly between the study sites and other PD centers.

After exiting the peritoneal cavity, catheters can be anchored in the subcutaneous space with either one or two cuffs. Two cuffs may more firmly anchor the catheter in the subcutaneous space. It has been suggested that a double-cuff catheter may also provide a better barrier to bacterial spread along the catheter tunnel. The largest randomized study to test this benefit enrolled 60 patients and randomized them to either a double-cuff or single-cuff catheter [5]. The study demonstrated no benefit in peritonitis, exit site infections, or catheter infection with the double-cuff catheter. A retrospective study did demonstrate a benefit to preventing peritonitis with the use of double-cuffed catheters; however, this effect is lost in the post-2000 era [6]. Alignment of the intercuff segment of a double-cuff catheter can also improve a catheter's success. Since plastic catheters will maintain "memory" and revert to the original position, aligning the intercuff segment in the original position may help maintain the intraperitoneal segment in the pelvis.

The catheter conformation in the subcutaneous segment may either be curved (swan neck) or straight. The swan-neck conformation is designed to maintain a low, pelvic location of the intra-abdominal component as well as a downward-facing exit site. If a straight catheter has a downward-facing exit site, catheter "memory" may increase the likelihood of the intraperitoneal segment migrating to the upper abdomen. As with the other modifications, the swan-neck or straight catheters have been compared in small, randomized trials [2]. The trials have shown no difference in infection rates or migration. However, observational studies have suggested that swan-neck catheters have fewer episodes of catheter dysfunction [7].

8.2.2 Implantation Technique

The implantation procedure is as important as catheter characteristics for long-term catheter performance. The surgical technique can be performed blindly, using a laparoscopic approach, or through an open surgical approach. The blind approach (using the Seldinger technique) may be associated with more complications, such as bowel injury. A major disadvantage to this approach is the inability to simultaneously repair hernias or perform omentopexy [8]. Both surgical approaches (open and laparoscopic) are safe and allow the simultaneous repair of hernias.

Regardless of the specific implantation technique, the catheter tip should lie in the true pelvis. If the tip is located higher in the peritoneal cavity, there is a much higher risk for omental entrapment and catheter dysfunction. It is thought that placement in the left pelvis may be preferred over the right pelvis as peristalsis may continue to push the catheter in a downward direction. After catheter placement, tip migration can certainly be seen, often with constipation. If relief of constipation does not revert the catheter tip into the pelvis, surgical correction can often return the tip to the pelvis without requiring surgical placement of a new catheter.

Since omental entrapment often impairs catheter drainage, there are numerous approaches that attempt to prevent this complication. One described approach has been prophylactic removal of omentum [9]. However, this procedure significantly increases the complexity of the surgery and may be too aggressive since most patients never have omental entrapment. Another approach to manage the omentum has been described by Crabtree [8]. In this approach, the surgeon first examines the omentum to see if it will border the catheter tip in the pelvis. If the exam does suggest that there could be omental–catheter interactions in the pelvis, an omentopexy is performed. Omentopexy involves tacking the omentum to the abdominal wall and can be performed more quickly than an omentectomy. Omentopexy has been demonstrated to be a safe procedure and appears to confer good long-term outcomes for peritoneal catheters [10–12].

8.2.3 Externalization Procedure

Catheter externalization may be done immediately at the time of catheter placement. Alternatively, the catheter may be placed several weeks to months prior to the anticipated need for dialysis (Moncrief–Popovich technique). Immediate catheter externalization is widely performed and has a number of advantages. The major advantage with externalization at the time of catheter placement is the ability to start dialysis immediately. In patients presenting with uremic symptoms or urgent dialysis needs, prompt PD catheter placement and dialysis initiation may obviate the need for a temporary hemodialysis catheter. The ability to perform urgent PD will allow patients with urgent dialysis needs to choose between hemodialysis and PD. It should be noted, however, that patients with a newly placed and immediately externalized peritoneal catheter may not tolerate large dialysate volumes as they are prone to dialysate leaks due to increased intra-abdominal pressure. Therefore, the major limitation to this approach is that dialysis is usually done in a recumbent position (overnight) with small drain volumes.

Delayed externalization offers certain advantages to the patient as well. At the time of catheter placement, after the catheter is flushed, the external portion of the catheter is buried in the subcutaneous space. Ideally, the patient will not need dialysis for at least 2 weeks and the catheter tunnel can heal in a sterile environment. For patients with chronic kidney disease (CKD) who choose PD, this proactive approach will likely preempt the need for a temporary hemodialysis catheter. When the patient develops a clinical need for dialysis, the catheter can be externalized via a small incision made under local anesthesia and full dose dialysis can be initiated. Burying PD catheters also eliminates the need for exit site care, supplies, and catheter flushes until the catheter is in use. The absence of an open exit site potentially lowers the infectious risk although that has not been clearly demonstrated in the literature. Whether or not prolonged period of embedding negatively affects catheter performance is unclear. Data from one PD center suggested that prolonged embedding does harm catheter performance, while another recent retrospective study did not show any deleterious effects from prolonged embedding [13, 14].

There has been one prospective study comparing the two externalization techniques. Danielsson et al. randomized patients at two centers to immediate catheter externalization or delayed externalization [15]. Sixty patients were enrolled in the study and infectious complications were compared. After 2 years of follow-up, there was no significant difference in exit site infections or peritonitis between the two groups. Rates of catheter dysfunction were not specifically quantified in the study.

8.2.4 Exit Site Characteristics

Creation of a good exit site will also improve the likelihood of success for a peritoneal catheter. After the catheter is externalized, providers should employ appropriate measures to maintain a sterile exit site. Sutures should be avoided at the exit site due to the risk of foreign body reaction; rather, Steri-Strips should be used. The exit site should be directed downwardly or laterally and away from the belt line or skin folds [7, 16]. Since patients will be responsible for caring for the exit site, it is crucial that the patients can see and reach the exit site.

For many patients, a presternal catheter is an appropriate choice. Presternal exit sites are created by connecting an extender catheter to the PD catheter and creating a presternal exit site. The catheter should not cross the sternum in case the patient will need cardiac surgery. Patients with morbid obesity are potential candidates for presternal catheters due to greater ease of catheter care. Other conditions that may warrant presternal catheters are the presence of abdominal stomas or urinary and fecal incontinence. Observational studies have shown that abdominal and presternal catheters have similar infection rates and overall survival [17, 18].

8.3 Dialysis Solutions

8.3.1 Dextrose-Based Solutions

Dextrose-containing solutions have been the most widely used dialysate solutions for decades. The electrolyte composition of the commonly used solutions is shown in Table 8.2. A high dextrose concentration provides an osmotic gradient favoring water movement into the peritoneal space. Lactate is used as the buffer since bicarbonate will precipitate with dialysate calcium. The pH of the solutions is acidic (5.0) to minimize production of glucose degradation products (GDPs) during sterilization.

The degree of solute and water removal with dextrose solutions depends on the characteristics of the individual patient's peritoneal membrane. These characteristics have been quantified using the peritoneal equilibration test (PET) [19]. During a standard PET, 2.5 % dextrose dialysate is instilled into peritoneal cavity for a 4-h period. The dialysate glucose concentration at 4 h is compared to the dialysate glucose concentration at the beginning of the dwell (D/D_0 glucose). The concentration of dialysate urea and creatinine are compared to their relative plasma concentration (D/P_{urea} and

Table 8.2 Composition of dextrose-based peritoneal dialysate solutions

Component	Concentration
Dextrose	1.5 %, 2.5 %, 4.25 %
Sodium	132 mEq/L
Calcium	2.5 or 3.5 mEq/L
Magnesium	0.5 mEq/L
Chloride	96 mEq/L
Lactate	40 mEq/L

$D/P_{creatinine}$). Patients designated as rapid transporters have rapid systemic absorption of dialysate glucose and quick equilibration of urea and creatinine. Most patients on PD are high- or low-average transporters [20]. In this patient population, approximately 40 % of dialysate glucose is absorbed after 4 h. Since urea is a small molecule, dialysate urea is roughly 90 % of plasma urea by 4 h, while dialysate creatinine is approximately 65 % of plasma creatinine.

Ultrafiltration with the use of dextrose solutions occurs by water transport down an osmotic gradient. Some water transport occurs concurrently with solute transport via the small pores in peritoneal capillaries. Another component of water transport is mediated by aquaporin-1 water channels and is independent of solute transport. In low- or high-average transporters, water will continue to enter the peritoneal cavity for more than 6 h after instillation of 2.5 % dextrose dwell. However, since there is a constant rate of lymphatic absorption of peritoneal dialysate, dextrose solutions may lead to net fluid reabsorption if an individual dwell remains in the peritoneal cavity for a prolonged period [21].

Both local and systemic adverse effects can be seen with dextrose-containing solutions. In some patients, infusion of the dextrose solutions can lead to pain, possibly as a result of the non-physiologic pH. The solutions can also be associated with adverse metabolic consequences. Systemic absorption of dextrose can increase the daily caloric load, potentially leading to hypertriglyceridemia and worsening control of diabetes mellitus. The increase in calories from dextrose may worsen obesity or, alternatively, may paradoxically lead to malnutrition by decreasing appetite and protein intake.

In addition to the clinical effects listed above, some research suggests that dextrose-containing solutions may negatively affect the health of the peritoneal membrane. Longitudinal studies have established that the peritoneal membrane thickens over years of PD with increased angiogenesis and vessel density [22, 23]. Studies have supported the hypothesis that the non-physiologic pH of the solutions as well as GDPs and advanced glycosylated end products (AGEs) may promote peritoneal thickening. In vitro and animal studies have demonstrated negative effects of dextrose solutions on mesothelial cells [24, 25]. Establishing a causal relationship between dialysate solutions and peritoneal membrane pathology is more difficult. Most studies have reported effluent levels of cancer antigen 125 (CA-125), vascular endothelial growth factor (VEGF), and interleukin-6 (IL-6) as surrogate markers of peritoneal health. CA-125 is used as marker for mesothelial cell mass although the relationship between mesothelial cell mass and effluent CA-125 has not been rigorously tested. Similarly, VEGF levels are assumed to be a proxy for angiogenesis and IL-6 is reported to measure inflammation. In some studies, there is discordance between the markers. Nonetheless, based on the above studies, the hypothesis that chronic use of dextrose solutions negatively affects membrane health seems probable.

In vitro studies have also suggested that the high GDP levels negatively affect the function of peritoneal immune cells and potentially increase the risk of peritonitis. High GDP levels and low pH decrease survival of peritoneal leukocytes [26, 27]. Retrospective, observational studies have detected an increase in peritonitis rates. However, the data from RCTs published to date has not consistently demonstrated that alternative dialysis solutions lead to an improvement in peritonitis rates.

8.3.2 Icodextrin

A solution with 7.5 % icodextrin is approved for use a single daily dwell (daytime dwell in patients on automated PD and nighttime dwell for patients performing continuous ambulatory PD). Icodextrin is an iso-osmolar solution of large molecular weight starch molecules. It is slowly metabolized to maltose, a monosaccharide that is subsequently absorbed. The electrolyte composition in an icodextrin solution matches that of the standard dextrose solutions.

Since icodextrin is a large molecule and is slowly absorbed, it provides for sustained peritoneal ultrafiltration. For the first 2–4 h of a dwell, icodextrin solutions provide similar ultrafiltration to 2.5 % dextrose solutions. While 4.25 % dextrose solutions deliver more rapid ultrafiltration than icodextrin, the latter solution allows for more ultrafiltration over a 12–14-h period. Furthermore, the amount of carbohydrate absorbed from icodextrin is less than that of a 4.25 % dextrose solution. Icodextrin solution also has fewer GDPs although the clinical significance of this difference is unknown. Clinical studies have shown that icodextrin provides equivalent ultrafiltration to 4.25 % dextrose solutions over 8–12 h, reduces glucose and hemoglobin A_{1C} levels, and possibly serum triglycerides [28–30].

In patients with rapid transporter status, icodextrin solutions offer a significant advantage over dextrose solutions [31–34]. In this patient population, dextrose is rapidly absorbed and fluid overload can be seen with long dwells; icodextrin can provide improved ultrafiltration with long dwells. A randomized, controlled trial in automated peritoneal dialysis (APD) patients with high-average or high transporter status demonstrated superior ultrafiltration, improved small solute clearance, and reduced carbohydrate absorption with icodextrin [31].

Patients with other transport characteristics may also benefit from icodextrin instillation during long dwells. Icodextrin can improve ultrafiltration and small solute clearance in low-average transporters although that has not been a universal finding [31, 32]. A small minority of PD patients exhibit a low transport status. Since dialysate glucose is absorbed slowly in low transporters, icodextrin would not be predicted to have a significant beneficial effect. In clinical trials, icodextrin has not demonstrated improved ultrafiltration in low transporters; however, no study has enrolled a large number of patients with low transporter status [31, 32, 35].

Although most studies evaluating icodextrin have been short-term studies, there is evidence that a sustained ultrafiltration benefit is maintained for up to 2 years. At 1 year, there is improved weight loss in patients on ultrafiltration. Patients treated with icodextrin for 1 year appear to have fewer episodes of volume overload [29, 35]. In one study, icodextrin improved technique survival by decreasing episodes of volume overload [35]. Most studies involving icodextrin have been short-term studies and were unable to study technique survival. In summary, the bulk of data from randomized controlled trials validates the hypothesis that icodextrin improves ultrafiltration and volume status in patients on PD, although this effect is most robust in high-average or high transporters.

While icodextrin is well tolerated in clinical studies, there are adverse effects associated with icodextrin. Icodextrin degradation products such as maltose are absorbed and serum amylase levels are reduced probably as an artifact of measurement methods. Whether either consequence directly causes harm is unknown but both do have implications for patients. There is a significant safety precaution that must be taken in patients with diabetes mellitus. Many glucometers used for home glucose monitoring do not differentiate between glucose and maltose, placing patients at risk for hypoglycemia if insulin doses are inappropriately raised [36]. It is therefore crucial that providers ensure that each diabetic patient receiving icodextrin has a glucometer compatible with this therapy. The incorrect levels of amylase suggest that a low serum amylase alone cannot exclude pancreatitis in patients for whom there is clinical suspicion [37]. Icodextrin has also been linked to an exfoliative rash on palms and soles [33]; patients with this complication should have icodextrin temporarily stopped.

8.3.3 Amino Acid Solutions

A 1.1 % amino acid (AA) solution is approved for exchanges in PD patients in Europe but not in the USA. AA solutions provide similar ultrafitration and small solute clearance to 1.5 % dextrose solutions but contain no dextrose. The pH of the AA solutions is higher than standard dextrose solutions and, given the lack of dextrose, the solutions contain no GDPs. Given the relatively high rate of protein-calorie malnutrition in patients on dialysis and the daily loss of AAs in dialysate, AA solutions were designed to prevent protein loss and improve measures of malnutrition.

There is limited data from controlled trials regarding outcomes with AA solutions. Substituting a dwell of dextrose dialysate with AA dialysate does not significantly change ultrafiltration or dialysis adequacy [38]. Short-term studies do demonstrate an improvement in surrogate markers of muscle anabolism, such as an increase in serum insulin-like growth factor-1 (IGF-1), serum albumin, and serum pre-albumin [39, 40]. Whether or not AA solutions can significantly modify endpoints such as technique survival or mortality has not been tested in adequately powered studies. Given the increase in AA and nitrogen absorption, AA solutions have the potential to provoke uremic symptoms in a dose-dependent manner [41].

8.3.4 Biocompatible Dextrose-Based Solutions

Since standard dextrose solutions contain low pH and GDPs, it has been hypothesized that, after use for long periods of time, these solutions can harm the peritoneal membrane and peritoneal immune function. Recently, many different "biocompatible" solutions characterized by normal pH and low GDPs have been studied. Some solutions have lactate buffer while others employ a dual chamber system with bicarbonate-based buffer. Recently, studies have been published using a low glucose-icodextrin hybrid solution [42].

As with most studies evaluating dialysate solutions, clinical trials with biocompatible solutions have been relatively small and short. A summary of large trials with low-GDP solutions is presented in Table 8.3 [43–49]. The biocompatible solutions appear to improve urine volume but have no significant effect on glomerular filtration rate [50]. However, the solutions also lead to lower ultrafiltration. The change in urine volume may not be due to a lower rate of GDP absorption but may be secondary to volume overload. Long-term studies have not demonstrated an improvement in volume status or left ventricular hypertrophy nor has there been reproducible data demonstrating an improvement in technique survival or the incidence of peritonitis.

Table 8.3 Selected trials studying low-GDP and neutral pH dialysate solutions

Reference	Experimental solution	Patient number/ duration (mos)	Outcomes
Choi et al. [43]	Lactate buffered, pH 7, low GDP (Fresenius, Balance)	104/12	Low-GDP solution with improved ultrafiltration and urea clearance. No change in residual kidney function (RKF)
Haag–Weber et al. (DIUREST) [44]	Lactate buffered, normal pH, multicompartment, low GDP (Gambro, Gambrosol Trio)	80/18	Low-GDP with improved urine volume and increased CA-125. Trend towards decreased UF with low-GDP solution
Johnson et al. (balANZ) [45]	Lactate buffered, pH 7, low GDP (Fresenius, Balance)	185/24	Experimental group with longer time to anuria, fewer episodes of peritonitis, and reduced ultrafiltration
Williams et al. (Euro-Balance) [46]	Lactate buffered, pH 7, low GDP (Fresenius, Balance)	86/3	Experimental group with increased effluent CA-125 and decreased hyaluronic acid
Kim et al. [47]	Lactate buffered, pH 7, low GDP (Fresenius, Balance)	91/12	Experimental group with higher glomerular filtration rate (GFR) and effluent CA-125 but lower peritoneal ultrafiltration
Rippe et al. [48]	Lactate based, multicompartment solution	80/24	Experimental group with increased CA-125 and decreased hyaluronic acid
Fan et al. [49]	Different bicarbonate-based solutions	93/12	No change in peritoneal solute transport. No change in solute clearance, urine volume, or peritoneal ultrafiltration
Li et al. (IMPENDIA and EDEN) [42]	Low glucose, icodextrin, amino acid solutions	251/6	Intervention group with improved glycated hemoglobin and triglycerides but increased volume overload and death

GDP glucose degradation products, *CA-125* cancer antigen 125, *UF* ultrafiltration

References

1. Riu S, Ruiz CG, Martinez-Vea A, Peralta C, Oliver JA. Spontaneous rupture of polyurethane peritoneal catheter. A possible deleterious effect of mupirocin ointment. Nephrol Dial Transpl. 1998;13(7):1870–1.
2. Hagen SM, Lafranca JA, Ijzermans JN, Dor FJ. A systematic review and meta-analysis of the influence of peritoneal dialysis catheter type on complication rate and catheter survival. Kidney Int. 2014;85(4):920–32.
3. Xie J, Kiryluk K, Ren H, Zhu P, Huang X, Shen P, et al. Coiled versus straight peritoneal dialysis catheters: a randomized controlled trial and meta-analysis. Am J Kidney Dis. 2011;58(6):946–55.
4. Johnson DW, Wong J, Wiggins KJ, Kirwan R, Griffin A, Preston J, et al. A randomized controlled trial of coiled versus straight swan-neck tenckhoff catheters in peritoneal dialysis patients. Am J Kidney Dis. 2006;48(5):812–21.
5. Eklund B, Honkanen E, Kyllonen L, Salmela K, Kala AR. Peritoneal dialysis access: prospective randomized comparison of single-cuff and double-cuff straight Tenckhoff catheters. Nephrol Dial Transpl. 1997;12(12):2664–6.
6. Nessim SJ, Bargman JM, Jassal SV. Relationship between double-cuff versus single-cuff peritoneal dialysis catheters and risk of peritonitis. Nephrol Dial Transpl. 2010;25(7):2310–4.
7. Flanigan M, Gokal R. Peritoneal catheters and exit-site practices toward optimum peritoneal access: a review of current developments. Perit Dial Int. 2005;25(2):132–9.
8. Crabtree JH. Selected best demonstrated practices in peritoneal dialysis access. Kidney Int Suppl. 2006;103:27–37.
9. Reissman P, Lyass S, Shiloni E, Rivkind A, Berlatzky Y. Placement of a peritoneal dialysis catheter with routine omentectomy—does it prevent obstruction of the catheter? Eur J Surg (Acta chirurgica). 1998;164(9):703–7.
10. Attaluri V, Lebeis C, Brethauer S, Rosenblatt S. Advanced laparoscopic techniques significantly improve function of peritoneal dialysis catheters. J Am Coll Surg. 2010;211(6):699–704.
11. Crabtree JH, Burchette RJ. Effective use of laparoscopy for long-term peritoneal dialysis access. Am J Surg. 2009;198(1):135–41.
12. Crabtree JH, Fishman A. Selective performance of prophylactic omentopexy during laparoscopic implantation of peritoneal dialysis catheters. Surg Laparosc Endosc Percutaneous Tech. 2003;13(3):180–4.
13. Brown PA, McCormick BB, Knoll G, Su Y, Doucette S, Fergusson D, et al. Complications and catheter survival with prolonged embedding of peritoneal dialysis catheters. Nephrol Dial Transpl. 2008;23(7):2299–303.
14. Elhassan E, McNair B, Quinn M, Teitelbaum I. Prolonged duration of peritoneal dialysis catheter embedment does not lower the catheter success rate. Perit Dial Int. 2011;31(5):558–64.
15. Danielsson A, Blohme L, Tranaeus A, Hylander B. A prospective randomized study of the effect of a subcutaneously "buried" peritoneal dialysis catheter technique versus standard technique on the incidence of peritonitis and exit-site infection. Perit Dial Int. 2002;22(2):211–9.
16. Crabtree JH, Burchette RJ. Prospective comparison of downward and lateral peritoneal dialysis catheter tunnel-tract and exit-site directions. Perit Dial Int. 2006;26(6):677–83.
17. Twardowski ZJ, Prowant BF, Nichols WK, Nolph KD, Khanna R. Six-year experience with Swan neck presternal peritoneal dialysis catheter. Perit Dial Int. 1998;18(6):598–602.
18. Crabtree JH, Fishman A. Laparoscopic implantation of swan neck presternal peritoneal dialysis catheters. J Laparoendosc Adv Surg Tech Part A. 2003;13(2):131–7.
19. Twardowski Z, Nolph KO, Khanna R, Prowant BF, Ryan LP, Moore HL, et al. Peritoneal equilibration test. Perit Dial Int. 1987;7(3):138–48.
20. Mujais S, Vonesh E. Profiling of peritoneal ultrafiltration. Kidney Int Suppl. 2002(81):S17–22.
21. Mactier RA, Khanna R, Twardowski Z, Moore H, Nolph KD. Contribution of lymphatic absorption to loss of ultrafiltration and solute clearances in continuous ambulatory peritoneal dialysis. J Clin Invest. 1987;80(5):1311–6.
22. Yanez-Mo M, Lara-Pezzi E, Selgas R, Ramirez-Huesca M, Dominguez-Jimenez C, Jimenez-Heffernan JA, et al. Peritoneal dialysis and epithelial-to-mesenchymal transition of mesothelial cells. N Engl J Med. 2003;348(5):403–13.
23. Aroeira LS, Aguilera A, Sanchez-Tomero JA, Bajo MA, del Peso G, Jimenez-Heffernan JA, et al. Epithelial to mesenchymal transi-

tion and peritoneal membrane failure in peritoneal dialysis patients: pathologic significance and potential therapeutic interventions. J Am Soc Nephrol. 2007;18(7):2004–13.
24. Witowski J, Korybalska K, Wisniewska J, Breborowicz A, Gahl GM, Frei U, et al. Effect of glucose degradation products on human peritoneal mesothelial cell function. J Am Soc Nephrol. 2000;11(4):729–39.
25. Mortier S, Faict D, Lameire NH, De Vriese AS. Benefits of switching from a conventional to a low-GDP bicarbonate/lactate-buffered dialysis solution in a rat model. Kidney Int. 2005;67(4):1559–65.
26. Catalan MP, Santamaria B, Reyero A, Ortiz A, Egido J, Ortiz A. 3,4-di-deoxyglucosone-3-ene promotes leukocyte apoptosis. Kidney Int. 2005;68(3):1303–11.
27. Plum J, Lordnejad MR, Grabensee B. Effect of alternative peritoneal dialysis solutions on cell viability, apoptosis/necrosis and cytokine expression in human monocytes. Kidney Int. 1998;54(1):224–35.
28. Cho Y, Johnson DW, Badve S, Craig JC, Strippoli GF, Wiggins KJ. Impact of icodextrin on clinical outcomes in peritoneal dialysis: a systematic review of randomized controlled trials. Nephrol Dial Transpl. 2013;28(7):1899–907.
29. Paniagua R, Ventura MD, Avila-Diaz M, Cisneros A, Vicente-Martinez M, Furlong MD, et al. Icodextrin improves metabolic and fluid management in high and high-average transport diabetic patients. Perit Dial Int. 2009;29(4):422–32.
30. Mistry CD, Gokal R, Peers E. A randomized multicenter clinical trial comparing isosmolar icodextrin with hyperosmolar glucose solutions in CAPD. MIDAS, study group. Multicenter investigation of icodextrin in ambulatory peritoneal dialysis. Kidney Int. 1994;46(2):496–503.
31. Wolfson M, Piraino B, Hamburger RJ, Morton AR, Icodextrin Study G. A randomized controlled trial to evaluate the efficacy and safety of icodextrin in peritoneal dialysis. Am J Kidney Dis. 2002;40(5):1055–65.
32. Lin A, Qian J, Li X, Yu X, Liu W, Sun Y, et al. Randomized controlled trial of icodextrin versus glucose containing peritoneal dialysis fluid. Clin J Am Soc Nephrol. 2009;4(11):1799–804.
33. Finkelstein F, Healy H, Abu-Alfa A, Ahmad S, Brown F, Gehr T, et al. Superiority of icodextrin compared with 4.25% dextrose for peritoneal ultrafiltration. J Am Soc Nephrol. 2005;16(2):546–54.
34. Davies SJ, Woodrow G, Donovan K, Plum J, Williams P, Johansson AC, et al. Icodextrin improves the fluid status of peritoneal dialysis patients: results of a double-blind randomized controlled trial. J Am Soc Nephrol. 2003;14(9):2338–44.
35. Takatori Y, Akagi S, Sugiyama H, Inoue J, Kojo S, Morinaga H, et al. Icodextrin increases technique survival rate in peritoneal dialysis patients with diabetic nephropathy by improving body fluid management: a randomized controlled trial. Clin J Am Soc Nephrol. 2011;6(6):1337–44.
36. Sloand JA. Dialysis patient safety: safeguards to prevent iatrogenic hypoglycemia in patients receiving icodextrin. Am J Kidney Dis. 2012;60(4):514–6.
37. Villacorta J, Rivera M, Alvaro SJ, Palomares JR, Ortuno J. Acute pancreatitis in peritoneal dialysis patients: diagnosis in the icodextrin era. Perit Dial Int. 2010;30(3):374–8.
38. Li FK, Chan LY, Woo JC, Ho SK, Lo WK, Lai KN, et al. A 3-year, prospective, randomized, controlled study on amino acid dialysate in patients on CAPD. Am J Kidney Dis. 2003;42(1):173–83.
39. Jones M, Hagen T, Boyle CA, Vonesh E, Hamburger R, Charytan C, et al. Treatment of malnutrition with 1.1% amino acid peritoneal dialysis solution: results of a multicenter outpatient study. Am J Kidney Dis. 1998;32(5):761–9.
40. Kopple JD, Bernard D, Messana J, Swartz R, Bergstrom J, Lindholm B, et al. Treatment of malnourished CAPD patients with an amino acid based dialysate. Kidney Int. 1995;47(4):1148–57.
41. Tjiong HL, Swart R, van den Berg JW, Fieren MW. Amino Acid-based peritoneal dialysis solutions for malnutrition: new perspectives. Perit Dial Int. 2009;29(4):384–93.
42. Li PK, Culleton BF, Ariza A, Do JY, Johnson DW, Sanabria M, et al. Randomized, controlled trial of glucose-sparing peritoneal dialysis in diabetic patients. J Am Soc Nephrol. 2013;24(11):1889–900.
43. Choi HY, Kim DK, Lee TH, Moon SJ, Han SH, Lee JE, et al. The clinical usefulness of peritoneal dialysis fluids with neutral pH and low glucose degradation product concentration: an open randomized prospective trial. Perit Dial Int. 2008;28(2):174–82.
44. Haag-Weber M, Kramer R, Haake R, Islam MS, Prischl F, Haug U, et al. Low-GDP fluid (Gambrosol trio) attenuates decline of residual renal function in PD patients: a prospective randomized study. Nephrol Dial Transpl. 2010;25(7):2288–96.
45. Johnson DW, Brown FG, Clarke M, Boudville N, Elias TJ, Foo MW, et al. Effects of biocompatible versus standard fluid on peritoneal dialysis outcomes. J Am Soc Nephrol. 2012;23(6):1097–107.
46. Williams JD, Topley N, Craig KJ, Mackenzie RK, Pischetsrieder M, Lage C, et al. The Euro-balance trial: the effect of a new biocompatible peritoneal dialysis fluid (balance) on the peritoneal membrane. Kidney Int. 2004;66(1):408–18.
47. Kim S, Oh J, Kim S, Chung W, Ahn C, Kim SG, et al. Benefits of biocompatible PD fluid for preservation of residual renal function in incident CAPD patients: a 1-year study. Nephrol Dial Transpl. 2009;24(9):2899–908.
48. Rippe B, Simonsen O, Heimburger O, Christensson A, Haraldsson B, Stelin G, et al. Long-term clinical effects of a peritoneal dialysis fluid with less glucose degradation products. Kidney Int. 2001;59(1):348–57.
49. Fan SL, Pile T, Punzalan S, Raftery MJ, Yaqoob MM. Randomized controlled study of biocompatible peritoneal dialysis solutions: effect on residual renal function. Kidney Int. 2008;73(2):200–6.
50. Cho Y, Johnson DW, Badve SV, Craig JC, Strippoli GF, Wiggins KJ. The impact of neutral-pH peritoneal dialysates with reduced glucose degradation products on clinical outcomes in peritoneal dialysis patients. Kidney Int. 2013;84(5):969–79.

9 Dosing of Peritoneal Dialysis

Dirk Gijsbert Struijk

9.1 Introduction

Peritoneal dialysis (PD) can be performed either manually (continuous ambulatory peritoneal dialysis, CAPD) or by using a cycler (automated peritoneal dialysis, APD). Ideally, adequate treatment of renal failure by PD should replace the normal renal function for both treatment modalities. Thus, adequate dialysis could be defined as a treatment that results in patients with an acceptable quality of life, no physical complaints, and a morbidity and mortality that equals that of the healthy population. Unfortunately, this objective cannot be reached. In the early days of dialysis, Scribner proposed to assess dialysis adequacy by using a combination of patient variables, dialysis system variables, and careful clinical observation of the patient [1]. However, many of these variables are subjective and/or difficult to quantify, so the focus has moved to indices of the removal of low-molecular weight solutes. At present, mainly Kt/V urea (urea clearance normalized to total body water) and to some extent weekly creatinine clearance (normalized to body surface area) are used as estimates of dialysis adequacy. These parameters can easily be calculated from a 24-h collection of dialysate and urine and used in retrospective and prospective analyses of dialysis outcome. However, an adequate control of the fluid status of the patient has often been neglected and is probably even more important than solute removal parameters [2, 3]. Dialysis adequacy should also involve many other aspects of the treatment, such as control of anemia and acidosis, mineral metabolism, treatment of comorbidity, and prevention of cardiovascular and infectious complications. Nevertheless, this chapter focuses on how to prescribe PD treatment to achieve adequate solute and fluid removal.

D. G. Struijk (✉)
Department of Nephrology, Dianet, Academic Medical Center, Amsterdam, The Netherlands
e-mail: d.g.struijk@amc.uva.nl

9.2 Current Recommendations and Targets for Peritoneal Solute Clearances

Recently, several guidelines have been published on adequate solute clearances in CAPD and APD [4–7]. In these guidelines, peritoneal and renal solute clearances are combined. This policy is questionable because the amount of urine production and the magnitude of residual glomerular filtration rate (GFR) are related to mortality, while the removal of urea and creatinine has no effect [8, 9]. Probably the effects of residual renal function overrule those of the dialysis dose. Nevertheless, there is a general agreement that the target Kt/V urea in PD patients should be 1.7 or higher. These recommendations are to a large extent based on two randomized controlled trials [10, 11]. These showed that increasing the dialysis dose from 1.65 to 2.0 had no effect on patient survival. To avoid insufficient dialysis for solutes larger than urea in APD due to incorrect use of short dwell times, either additional opinion-based targets have been formulated for creatinine clearance (>45 L/week/1.73 m^2) [4, 5], or the recommendation is given to take into account membrane transport characteristics [7]. An analysis in anuric patients showed that minimum values, below which mortality was increased, were 1.5/week for Kt/V urea and 40 L/week for creatinine clearance [12]. How to measure peritoneal transport, its impact on solute and fluid removal, and its importance for an optimal dialysis prescription is discussed later in this chapter.

9.3 Current Recommendations and Targets for Peritoneal Fluid Removal

Only the European Best Practice Guidelines on Peritoneal Dialysis recommend a minimum ultrafiltration target in anuric patients of 1000 mL/24 h [4]. These recommendations are based upon several retrospective and prospective studies showing that mortality is higher when net ultrafiltration is lower [4]. In the absence of a well-conducted randomized

A. K. Singh et al. (eds.), *Core Concepts in Dialysis and Continuous Therapies*, DOI 10.1007/978-1-4899-7657-4_9

Table 9.1 Treatment recommendations based on peritoneal transport characteristics

	Transport velocity			
	Very slow	Slow	Fast	Very fast
Expected UF	Excellent	Good	Sufficient	Poor
Expected solute transport	Low, maybe inadequate	Sufficient	Good	Very good, providing treatment is adjusted for loss of UF
Treatment of choice	CAPD or APD with additional daily exchange	CAPD/APD	APD/CAPD	APD with icodextrin for long dwell

UF ultrafiltration, *CAPD* continuous ambulatory peritoneal dialysis, *APD* automated peritoneal dialysis

controlled trial, other guidelines merely recommend achieving euvolemia and monitoring the peritoneal ultrafiltration [5–7]. The determination of the dry weight of a patient remains difficult as long as reliable clinical tools are missing. As overhydration is frequently present in dialysis patients [13, 14], the volume status of the patient is an important factor in the daily prescription of PD patients.

9.4 Peritoneal Transport Characteristics and Its Consequences for the Treatment

Unlike the specifications of an artificial kidney, the properties of the peritoneal membrane for solute and water transport vary individually and can change in time. Several tests are available for monitoring the peritoneal function, and it is recommended to repeat the test at least once a year [15]. The majority of these tests are based upon the appearance of low-molecular weight solutes during a 4-h dwell. According to the speed of low-molecular weight solute transport from blood to the dialysate, patients can be categorized into four groups of slow, slow-average, fast-average, and fast transport. Slow transport is defined by a dialysate to plasma creatinine ratio (D/PCr) less than the mean − 1 standard deviation (SD) or a dialysate glucose to initial dialysate glucose ratio (D/Do) exceeding the mean + 1 SD. Slow-average transport means a D/PCr between the mean and mean − 1 SD or a D/Do between the mean and mean + 1 SD. Analogously, the other two groups are defined. Fluid transport should be measured using the most hypertonic solution, glucose concentration (3.86:4.25 %), during a standardized dwell of 4 h. Ultrafiltration failure is defined as net ultrafiltration > 400 mL [16].

Recommendations have been made on the mode and quantity of PD according to the solute transport velocity of the patients [17, 18]. This is illustrated in Table 9.1. By and large, these recommendations can be summarized into two rules:

1. For adequate solute removal, the dwell time should be inversely related to the transport velocity of low-molecular weight solutes. This implies that in patients with a slow transport, long dwell times are needed to accommodate sufficient time for equilibration for solute removal, while in patients with a fast transport, the dwell time can be reduced due to the more rapid saturation of the dialysate.
2. For adequate fluid removal in patients with fast-average or fast transport, long dwell times should be avoided due to the rapid dissipation of the osmotic gradient of glucose. Alternatively, high-molecular weight solutes (such as icodextrin) could be used for the long dwells.

9.5 Modifiable Treatment Variables in Peritoneal Dialysis

The number of variables that can be modified in PD treatment are limited (Table 9.2). Most variables are one way or the other interrelated. As an example, to increase the total dialysate volume either the number of dwells can be increased or the dwell fill volume.

9.6 Fill Volume

In adult patients, only few data are available on the role of the fill volume on solute and fluid transport. In theory, three mechanisms can play a role, namely the impact of volume on the contact area between dialysate and peritoneal membrane, the effect of volume on the total amount of solute transport, and the effect of volume on net ultrafiltration.

9.6.1 The Relation Between Fill Volume and Dialysate/Membrane Contact

It is obvious that a lower threshold of the intraperitoneal volume does exist for optimal recruitment of the peritoneal membrane surface area. A study in ten patients using incremental fill volumes up to 3.5 L demonstrated that diffusive capacity nearly doubled from 0.5 to 2 L but increased only marginally thereafter [19]. This implies that for adequate recruitment of the membrane surface in clinical practice 2 L are sufficient.

Table 9.2 Treatment variables, interconnections, and influencing factors

Treatment variables	Related treatment variables	Other influencing factors
Total treatment time		
Total dialysis volume	Fill volume	
	Dwell time	
	Number of dwells	
Fill volume		Intraperitoneal pressure
Dwell time	Number of dwells	Peritoneal transport characteristics
Number of dwells	Dwell time	
Dialysate		Peritoneal transport characteristics
Ultrafiltration volume	Dialysate	Intraperitoneal pressure
	Fill volume	Peritoneal transport characteristics
	Dwell time	

9.6.2 The Effect of Fill Volume on Total Solute Removal

Apart from the above-described mechanism, a larger volume will result in an increased solute removal as more solute will be transferred before equilibrium is reached. As expected, low-molecular solute removal is enhanced when the volume is increased [20, 21].

9.6.3 The Effect of Fill Volume on Fluid Removal

The impact of increasing the fill volume on fluid removal is difficult to predict in the individual patient, as it is the resultant of two counteracting mechanisms. A larger volume will result in a longer maintenance of the osmotic gradient and therefore an increase in the transcapillary ultrafiltration. However, increasing the dwell volume will also result in a higher intraperitoneal pressure leading to an increased peritoneal fluid absorption [22, 23]. So, net ultrafiltration can either increase or decrease when dwell volume increases [20, 21]. Finally, most if not all studies that measured the effect of volume on intraperitoneal pressure were acute experiments. Whether patients might adapt to the increased volume and the effects of increasing the volume during longer periods of time is not known.

9.6.4 Measurement of Intraperitoneal Pressure and Clinical Implications

Larger volumes than 2 L are often well tolerated, and patients even cannot always tell the difference among 2, 2.5, or 3 L [24–26]. To determine the maximum tolerable volume, intraperitoneal pressure can be measured. It is determined easily by measuring the height of the dialysis fluid in the drain tubing [27]. To avoid clinical symptoms, it is advised to keep the intraperitoneal pressure lower than 18 cmH_2O [28]. In a group of 61 APD patients in which the dwell volume was chosen to avoid an intraperitoneal pressure >16 cmH_2O, no relation was found between intraperitoneal pressure and the occurrence of hernias, late leakage, and gastroesophageal reflux [29]. Only an association between intraperitoneal pressure and enteric peritonitis was found.

9.7 Total Drained Volume

Total drained volume is the result of fill volume, number of dwells, dwell time per fill, and ultrafiltration volume. For low-molecular weight solutes such as urea, total drained volume is the only determinant of its peritoneal clearance as long as the dwell time for each dwell is long enough to reach equilibrium [30]. When the dialysis is performed manually, this is usually the case. In view of the above, all guidelines for CAPD only advise to measure Kt/V of urea to determine the dialysis adequacy.

9.8 Dwell Time and Number of Dwells

The dwell time (and thereby also its intertwined variable number of dwells) is for short dwells probably the most critical parameter in the prescription of PD treatment. It is evident that solute transport decreases when the dwell time is reduced due to the lower dialysate saturation. However, for short dwells the transport characteristics of the individual patient have a major impact on the degree of saturation, and thereby total low-molecular weight solute removal. When the majority of the dwells during 24 h are short dwells, patients with a slow- or slow-average peritoneal transport might not reach the targets for adequate dialysis. Also the amount of ultrafiltration depends on the dwell time and transport type of the patient. The peak of the intraperitoneal volume is reached earlier when the peritoneal transport is faster.

As long as the dwell time is long (>4 h) and the number of dwells is low (3–5 exchanges), dialysis adequacy is only determined by the earlier discussed total drained volume and the net fluid removal by the osmotic agent in the dialysate. In a study of 50 patients, one additional daytime 2-L exchange was added to a regimen of 3 or 4 exchanges a day [31]. As can be expected, Kt/V increased about 20%.

Only limited data are available on the effect of increasing the number of exchanges when patients are treated with a cycler during the night. Most published data are based on mathematic modeling and not tested in clinical studies. In one study assuming net ultrafiltration was negligible, it was calculated that using 2 L exchanges for 5–6 cycles was optimal for urea removal when D/P of urea was 0.6 or lower, and 8–9 exchanges when the D/P urea was 0.7 or higher [32]. However, urea removal only very moderately increased when more than six exchanges were used. Another study modeled fluid removal and found that when the number of dwells exceeded five this had a negative impact on net fluid removal during the night [33]. In PD patients, the effects of 5×2 L, 7×2 L, and 9×2 L (average glucose concentrations around 2.25%) were studied on urea clearance, creatinine clearance, and net ultrafiltration [34]. In slow and slow-average transport patients, urea clearance increased 4%, creatinine clearance 11%, and net fluid removal 14% when seven instead of five exchanges were used. Adding two more dwells resulted in a further increase of urea clearance of 14%, creatinine clearance of 13%, and net ultrafiltration of 22%. In fast-average and fast-transport patients, these data were for urea clearance 18 and 5%, creatinine clearance 23 and 3%, and net ultrafiltration 51 and 1%. The authors concluded that 5×2 L significantly underutilizes the potential for APD to deliver high clearances.

9.9 Dialysate

For the dosing of PD only, the capacity to attract fluid from the circulation is important. For the removal of fluid only glucose, amino acids, and icodextrin are available. Apart from the removal of surplus of fluid, this also contributes to the removal of solutes by convection.

Glucose has been used as an osmotic agent since the introduction of PD. It is available in three concentrations (1.36:1.5%, 2.27:2.5%, and 3.86:4.25%). Due to its low molecular weight of 180 Da, it disappears rapidly out of the peritoneal cavity by diffusion. So, it is most effective for fluid removal during short dwells. During a 4-h dwell comparing 1.36–3.86% in ten patients, net ultrafiltration increased from an average of −55 to 500 ml, which resulted in an increase in peritoneal clearance of urea of 25% [34]. However, net ultrafiltration can vary markedly in individual patients depending on their peritoneal membrane characteristics as mentioned earlier. An example of fluid kinetic modeling in patients with a fast-average peritoneal transport is shown in Fig. 9.1. As a causal relationship between glucose and/or glucose degradation products and peritoneal morphological changes has been suggested [35–38], high glucose concentrations in the dialysate should be avoided when possible.

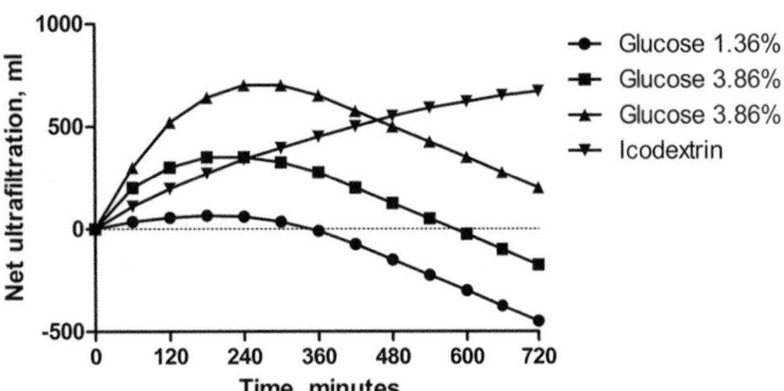

Fig. 9.1 Profiles of net ultrafiltration for glucose-containing solutions and icodextrin using kinetic modeling in ten patients with a fast-average peritoneal transport. (Unpublished data)

Amino acids can be used once a day to reduce the glucose exposure to the patient. Net ultrafiltration is similar to glucose 1.36% dialysate [39]. It can also be used to supplement protein intake in malnourished patients [40].

The glucose polymer icodextrin is a high molecular weight osmotic agent with an average molecular weight of 16,800 Da. Its disappearance from the peritoneal cavity will mainly be by uptake into the lymphatic system due to its high molecular weight. As its absorption is only 16–20% during 6–12-h dwells, icodextrin is effective in the removal of fluid during long dwells (Fig. 9.1). During an 8-h dwell in ten patients, average net ultrafiltration was 344 mL [41]. Again, in individual patients a wide range existed of −65 to 673 ml. Recently, a few studies in patients with ultrafiltration failure showed a beneficial effect when icodextrin was used twice daily [42].

9.10 Treatment Modalities

PD can be performed either manually or automatically using a cycler. Both treatments are equal in terms of clinical outcome [3]. When needed both modes can be used in the same patient. Usually the treatment is given during 24 h. In general, when residual renal function has disappeared, only in patients with a fast transport is a dry day feasible [43].

9.10.1 Continuous Ambulatory Peritoneal Dialysis

The dosing of PD in CAPD is straightforward. The number of manual exchanges is limited to 3–5 times a day (Fig. 9.2). Due to the burden of the treatment, more exchanges are scarcely ever acceptable for a patient. Because of the long dwells, only the total drained volume, and not the peritoneal membrane characteristics, is relevant for dialysate adequacy. Increasing the dwell volume (taking into account the effect of fill volume on fluid removal) and thereby decreasing the number of dwells is advantageous for the treatment burden of the patient and is cost effective.

The initial prescription when some residual renal function is still present usually consists of 3–4 exchanges with 1.5–2 L of low-glucose-containing dialysate. When a glucose-sparing regimen is followed, one of the short dwells with glucose can be replaced by amino acids. When more ultrafiltration

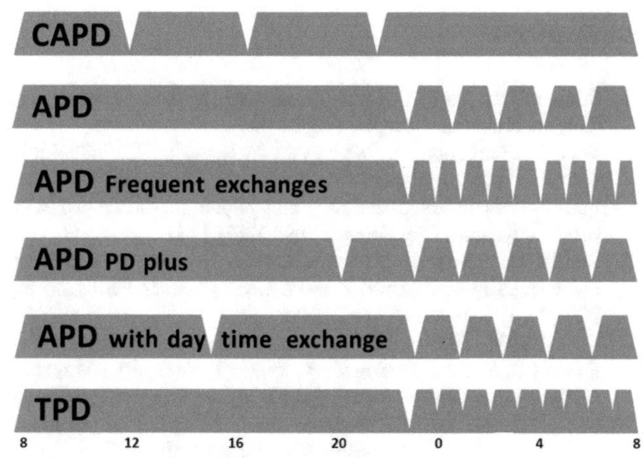

Fig. 9.2 Treatment schedules of continuous ambulatory peritoneal dialysis *(CAPD),* automated peritoneal dialysis *(APD),* and tidal peritoneal dialysis *(TPD)*. *PD* peritoneal dialysis

is needed, to avoid high glucose concentrations, icodextrin should be introduced for the long dwell first. Until now, only scarce evidence existed that glucose-sparing strategies are beneficial either for preservation of the peritoneal membrane [44] or for the metabolic control of diabetic patients [45].

To increase the dialysis dose, the only available options are increasing the volume to the maximum the patient can tolerate (taken into account the impact on net ultrafiltration) and increasing the volume to five exchanges a day.

9.10.2 Automated Peritoneal Dialysis

The dosing of APD is more complex compared to CAPD as many variables can be modified and patient characteristics have to be taken into account. Nevertheless, most patients are probably treated with a treatment scheme of 4–5 dwell during the night and one long daily dwell [46].

The initial prescription when some residual renal function is still present usually consists of 4–5 exchanges during 8–9 h with 1.5–2 L of low-glucose-containing dialysate during the night (Fig. 9.2). When a glucose-sparing regimen is followed, one of the short dwells with glucose can be replaced by amino acids. For the long dwell also, low-glucose-containing dialysate can be used. When more ultrafiltration is needed to avoid high glucose concentrations, icodextrin should be introduced for the long dwell.

Before increasing the dose in APD, it is essential to assess the peritoneal membrane characteristics of the patient. These data are needed to judge the effect of the various modifiable factors on dialysate adequacy and net ultrafiltration. The data can also be used to predict the effect of the treatment changes by kinetic modeling using computer programs [47–49]. Such a program is also used as a tool to recommend clinical practices for maximizing the treatment [43]. Taking into account the earlier described effects of changing treatment variables, in general the first step should be to increase the fill volume. When acceptable then the nightly treatment time can be prolonged with 1–2 h. Third, when both increasing the nightly number of dwells and adding additional daily exchange are feasible (Fig. 9.2), the latter is usually more effective and/or cost saving [43, 50]. An extra exchange given by the cycler before connecting for the nightly treatment can be chosen alternatively [51, 52].

To reduce the glucose exposure, two recently published strategies can be followed. Icodextrin can be used to replace one of the night dwells [53], or it can be added as an additional daily exchange in combination with simultaneously reducing the night dwells in one cycle [54] .

9.10.3 Tidal Peritoneal Dialysis

To enhance the efficacy of APD, tidal peritoneal dialysis (TPD) was introduced in the late 1970s. In tidal dialysis, only part of the initial inflow volume (usually 50–75 %) is exchanged during each following dwell (Fig. 9.2). The theory behind this concept is based on two principles. Firstly, down time, that is the time the peritoneal cavity is almost empty during draining, is avoided by TPD resulting in longer dialysate—membrane contact. Secondly, as the outflow of dialysate slows down after about 80 % of the drained volume as can be seen in Fig. 9.3 [55], more exchanges can be done within the same total treatment time. However, incomplete drainage also results in loss of the concentration gradient needed for diffusive solute transport. After reviewing the literature, it has been concluded that in home PD patients, TPD generally provides no advantage of improved small-solute and middle-molecule clearances and no better fluid removal as compared to conventional nontidal APD [56]. It is nowadays mostly used to reduce abdominal discomfort

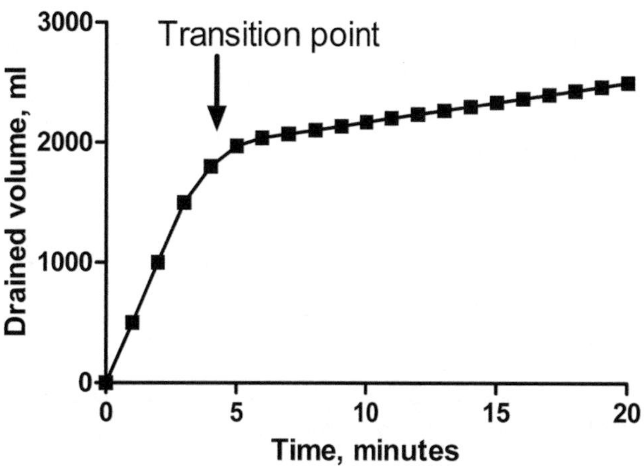

Fig. 9.3 Typical drainage pattern of the peritoneal cavity showing an initial fast outflow, followed by a decrease in outflow velocity

and nightly alarms during the treatment in case of catheter outflow problems or abdominal complaints during complete drainage.

In the prescription for TPD, net ultrafiltration has to be predicted in order to keep the intraperitoneal volume constant during the treatment. Although events caused by an increased intraperitoneal volume are also reported during APD, its incidence is highest in TPD [57].

9.11 Sodium Removal During Peritoneal Dialysis

The removal of sodium by diffusion is limited due to the small concentration gradient for sodium between plasma and dialysate (around 10 m mol/L). So, convective transport is important for sodium removal from the circulation. With hypertonic solutions, sodium sieving occurs early in the dwell due to aquaporin-1-mediated transcellular water transport. The dialysate concentration of sodium decreases during the initial phase of the dwell using hypertonic solutions followed by a gradual rise. The minimum value is usually reached after 1–2 h, and the decrease is more pronounced with a more hypertonic solution (Fig. 9.4). In short dwells, this results in peritoneal removal of relatively more water than sodium [58]. When dwells are prolonged, diffusive and convective sodium transport into the peritoneal cavity increases continuously until equilibrium between plasma and dialysate is reached. The consequence of this phenomenon is that the removal of sodium is impaired in APD as compared to CAPD [59, 60]. Although sodium removal increased after introducing icodextrin in APD, it remained lower compared to CAPD [59]. Thus, special attention should be given to the fluid status in APD when using many short dwells.

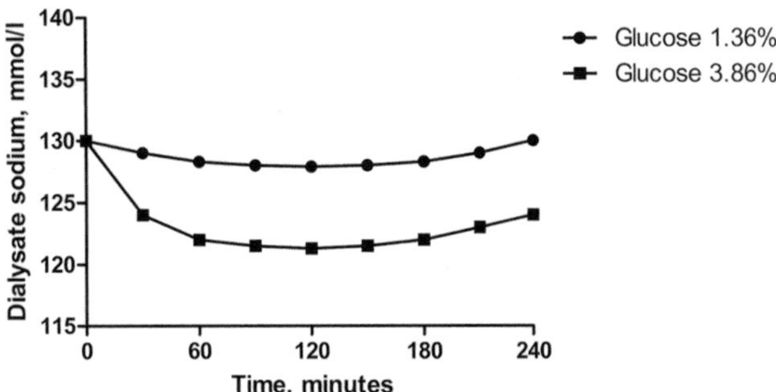

Fig. 9.4 The change in dialysate sodium concentration using dialysate with 1.36 and 3.86% glucose during a 4-h dwell

References

1. Scribner BH. Some thoughts on research to define adequacy of dialysis. Kidney Int Suppl. 1975;2:3–6.
2. Wang T, Heimburger O, Waniewski J, Bergström J, Lindholm B. Increased peritoneal permeability is associated with decreased fluid and small solute removal and higher mortality in CAPD patients. Nephrol Dial Transpl. 1998;13(5):1242–9.
3. Struijk DG. Volume status in CAPD and APD: does treatment modality matter and is more always better? Perit Dial Int. 2007;27(6):641–4.
4. Dombros N, Dratwa M, Feriani M, Gokal R, Heimbürger O, Krediet R, Plum J, Rodrigues A, Selgas R, Struijk D, Verger C, EBPG Expert Group on Peritoneal Dialysis. European best practice guidelines for peritoneal dialysis. 7 Adequacy of peritoneal dialysis. Nephrol Dial Transpl. 2005;20(Suppl 9):24–7.
5. Lo WK, Bargman JM, Burkart J, Krediet RT, Pollock C, Kawanishi H, Blake PG. ISPD Adequacy of Peritoneal Dialysis Working Group. Guideline on targets for solute and fluid removal in adult patients on chronic peritoneal dialysis. Perit Dial Int. 2006;26(5):520–2.
6. Peritoneal Dialysis Adequacy Work Group. Clinical practice guidelines for peritoneal dialysis adequacy. Am J Kidney Dis. 2006;48(Suppl 1):98–129.
7. Blake PG, Bargman JM, Brimble KS, Davison SN, Hirsch D, McCormick BB, Suri RS, Taylor P, Zalunardo N, Tonelli M. Canadian Society of Nephrology Work Group on adequacy of peritoneal dialysis. Perit Dial Int. 2011;31(2):218–39.
8. Bargman JM, Thorpe KE, Churchill DN, CANUSA Peritoneal Dialysis Study Group. Relative contribution of residual renal function and peritoneal clearance to adequacy of dialysis: a reanalysis of the CANUSA study. J Am Soc Nephrol. 2001;12(10):2158–62.
9. Termorshuizen F, Korevaar JC, Dekker FW, van Manen JG, Boeschoten EW, Krediet RT, NECOSAD Study Group. The relative importance of residual renal function compared with peritoneal clearance for patient survival and quality of life: an analysis of the Netherlands cooperative study on the adequacy of dialysis (NECOSAD)-2. Am J Kidney Dis. 2003;41(6):1293–302.
10. Paniagua R, Amato D, Vonesh E, Correa-Rotter R, Ramos A, Moran J, et al. On behalf of the Mexican nephrology collaborative study group. Effects of increased peritoneal clearances on mortality rates in peritoneal dialysis: ADEMEX, a prospective, randomized, controlled trial. J Am Soc Nephrol. 2002;13(5):1307–20.
11. Lo WK, Ho YW, Li CS, Wong KS, Chan TM, Yu AW, et al. Effect of Kt/V on survival and clinical outcome in CAPD patients in a randomized prospective study. Kidney Int. 2003;64(2):649–56.
12. Jansen MA, Termorshuizen F, Korevaar JC, Dekker FW, Boeschoten E, Krediet RT, NECOSAD Study Group. Predictors of survival in anuric peritoneal dialysis patients. Kidney Int. 2005;68(3):1199–205.
13. Konings CJ, Kooman JP, Schonck M, Dammers R, Cheriex E, Palmans Meulemans AP, et al. Fluid status, blood pressure, and cardiovascular abnormalities in patients on peritoneal dialysis. Perit Dial Int. 2002;22(4):477–87.
14. Enia G, Mallamaci F, Benedetto FA, Panuccio V, Parlongo S, Cutrupi S, et al. Long-term CAPD patients are volume expanded and display more severe left ventricular hypertrophy than haemodialysis patients. Nephrol Dial Transpl. 2001;16(7):1459–64.
15. Coester AM, Smit W, Struijk DG, Krediet RT. Peritoneal function in clinical practice: the importance of follow-up and its measurement in patients. Recommendations for patient information and measurement of peritoneal function. NDT Plus. 2009;2(2):104–10.

16. Mujais S, Nolph K, Gokal R, Blake P, Burkart J, Coles G, et al. Evaluation and management of ultrafiltration problems in peritoneal dialysis. International Society for Peritoneal Dialysis Ad Hoc Committee on ultrafiltration management in peritoneal dialysis. Perit Dial Int. 2000;20(Suppl 4):5–21.
17. Twardowski ZJ, Nolph KD, Khanna R, Prowant BF, Ryan LP, Moore HL, Nielsen MP. Peritoneal equilibration test. Perit Dial Bull. 1987;7:138–47.
18. Davies SJ, Brown B, Bryan J, Russell GI. Clinical evaluation of the peritoneal equilibration test: a population-based study. Nephrol Dial Transpl. 1993;8(1):64–70.
19. Keshaviah P, Emerson PF, Vonesh EF, Brandes JC. Relationship between body size, fill volume, and mass transfer area coefficient in peritoneal dialysis. J Am Soc Nephrol. 1994;4(10):1820–6.
20. Krediet RT, Boeschoten EW, Struijk DG, Arisz L. Differences in the peritoneal transport of water, solutes and proteins between dialysis with two- and with three-litre exchanges. Nephrol Dial Transpl. 1988;3(2):198–204.
21. Paniagua R, Ventura Mde J, Rodríguez E, Sil J, Galindo T, Hurtado ME, Alcántara G, Chimalpopoca A, González I, Sanjurjo A, Barrón L, Amato D, Mujais S. Impact of fill volume on peritoneal clearances and cytokine appearance in peritoneal dialysis. Perit Dial Int. 2004;24(2):156–62.
22. Durand PY, Chanliau J, Gamberoni J, Hestin D, Kessler M. Intraperitoneal pressure, peritoneal permeability and volume of ultrafiltration in CAPD. Adv Perit Dial. 1992;8:22–5.
23. Imholz AL, Koomen GC, Struijk DG, Arisz L, Krediet RT. Effect of an increased intraperitoneal pressure on fluid and solute transport during CAPD. Kidney Int. 1993;44(5):1078–85.
24. Sarkar S, Bernardini J, Fried L, Johnston JR, Piraino B. Tolerance of large exchange volumes by peritoneal dialysis patients. Am J Kidney Dis. 1999;33(6):1136–41.
25. de Jesús VM, Amato D, Correa-Rotter R, Paniagua R. Relationship between fill volume, intraperitoneal pressure, body size, and subjective discomfort perception in CAPD patients. Mexican nephrology collaborative study group. Perit Dial Int. 2000;20(2):188–93.
26. Harris KP, Keogh AM, Alderson L. Peritoneal dialysis fill volume: can the patient tell the difference? Perit Dial Int. 2001;21(Suppl 3):144–7.
27. Durand PY, Chanliau J, Gamberoni J, Hestin D, Kessler M. Routine measurement of hydrostatic intraperitoneal pressure. Adv Perit Dial. 1992;8:108–12.
28. Durand PY, Chanliau J, Gamberoni J, Hestin D, Kessler M. APD: clinical measurement of the maximal acceptable intraperitoneal volume. Adv Perit Dial. 1994;10:63–7.
29. Dejardin A, Robert A, Goffin E. Intraperitoneal pressure in PD patients: relationship to intraperitoneal volume, body size and PD-related complications. Nephrol Dial Transpl. 2007;22(5):1437–44.
30. Krediet RT, Douma CE, van Olden RW, Ho-dac-Pannekeet MM, Struijk DG. Augmenting solute clearance in peritoneal dialysis. Kidney Int. 1998;54(6):2218–25.
31. Szeto CC, Wong TY, Chow KM, Leung CB, Wang AY, Lui SF, Li PK. The impact of increasing the daytime dialysis exchange frequency on peritoneal dialysis adequacy and nutritional status of Chinese anuric patients. Perit Dial Int. 2002;22(2):197–203.
32. Kumano K, Yamashita A, Sakai T. Optimal number of dialysate exchanges in automated peritoneal dialysis. Adv Perit Dial. 1993;9:110–3.
33. Abu-Alfa AK, Burkart J, Piraino B, Pulliam J, Mujais S. Approach to fluid management in peritoneal dialysis: a practical algorithm. Kidney Int Suppl. 2002;81:8–16.
34. Perez RA, Blake PG, McMurray S, Mupas L, Oreopoulos DG. What is the optimal frequency of cycling in automated peritoneal dialysis? Perit Dial Int. 2000;20(5):548–56.
35. Imholz AL, Koomen GC, Struijk DG, Arisz L, Krediet RT. Effect of dialysate osmolarity on the transport of low-molecular weight solutes and proteins during CAPD. Kidney Int. 1993;43(6):1339–46.
36. Hendriks PM, Ho-dac-Pannekeet MM, van Gulik TM, Struijk DG, Phoa SS, Sie L, Kox C, Krediet RT. Peritoneal sclerosis in chronic peritoneal dialysis patients: analysis of clinical presentation, risk factors, and peritoneal transport kinetics. Perit Dial Int. 1997;17(2):136–43.
37. Davies SJ, Philips L, Naish PF, Russell GI. Peritoneal glucose exposure and changes in membrane solute transport with time on peritoneal dialysis. J Am Soc Nephrol. 2001;12(5):1046–51.
38. Krediet RT, Struijk DG. Peritoneal changes in patients on long-term peritoneal dialysis. Nat Rev Nephrol. 2013;9(7):419–29.
39. Li FK, Chan LY, Woo JC, Ho SK, Lo WK, Lai KN, Chan TM. A 3-year, prospective, randomized, controlled study on amino acid dialysate in patients on CAPD. Am J Kidney Dis. 2003;42(1):173–83.
40. Kopple JD, Bernard D, Messana J, Swartz R, Bergström J, Lindholm B, Lim V, Brunori G, Leiserowitz M, Bier DM, et al. Treatment of malnourished CAPD patients with an amino acid based dialysate. Kidney Int. 1995;47(4):1148–57.
41. Douma CE, Hiralall JK, de Waart DR, Struijk DG, Krediet RT. Icodextrin with nitroprusside increases ultrafiltration and peritoneal transport during long CAPD dwells. Kidney Int. 1998;53(4):1014–21.
42. Dousdampanis P, Trigka K, Bargman JM. Bimodal solutions or twice-daily icodextrin to enhance ultrafiltration in peritoneal dialysis patients. Int. J Nephrol. 2013;2013:424915. doi:10.1155/2013/424915.
43. Blake P, Burkart JM, Churchill DN, Daugirdas J, Depner T, Hamburger RJ, Hull AR, Korbet SM, Moran J, Nolph KD. Recommended clinical practices for maximizing peritoneal dialysis clearances. Perit Dial Int. 1996;16(5):448–56.
44. Davies SJ, Brown EA, Frandsen NE, Rodrigues AS, Rodriguez-Carmona A, Vychytil A, Macnamara E, Ekstrand A, Tranaeus A, Filho JC, EAPOS Group. Longitudinal membrane function in functionally anuric patients treated with APD: data from EAPOS on the effects of glucose and icodextrin prescription. Kidney Int. 2005;67(4):1609–15.
45. Li PK, Culleton BF, Ariza A, Do JY, Johnson DW, Sanabria M, Shockley TR, Story K, Vatazin A, Verrelli M, Yu AW, Bargman JM; IMPENDIA and EDEN Study Groups. Randomized, controlled trial of glucose-sparing peritoneal dialysis in diabetic patients. J Am Soc Nephrol. 2013;24(11):1889–900.
46. Mujais S, Childers RW. Profiles of automated peritoneal dialysis prescriptions in the US 1997–2003. Kidney Int Suppl. 2006;103:84–90.
47. Vonesh EF, Keshaviah PR. Applications in kinetic modeling using PD ADEQUEST. Perit Dial Int. 1997;17(Suppl 2):S119–25.
48. Vonesh EF, Story KO, O'Neill WT. A multinational clinical validation study of PD ADEQUEST 2.0. PD ADEQUEST international study group. Perit Dial Int. 1999;19(6):556–71.
49. Vonesh EF, Story KO, Douma CE, Krediet RT. Modeling of icodextrin in PD Adequest 2.0. Perit Dial Int. 2006;26(4):475–81.
50. Demetriou D, Habicht A, Schillinger M, Hörl WH, Vychytil A. Adequacy of automated peritoneal dialysis with and without manual daytime exchange: a randomized controlled trial. Kidney Int. 2006;70(9):1649–55.
51. Diaz-Buxo JA. Enhancement of peritoneal dialysis: the PD Plus concept. Am J Kidney Dis. 1996;27(1):92–8.
52. Freida P, Issad B. Continuous cyclic peritoneal dialysis prescription and power. Contrib Nephrol. 1999;129:98–108.
53. Rodríguez-Carmona A, Pérez Fontán M, García López E, García Falcón T, Díaz Cambre H. Use of icodextrin during nocturnal automated peritoneal dialysis allows sustained ultrafiltration while reducing the peritoneal glucose load: a randomized crossover study. Perit Dial Int. 2007;27(3):260–6.
54. Gobin J, Fernando S, Santacroce S, Finkelstein FO. The utility of two daytime icodextrin exchanges to reduce dextrose exposure

in automated peritoneal dialysis patients: a pilot study of nine patients. Blood Purif. 2008;26(3):279–83.
55. Brandes JC, Packard WJ, Watters SK, Fritsche C. Optimization of dialysate flow and mass transfer during automated peritoneal dialysis. Am J Kidney Dis. 1995;25(4):603–10.
56. Vychytil A, Hörl WH. The role of tidal peritoneal dialysis in modern practice: A European perspective. Kidney Int Suppl. 2006;103:96–103. Review.
57. Cižman B, Lindo S, Bilionis B, Davis I, Brown A, Miller J, Phillips G, Kriukov A, Sloand JA. The occurrence of increased intraperitoneal volume events in automated peritoneal dialysis in the US: role of programming, patient/user actions and ultrafiltration. Perit Dial Int. 2014;34(4):434–42. doi:10.3747/pdi.2013.01157.
58. Struijk DG, Krediet RT. Sodium balance in automated peritoneal dialysis. Perit Dial Int. 2000;20(Suppl 2):S101–5.
59. Rodríguez-Carmona A, Fontán MP. Sodium removal in patients undergoing CAPD and automated peritoneal dialysis. Perit Dial Int. 2002;22(6):705–13.
60. Rodriguez-Carmona A, Pérez-Fontán M, Garca-Naveiro R, Villaverde P, Peteiro J. Compared time profiles of ultrafiltration, sodium removal, and renal function in incident CAPD and automated peritoneal dialysis patients. Am J Kidney Dis. 2004;44(1):132–45.

10 Complications of Peritoneal Dialysis

Alice Kennard, David W. Johnson and Carmel M. Hawley

10.1 Introduction

Peritoneal dialysis (PD) is the dominant modality for home dialysis in end-stage kidney failure (ESKF), although its uptake varies enormously worldwide, ranging between 2 and 74% of dialysis populations [1]. Despite proven economic advantage [2–4], improved quality of life [5, 6], higher levels of satisfaction with treatment [7], early survival advantage [8, 9], delayed need for vascular access procedures [10, 11], reduced blood transfusion requirements [12], reduced hepatitis virus transmission rates [13] and better preservation of residual renal function [14, 15], PD is a greatly underutilised dialysis modality [16], and there is decreased uptake across North America, Australia and New Zealand, with greater variability within Europe [16–18]. Infection risk and concern about inferior outcomes are the most commonly cited reasons for preferential uptake of haemodialysis (HD) [16, 18]. Despite this impression, research indicates that HD and PD patients have similar overall infection risk [19] and that improvements in PD outcome have outperformed those seen with in-centre HD [20]. Nonetheless, the complications of PD represent barriers to its widespread implementation, and their management and prevention are key to maintaining PD technique and overcoming clinicians' prejudices.

10.2 Infectious Complications

10.2.1 Peritonitis

10.2.1.1 Epidemiology and Risk Factors

PD-related peritonitis is the most frequent, serious complication of PD and is the most common reason for transfer to HD [21]. PD peritonitis contributes to about 20% of PD technique failure [21] via increased risks of catheter removal and permanent HD transfer. Long-term peritonitis damages the peritoneal membrane, resulting in ultrafiltration failure and dialysis inadequacy and may contribute to the most feared complication—encapsulating peritoneal sclerosis [22]. PD-related peritonitis increases mortality risk, accounting for 16% of PD deaths [23–25] and increases morbidity in terms of hospitalisation and reduction in residual renal function [26].

Rates of PD-related peritonitis vary enormously across different centres and countries. Reported rates range from 0.06 to 1.66 episodes per patient-year [27], although the literature suffers from a paucity of well-performed studies dominated by single-centre reports. Even within the same country, there is considerable variation in the rates of PD peritonitis regardless of centre size. The Australian and New Zealand Dialysis and Transplant (ANZDATA) Registry has demonstrated a tenfold variation in PD peritonitis rates among centres [21] (Fig. 10.1), epidemiological studies performed in Scotland and the UK irrespective of centre size, patient-to-staff ratio or duration of PD training time [28]. Poor PD outcomes reflect variations in clinical practice and deviations from international guidelines, particularly with respect to prophylaxis practices with exit-site mupirocin and antifungal therapy during episodes of bacterial peritonitis [21].

Contributing to this observed variation in peritonitis rates are inconsistencies in the definitions adopted by heterogeneous studies. The International Society of Peritoneal Dialysis (ISPD) has standardised diagnostic criteria along with the definitions for recurrent, relapsing, repeat, refractory and catheter-related infections [24]. Peritonitis patients presenting with cloudy effluent should be presumed to have peritonitis, which is confirmed by obtaining effluent cell count, differential and culture. Peritonitis should, however, always be included in the differential diagnosis of any PD patient with abdominal pain or fever, even if the effluent is clear. An

D. W. Johnson (✉) · A. Kennard · C. M. Hawley
Department of Nephrology, Princess Alexandra Hospital, Brisbane, QLD, Australia
e-mail: david.johnson2@health.qld.gov.au

A. K. Singh et al. (eds.), *Core Concepts in Dialysis and Continuous Therapies*, DOI 10.1007/978-1-4899-7657-4_10

Peritonitis rates by treating unit

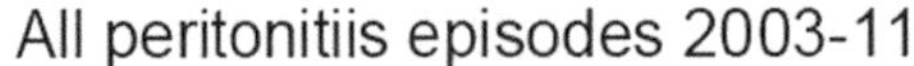

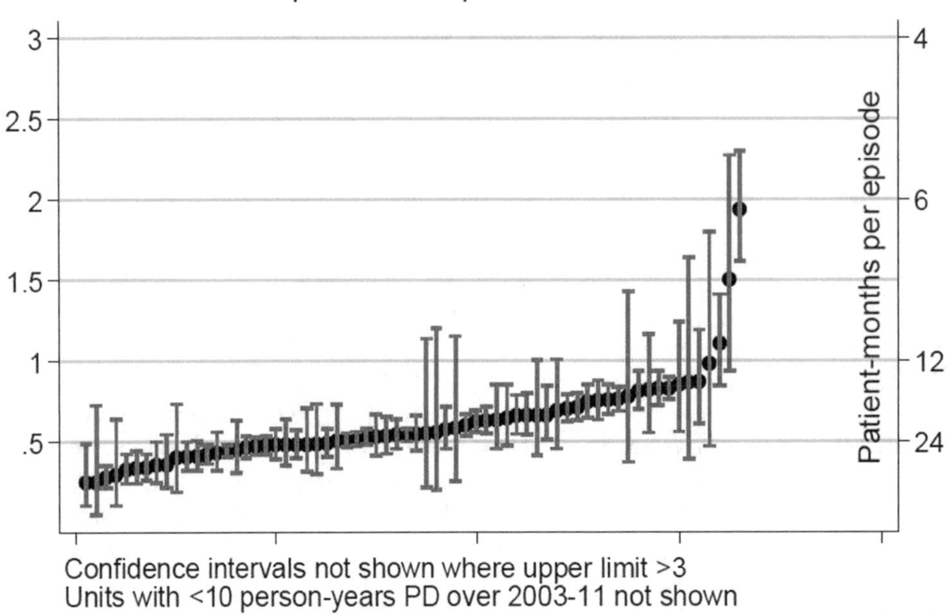

Fig. 10.1 Peritoneal dialysis rates by treating centre in Australia and New Zealand in 2011, as captured by the ANZDATA registry. (ANZDATA 2012 Annual Report)

effluent cell count with white blood cells numbering more than 100/μL following a dwell time of at least 2 h with at least 50 % polymorphonuclear neutrophilic cells reflects significant peritoneal inflammation and peritonitis is the most likely cause. The ISPD guidelines emphasise the percentage of polymorphonuclear cells rather than the absolute number of white cells to diagnose peritonitis and endorse an empirical approach to antibiotic therapy largely irrespective of the initial Gram stain as it is frequently negative or misleading [24, 29]. The role of the Gram stain is primarily to identify the presence of yeast or other fungal elements and thereby prompt early initiation of antifungal therapy and removal of the Tenckoff catheter [24]. Effluent samples should be inoculated into two blood culture bottles at the bedside and brought within 6 hours to the laboratory. Identification of causative organisms is not only important for determining antibiotic sensitivities and guiding antibiotic selection, but also for assisting in elucidating the source of contamination and risk stratifying the patient with regards to relapsing, recurrent and repeat infection. Questioning the patient about lapses in technique and, in particular, contamination or disconnection, may frame re-education attempts following resolution of the infection. Likewise, clinical features that suggest a gastroenterological source, such as recent endoscopy, constipation and the presence of localised tenderness suggestive of appendicitis or cholecystitis, may indicate the presence of an underlying surgical issue. The catheter should be inspected for evidence of exit-site and tunnel infection.

There is currently inadequate evidence to recommend the use of flow cytometry or multiple enzyme-linked immunosorbent assay to distinguish between Gram-positive and Gram-negative infections [28]. This novel development, however, suggests a future possibility for point of care testing and the emergence of more timely and targeted peritonitis therapy [30].

The ISPD guidelines state that rates of culture-negative peritonitis should not be greater than 20 % of episodes and could be further improved by culturing the sediment after centrifuging 50 mL of effluent [24]. The species cultured is useful for prognostication purposes. Relapsing peritonitis is an infection with the same organism or a sterile episode occurring within 4 weeks of completion of therapy, whereas recurrent peritonitis involves a different causative organism, still within 4 weeks of completion of therapy. Relapsing and recurrent peritonitis complicate 14 and 5 % of peritonitis episodes, respectively, and carry increased risk of catheter removal and permanent transfer to HD therapy [31]. By contrast, repeat peritonitis, defined as infection caused by the same organism after 4 weeks of completion of therapy, has more benign implications [32]. The detection of bacterial

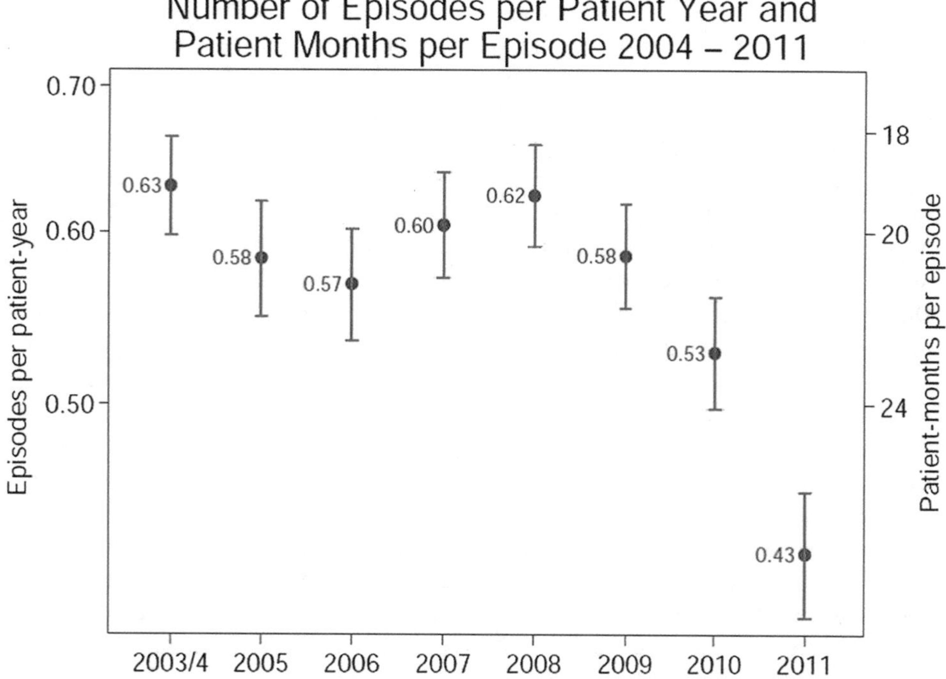

Fig. 10.2 Improved rates of peritoneal dialysis (PD)-related peritonitis following the "Call to Action" initiative and the launch of the PD Academy educational program. (ANZDATA Registry annual report 2012)

fragments in PD effluent following an episode of peritonitis may predict relapse or repeat peritonitis but has not yet been adopted into clinical practice [33].

Rates of peritonitis escalate where units deviate from ISPD guidelines [34]. A rate of 1 episode every 18 months (0.67/year at risk) has been deemed acceptable [24], although units should strive to improve beyond this. PD peritonitis rates as low as 0.36 episodes per patient-year (1 episode every 33 patient-months at risk) are considered achievable with adoption of best practice [29]. Departures from ISPD guidelines predict inferior PD outcomes and reduced technique survival [34, 35]. In Australia, the most recent official overall peritonitis rate is 0.43 episodes per patient-year (1 episode per 28 patient-months; Fig. 10.2). Surveys however indicate poor adherence (<50%) to evidence-based practices, such as administering prophylactic antibiotics at the time of Tenckoff catheter insertion, prescribing topical antimicrobial prophylaxis [36] or selecting appropriate antibiotics for treatment of peritonitis [37]. PD peritonitis rates in other parts of the world are likewise suboptimal [24, 34]. Although implementation of ISPD guideline recommendations into clinical practice remains suboptimal, the "Call to Action" initiative in Australia has demonstrated that the systematic adoption of standardised unit protocols based on ISPD Guidelines, education of young nephrologists in PD management, establishment of national peritonitis registry, introduction of a national key performance indicator project based on benchmarked peritonitis rates and conduct of ongoing surveillance of PD practice and patient outcomes [34] has achieved dramatic reductions in PD peritonitis rates across Australia [21] (Fig. 10.2).

Risk factors for PD peritonitis include advanced age, frailty and comorbidity along with lower socioeconomic status and indigenous racial origin [21, 28]. Smoking and obesity increase risk of infection generally and PD peritonitis more specifically, while pets and rural living emphasise the importance of good hygiene to successful PD technique [21]. Preserved residual renal function and the prior use of HD also increase risk [35, 38]. Patient preference for PD predicts technique success [39], while depression and anxiety predict higher rates of PD peritonitis [29]. In their discussion of PD peritonitis risk factors, Cho and Johnson [28] emphasise that there is no high-level evidence that modifying these risk factors will lead to reduced peritonitis rates, nor that for patients with nonmodifable risk factors increased home support, increased training frequency or more intensive infection prophylaxis mitigate peritonitis risk.

10.2.1.2 Empirical Management

The mainstay of peritonitis management is the timely initiation of empirical antimicrobial agents that are likely to eradicate the most common causative organisms, as endorsed by ISPD. Empiric antibiotics must cover both Gram-positive and Gram-negative organisms and should be based on local antimicrobial susceptibility data [24, 33, 35]. Vancomycin or cephalosporins may be used for Gram-positive organism cover along with third-generation cephalosporin, aminoglycoside or carbopenam for Gram-negative organism cover. First-generation cephalosporins, such as cefazolin or cephalothin, demonstrate generally equivalent outcomes to glycopeptides (e.g. vancomycin), although glycopeptide regimens were more likely to achieve a complete cure (3 studies, 370 episodes: risk ratio (RR) 1.66, 95 % confidence interval (CI) 1.01–2.72) [40]. On the other hand, cephalosporin administration may be associated with a lower risk of selecting for multiresistant organisms [41]. Short-term use of gentamicin (<5 days) has not been shown to be associated with more rapid decline of residual renal function [26, 42]. This factor, together with the risk of ototoxicity, should, however, be considered during prolonged courses of more than 1–2 weeks duration where alternative agents should be sought [40].

Intraperitoneal (IP) administration of antibiotics is superior to intravenous (IV) dosing for treating peritonitis [40]. Intermittent versus continuous IP antibiotic dosing results in comparable clinical outcomes [40]. Rapid exchanges in automated peritoneal dialysis (APD) may lead to inadequate time to establish effective dialysate concentrations of antibiotics [24], although it is presently unknown whether or not APD patients with peritonitis should be temporarily switched from APD to continuous ambulatory peritoneal dialysis (CAPD) for the duration of their peritonitis treatment. One retrospective, observational study reported no differences in peritonitis-related relapse rates, catheter removal rates or death in 239 PD patients continued on APD during peritonitis treatment compared with 269 patients managed on CAPD [43]. Although further research in the area is clearly warranted, the ISPD Guidelines recommend that APD patients treated for PD-related peritonitis using an intermittent IP dosing regimen should dwell their antibiotic-loaded dialysis fluids for at least 6 h to facilitate adequate antimicrobial concentrations and effect [24].

Monitoring of serum antibiotic levels (vancomycin, gentamicin) during treatment of PD peritonitis has not been clearly demonstrated to result in improved efficacy or safety, but is often performed [44–46]. Re-dosing is generally advised when serum vancomycin levels fall below 15 μg/mL and serum gentamicin levels fall below 0.5 μg/mL.

It is imperative that antifungal prophylaxis, in the form of either nystatin or daily fluconazole, is administered during antibiotic therapy based on previous randomised controlled studies that such an approach reduces the risk of subsequent fungal peritonitis [47–50]. Unfortunately, registry data suggest that less than one in ten patients in Australia and New Zealand receive antifungal prophylaxis and risk-adverse outcomes following severe fungal peritonitis [35, 49].

Once culture results and sensitivities are known, antibiotic therapy should be adjusted to appropriate specific therapy. Efficacy of therapy should be assessed on clinical grounds; most patients with PD peritonitis show considerable improvement with 48 h of commencement of therapy. Repeated cell counts of $\geq 1090/\text{mm}^2$ within dialysis effluent predict treatment failure and catheter removal is indicated [51]. Refractory peritonitis, defined as failure of PD effluent to clear after 5 days of appropriate antibiotic treatment, should be treated with immediate catheter removal, as per ISPD Guidelines [24]. Prolonged attempts to treat refractory peritonitis with antimicrobial agents but without catheter removal result in extended hospital stay, peritoneal membrane damage and increased risks of fungal peritonitis and death. Catheter removal is also indicated in all cases of fungal peritonitis and many cases of *Pseudomonas* and relapsing peritonitis [31, 49, 52]. Following catheter removal and transfer to HD, patients who subsequently return to PD have comparable peritonitis-free, technique and patients survival rates to those PD patients who experienced peritonitis and did not have a catheter removed [53]. The survival of such patients was also comparable to those of PD patients who permanently transferred to HD following catheter removal for peritonitis [53]. Thus, patients who transfer to HD following a severe peritonitis episode should not be discouraged from returning to PD. The optimal timing of return to PD is not known at present.

For PD peritonitis that does respond promptly to IP antibiotic therapy (typically 70–80 % of cases), the ISPD guidelines endorse a minimum duration of antimicrobial therapy for peritonitis of 2 weeks for mild infections but 3 weeks for moderate-to-severe infection (e.g. *Staphylococcus aureus*, Gram-negative organism, enterococci, polymicrobial).

10.2.1.3 Microbiology

Gram-Positive Peritonitis

Historically, Gram-positive organisms and particularly Coagulase-negative *Staphylococcus* account for the majority of PD peritonitis cases. Such infections are typically of milder severity and generally reflect touch contamination and a break in technique. The introduction of disconnect systems rather than standard spike systems particularly improved the rates of Gram-positive contamination-related PD peritonitis [54–58]. Such infections typically respond rapidly to antibiotic therapy and may be appropriate for outpatient therapy. In some units, there is a very high rate of methicillin-resistance, which may necessitate the use of vancomycin as empiric therapy. Relapsing coagulase-negative peritonitis is suggestive of biofilm formation, which can be addressed through catheter replacement under antibiotic coverage as a single procedure [28]. A recent Cochrane systematic review demonstrated that, based on a single small study, simultaneous catheter removal and replacement was better than urokinase at reducing treatment failure rates (RR 2.35, 95 % CI 1.13–4.91) in the setting of relapsing or persistent peritonitis [40]. *Streptococcus* and *Enterococcus* peritonitis tend to present with more severe and painful infection and may reflect a metastatic source such as gastrointestinal tract, genitourinary tract, exit-site or tunnel infection, or dental abscess. Touch contamination should also be considered. Enterococccal infections carry a high risk of catheter removal (52 %), permanent transfer to HD (52 %) and death, which may be averted by timely removal of the PD catheter [24, 28]. Ampicillin remains the antibiotic of choice in vancomycin-resistant enterococcal (VRE) infection, but linezolid or quinupristin/dalfpristin may be required if ampicillin resistance is detected. *S. aureus* causes severe peritonitis and is frequently accompanied by exit-site or tunnel infection. *S. aureus* infection with concurrent exit-site or tunnel infection is frequently refractory and requires catheter removal and a rest period of at least 2 weeks off PD. Methicillin-resistant *S. aureus* infections are typically refractory and carry a high risk of permanent transfer to HD. Both vancomycin and rifampicin can be used intraperitoneally.

Gram-Negative Peritonitis

The most common causes of Gram-negative peritonitis episodes are *Pseudomonas, E. coli* and *Klebsiella* and clinically manifest as severe peritonitis with high rates of hospitalisation, catheter removal and permanent transfer to HD. Catheter removal is indicated if there is accompanying catheter infection. A review of 210 episodes of Enterobacteriaceae peritonitis found that recent antibiotic use and concurrent exit-site infection were predictors of this type of peritonitis with 10 % of patients dying within a month of peritonitis onset [59]. This emphasises the need for aggressive and appropriate therapy to prevent mortality and catheter loss. An assessment should be made for constipation, diverticulitis and colitis, which allow the transmural migration of coliforms. Gram-negative organisms have a high risk of relapse due to biofilm formation and require a longer duration of therapy. *Pseudomonas* infections should always be managed with two antipseudomonal antibiotics and must be continued for 2 weeks while the patient is temporarily transferred to HD. *Stenotrophomonas* peritonitis may follow the use of carbapenems, fluoroquinolones and late-generation cephalosporins, which select for this multiresistant organism. Therapy must be prolonged (3–4 weeks) and utilise two drugs; usually a combination of trimethoprim/sulphamethoxazole, ticarcillin/clavulanate and/or oral minocycline [24].

Polymicrobial Peritonitis

Polymicrobial infections, particularly those involving the presence of anaerobic organisms, carry a high risk of death and should prompt surgical evaluation for the possibility of underlying intra-abdominal pathology, such as cholecystitis, ischaemic bowel, appendicitis or abscess. Nevertheless, most recent reports suggest that polymicrobial peritonitis is associated with a relatively low incidence of catastrophic surgical pathology, ranging from 2.8 to 9 % [60–63]. Underlying surgical peritonitis should be suspected if patients present with haemodynamic instability, sepsis, lactic acidosis or elevations in peritoneal fluid amylase. The Gram stain may identify a mixed bacterial population and should prompt early surgical opinion, abdominal imaging and management with ampicillin, metronidazole and aminoglycoside in the recommended IV doses. Early catheter removal should be considered.

Fungal Peritonitis

Fungal peritonitis occurs in 1–23 % of peritonitis episodes [64]. Risk factors include multiple episodes of bacterial peritonitis, particularly polymicrobial, and recent (within 1 month) treatment with broad-spectrum antibiotics in the absence of adequate fungal prophylaxis [49, 60]. Outcomes following fungal peritonitis are generally poor with a risk of death as high as 25 % [51]. Fungal peritonitis necessitates immediate removal of the catheter and empirical management with amphotericin B or flucytosine and thereafter based on culture and susceptibility results [24].

Tuberculous Peritonitis

Peritonitis due to mycobacteria is a rare occurrence, but should be considered when peritonitis persists or relapses despite antimicrobial therapy, in patients with systemic features and when the peritoneal effluent demonstrates a lymphocytosis. Outcomes are poor with very high rates of catheter loss (80 %) and significant mortality (40 %) [40]. Smears should be examined for acid fast bacteria with Ziehl-Neelsen stain but smear-negative disease is common. Although examination of dialysate effluent for mycobacterial DNA and/or adenosine deaminase is useful, exploratory laparoscopy with biopsy of the peritoneum has a higher diagnostic yield and should be considered when tuberculous peritonitis is suspected. Treatment reflects general tuberculosis protocols with the avoidance of ethambutol due to increased risk of optic neuritis in end-stage renal failure. Typical regimens include rifampicin, isoniazid, pyrazinamide and ofloxacin. Catheter removal is usually advised.

Culture-Negative Peritonitis

As previously indicated, rates of culture-negative peritonitis can be minimised by improved PD fluid sampling and culture techniques and should be below 20 % in all PD units. A history of previous antibiotic use is a recognised risk factor and should be sought on presentation. Outcomes following culture-negative peritonitis are relatively benign with higher rates of cure with antibiotics alone, less need for hospitalisation, less mortality, less catheter removal and increased maintenance of PD modality [65, 66]. Special culture techniques may identify lipid-dependent yeast, *Mycobacteria*, fungi, *Campylobacter, Legionella* and other fastidious bacteria. In clinical practice, if a patient is improving clinically on empirical therapy, it can be continued for duration of 2 weeks provided the effluent clears rapidly.

10.2.1.4 Outcomes Following PD Peritonitis

The majority of patients who suffer an episode of PD peritonitis will respond to therapy and continue with this dialysis modality. Studies indicate 80–85 % of peritonitis episodes are successfully treated [39]. In certain areas, including Australia, rates of suboptimal outcomes are higher and include a 14 % risk of relapse, 5 % risk of recurrence, 22 % risk of catheter removal and 18 % rate of permanent HD transfer [35, 49, 50, 52, 67, 68]. In their recent Cochrane Review, Ballinger and colleagues considered catheter removal to be equivalent to treatment failure [40]. Other bodies regard the need for catheter removal as a marker of the severity of the episode [69]. Certainly, a delay in catheter removal is associated with high rates of transfer to permanent HD and should be considered early in peritonitis cases caused by *S. aureus* [35, 69], *Pseudomonas* [35, 69], *Enterococci* [68], fungi [49] and multiple organisms [35, 60]. In their study of patients with severe peritonitis requiring catheter removal, Szeto and colleagues concluded that PD can be resumed in only a small number of patients and, when successful, predicts both patient and technique survival [69]. Other studies have likewise reported a low rate (about 20 %) [70] of successful reinsertion and resumption of PD following peritonitis. The timing of reinsertion is not clear but anecdotal recommendations endorsed by the Caring for Australasians with renal impairment (CARI) guidelines range from simultaneous removal and reinsertion to waiting a minimum of 3 weeks [71].

Peritoneal transport characteristics are dramatically altered by an episode of severe peritonitis with marked decline in ultrafiltration and increase in D/P creatinine ratio at 4 h, but dialysis adequacy and nutritional status can be maintained regardless of this [69]. It is interesting to that note that, in general, Asian patients enjoy better post-PD peritonitis outcomes than do Caucasian patients [34, 37, 69].

Epidemiological studies of cases of PD peritonitis report an association with PD peritonitis and mortality with highest risk in the first 30 days but extending until 120 days following an episode of infection [25, 27]. Low serum albumin predicts technique failure and death in patients on PD [72], which likely reflects its role as an acute phase reactant and marker of inflammation but may also reflect malnutrition. Hypoalbuminaemia also predicts catheter loss in PD peritonitis [73].

10.2.2 Exit-Site and Tunnel Infections

Exit-site infection is suggested by the presence of erythematous skin surrounding the catheter and definite in the presence of purulent drainage. A positive culture in the absence of these clinical findings may reflect simple colonisation rather than infection. Thus, the diagnosis requires experience and clinical judgement. Tunnel infection may occur with or without accompanying exit-site infection and manifests as erythema, oedema and tenderness, although is frequently clinically occult. Tunnel infection may be confirmed with the use of ultrasound. Aggressive management is recommended for *S. aureus* and *Pseudomonas* exit-site infection as there is often concomitant tunnel infection. Empirical antibiotic therapy may be initiated immediately and should always cover *S. aureus* or may be deferred until culture and sensitivity results become available to guide therapy. Oral antibiotic therapy is as effective as intraperitoneal antibiotic therapy. Gram-positive exit-site and tunnel infection can be managed with a first-generation cephalosporin, such as cephalexin. Alternatives include clindamycin, doxycycline and minocycline. These drugs do not require dose adjustment for renal failure. In slowly resolving or severe *S. aureus* infection, rifampicin 600 mg daily should be added. *Pseudomonas* exit-site infections are particularly difficult to treat and require prolonged duration of therapy. Oral fluoroquinolones as monotherapy may be a reasonable treatment option for mild cases. However, severe, refractory or recurrent pseudomonal exit-site infection requires a second antipseudomonal drug. Antibiotic therapy should be continued until the exit site appears normal. ISPD guidelines recommend a duration of 2 weeks for most exit-site infections, which is extended to 3 weeks in the case of pseudomonal exit-site infection [24]. Progression to peritonitis or concomitant peritonitis is an indication for catheter removal.

10.2.2.1 Prevention of Peritoneal Dialysis-Related Peritonitis and Exit-Site Infection

Practices to reduce infection risk in PD patients include a number of interventions already mentioned, including appropriate selection of patients, training and retraining of patients and staff education to increase professional confidence in PD and to champion its role in renal replacement therapy. The role of hand hygiene cannot be overemphasised. Patient education should teach routine exit-site care with water and antibacterial soap or non-cytotoxic antiseptics. Furthermore, units should establish ongoing surveillance of their infection rates and perform root cause analysis of all episodes of peritonitis [34]. Nasal carriage status of *S. aureus* should be sought and documented on all patients entering a PD program and eradication attempted. Nasal carriage of *S. aureus* is associated with an increased risk of catheter exit-site infection and its eradication with mupirocin has been shown to improve rates of both exit-site infection and PD peritonitis [74, 75].

There is currently no evidence to support the use of any particular catheter other than the standard silicone Tenckoff catheter for the prevention of peritonitis. The use of double-cuff catheters initially showed promise, but with the widespread adoption of prophylactic intranasal and exit-site ointments their role has diminished [28]. Prior to catheter placement, proper bowel preparation and skin cleansing, including removal of hair where indicated, can improve rates of peritonitis and exit-site infection [27, 76]. Catheter placement by an experienced surgeon with prophylactic single-dose IV antibiotics decreases the risk of subsequent infection [77]. There is some evidence that vancomycin may be superior to cephalosporin [27]. Newly inserted catheters should be immobilised but sutures at the exit site increase infection and are contraindicated [75].

Disconnect systems utilising twin-bag and Y-sets are superior to spiking of dialysis bags, and this is supported by randomised control trial evidence and systematic review [77, 78]. There are equivalent rates of PD peritonitis among APD and CAPD patients [79].

Exit-site infection and peritonitis caused by *S. aureus* and other Gram-positive organisms are prevented by the use of topical exit-site mupirocin. A number of studies have demonstrated efficacy, while meta-analysis data reveal reductions in the rates of peritonitis by 40–66% and exit-site infection by 62–77% [74]. Hence, the use of topical exit-site mupirocin is endorsed by the ISPD [29]. Gentamicin and Polysporin Triple ointment were also found to be effective in preventing bacterial exit-site and peritoneal infection at the cost of increased rates of fungal infection at these sites [80–82]. The ISPD guidelines recommend against their use and raise concern over the particular risk of inducing gentamicin resistance, which remains a useful drug for treatment of PD peritonitis [27]. Likewise, mupirocin resistance has been documented and it is expected that high-level resistance will eventually result in clinical failure or unacceptable relapse rate. The HONEYPOT trial proposed that medical grade, antibacterial honey has antimicrobial properties without inducing antimicrobial resistance and may have a role in preventing exit-site infections and hence PD peritonitis [83]. This multicentre open-label trial randomly assigned 371 patients to either topical exit-site honey or intranasal mupirocin. The rate of infection within the honey group was equivalent to that seen in the mupirocin group. Diabetics randomised to honey, however, had increased rates of exit-site and peritoneal infection and use of honey was poorly tolerated and greater numbers of patients withdrew from this arm compared to the mupirocin group. Thus, current evidence does not support the use of honey in PD patients.

Fungal peritonitis is predicted by the use of antibiotics for both bacterial peritonitis and nonperitoneal infections [49]. Fungal prophylaxis with oral fluconazole or nystatin has demonstrated benefit and should be routinely employed, particularly during prolonged courses of antibiotics for conditions, such as foot ulcer or osteomyelitis.

Severe constipation and diarrhoea may precipitate episodes of PD peritonitis via the transmigration of microorganisms across the bowel wall [84]. Hypomotility and gastroparesis likewise increase risk, and constipation is a common clinical problem that is often poorly recognised by the chronic PD patient. These disorders should be sought and managed appropriately to prevent PD peritonitis. Gastrointestinal pathology, such as cholecystitis, ischaemic bowel, diverticulitis and colitis, can cause an enteric peritonitis, which is frequently polymicrobial. Many nephrologists consider inflammatory bowel disease to be a contraindication to PD. The occurrence of surgical issues such as these may be an indication for catheter removal and transfer to HD.

Invasive procedures, such as colonoscopy, hysteroscopy and performance of dental work, can also lead to peritonitis at a rate of up to 6 in every 100 patients [85]. Ampicillin prophylaxis eradicated all cases of post-procedural peritonitis, although the difference was not statistically significant due to the relatively low event rates. The ISPD guidelines recommend emptying the abdomen of fluid prior to the procedure and giving consideration to pre-procedural antibiotic prophylaxis [27].

Combining and implementing all of the above prevention strategies in "bundle-of-care" programs delivered by experienced units with regularly trained doctors, nurse and patients can help to ensure adherence to evidence-based best practices, thereby effectively reducing peritonitis rates in continuous cycles of quality improvement [76].

The BalANZ trial recently demonstrated a potential role for neutral pH, low glucose degradation product (GDP), and "biocompatible" PD fluids in preventing PD peritonitis [86, 87]. This multicentre open-label randomised controlled trial assigned 185 incident PD patients with residual renal function to pH-neutral, low GDP dialysis solution or conventional dialysis solution for 2 years. The biocompatible group exhibited significantly longer times to first peritonitis episode and lower rates of peritonitis as well as longer times to the development of anuria. This same study also observed that use of novel dialysis solutions resulted in shorter peritonitis-related duration of hospitalisation, suggesting that biocompatible solutions reduced both the likelihood and severity of peritonitis. This finding has not been upheld in a recent Cochrane review of biocompatible dialysis fluids, but identified limitations in trial heterogeneity, definitions of peritonitis and high rates of attrition bias in included studies other than the BalANZ trial [88].

10.3 Noninfectious Complications

10.3.1 Catheter Complications

The success of chronic PD depends upon safe and permanent access to the peritoneal cavity [89]. A review of recent literature reveals catheter failure rates of up to 35 % at 1 year [90]. Catheter-related problems contribute to a significant proportion of failed PD cases and necessitate transfer to HD within the first year in up to 20 % of cases [91, 92]. Prevention, early recognition and appropriate management of these complications are important to avoid patient morbidity and disillusionment with the PD technique, which may undermine a patient's willingness to persevere with PD [91].

A number of different variations to the standard Tenckoff catheter have been developed, including variation on the number of cuffs (one vs two), the design of the subcutaneous pathway (bent or "swan neck" vs straight) and the profile of the intraperitoneal portion (straight vs coiled). Systemic review and meta-analysis data reveal an advantage in favour of straight compared to coiled catheters [90]. There is inadequate evidence to recommend single versus double cuff catheters [89]. The use of a "swan neck" catheter is associated with the lowest rates of drainage dysfunction [90] and is endorsed by the ISPD [89].

Presurgical evaluation should include assessment for preexisting abdominal wall herniation, as this will likely worsen when subjected to increased intraperitoneal pressures. A history of prior abdominal surgeries and most particularly abdominal catastrophe should be sought [89]. Skin and bowel preparation has been covered elsewhere. Insertion technique, either by laparoscopic route or open procedure, does not predict infectious outcome nor catheter survival [77]. The experience of the surgeon, however, is critical in optimising catheter outcomes [34, 89]. The catheter tip should sit deep in the pelvis and ideally within the left lower quadrant to minimise risk of incomplete drainage [89]. Some groups describe an advanced laparoscopic technique with rectus sheath tunnelling, prophylactic adhesiolysis and prophylactic omentopexy to fix redundant omentum to the upper abdomen via a suture [93]. They report reduction in the rate of catheter flow complications to <1 % compared with 12 % with standard laparoscopic technique [93]. The advanced laparoscopic technique may be employed in patients with risk of catheter malfunction, such as prior abdominal surgery [91]. ISPD guidelines suggest catheter survival of >80 % at 1 year is a reasonable goal [89].

10.3.2 Inflow Pain

Pain on dialysate infusion may occur in the absence of infection and is a common occurrence in PD patients. The pain typically diminishes with the duration of the dwell period and usually improves with increasing time on PD as the peritoneal membrane adapts. Some patients, however, experience severe and persistent pain that necessitates the discontinuation of PD. The pain is attributed to the acidic pH of conventional lactate-buffered dialysate (usually pH 5.2–5.5) and bioincompatible hypertonic, high glucose concentration and dialysate temperature as well as catheter tip position. In their systematic review of biocompatible PD fluids, Cho and colleagues concluded that there was a significant reduction in inflow pain with the adoption of bicarbonate-buffered pH neutral, low glucose dialysate [94] and this was supported by meta-analysis [88]. Slowing the rate of infusion may also alleviate pain. It has been hypothesised that other sequelae of non-physiologic dialysate fluids, such as loss of peritoneal mesothelial cell viability and function, compromised peritoneal immune function, promotion of fibrosis and vascular remodelling within the peritoneal membrane are also reversible with the adoption of biocompatible fluids [94].

10.3.3 Outflow Failure

Outflow failure is defined as the incomplete recovery of instilled dialysate fluid within a reasonable time frame (30–45 min), which may be precipitated by constipation, catheter migration, intraluminal catheter obstruction by thrombus or fibrin, catheter kinking or catheter occlusion (e.g. by redundant omentum or adhesions). This issue complicates approximately 10 % of PD cases. It is not explained by catheter type (straight vs coiled intraperitoneal segment) [90], although may be amenable to advanced laparoscopic technique (described above) [93]. A kinked catheter usually demonstrates resistance to both inflow and outflow of dialysate and may be identified by plain abdominal radiograph. Likewise, the presence of constipation can be assessed by abdominal imaging. Catheter malposition is usually apparent within days of first using the catheter, while omental occlusion complicates PD several weeks after catheter placement. Physical examination can exclude leakage as a differential to outflow failure.

Management of outflow failure depends primarily on the cause identified. Liberal use of laxatives including suppositories and enemas can be used to treat constipation, and the resumption of bowel movement cures the majority of cases of outflow failure [95]. Intraluminal instillation of heparin and thrombolytics [96] may resolve both inflow and outflow obstruction, and guide-wire manipulation [97–99] can be considered when there is radiographic evidence of migration. Studies report an initial good success rate (85 %) but warn this is short-lived and prone to recurrence in the long term [97]. Laparoscopic repositioning and/or replacement of a nonfunctioning catheter remains a valuable recourse for long-term patency [97, 99] and is usually required if a catheter fails to flip down or unblock after 2–3 days of aperients and when no other cause has been identified. Occluded catheters may need to be managed by adhesiolysis, omentectomy or catheter replacement, as necessary.

10.3.4 PD Fluid Leakage

Leakage of dialysate may occur around the catheter (manifest as an accumulation of high glucose-containing fluid around the PD catheter exit site, subcutaneous swelling, genital oedema and/or apparent ultrafiltration failure), into the genitalia via a patent processus vaginalis, or into the pleural cavity (manifesting as dyspnoea, weight gain and ultrafiltration failure). The incidence (5 %) appears higher in CAPD, presumably related to upright posture and increased pressures on the abdominal wall but is widely under-reported [100]. Risk factors for pericatheter leaks include weak abdominal wall musculature following pregnancy or multiple abdominal surgeries, early initiation of PD following catheter placement, use of large intraperitoneal exchange volumes and factors impairing wound healing (e.g. diabetes mellitus, obesity, corticosteroid therapy, etc.) [95, 100]. There is no consensus on catheter choice for the avoidance of this complication but the use of a laparoscopic technique may reduce its incidence [95, 101]. Evidence favours a 14-day rest period following surgical catheter placement to allow postoperative healing [100], but urgent-start PD may employ low volumes in the supine position using a cycler [102].

Management of pericatheter leaks consists of decreased upright posture, temporary adoption of nocturnal APD, reduction in dialysis volumes and surgical repair. Genital oedema responds to surgical ligation of the patent processus vaginalis. Pleural leaks are more resistant to intervention and often necessitate transfer to HD [103, 104]. Some centres report success with chemical pleurodesis using either talc [105, 106] or tetracycline [107]. Systemic volume overload and congestive cardiac failure should be excluded [103, 104].

10.3.5 Abdominal Wall Herniation

Abdominal wall herniation can be a troublesome complication of CAPD and its risk is increased by female gender, parity, small body size, increasing age, longer time on PD, autosomal dominant polycystic kidney disease, diabetes and prior abdominal surgery [108–110]. Sites of occurrence include the inguinal canal and patent processus vaginalis, umbilicus, linea alba and site of prior abdominal incisions [111]. Symptoms include swelling and disfigurement and can be complicated by intestinal obstruction, bowel incarceration and strangulation. Diagnosis is made by physical examination and ultrasound imaging. Management consists of surgical repair employing a polypropylene mesh prosthesis, which allows the resumption of PD within several days of hernia repair, usually via low-volume supine rapid cycling PD and graduated return to the former PD regimen [110, 111]. The Bargman protocol for postoperative management of PD following hernia repair avoids interim transfer to HD while avoiding underdialysis and re-herniation [112].

10.3.6 Intestinal Perforation

Intestinal perforation can complicate catheter implantation due to direct injury or may occur later due to bowel wall erosion and ulceration. In patients with advanced vascular disease, intestinal perforation may be precipitated by ischaemia of the bowel wall. It is an uncommon complication that reflects the experience of the surgeon. Clues to presentation are the occurrence of polymicrobial peritonitis, bloody or feculent dialysate and diarrhoea following dialysate instillation. Management includes cessation of PD with catheter removal and surgical repair of the bowel under antibiotic coverage [95].

10.3.7 Haemoperitoneum

Bloody peritoneal dialysate is an infrequent occurrence and may reflect a range of intra-abdominal events with both benign and harmful significance. It should be remembered that a very small amount (<1 ml of blood) can make peritoneal fluid appear blood tinged and that in the absence of PD many of these events may be clinically silent.

Benign causes of haemoperitoneum include menstrual bleeding, likely secondary to ovulation, retrograde menstruation and endometriosis. Rapid flushes and the instillation of heparin can prevent obstruction of the PD catheter due to clots. Mild and spontaneously resolving bleeding can also follow catheter manipulation or insertion. To date, there is no evidence favouring coiled catheters over straight tip catheters with respect to the complication of catheter-related haemoperitoneum.

Intra-abdominal pathology, such as rupture of liver cysts and splenic injury, may cause intra-abdominal bleeding, sometimes with surgical implications. Retroperitoneal events including rupture of kidney cysts may uncommonly cause haemoperitoneum accompanied by haematuria [113]. Intra-abdominal malignancy including liver carcinomatosis [114] and renal cell carcinoma [115] may potentially cause haemoperitoneum in PD. This possibility can be evaluated further with PD fluid cytology and computed tomography (CT) of abdomen.

10.3.8 Encapsulating Peritoneal Sclerosis

Encapsulating peritoneal sclerosis (EPS; formerly sclerosing encapsulating peritonitis) is a complication of PD characterised by persistent, intermittent or recurrent adhesive bowel obstruction with peritoneal fibrosis and malnutrition. Its incidence varies from 0.3 to 3.3 % and increases with time on PD with occurrences as high as 6.4 and 19.4 % in Australia and 2.1 and 5.9 % in Japan at 5 and 8 years, respectively [22]. Mortality rates have been reported to be as high as 50 % but more recent data from an Australian study suggest a considerably lower mortality risk [116]. The ISPD guidelines emphasise that EPS is infrequent and its risk of occurrence should not time limit the delivery of PD [22]. In this way, it is comparable to the risk of infectious endocarditis or osteomyelitis in the HD population. Risk factors for EPS include time on dialysis [22, 117, 118], bioincompatible dialysate [120], dialysate contamination [119, 120, 122], catheter type and episodes of severe peritonitis [116–118, 121].

Clinical manifestations vary widely and there are no reliable biochemical or radiological screening tests. It is frequently recognised following the cessation of PD. Patients present with clinical features of bowel obstruction, including anorexia, nausea, vomiting and weight loss. Other presentations include haemoperitoneum and sterile nonresolving PD peritonitis. Inflammatory markers may be present, such as raised serum C-reactive protein concentrations, anaemia and hypoalbuminaemia. Suggestive CT features include peritoneal calcification, bowel thickening, bowel tethering and bowel dilatation. Laparotomy is required for a definitive diagnosis [22].

Membrane transport characteristics may reflect a decline in ultrafiltration capacity and increase in peritoneal membrane small solute transport over time, similar to that seen following episodes of severe peritonitis (see above) and with long-term PD [120]. However, screening for a rise in transport characteristics is not helpful in risk-stratifying patients, as EPS can occur in patients with slow transport characteristics.

Management consists of cessation of PD, removal of the catheter and transfer to HD. Nutritional support via parenteral nutrition may be necessary and many patients will recover with conservative therapy. Drug therapies include corticosteroids, tamoxifen and immunosuppression, although the evidence for these treatments is scant. Surgical enterolysis by an experienced surgeon may improve symptom burden and survival [22].

10.4 Conclusion

Peritonitis is a major complication that undermines the significant lifestyle, survival and economic benefits of PD. It represents a major disincentive to uptake this dialysis modality and has profound morbidity, mortality and healthcare consequences. Central to the management of peritonitis is the adoption of appropriate prophylaxis strategies, continuous quality improvement programs and the implementation of evidence-based practice and retraining programs. Noninfectious complications of PD are likewise amenable to thoughtful presurgical evaluation and management based on best practice. Further collaborative research is required in this area to overcome the barriers to maintaining long-term PD.

References

1. Jain AK, Blake P, Cordy P, Garg AX. Global trends in rates of peritoneal dialysis. J Am Soc Nephrol. 2012;23(3):533–44.
2. Van Biesen W, Vanholder R, Lameire N. The role of peritoneal dialysis as the first-line renal replacement modality. Perit Dial Int. 2000;20(4):375–83.
3. Klarenbach S, Manns B. Economic evaluation of dialysis therapies. Semin Nephrol. 2009;29(5):524–32.
4. Cass A, Chadban S, Craig J, Howard H, McDonald S, Salkeld G, White S. The economic impact of end-stage kidney disease in Australia. Melbourne: Kidney Health Australia; 2006.
5. Wu AW, Fink NE, Marsh-Manzi JV, Meyer KB, Finkelstein FO, Chapman MM, Powe NR. Changes in quality of life during hemodialysis and peritoneal dialysis treatment: generic and disease specific measures. J Am Soc Nephrol. 2004;15(3):743–53.
6. Noshad H, Sadreddini S, Nezami N, Salekzamani Y, Ardalan MR. Comparison of outcome and quality of life: haemodialysis versus peritoneal dialysis patients. Singapore Med J. 2009;50(2):185–92.
7. Rubin HR, Fink NE, Plantinga LC, Sadler JH, Kliger AS, Powe NR. Patient ratings of dialysis care with peritoneal dialysis vs hemodialysis. JAMA. 2004;291(6):697–703.
8. Vonesh EF, Snyder JJ, Foley RN, Collins AJ. Mortality studies comparing peritoneal dialysis and hemodialysis: what do they tell us? Kidney Int. 2006;103(Supplement):3–11.
9. Mehrotra R, Chiu YW, Kalantar-Zadeh K, Bargman J, Vonesh E. Similar outcomes with hemodialysis and peritoneal dialysis in patients with end-stage renal disease. Arch Intern Med. 2011;171(2):110–8.
10. Perl J, Wald R, McFarlane P, Bargman JM, Vonesh E, Na Y, Jassal SV, Moist L. Hemodialysis vascular access modifies the association between dialysis modality and survival. J Am Soc Nephrol. 2011;22(6):1113–21.
11. Polkinghorne KR, McDonald SP, Atkins RC, Kerr PG. Vascular access and all-cause mortality: a propensity score analysis. J Am Soc Nephrol. 2004;15(2):477–86.
12. House AA, Pham B, Pagé DE. Transfusion and recombinant human erythropoietin requirements differ between dialysis modalities. Nephrol Dial Transpl. 1998;13(7):1763–9.
13. Johnson DW, Dent H, Yao Q, Tranaeus A, Huang CC, Han DS, Jha V, Wang T, Kawaguchi Y, Qian J. Frequencies of hepatitis B, and C infections among haemodialysis and peritoneal dialysis patients in Asia-Pacific countries: analysis of registry data. Nephrol Dial Transpl. 2009;24(5):1598–603.
14. Tam P. Peritoneal dialysis and preservation of residual renal function. Perit Dial Int. 2009;9(Suppl 2):108–10.
15. Lang SM, Bergner A, Töpfer M, Schiffl H. Preservation of residual renal function in dialysis patients: effects of dialysis-technique-related factors. Perit Dial Int. 2001;21(1):52–7.
16. Jiwakanon SC, Yi-Wena K-Z, Kamyara M, Rajnisha. Peritoneal dialysis: an underutilized modality. Curr Opin Nephrol Hypertens. 2010;19(6):573–7.
17. Mehrotra R, Kermah D, Fried L, Kalantar-Zadeh K, Khawar O, Norris K, Nissenson A. Chronic peritoneal dialysis in the United States: declining utilization despite improving outcomes. J Am Soc Nephrol. 2007;18(10):2781–8.

18. Khawar O, Kalantar-Zadeh K, Lo WK, Johnson D, Mehrotra R. Is the declining use of long-term peritoneal dialysis justified by outcome data? Clinical. J Am Soc Nephrol. 2007;2(6):1317–28.
19. Aslam N, Bernardini J, Fried L, Burr R, Piraino B. Comparison of infectious complications between incident hemodialysis and peritoneal dialysis patients. Clin J Am Soc Nephrol. 2006;1(6):1226–33.
20. Chiu YW, Jiwakanon S, Lukowsky L, Duong U, Kalantar-Zadeh K, Mehrotra R. An update on the comparisons of mortality outcomes of hemodialysis and peritoneal dialysis patients. Semin Nephrol. 2011;31(2):152–8.
21. Brown FG, Dent AH, McDonald S, Hurst K. Chapter 6: Peritoneal dialysis. 2012.
22. Brown EA, Van Biesen W, Finkelstein FO, Hurst H, Johnson DW, Kawanishi H, Pecoits-Filho R, Woodrow G, ISPD Working Party. Length of time on peritoneal dialysis and encapsulating peritoneal sclerosis; position paper for ISPD. Perit Dial Int. 2009;29(6):595–600.
23. Odudu A, Wilkie M. Controversies in the management of infective complications of peritoneal dialysis. Nephron Clin Pract. 2011;118(3):301–8.
24. Li PK, Szeto CC, Piraino B, Bernardini J, Figueiredo AE, Gupta A, Johnson DW, Kuijper EJ, Lye WC, Salzer W, Schaefer F Struijk DG, International Society for Peritoneal Dialysis. Peritoneal dialysis-related infections recommendations: 2010 update. Perit Dial Int. 2010;30(4):393–423.
25. Boudville N, Kemp A, Clayton P, Lim W, Badve SV, Hawley CM, McDonald SP, Wiggins KJ, Bannister KM, Brown FG, Johnson DW. Recent peritonitis associates with mortality among patients treated with peritoneal dialysis. J Am Soc Nephrol. 2012;23(8):1398–405.
26. Badve SV, Hawley CM, McDonald SP, Brown FG, Boudville NC, Wiggins KJ, Bannister KM, Johnson DW. Use of aminoglycosides for peritoneal dialysis-associated peritonitis does not affect residual renal function. Nephrol Dial Transpl. 2012;27(1):381–7.
27. Piraino BB, Bernardini J, Brown E, Figueiredo A, Johnson DW, Lye W-C, Price V, Ramalakshmi S, Szeto C-C. ISPD position statement on reducing the risks of peritoneal dilaysis-related infections. Perit Dial Int. 2011;31(6):614–30.
28. Cho Y, Johnson DW. Peritoneal dialysis-related peritonitis: towards improving evidence, practices, and outcomes. Am J Kidney Dis. 2014;64:278–89.
29. Peritoneal dialysis—best practice—peritonitis prevention and management [press release]. 2013.
30. Lin CY, Roberts GW, Kift-Morgan A, Donovan KL, Topley N, Eberl M. Pathogen-specific local immune fingerprints diagnose bacterial infection in peritoneal dialysis patients. J Am Soc Nephrol. 2013;24(12):2002–9.
31. Burke M, Hawley CM, Badve SV, McDonald SP, Brown FG, Boudville N, Wiggins KJ, Bannister KM, Johnson DW. Relapsing and recurrent peritoneal dialysis-associated peritonitis: a multicenter registry study. Am J Kidney Dis. 2011;58(3):429–36.
32. Thirugnanasambathan T, Hawley CM, Badve SV, McDonald SP, Brown FG, Boudville N, Wiggins KJ, Bannister KM, Clayton P, Johnson DW. Repeated peritoneal dialysis-associated peritonitis: a multicenter registry study. Am J Kidney Dis. 2012;59(1):84–91.
33. Szeto CC, Lai KB, Kwan BC, Chow KM, Leung CB, Law MC, Yu V, Li PK. Bacteria-derived DNA fragment in peritoneal dialysis effluent as a predictor of relapsing peritonitis. Clinical. J Am Soc Nephrol. 2013;8(11):1935–41.
34. Jose MD, Johnson DW, Mudge DW, Tranaeus A, Voss D, Walker R, Bannister KM. Peritoneal dialysis practice in Australia and New Zealand: a call to action. Nephrology. 2011;16(1):19–29.
35. Ghali JR, Bannister KM, Brown FG, Rosman JB, Wiggins KJ, Johnson DW, McDonald SP. Microbiology and outcomes of peritonitis in Australian peritoneal dialysis patients. Perit Dial Int. 2011;31(6):651–62.
36. Badve SV, Smith A, Hawley CM, Johnson, David W. Adherence to guideline recommendations for infection prophylaxis in peritoneal dilaysis patients. Nephrol Dial Transpl. 2009;2(6):508.
37. Piraino B, Bailie GR, Bernardini J, Boeschoten E, Gupta A, Holmes C, Kuijper EJ, Li PK, Lye WC, Mujais S, Paterson DL, Fontan MP, Ramos A, Schaefer F, Uttley L, ISPD Ad Hoc Advisory Committee. Peritoneal dialysis-related infections recommendations: 2005 update. Perit Dial Int. 2005;25(2):107–31.
38. Johnson DW, Livingston B, Bannister K, McDonald S. Chapter 6; Peritoneal dialysis. 2008.
39. Troidle L, Finkelstein F. Treatment and outcome of CPD-associated peritonitis. Ann Clin Microbiol Antimicrob. 2006;5:6.
40. Ballinger AE, Palmer SC, Wiggins KJ, Craig JC, Johnson DW, Cross NB, Strippoli, Giovanni F. Treatment for peritoneal dialysis-associated peritonitis. Cochrane Database Syst Rev. 2014;4:CD005284. doi:10.1002/14651858.CD005284.pub3(4).
41. Ariano RE, Franczuk C, Fine A, Harding GK, Zelenitsky SA. Challenging the current treatment paradigm for methicillin-resistant Staphylococcus epidermidis peritonitis in peritoneal dialysis patients. Perit Dial Int. 2002;22(3):335–8.
42. Mulhern JG, Braden GL, O'Shea MH, Madden RL, Lipkowitz GS, Germain MJ. Trough serum vancomycin levels predict the relapse of gram-positive peritonitis in peritoneal dialysis patients. Am J Kidney Dis. 1995;25(4):611–5.
43. Rüger W, van Ittersum FJ, Comazzetto LF, Hoeks SE, ter Wee PM. Similar peritonitis outcome in CAPD and APD patients with dialysis modality continuation during peritonitis. Perit Dial Int. 2011;31(1):39–47.
44. Johnson DW. Do antibiotic levels need to be followed in treating peritoneal dialysis-associated peritonitis? Semin Dial. 2011;24(4):445–6.
45. Stevenson S, Tang W, Cho Y, Mudge DW, Hawley CM, Badve SV, Johnson DW. The role of monitoring vancomycin levels in patients with peritoneal dialysis-associated peritonitis. Perit Dial Int. 2014.
46. Tang W, Cho Y, Hawley CM, Badve SV, Johnson DW. The role of monitoring gentamicin levels in patients with gram-negative peritoneal dialysis-associated peritonitis. Perit Dial Int. 2014;34(2):219–26.
47. Wang AY, Yu AW, Li PK, Lam PK, Leung CB, Lai KN, Lui SF. Factors predicting outcome of fungal peritonitis in peritoneal dialysis: analysis of a 9-year experience of fungal peritonitis in a single center. Am J Kidney Dis. 2000;36(6):1183–92.
48. Goldie SJ, Kiernan-Tridle L, Torres C, Gorban-Brennan N, Dunne D, Kliger AS, Finkelstein FO. Fungal peritonitis in a large chronic peritoneal dialysis population: a report of 55 episodes. Am J Kidney Dis. 1996;28(1):86–91.
49. Miles R, Hawley CM, McDonald SP, Brown FG, Rosman JB, Wiggins KJ, Bannister KM, Johnson DW. Predictors and outcomes of fungal peritonitis in peritoneal dialysis patients. Kidney Int. 2009;76(6):622–8.
50. Restrepo C, Chacon J, Manjarres G. Fungal peritonitis in peritoneal dialysis patients: successful prophylaxis with fluconazole, as demonstrated by prospective randomized control trial. Perit Dial Int. 2010;30(6):619–25.
51. Chow KM, Szeto CC, Cheung KK, Leung CB, Wong SS, Law MC, Ho YW, Li PK. Predictive value of dialysate cell counts in peritonitis complicating peritoneal dialysis. Clin J Am Soc Nephrol. 2006;1(4):768–73.
52. Cho Y, Badve SV, Hawley CM, McDonald SP, Brown FG, Boudville N, Clayton P, Johnson DW. Peritoneal dialysis outcomes after temporary haemodialysis transfer for peritonitis. Nephrol Dial Transpl. 2014;29(10):1940–7.
53. Han SH, Lee SC, Ahn SV, Lee JE, Choi HY, Kim BS, Kang SW, Choi KH, Han DS, Lee HY. Improving outcome of CAPD: twenty-five years' experience in a single Korean center. Perit Dial Int. 2007;27(4):432–40.

54. Moraes TP, Pecoits-Filho R, Ribeiro SC, Rigo M, Silva MM, Teixeira PS, Pasqual DD, Fuerbringer R, Riella MC. Peritoneal dialysis in Brazil: twenty-five years of experience in a single center. Perit Dial Int. 2009;29(5):492–8.
55. Rocha A, Rodrigues A, Teixeira L, Carvalho MJ, Mendonça D, Cabrita A. Temporal trends in peritonitis rates, microbiology and outcomes: the major clinical complication of peritoneal dialysis. Blood Purif. 2012;33(4):284–91.
56. Huang JW, Hung KY, Yen CJ, Wu KD, Tsai TJ. Comparison of infectious complications in peritoneal dialysis patients using either a twin-bag system or automated peritoneal dialysis. Nephrol Dial Transpl. 2001;16(3):604–7.
57. Kiernan L, Kliger A, Gorban-Brennan N, Juergensen P, Tesin D, Vonesh E, Finkelstein F. Comparison of continuous ambulatory peritoneal dialysis-related infections with different "Y-tubing" exchange systems. J Am Soc Nephrol. 1995;5(10):1835–8.
58. Szeto CC, Chow VC, Chow KM, Lai RW, Chung KY, Leung CB, Kwan BC, Li PK. Enterobacteriaceae peritonitis complicating peritoneal dialysis: a review of 210 consecutive cases. Kidney Int. 2006;69(7):1245–52.
59. Barraclough K, Hawley CM, McDonald SP, Brown FG, Rosman JB, Wiggins KJ, Bannister KM, Johnson DW. Polymicrobial peritonitis in peritoneal dialysis patients in Australia: predictors, treatment, and outcomes. Am J Kidney Dis. 2010;55(1):121–31.
60. Kim GC, Korbet SM. Polymicrobial peritonitis in continuous ambulatory peritoneal dialysis patients. Am J Kidney Dis. 2000;36(5):1000–8.
61. Holley JL, Bernardini J, Piraino B. Polymicrobial peritonitis in patients on continuous peritoneal dialysis. Am J Kidney Dis. 1992;19(2):162–6.
62. Szeto CC, Chow KM, Wong TY, Leung CB, Li PK. Conservative management of polymicrobial peritonitis complicating peritoneal dialysis—a series of 140 consecutive cases. Am J Med. 2002;113(9):728–33.
63. Akoh J. Peritoneal dialysis associated infections; an update in diagnosis and management. World J Nephrol. 2012;1(4):106–22.
64. Johnson DW, Gray N, Snelling P. A peritoneal dialysis patient with fatal culture-negative peritonitis. Nephrology. 2003;8(1):49–55.
65. Fahim M, Hawley CM, McDonald SP, Brown FG, Rosman JB, Wiggins KJ, Bannister KM, Johnson DW. Culture-negative peritonitis in peritoneal dialysis patients in Australia: predictors, treatment, and outcomes in 435 cases. Am J Kidney Dis. 2010;55(4):690–7.
66. Siva B, Hawley CM, McDonald SP, Brown FG, Rosman JB, Wiggins KJ, Bannister KM, Johnson DW. Pseudomonas peritonitis in Australia: predictors, treatment, and outcomes in 191 cases. Clin J Am Soc Nephrol. 2009;4(5):957–64.
67. O'Shea S, Hawley CM, McDonald SP, Brown FG, Rosman JB, Wiggins KJ, Bannister KM, Johnson DW. Streptococcal peritonitis in Australian peritoneal dialysis patients: predictors, treatment and outcomes in 287 cases. BMC Nephrol. 2009;10:19.
68. Edey M, Hawley CM, McDonald SP, Brown FG, Rosman JB, Wiggins KJ, Bannister KM, Johnson DW. Enterococcal peritonitis in Australian peritoneal dialysis patients: predictors, treatment and outcomes in 116 cases. Nephrol Dial Transpl. 2010;25(4):1272–8.
69. Szeto CC, Chow KM, Wong TY, Leung CB, Wang AY, Lui SF, Li PK. Feasibility of resuming peritoneal dialysis after severe peritonitis and Tenckhoff catheter removal. J Am Soc Nephrol. 2002;13(4):1040–5.
70. Troidle L, Gorban-Brennan N, Finkelstein FO. Outcome of patients on chronic peritoneal dialysis undergoing peritoneal catheter removal because of peritonitis. Adv Perit Dial. 2005;21:98–101.
71. George C. Catheter removal, adjunct therapies and timing of reinsertion of peritoneal dialysis catheter after peritonitis. The CARI Guidelines—Caring for Australasians with Renal Impairment. 2013.
72. Blake PG, Flowerdew G, Blake RM, Oreopoulos DG. Serum albumin in patients on continuous ambulatory peritoneal dialysis—predictors and correlations with outcomes. J Am Soc Nephrol. 1993;3(8):1501–7.
73. Yang CY, Chen TW, Lin YP, Lin CC, Ng YY, Yang WC, Chen JY. Determinants of catheter loss following continuous ambulatory peritoneal dialysis peritonitis. Perit Dial Int. 2008;28(4):361–70.
74. Group MS. Nasal mupirocin prevents Staphylococcus aureus exit-site infection during peritoneal dialysis. J Am Soc Nephrol. 1996;7(11):2403–8.
75. Xu G, Tu W, Xu C. Mupirocin for preventing exit-site infection and peritonitis in patients undergoing peritoneal dialysis. Nephrol Dial Transpl. 2010;25(2):587–92.
76. Mactier R. Peritonitis is still the achilles' heel of peritoneal dialysis. Perit Dial Int. 2009;29(3):262–6.
77. Strippoli GF, Tong A, Johnson D, Schena FP, Craig JC. Catheter type, placement and insertion techniques for preventing peritonitis in peritoneal dialysis patients. Cochrane Database Syst Rev. 2004;4:CD004680.
78. Li PK, Szeto CC, Law MC, Chau KF, Fung KS, Leung CB, Li CS, Lui SF, Tong KL, Tsang WK, Wong KM, Lai KN. Comparison of double-bag and Y-set disconnect systems in continuous ambulatory peritoneal dialysis: a randomized prospective multicenter study. Am J Kidney Dis. 1999;33(3):535–40.
79. Lan PG, Johnson DW, McDonald SP, Boudville N, Borlace M, Badve SV, Sud K, Clayton PA. The association between peritoneal dialysis modality and peritonitis. Clin J Am Soc Nephrol. 2014;9(6):1091–7.
80. McQuillan RF, Chiu E, Nessim S, Lok CE, Roscoe JM, Tam P, Jassal SV. A randomized controlled trial comparing mupirocin versus polysporin triple for the prevention of catheter-related infections in peritoneal dialysis patients (the MP3 study). Perit Dial Int. 2008;28(1):67–72.
81. Bernardini J, Bender F, Florio T, Sloand J, Palmmontalbano L, Fried L, Piraino B. Randomized, double-blind trial of antibiotic exit site cream for prevention of exit site infection in peritoneal dialysis patients. J Am Soc Nephrol. 2005;16(2):539–45.
82. Chu KH, Choy WY, Cheung CC, Fung KS, Tang HL, Lee W, Cheuk A, Yim KF, Chan WH, Tong KL. A prospective study of the efficacy of local application of gentamicin versus mupirocin in the prevention of peritoneal dialysis catheter-related infections. Perit Dial Int. 2008;28(5):505–8.
83. Johnson DW, Badve SV, Pascoe EM, Beller E, Cass A, Clark C, de Zoysa J, Isbel NM, McTaggart S, Morrish AT, Playford EG, Scaria A, Snelling P, Vergara LA, Hawley CM, HONEYPOT Study Collaborative Group. Antibacterial honey for the prevention of peritoneal-dialysis-related infections (HONEYPOT): a randomised trial. Lancet Infect Dis. 2014;14(1):23–30.
84. Singharetnam W, Holley JL. Acute treatment of constipation may lead to transmural migration of bacteria resulting in gram-negative, polymicrobial, or fungal peritonitis. Perit Dial Int. 1996;16(4):423–5.
85. Yip T, Tse KC, Lam MF, Cheng SW, Lui SL, Tang S, Ng M, Chan TM, Lai KN, Lo WK. Risks and outcomes of peritonitis after flexible colonoscopy in CAPD patients. Perit Dial Int. 2007;27(5):560–4.
86. Johnson DW, Brown FG, Clarke M, Boudville N, Elias TJ, Foo MW, Jones B, Kulkarni H, Langham R, Ranganathan D, Schollum J, Suranyi M, Tan SH, Voss D, balANZ Trial Investigators. Effects of biocompatible versus standard fluid on peritoneal dialysis outcomes. J Am Soc Nephrol. 2012;23(6):1097–107.
87. Johnson DW, Brown FG, Clarke M, Boudville N, Elias TJ, Foo MW, Jones B, Kulkarni H, Langham R, Ranganathan D, Schollum J, Suranyi MG, Tan SH, Voss D; balANZ Trial Investigators. The effects of biocompatible compared with standard peritoneal dialysis solutions on peritonitis microbiology, treatment, and outcomes: the balANZ trial. Perit Dial Int. 2012;32(5):497–506.

88. Cho Y, Johnson DW, Craig JC, Strippoli GF, Badve SV, Wiggins KJ. Biocompatible dialysis fluids for peritoneal dialysis. Cochrane Database Syst Rev. 2014;3:CD007554.
89. Flanigan M, Gokal R. Peritoneal catheters and exit-site practices toward optimum peritoneal access: a review of current developments. Perit Dial Int. 2005;25(2):132–9.
90. Hagen SM, Lafranca JA, IJzermans JN, Dor FJ. A systematic review and meta-analysis of the influence of peritoneal dialysis catheter type on complication rate and catheter survival. Kidney Int. 2014;85(4):920–32.
91. McCormick BB, Bargman JM. Noninfectious complications of peritoneal dialysis: implications for patient and technique survival. J Am Soc Nephrol. 2007;18(12):3023–3.
92. Mujais S, Story K. Peritoneal dialysis in the US: evaluation of outcomes in contemporary cohorts. Kidney Int. 2006;103(Suppl):21–6.
93. Crabtree JH, Fishman A. A laparoscopic method for optimal peritoneal dialysis access. Am Surg. 2005;71(2):135–43.
94. Cho Y, Badve SV, Hawley CM, Wiggins K, Johnson DW. Biocompatible peritoneal dialysis fluids: clinical outcomes. Int J Nephrol. 2012;2012:812609. doi:10.1155/**2012**/812609.
95. Schmidt R, Holley JL. Noninfectious complications of peritoneal dialysis catheters. UpToDate. 2014.
96. Shea M, Hmiel SP, Beck AM. Use of tissue plasminogen activator for thrombolysis in occluded peritoneal dialysis catheters in children. Adv Perit Dial. 2001;17:249–52.
97. Moss JS, Minda SA, Newman GE, Dunnick NR, Vernon WB, Schwab SJ. Malpositioned peritoneal dialysis catheters: a critical reappraisal of correction by stiff-wire manipulation. Am J Kidney Dis. 1990;15(4):305–8.
98. Kim HJ, Lee TW, Ihm CG, Kim MJ. Use of fluoroscopy-guided wire manipulation and/or laparoscopic surgery in the repair of malfunctioning peritoneal dialysis catheters. Am J Nephrol. 2002;22(5–6):532–8.
99. Miller M, McCormick B, Lavoie S, Biyani M, Zimmerman D. Fluoroscopic manipulation of peritoneal dialysis catheters: outcomes and factors associated with successful manipulation. Clin J Am Soc Nephrol. 2012;7(5):795–800.
100. Leblanc M, Ouimet D, Pichette V. Dialysate leaks in peritoneal dialysis. Semin Dial. 2001;14(1):50–4.
101. Gadallah MF, Pervez A, El-Shahawy MA, Sorrells D, Zibari G, McDonald J, Work J. Peritoneoscopic versus surgical placement of peritoneal dialysis catheters: a prospective randomized study on outcome. Am J Kidney Dis. 1999;33(1):118–22.
102. Arramreddy R, Zheng S, Saxena AB, Liebman SE, Wong L. Urgent-start peritoneal dialysis: a chance for a new beginning. Am J Kidney Dis. 2014;63(3):390–5.
103. Chow KM, Szeto CC, Li PK. Management options for hydrothorax complicating peritoneal dialysis. Semin Dial. 2003;16(5):389–94.
104. Lew S. Hydrothorax: pleural effusion associated with peritoneal dialysis. Perit Dial Int. 2012;30(1):13–8.
105. Jagasia MH, Cole FH, Stegman MH, Deaton P, Kennedy L. Video-assisted talc pleurodesis in the management of pleural effusion secondary to continuous ambulatory peritoneal dialysis: a report of three cases. Am J Kidney Dis. 1996;28(5):772–4.
106. Okada H, Ryuzaki M, Kotaki S, Nakamoto H, Sugahara S, Kaneko K, Yamamoto T, Kawahara H, Suzuki H. Thoracoscopic surgery and pleurodesis for pleuroperitoneal communication in patients on continuous ambulatory peritoneal dialysis. Am J Kidney Dis. 1999;34(1):170–2.
107. Bakkaloglu SA, Ekim M, Tümer N, Güngör A, Yilmaz S. Pleurodesis treatment with tetracycline in peritoneal dialysis-complicated hydrothorax. Pediatr Nephrol. 1999;13(7):637–8.
108. Del Peso G, Bajo MA, Costero O, Hevia C, Gil F, Díaz C, Aguilera A, Selgas R. Risk factors for abdominal wall complications in peritoneal dialysis patients. Perit Dial Int. 2003;23(3):249–53.
109. Tokgöz B, Dogukan A, Güven M, Unlühizarci K, Oymak O, Utas C. Relationship between different body size indicators and hernia development in CAPD patients. Clin Nephrol. 2003;60(3):183–6.
110. Martínez-Mier G, Garcia-Almazan E, Reyes-Devesa HE, Garcia-Garcia V, Cano-Gutierrez S, Mora Y, Fermin R, Estrada-Oros J, Budar-Fernandez LF, Avila-Pardo SF, Mendez-Machado GF. Abdominal wall hernias in end-stage renal disease patients on peritoneal dialysis. Perit Dial Int. 2008;28(4):391–6.
111. García-Ureña MA, Rodríguez CR, Vega Ruiz V, Carnero Hernández FJ, Fernández-Ruiz E, Vazquez Gallego JM, Velasco García M. Prevalence and management of hernias in peritoneal dialysis patients. Perit Dial Int. 2006;26(2):198–202.
112. Shah H, Chu M, Bargman JM. Perioperative management of peritoneal dialysis patients undergoing hernia surgery without the use of interim hemodialysis. Perit Dial Int. 2006;26(6):684–7.
113. Borràs M, Valdivielso JM, Egido R, Vicente de Vera P, Bordalba JR, Fernández E. Haemoperitoneum caused by bilateral renal cyst rupture in an ACKD peritoneal dialysis patient. Nephrol Dial Transplant. 2006;21(3):789–91.
114. Fine A, Novak C. Hemoperitoneum due to carcinomatosis in the liver of a CAPD patient. Perit Dial Int. 1996;16(2):181–3.
115. Bleyer A, Burkart JM. Bloody peritoneal dialysate (hemoperitoneum). UpToDate. 2014.
116. Johnson DW, Cho Y, Livingston BE, Hawley CM, McDonald SP, Brown FG, Rosman JB, Bannister KM, Wiggins KJ. Encapsulating peritoneal sclerosis: incidence, predictors, and outcomes. Kidney Int. 2010;77(10):904–12.
117. Brown MC, Simpson K, Kerssens JJ, Mactier RA, Scottish Renal Registry. Encapsulating peritoneal sclerosis in the new millennium: a national cohort study. Clin J Am Soc Nephrol. 2009;4(7):1222–9.
118. Rigby RJ, Hawley CM. Sclerosing peritonitis: the experience in Australia. Nephrol Dial Transpl. 1998;13(1):154–9.
119. Dobbie JW. Serositis: comparative analysis of histological findings and pathogenetic mechanisms in nonbacterial serosal inflammation. Perit Dial Int. 1993;13(4):256–69.
120. Yamamoto R, Nakayama M, Hasegawa T, Miwako N, Yamamoto H, Yokoyami K, Ikeda M, Kato N, Hayakawa H, Takahashi H, Otsuka Y, Kawaguchi Y, Hosoya T. High-transport membrane is a risk factor for encapsulating peritoneal sclerosis developing after long-term continuous ambulatory peritoneal dialysis treatment. Adv Perit Dial. 2002;18:131–4.
121. Lee HY, Kim BS, Choi HY, Park HC, Kang SW, Choi KH, Ha SK, Han DS. Sclerosing encapsulating peritonitis as a complication of long-term continuous ambulatory peritoneal dialysis in Korea. Nephrology. 2003;8(Suppl):33–9.
122. Snyder JJ, Kasiske BL, Gilbertson DT, Collins AJ. A comparison of transplant outcomes in peritoneal and hemodialysis patients. Kidney Int. 2002;62(4):1423–30.

11 Peritoneal Dialysis in Children

Keia Sanderson, Joshua Zaritsky and Bradley A. Warady

11.1 Introduction

Pediatric end-stage renal disease (ESRD) is a rare medical disorder, but with an exponentially increasing prevalence over the past 20 years. While the preferred treatment for pediatric ESRD patients is renal transplantation, the majority of children receive dialysis prior to transplant. Peritoneal dialysis (PD) is the dialysis modality most commonly prescribed to pediatric patients with ESRD worldwide, in large part due its ease of administration to infants, children, and adolescents and the cost-effective nature of the therapy. It also still has a substantial role in the treatment of acute kidney injury (AKI) around the globe. The widespread usage of the therapy underlies the importance of medical providers caring for pediatric patients with kidney disorders to have an understanding of key aspects of the clinical application of PD. In turn, this chapter will provide an overview of PD usage in the pediatric patient, with an emphasis on catheter selection, prescription, and the diagnosis and management of PD-related complications.

11.2 History of Pediatric Peritoneal Dialysis

The use of the peritoneum for saline injections as fluid resuscitation in children was first described at the beginning of the twentieth century [1]. Approximately 40 years later, the first descriptions of attempts to use the peritoneum to treat children with renal failure were published [2, 3]. Pediatric surgeons Swan and Gordon described what was considered the first successful demonstration of PD using continuous peritoneal lavage in three children with acute anuric kidney injury in 1949 [3]. The use of intermittent PD followed continuous peritoneal lavage and was soon found to be well tolerated and effective for children of all ages, in part because of the lack of need for the large extracorporeal blood circuits required of hemodialysis (HD) . Subsequently, acute PD became the preferred renal replacement therapy (RRT) in children with AKI.

In the 1960s, Henry Tenckhoff developed the permanent indwelling peritoneal catheter and thereafter, the first home PD regimen was developed [4]. However, it was not until the description of continuous ambulatory peritoneal dialysis (CAPD) by Moncrief and Popovich in 1976 that PD flourished as a chronic dialytic therapy for pediatric patients [5]. CAPD was first used in a 3-year-old child in 1978 in Toronto and offered an RRT option for infants with ESRD, previously considered too small for chronic dialysis.

At the beginning of the 1980s, automated machines were developed for use with intermittent PD. Automated PD (APD) was first used in a child in 1981 by Price and Suki and became the preferred modality of pediatric programs in North America [6]. Before the 1980s, fewer than 100 pediatric patients were reported to have been treated with CAPD worldwide. Currently, the 2013 United States Renal Data System (USRDS) Annual Data Report (ADR) describes more than 900 patients <19 years on chronic PD and the International Pediatric Peritoneal Dialysis Network (IPPN) registry has voluntary enrollment of >2500 pediatric PD patients worldwide [7, 8].

B. A. Warady (✉)· K. Sanderson
Division of Nephrology, Children's Mercy Hospital, Kansas City, MO, USA
e-mail: bwarady@cmh.edu

B. A. Warady
University of Missouri–Kansas City School of Medicine, Kansas City, USA

J. Zaritsky
Department of Pediatrics, Division of Nephrology, A. I. duPont Hospital for Children, Wilmington, DE, USA

A. K. Singh et al. (eds.), *Core Concepts in Dialysis and Continuous Therapies,* DOI 10.1007/978-1-4899-7657-4_11

11.3 Principles of Peritoneal Dialysis

11.3.1 Physiologic and Anatomic Concepts of the Peritoneal Membrane in Children

Early studies by Putiloff more than 100 years ago revealed that the pediatric peritoneum possessed a greater surface area per scaled body weight when compared to adults [9]. Following this anatomic discovery, studies of the function of the peritoneum suggested that the pediatric peritoneal membrane was also more efficient than the adult peritoneal membrane related to the greater pediatric peritoneal surface area [10]. However, these early kinetic studies were flawed with inconsistencies in dialysis mechanics and research methods. Studies conducted over the past 25 years have instead established a similar functionality of the pediatric and adult peritoneum [11].

The peritoneal exchange process involves two transport mechanisms, diffusion and convection. Diffusion refers to the exchange of solute down a concentration gradient between two solutions separated by a semipermeable membrane. Convection refers to the movement of solute along with water across a semipermeable membrane down a pressure gradient led by ultrafiltration (UF). The recruitment of the functional peritoneum for these forms of transport in children, as in adults, is dependent upon several physiologic factors, most notably the peritoneal capillary microcirculation. It is currently proposed that the peritoneal membrane and the peritoneal microcirculation permit solute and water transport via a three-pore model [12]. The ultrasmall pores of the peritoneal capillary bed make up 1–2% of the total pore area and are involved with approximately 40% of the sodium-free water exchange. Small pores comprise 90% of the total pore area and participate primarily in low molecular weight compound exchange (i.e., urea) via diffusive transport as well as some convective transport. Finally, large pores comprise 5–7% of the total pore area and allow higher molecular weight compound (i.e., proteins, albumin) transport driven by solvent drag associated with convective forces [12].

11.3.2 Diffusive Transport

Studies of diffusive transport demonstrate that the rate of diffusive transfer is directly related to the functional membrane size, the dialysate concentration gradient, and a parameter known as the mass transfer area coefficient (MTAC). This parameter is essentially independent of dialysis mechanics and is an expression of the diffusive permeability of the functional peritoneal membrane in the absence of an osmotic gradient between blood and dialysate [13]. Calculation of the MTAC is quite rigorous, and the studies in which the MTAC values were measured in pediatric patients have yielded mixed results. In the largest study, Warady et al. found that MTACs for potassium, glucose, and creatinine decreased inversely with increasing age, suggesting either an inverse relationship between age and the functional peritoneal surface area or an age-related inverse relationship with the peritoneal permeability [14]. It should be noted that although the age-related differences in the MTAC values obtained by Warady et al. were statistically significant, the differences were small and of arguable clinical importance.

In addition to the MTAC, the transmembrane concentration gradient, the peritoneal permeability, and any residual peritoneal volume also affect the rate of diffusive transport. The concentration gradient between blood and dialysate diminishes over time and is influenced by factors including cycle frequency and dialysate volume. The impact of dialysate volume rests on the principle of geometry of diffusion, which states that the larger the volume of dialysate, the longer the transmembrane concentration gradient will persist and thereby drive diffusion. In children, this principle has been a confounding variable in many early PD studies in which exchange volumes were scaled to body weight as opposed to body surface area (BSA). Given that infants have a greater ratio of BSA to body weight compared to adults, earlier studies in pediatric PD patients in which exchange volumes were scaled to body weight resulted in relatively small dialysate volumes in the youngest patients and thus an inaccurate interpretation of enhanced membrane transport capacity [10]. Finally, the presence of residual exchange volume from previous exchanges diminishes the concentration gradient and thus limits solute transport. Studies have shown that the residual volume can be substantial in children [14].

11.3.3 Convective Transport

Convection involves the transfer of dissolved solute across the peritoneal membrane in association with ultrafiltered water, a process also known as solvent drag. Determination of the exact fraction of solute transport which occurs due to convection is complex due to the relationship with transperitoneal UF and peritoneal membrane permeability. Transperitoneal UF is a time-dependent process, which occurs simultaneously with fluid absorption and can dilute the dialysate solute concentration, enhancing diffusive transport [15]. Therefore, mathematical models are often necessary to differentiate the amount of diffusive and convective solute transport that occurs during PD [16].

The membrane permeability is expressed as a sieving coefficient, which is the ratio of the dialysate concentration of solute and its plasma water concentration in the absence of diffusive transport. A study conducted by Pyle estimated that in a 4-h CAPD exchange with 4.25% dextrose dialysis solution, the contribution of convection to urea removal was 12 %, 45 % for inulin, and 86 % for protein [17]. Thus, in the context of solute removal, convection is thought to contribute to a lesser degree to removal of small solutes and is primarily responsible for most large solute removal [18].

11.3.4 Ultrafiltration

UF describes the movement of fluid across the peritoneal membrane. It is a complex process that is primarily driven by the balance between osmotic pressures created by dextrose within the dialysis solution, most notably, and the uptake of fluid into the peritoneal and lymphatic tissues. Early studies of UF in infants and younger children suggested that adequate UF was difficult to achieve because researchers noted a more rapid dissipation of the dialysate dextrose concentration in this population [19]. However, as noted above, earlier studies used exchange volumes scaled to body weight. Subsequent pediatric PD studies with exchange volumes scaled to BSA demonstrated an age-independent UF capacity [20].

11.3.5 Peritoneal Lymphatic Absorption

Peritoneal lymphatic absorption involves the movement of fluid into the peritoneal interstitium driven by hydraulic pressure. It has been estimated to account for nearly a 20 % reduction of net UF. While there are limited studies on the contribution of lymphatic absorption to net UF in children receiving PD, studies by Schroder et al. and de Boer et al. found that net UF and lymphatic absorption were not age dependent [21, 22]. When lymphatic absorption rates were scaled to BSA in children, there were no differences when compared to adult reference values [23].

11.3.6 Peritoneal Dialysis for Acute Kidney Injury

PD was the first RRT used for the management of AKI in children. Although there have been many advancements in vascular access techniques as well as improvements in HD and continuous renal replacement therapies (CRRT) for the treatment of AKI, acute PD remains the modality of choice in many parts of the world, particularly in infants and small children [24]. Its advantages include its wide availability, the avoidance of the need for vascular access and large extracorporeal blood volume requirements, and its slow and well-tolerated solute and fluid removal. Furthermore, while there have been no randomized clinical trials comparing the different dialysis modalities for the treatment of pediatric AKI, observational studies have not demonstrated a difference in mortality between children treated with PD and those treated with CRRT [25].

11.3.7 Indications for the Initiation of Acute Peritoneal Dialysis

In general, most of the indications for acute PD in the pediatric age group mirror those seen in adults. Although the majority of cases of AKI can be managed conservatively, severe metabolic disturbances, particularly hyperkalemia that is not responsive to medical management, mandate prompt initiation of dialysis. Additionally, there is accumulating evidence that fluid overload in the setting of AKI is associated with adverse outcomes, particularly in the pediatric population [26–30]. A multicenter, prospective study of children demonstrated that the percent fluid accumulation prior to starting RRT was significantly lower in survivors versus non-survivors [29].

11.3.8 Acute Peritoneal Dialysis Access

The two most commonly used accesses for acute PD are the percutaneously placed Cook catheter and the surgically placed Tenckhoff catheter. The Cook catheter offers the advantage of bedside placement by a nephrologist or intensivist via the Seldinger technique. Since only local anesthesia is required, it can be placed promptly, even in an unstable patient [31, 32]. However, its use is hampered by a very high rate of complications such as obstruction from omentum and leakage of dialysate from the catheter entry site on the abdominal wall. Chadha et al. [33] in a single-center retrospective study of infants and young children with AKI found that by day 6 of dialysis, only 46 % of the Cook catheters were functioning without complications. In comparison, they found that over 90 % of surgically placed Tenckhoff catheters were free of complications at the same time point. Thus, the authors suggested that if dialysis is expected to be required for more than 5 days, a Tenckhoff catheter should either be placed initially or elective replacement of the Cook catheter with a Tenckhoff catheter should be performed in a timely manner. More recently, a multipurpose percutaneous catheter (Cook Mac-Loc Multipurpose Drainage catheter) showed promising results in a small cohort of infants with AKI with a mean complication-free survival of approximately 11 days [32].

Current pediatric recommendations from the International Society of Peritoneal Dialysis (ISPD) reflect the published data and support a surgically placed Tenckhoff catheter as the "catheter of choice" for acute PD [34]. Additionally, the guidelines recommend that the catheter be inserted laparoscopically, given the reduced chance for leakage compared to placement by laparotomy. Methods to decrease the risk of dialysate leakage are particularly important when dialysis is to be initiated emergently. There is preliminary evidence that the application of fibrin sealant (glue) at the peritoneum can be used to treat leaks that occur soon after the placement of a Tenckhoff catheter and the implementation of PD. Rusthoven et al. demonstrated in eight infants, ages 0.8–57 months that application of fibrin glue into the subcutaneous catheter tunnel through the exit site was able to successfully correct leaks that occurred within 48 h of initiating therapy while using a single-cuff Tenckhoff catheter [35]. Additionally, Sojo et al. demonstrated that application of fibrin glue to the peritoneal cuff suture at the time of implantation reduced the incidence of leakage in the early postoperative period [36]. Dialysate leakage only occurred in 9% of the fibrin glue group versus 57% of the control group.

11.3.9 Acute Peritoneal Dialysis Prescription

Much like the chronic PD prescription (see below), there are four main components of the acute PD prescription: fill volume, dialysate composition, dwell times, and total length of dialysis therapy. The initial fill volume of 10 ml/kg should be used for at least the first 24–48 h to minimize the risk of dialysate leakage through the catheter insertion site. The fill volume can be gradually increased to a target volume of 30–40 ml/kg (800–1100 ml/m^2 BSA) to achieve adequate fluid and solute removal goals [34]. Whether performing manual exchanges or automated exchanges, the initial dwell time should be at least 30–60 min, with gradual prolongation as the patient is stabilized and fluid and solute removal targets are achieved. Acute PD should be continuous for the first 1–3 days with gradual shortening of the total daily duration of dialysis as tolerated by the patient [34]. Given the use of rapid exchanges, often with higher dialysate dextrose concentrations, along with the continuous nature of the dialysis, close monitoring of electrolytes is mandatory. Patients undergoing acute PD are at risk for hypernatremia secondary to sodium sieving, a consequence of disproportionately greater water to sodium transport via aquaporin-mediated pores, and hyperglycemia secondary to substantial dextrose absorption [37].

11.3.10 Causes of End-Stage Renal Disease in Children

While a variety of disorders result in ESRD during childhood, approximately one half are congenital in origin and one half are acquired lesions. The largest source of data on primary diagnoses comes from the dialysis registry of the North American Pediatric Renal Trials and Collaborative Studies (NAPRTCS) [38]. The most common diagnoses in the registry's cohort of >7000 patients are focal segmental glomerulosclerosis, congenital aplasia/hypoplasia/dysplasia, and obstructive uropathy, accounting for 14.4, 14.2 and 12.6% of cases, respectively (Table 11.1) [38].

Table 11.1 Primary renal disorders [38]

	N	%
All dialysis patients	*7039*	*100.0*
Primary diagnosis		
FSGS	1016	14.4
A/hypo/dysplastic kidney	998	14.2
Obstructive uropathy	888	12.6
Reflux nephropathy	244	3.5
SLE nephritis	226	3.2
HUS	216	3.1
Chronic GN	214	3.0
Polycystic disease	201	2.9
Congenital nephrotic syndrome	182	2.6
Prune belly	144	2.0
Medullary cystic disease	140	2.0
Idiopathic crescentic GN	130	1.8
Familial nephritis	130	1.8
MPGN—Type I	116	1.6
Pyelo/interstitial nephritis	101	1.4
Cystinosis	99	1.4
Renal infarct	90	1.3
Berger's (IgA) nephritis	86	1.2
Henoch-Schönlein nephritis	67	1.0
MPGN—Type II	64	0.9
Wilms tumor	55	0.8
Wegener's granulomatosis	49	0.7
Drash syndrome	39	0.6
Other systemic immunologic disease	37	0.5
Oxalosis	32	0.5
Membranous nephropathy	29	0.4
Sickle cell nephropathy	21	0.3
Diabetic GN	10	0.1
Other	887	12.6
Unknown	528	7.5

FSGS focal segmental glomerulosclerosis, *SLE* systemic lupus erythematosus, *HUS* hemolytic uremic syndrome, *GN* glomerulonephritis, *MPGN* membranoproliferative glomerulonephritis, *IgA* immunoglobulin A

11.3.11 Indications and Contraindications for Chronic Peritoneal Dialysis

In many cases, the choice of PD as the initial dialytic modality is based on patient/family preference and center philosophy. In addition, however, an important aspect of the selection process for PD is a thorough evaluation of the family's social, psychological, and economic background so as to best determine the likely ability of the family to cope with the "burden of care" associated with the provision of home dialysis therapy on a daily basis [39]. An evaluation of the parent or caregiver's educational background and learning capacity is also desirable so that a realistic assessment of their ability to process the information necessary to carry out home dialysis can be made. All that being said, the absolute indications for PD in children with ESRD are a very small patient, lack of a vascular access, and the presence of contra-indications to anticoagulation [40–45].

With recognition that the performance of PD requires a patent abdominal cavity and a functioning peritoneal membrane, the only absolute contraindications to PD consists of the presence of one of the following: omphalocele, gastroschisis, bladder extrophy, diaphragmatic hernia, or an obliterated peritoneal cavity. While the lack of an appropriate caregiver for home therapy is a relative contraindication, the presence of a colostomy, gastrostomy, ureterostomy, and/or pyelostomy or a ventriculoperitoneal shunt does not preclude chronic PD [46].

11.3.12 Chronic Peritoneal Dialysis Usage

Data on the use of chronic PD by children with ESRD are derived from a number of different registries from around the globe. The NAPRTCS has demonstrated that chronic PD was the initial dialysis modality prescribed to 62.9 % of more than 7000 patients, most commonly through the use of APD (see below) [1]. Noteworthy is the fact that 85 % of the children <5 years were prescribed chronic peritoneal dialysis (CPD) versus 51 % of those >12 years. The USRDS ADR provides data on all patients 0–19 years old and on dialysis, in contrast to only those cared for in pediatric centers, as reported by the NAPRTCS [8]. In turn, the ADR recently reported that only 28 % of 1410 incident patients received PD, in contrast to the 49 % who were prescribed HD. A decade-old compilation of data from 12 European registries revealed that 34 % of the incident patients received PD (vs. 48 % HD), whereas European data published in 2013 showed that 50 % of the pediatric patients initiated therapy with PD and 34 % with HD, with patient/family choice and patient size being the most influential factors regarding modality selection [47, 48].

11.4 Chronic Peritoneal Dialysis Prescription

11.4.1 Choice of Modality

In centers where APD is freely available and without financial constraints, this PD modality is generally preferred in the pediatric population. It is the modality used by 82.9 % of the infant, child, and adolescent PD patients in the USA [49, 50]. The preference for APD is in large part because of the manual nature and daytime requirements of CAPD, in contrast to the nocturnal provision of multiple exchanges with APD, as well as the greater ability to tailor the PD prescription to the patient's needs. The peritoneal membrane transport capacity can also influence the PD modality choice, with those individuals demonstrating high membrane transport capacity more likely to require either continuous cycling peritoneal dialysis (CCPD) in which the dialysate is left in the abdomen following nocturnal cycling or nocturnal intermittent PD (NIPD) in which the abdomen is left dry during the daytime to achieve adequate UF. Recent data from the IPPN have, in fact, revealed that 37.4 % of the patients were prescribed CCPD, 37.5 % NIPD, and 23.8 % CAPD. Finally, tidal PD, an APD variant in which only a portion of each exchange is drained until completion of the entire dialysis session, has been used to alleviate "drain pain" in children on PD [51].

11.4.2 Chronic Peritoneal Dialysis Access

The most important consideration for the successful placement and long-term function of a Tenckhoff catheter in the pediatric patient with ESRD is the experience of the surgeon [52]. This can be particularly problematic at centers caring for a small number of patients, where the need to provide chronic dialysis to very young children may be a rare event. Because of the importance of the access and the desire for the outcome of placement to be complication free, surgical placement should ideally be limited to only a few surgeons per center and on rare occasion, it may be preferable to refer the patient to another, more experienced center for access placement, in a manner similar to what has been recommended for vascular access [53].

There are a variety of configurations of pediatric-sized Tenckhoff catheters available from several manufactures (Baxter, USA; Medionics, Canada; Covidien, USA). Current data from the IPPN show that ~70 % and 30 % of 2290 pediatric PD patients (median age 10.5 years) have curled versus straight catheters, respectively [54]. A majority of these catheters (86 %) had two cuffs with a downward or lateral exit-site orientation. Although there are limited data available to permit determination of the "best" configuration, observational data from the NAPRTCS suggest that a dual-cuffed, swan-neck (allows for downward facing exit site) catheter is associated with a reduction in infectious complications compared with other catheter configurations (Fig. 11.1) [55]. This information is especially relevant in infants and young children because of their increased rates of peritonitis compared to older children [55]. The exit site should also be placed outside of the groin area and away from the diaper region and any potential gastrostomy site, with the superficial cuff located approximately 2 cm from the skin surface [56]. While the catheter must be immobilized to minimize the risk

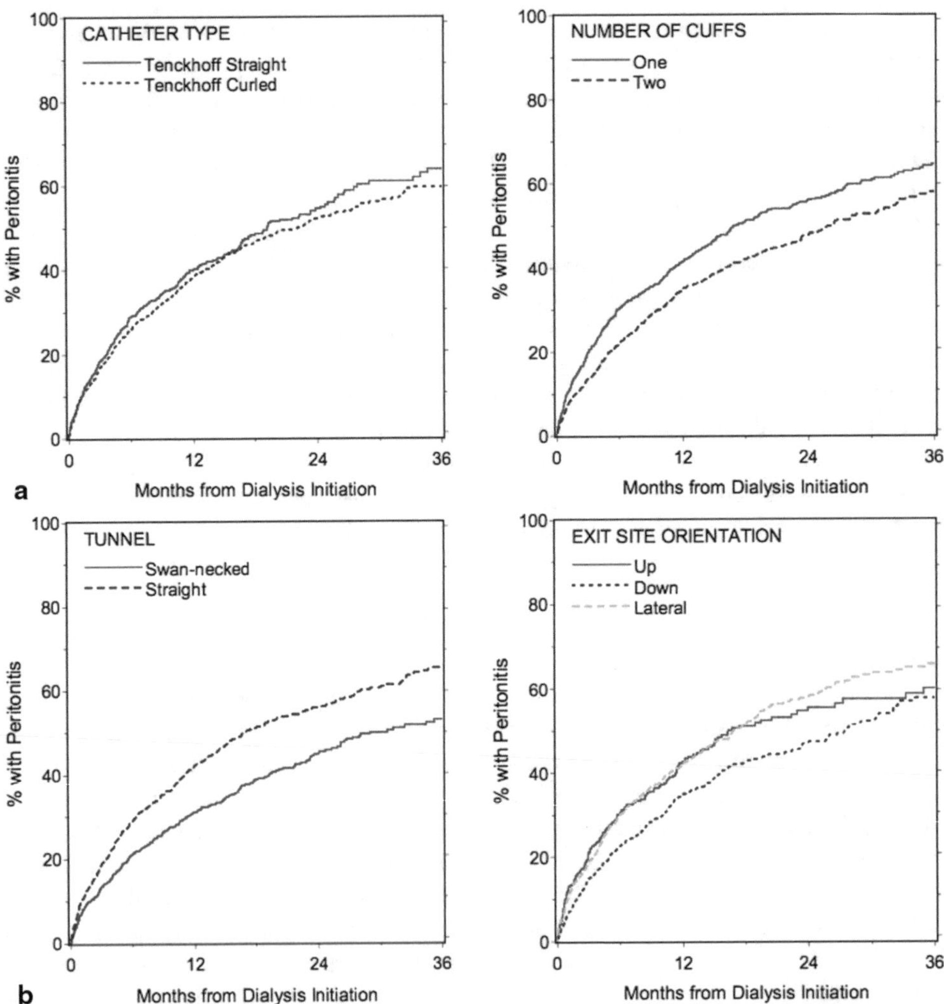

Fig. 11.1 Time to first peritonitis infection by peritoneal dialysis *(PD)* access characteristics [38]

of exit-site trauma, no sutures should be placed at the exit site as they increase the risk of bacterial colonization [57].

A somewhat controversial aspect of catheter placement is the decision whether or not to routinely perform an omentectomy. A survey of pediatric surgeons indicated that an omentectomy was performed routinely in 53 % of the participating centers at the time of catheter placement [58]. The basis for its performance in children is that catheter obstruction (usually due to omental wrapping) is second only to peritonitis in terms of major catheter complications in this age group [59]. Ironically, most of the data in support of omentectomy come from the adult literature [60]. One retrospective study of children by Cribbs et al. demonstrated a decreased risk of early catheter failure with omentectomy, and Rinaldi et al. noted improved catheter survival with omentectomy, especially in children less than 2 years of age [61, 62]. Additionally, in a retrospective study of 92 pediatric patients (mean age 5 years), Conlin et al. demonstrated that the outflow obstruction rate was 5 % in patients who received an omentectomy versus 10 % in patients who did not [63]. Finally, another single-center retrospective review of 207 patients (median age 10 years) revealed that failure to perform an omentectomy was associated with a higher rate of catheter failure [64].

One additional unique consideration for catheter placement in the pediatric age group is the timing and location of placement relative to the common need for gastrostomy tube (G-tube) placement in order to accommodate nutritional requirements (see below). As noted above, the catheter exit site should ideally be placed at a distance (often the contralateral side) from the site of a current or potential G-tube to decrease the risk of contamination and possible peritonitis. Likewise, it is recommended that when possible, the PD catheter should be placed either simultaneously or after placement of a G-tube to avoid contamination of the peritoneum from gastric contents [65]. When the catheter placement precedes G-tube placement, the latter procedure should take place under prophylactic antibiotic and antifungal therapy. Whereas percutaneous G-tube placement while on PD should not be performed due to the high risk of infection and mechanical failure; placement via an open Stamm gastrostomy procedure is possible [66]. Conversely, PD catheter placement is possible in the setting of a well-established G-tube with no increased risk of bacterial or fungal peritonitis [67–69].

Ideally, the use of a PD catheter for chronic dialysis should be postponed until the exit site is completely healed with dressing changes avoided during the first postoperative week, unless they are required because of soiling or bleeding. Generally, a minimum of 2–3 weeks delay is preferred, although the exact timing will vary from patient to patient with complete healing taking up to 6 weeks in some patients [57].

A quality transformation effort, *Standardizing Care to Improve Outcomes in Pediatric End Stage Renal Disease* (SCOPE), is currently examining the impact of standardizing PD catheter care on infectious complications in 29 pediatric dialysis centers in the USA [70].

11.4.3 Peritoneal Dialysis Solutions

The peritoneal dialysis solutions (PDS) used are the same for children and adults. The composition of the PD solutions is aimed at promoting removal of water and solute waste products while maintaining electrolyte homeostasis and the long-term stability of the peritoneal membrane. Therefore, standard PD solutions contain an osmotic agent necessary to maintain a transmembrane osmotic gradient, a buffer to correct metabolic acidosis, magnesium, calcium, and electrolytes. However, over the past decade, we have come to better understand the harmful effects of prolonged exposure of the peritoneum to the high glucose, lactate, and osmolar concentrations found in many of the commercially available PD solutions. Glucose concentrations used in PD solutions are particularly nonphysiologic, and the glucose degradation products (GDPs) generated during the heat sterilization process are directly toxic to the peritoneal membrane and vasculature. These have been shown to induce production of and crosslink with advanced glycation end products (AGE), all of which can contribute to diabetiform vascular changes, ultrafitration failure, and purification loss of the peritoneum [71].

The biocompatibility of PD solutions is of particular significance in the pediatric population who might require frequent, repeated, and a longer overall duration of exposure to PD solutions over a lifetime.

New PD solutions, which offer greater biocompatibility, are now available and offer lower GDP concentrations and are more pH neutral with a bicarbonate or bicarbonate/lactate buffer (Table 11.2). In children, the use of biocompatible PD solutions has been associated with equally good acidosis control and better membrane preservation [72]. Additionally, the neutral pH of these PD solutions has been shown to induce less pain at peritoneal filling.

Icodextrin, an isosmotic glucose polymer, is also a commercially available alternative PD solution which offers a slower, sustained UF by means of colloid osmotic pressure [72, 73]. A 7.5% icodextrin solution produces sustained UF over a 12–14 h dwell similar to that obtained with a 3.86% glucose-containing solution [74]. The use of icodextrin in pediatric patients has been shown to significantly increase solute and water removal during long dwell periods and is generally used in instances of UF failure. Long-term experience with icodextrin is, however, limited in pediatrics, and the results in infants have been poorer than in older children [72, 75]. Its application should be generally limited to one exchange per day [73, 76].

11.4.4 Fill Volume

As mentioned previously, initial recommendations that fill volumes in children be prescribed per kilogram of body weight led to PD prescriptions with small, suboptimal fill volumes, particularly in infants and young children. The small fill volumes lead to premature loss of the osmotic gradient and impaired UF capacity [20]. Given the age-independent relationship between the peritoneal membrane surface area and BSA, it was subsequently determined that the fill volumes in children should be based on BSA rather than weight [77]. In turn, the KDOQI clinical practice guidelines recommend that for children >2 years of age, the fill volume should be 1100–1200 ml/m^2 BSA (Fig. 11.2) [78]. This volume can be increased to an upper limit of 1400 ml/m^2 as tolerated to achieve maximum recruitment of the peritoneal membrane vascular pore area [12]. In children <2 years of age, a lower fill volume of 600–800 ml/m^2 is recommended based more on tolerance [79]. Measurement of the intraperitoneal pressure (IPP) can be useful in determining the optimum PD volume to maintain a target IPP between 7 and 14 cm H_2O [80]. A fill volume that is too large and generates an IPP of > 18 cm H_2O may contribute to complications such as abdominal pain, dyspnea, hydrothorax, hernia formation, GERD, and loss of UF due to increased lymphatic uptake.

11.4.5 Dwell Time

Determination of the length of each dialysis exchange, or dwell time, should also be selected based upon individual patient needs [12]. Long dwell times, as seen with CAPD, can be associated with insufficient UF, but are best for achieving phosphate purification. Most children, however, are treated

Table 11.2 Characteristics of currently available peritoneal dialysis solutions (PDS) [12]. (Source: Used with permission from Fischbach [12])

	Manufacturer	Potential drawbacks	Potential benefits
Lactate buffered: Balance®, Gambrosol Tri®	Fresenius Gambro	More physiological pH, but not neutral. Local and systemic glucose exposure	Lower GDP levels
			More physiological pH (5.5–6.5)
			Improved-peritoneal membrane biocompatibility
			Preserved-membrane defense
Lactate/bicarbonate buffered: Physioneal®	Baxter	Local and systemic glucose exposure. Does not eliminate peritoneal lactate exposure	Lower GDP levels
			More physiological pH (7.4)
			Improved-peritoneal membrane biocompatibility
			Preserved-membrane defense
			Reduced-infusion pain
Bicarbonate buffered: BicaVera®	Fresenius	Local and systemic glucose exposure	Lower GDP levels
			More physiological pH(7.4)
			More peritoneal membrane biocompatibility
			Preserved-membrane defense
			Improved correction of acidosis
Lactate-buffered glucose containing Dianeal®	Baxter	Low pH (5.5)	Ease of manufacture; low cost
		High GDP content	
		Poor peritoneal membrane biocompatibility	
		Infusion pain	
		Local and systemic glucose exposure	
Icodextrin-containing; lactate buffered	Baxter	Hypersensitivity	Sustained ultrafiltration
		Low pH (5.5)	Preservation of RRF
		Licensed for single daily use only	Hypertonic glucose replacement
		Lactate containing	Reduced hyperglycemia
			Improved short-term systemic hemodynamic profile
			Desirable effects on metabolic profile and body composition
Amino-acid containing: Nutrineal®	Baxter	Low pH (6.7)	No GDPs
		Licensed for single daily use only (avoid exacerbation of uremic symptoms and acidosis)	Avoid systemic and peritoneal glucose exposure
			Peritoneal membrane protection
			Enhance nutrition

GDP glucose degradation product, RRF residual renal function

with APD, in which the dwell times can be manipulated to optimize both solute and fluid removal.

The majority of children on APD are prescribed an initial regimen of 6–12 exchanges over 8–10 h per night with a daytime fill volume for patients on CCPD consisting of approximately 50% of the nighttime volume [38, 81] (Fig. 11.2). Thus, the typical choice for an initial APD dwell time is approximately 1 h. However, the dwell time (as well as the fill volume) should be reevaluated periodically to ensure that the prescription is meeting the needs of the individual patient in terms of solute clearance and UF. The use of multiple short exchanges can also result in hypernatremia secondary to sodium sieving, as noted in the discussion of AKI management [37]. Additionally, short exchanges can contribute to poor phosphate clearance and the inherent increased risk for cardiovascular and metabolic bone disorders in children [12]. A clinically useful way to individualize dwell duration in pediatric patients on CPD is by determining the peritoneal membrane transport capacity with the peritoneal equilibration test (PET) .

11.4.6 Peritoneal Equilibration Test Evaluation in Children

PET was developed by Twardowski et al. to evaluate peritoneal membrane function in the clinical arena [82]. Reference curves were constructed for adults based upon the kinetics of solute equilibration of creatinine and glucose between dialysate and plasma (D:P ratio), which made possible the categorization of adult PD patients into those with high, high average, low average, and low peritoneal membrane solute transport rates. Thus, PET data provide information which can guide the application of the most appropriate dialysis prescription in terms of dwell time [81]. It is recommended that an initial PET evaluation should be conducted

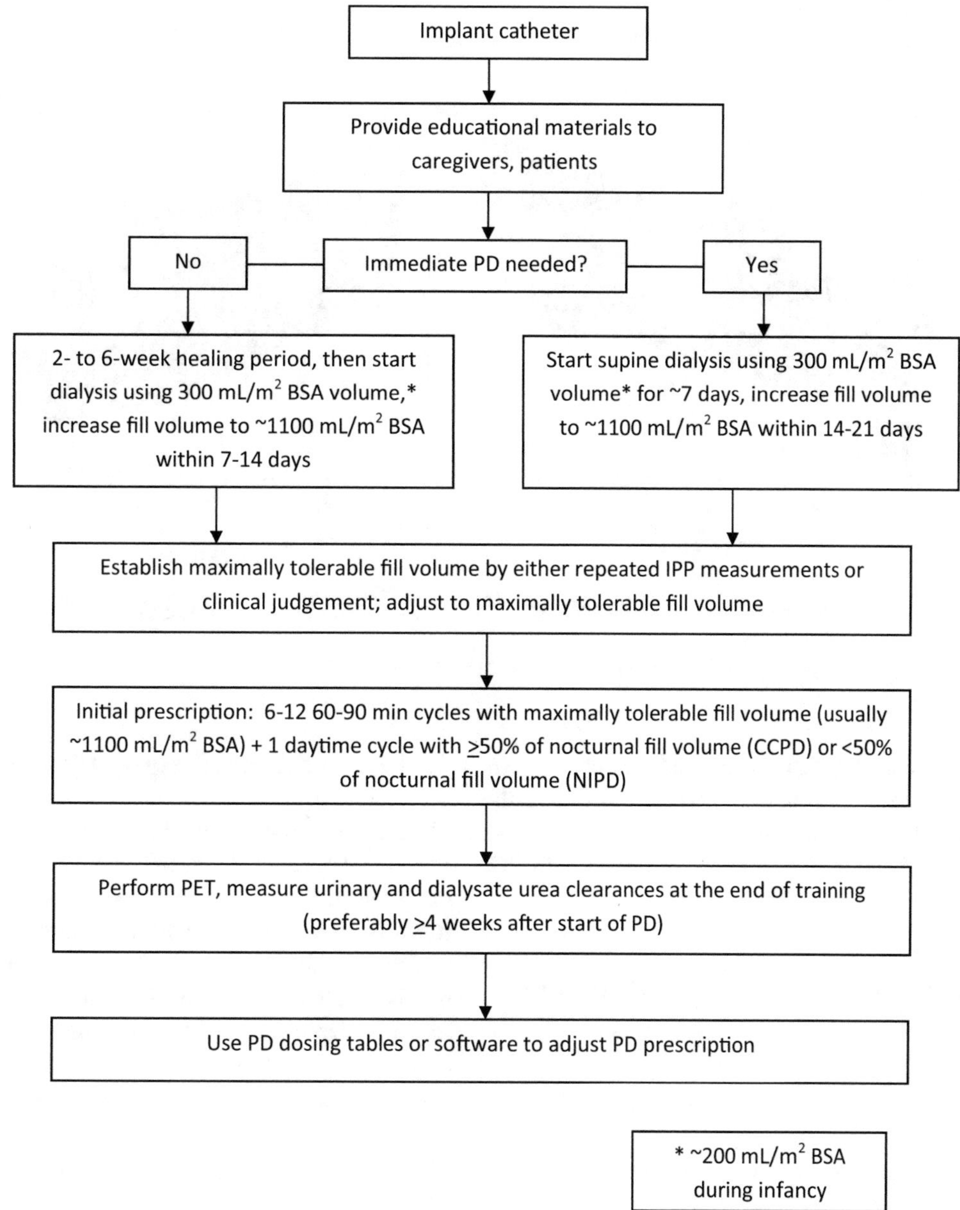

Fig. 11.2 Algorithm for initiation of chronic peritoneal dialysis *(PD)*. (Source: Used with permission from Warady [42])

4–8 weeks following the initiation of PD for most accurate results [81, 83, 84]. The PET should be repeated following clinical events known to alter peritoneal membrane transport (i.e., peritonitis), following the clinical demonstration of UF deterioration (i.e., worsening hypertension, increasing need for hypertonic dialysate, persistent fluid overload, erythropoietin-stimulating agents (ESA)-resistant anemia), or following worsening solute removal.

The PET for adults was designed to be performed during a 4-h dwell with a 2-L fill volume. However, in children, appreciation of the age-independent relationship between BSA and the peritoneal membrane surface area mandates use of a fill volume scaled to BSA when conducting studies of pediatric peritoneal transport kinetics. The Pediatric Peritoneal Dialysis Study Consortium (PPDSC) and the Mid-European Pediatric Peritoneal Dialysis Study Group (MEPPS) have both conducted large multicenter trials using a 2.5% or 2.3–2.4% dextrose dialysis solution and a fill volume of 1000–1100 ml/m^2 BSA to develop reference kinetic data (i.e., D:P ratios and D:D0 ratios), which can be used to categorize a pediatric patient's peritoneal membrane transport characteristics and contribute to the prescription process (Fig. 11.3) [5, 85]. Commercially available modeling programs which use these data for PD prescription have been validated in children [86]. In infants <2 years of age, however, the fill volume used for the PET evaluation is typically the current clinically prescribed volume due to the infant's limited tolerance of high fill volumes. The 4-h PET procedure in children

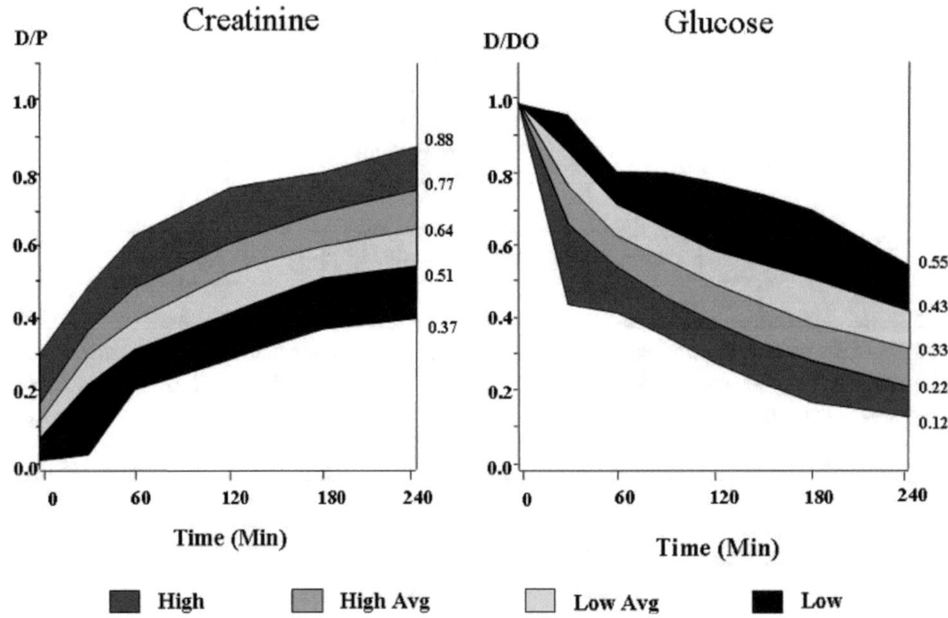

Fig. 11.3 Pediatric peritoneal equilibration test *(PET)* reference curves for creatinine and glucose

is described in Table 11.3. Finally, recent research suggests that a 2-h PET procedure in children performs as well as the 4-h procedure. The shortened version of the study is less labor intensive and less costly than the 4-h procedure [87, 88].

Table 11.3 The peritoneal equilibration test (PET) procedure in children

Dwell period: 4 h
Fill volume: 1100 mL/m² BSA[a]
2.3–2.4 % anhydrous glucose dialysis solution (Europe)
2.5 % dextrose dialysis solution (North America, Japan)
Test exchange after prolonged (8 h) dwell, if possible as follows:
Drain the overnight dwell
Record the length of the dwell and the volume drained. Also note the dextrose concentration and volume infused
Infuse the calculated fill volume, note infusion time
Keep patient in supine position
Drain < 10 % of dialysate solution into the drain bag at 0, 120, and 240 min
Invert bag for mixing and obtain sample. Reinfuse any remaining effluent
Obtain blood sample after 120 min
Measure creatinine and glucose in each sample
Calculate dialysate to plasma (D/P) creatinine and dialysate glucose to baseline dialysate glucose (D/DO) concentration ratios
Determine transporter state by comparing creatinine and glucose equilibration curves with pediatric reference percentiles

BSA body surface area

[a] In early infancy, volume may not be tolerable; in these cases, conduct PET with regular daily exchange volume for evaluation

11.4.7 Peritoneal Dialysis Adequacy

PD adequacy in children should be characterized by a prescription that results in the achievement of optimal UF, sodium balance, and solute clearance so that the patient's clinical status is characterized by sufficient growth, blood pressure control, avoidance of hypo- or hypervolemia, and adequate psychomotor development. Care must always be taken to individualize therapy with these considerations in mind because of the absence of definitive data linking patient outcome to measures such as urea clearance in pediatrics [87].

Despite the appropriate emphasis on clinical parameters, small solute (urea) clearance has historically been used as a surrogate for PD adequacy. Urea removal scaled for the urea volume of distribution or $Kt/V_{urea,}$ is this recommended measure of urea clearance and PD adequacy [89]. This measure includes evaluation of urea removal via residual renal function combined with urea removal via dialysis. Whereas data in adults support a target total (peritoneal and kidney) Kt/V_{urea} of at least 1.7/week, there is very little data correlating Kt/V_{urea} with outcomes in pediatrics [90, 91]. In turn, current KDOQI guidelines support the recommendation that the pediatric population should use clearance goals that meet or exceed current KDOQI adult standards, or a minimal delivered total Kt/V_{urea} of at least 1.8/week [81]. The total weekly Kt/V_{urea} is calculated as follows:

$$\text{Weekly}\,Kt/V_{urea} = \frac{(D_{ur} \cdot V_D)(U_{ur} \cdot V_u)}{P_{ur} \cdot V} \cdot 7$$

where D_{ur}, U_{ur}, and P_{ur} are the dialysate, urinary, and plasma concentrations of urea, V_D and V_U are the 24-h dialysate and urine volumes, and V is the urea distribution volume. The ability to accurately estimate V, or the patient's total body water (TBW) volume in children can be accomplished by using validated gender specific formulas [92]. The formulae are as follows:

$$\text{Boys}: \text{TBW} = 0.10 \times (\text{HtWt})^{0.68} - 0.37 \times \text{weight}$$

$$\text{Girls}: \text{TBW} = 0.14 \times (\text{HtWt})^{0.65} - 0.35 \times \text{weight}$$

It is recommended that a 24-h collection of urine and dialysis fluid should be obtained within the first month after the initiation of dialysis for Kt/V_{urea} evaluation. Following this initial clearance, pediatric PD patients should reassess Kt/V_{urea} a minimum of twice yearly or following any change in clinical status that could alter dialysis performance and may mandate a modification of the dialysis prescription.

Finally, and as mentioned above, fluid removal is also an important measure of PD adequacy and should be optimized to prevent fluid overload. Overhydration represents an important clinical problem in pediatric PD patients because of its contribution to hypertension and an increased risk of adverse cardiovascular outcomes [93]. Data from the NAPRTCS have demonstrated that 57% of 4000 pediatric PD patients in the registry had hypertension. In another study, 68% of the pediatric patients on chronic PD were found to have left ventricular hypertrophy [94, 95]. Therefore, routine monitoring of volume status including repeated assessment of target dry weight and measurement of residual urine output are important components of PD adequacy evaluation. A modified PET using 4.25% dextrose dialysate can be used to evaluate UF kinetics in the patient with evidence of UF failure [90]. In patients experiencing decreased UF, therapeutic interventions may include use of a long daytime exchange with icodextrin, an increase in the number of exchanges or an increased overall treatment time, and/or an increase in the dialysate glucose concentration [12]. Failure of these interventions to optimize fluid management may mandate transition to HD.

11.5 Infectious Complications of Peritoneal Dialysis

Records from the USRDS reveal that infection is the most common cause for hospitalization among children receiving PD with a hospitalization rate of >600 admissions per 1000 patient-years [8] (Fig. 11.4). Infection is also the most common reason for modality change for pediatric patients on PD [38].

11.5.1 Peritonitis

Peritonitis remains the most significant complication of chronic PD in the pediatric population, and one that can compromise the long-term viability of PD as a dialytic option. However, reductions in peritonitis rates have been reported in children in association with treatment of *Staphylococcus aureus* nasal carriage or application of topical antibiotics (e.g., mupirocin or gentamicin) at the catheter exit site, as well as with technical developments such as disconnect systems and the flush-before-fill technique [96–98]. The practice of prolonged training with an emphasis on hand hygiene has also proven beneficial [70].

11.5.1.1 Incidence

Data from the NAPRTCS include information on 4248 episodes of peritonitis, which reflects an annualized peritonitis rate of 0.64 or 1 infection every 18.8 patient-months [38]. Similar to previous reports, the data reveal an inverse rela-

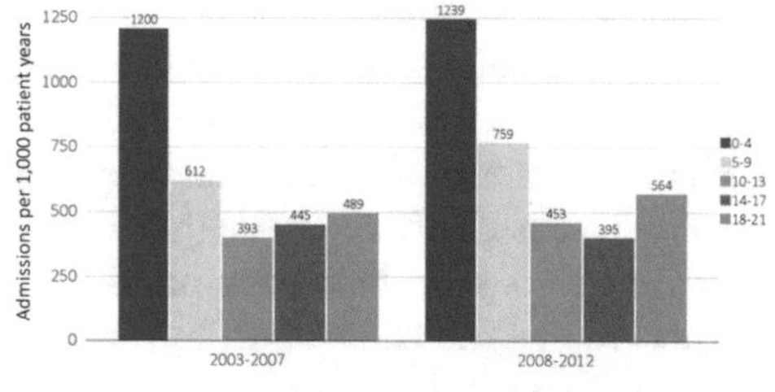

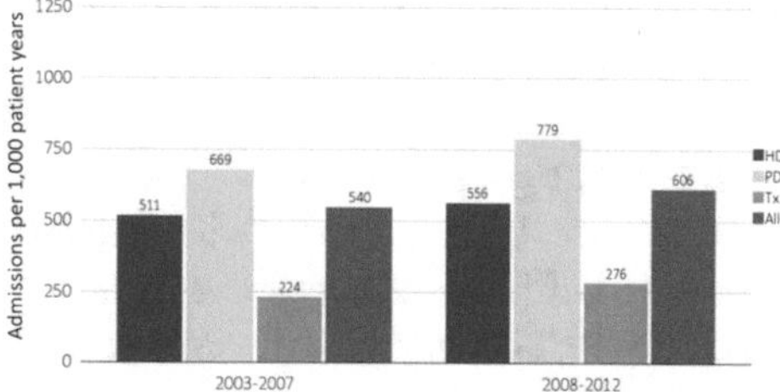

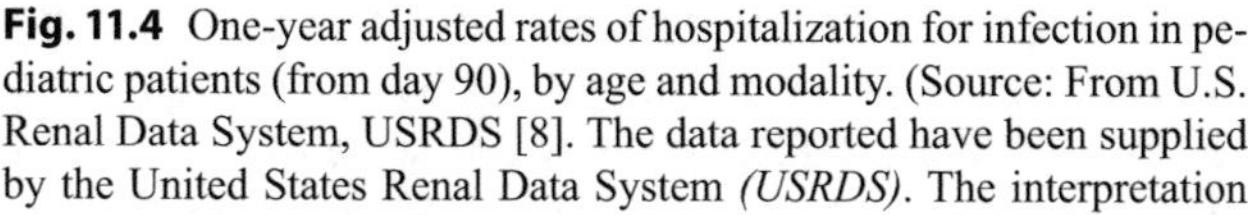

Fig. 11.4 One-year adjusted rates of hospitalization for infection in pediatric patients (from day 90), by age and modality. (Source: From U.S. Renal Data System, USRDS [8]. The data reported have been supplied by the United States Renal Data System *(USRDS)*. The interpretation and reporting of these data are the responsibility of the author(s) and in no way should be seen as an official policy or interpretation of the US government. http://www.usrds.org/faq.aspx)

Table 11.4 Peritoneal dialysis (PD) peritonitis rates in pediatric patients [38]

	No. of episodes	Years of FU	Annualized rate		Expected months between infections	
			Rate	95 % CI	Months	95 % CI
Total	4248	6658	0.64	(0.62–0.66)	18.8	(18.3–19.4)
Age						
0–1 years	938	1193	0.79	(0.74–0.84)	15.3	(14.3–16.3)
2–5 years	552	821	0.67	(0.62–0.73)	17.9	(16.5–19.5)
6–12 years	1345	2145	0.63	(0.59–0.66)	19.1	(18.2–20.2)
> 12 years	1413	2499	0.57	(0.54–0.59)	21.2	(20.2–22.4)
Catheter						
Straight	1180	1668	0.71	(0.67–0.75)	17.0	(16.0–18.0)
Curled	2697	4137	0.65	(0.63–0.68)	18.4	(17.7–19.1)
Presternal	225	420	0.54	(0.47–0.61)	22.4	(19.8–25.8)
Cuff						
One	2553	3440	0.74	(0.71–0.77)	16.2	(15.6–16.8)
Two	1620	2912	0.56	(0.53–0.58)	21.6	(20.6–22.7)
Tunnel						
Swan necked/curved	1161	2317	0.50	(0.47–0.53)	23.9	(22.6–25.4)
Straight	2995	4032	0.74	(0.72–0.77)	16.2	(15.6–16.8)
Exit-site orientation						
Up	702	850	0.83	(0.76–0.89)	14.5	(13.5–15.7)
Down	1181	2221	0.53	(0.50–0.56)	22.6	(21.4–23.9)
Lateral	1828	2466	0.74	(0.71–0.78)	16.2	(15.5–17.0)

CI confidence interval, *FU* follow up

tionship between the age of the patient and the peritonitis rate, with the highest rate (annualized rate: 0.79 or 1 infection every 15.3 months) seen in patients 0–1 year of age, in contrast to an annualized rate of 0.57 or 1 infection every 21.2 patient-months, in children more than 12 years of age (Table 11.4).

Noteworthy is a significant improvement in the overall annualized infection rate from 0.79 in 1992–1996 to 0.44 in recent years, likely related to the prophylactic measures described above, in addition to a greater use of PD catheters characterized by two cuffs and a downward pointed exit site and prophylactic antibiotic usage at the time of PD catheter placement and prior to invasive procedures, as described in the *Consensus Guidelines for the Prevention and Treatment of Catheter-Related Infections and Peritonitis in Pediatric Patients Receiving Peritoneal Dialysis* [57].

11.5.1.2 Presentation and Diagnosis

Peritonitis should be suspected in any patient with abdominal pain and/or cloudy PD effluent, accompanied by an effluent white blood cell (WBC) count > 100/mm^3 and at least 50 % polymorphonuclear leukocytes. For patients on APD, the PD effluent WBC count should be obtained from a dwell instilled for at least 1–2 h. In those cases, the percentage of neutrophils may meet diagnostic criteria when the total WBC count does not, and still be indicative of peritonitis.

11.5.1.3 Microbiology

The successful prophylaxis of exposure to *S. aureus* has resulted in a decrease in the incidence of gram-positive peritonitis and an associated increase in the incidence of gram-negative infections. Data from the International Pediatric Peritoneal Dialysis Registry (IPPR) revealed that 44 % of peritonitis episodes in children are secondary to gram-positive organisms, 25 % to gram-negative organisms, 2 % to fungi, and a remarkable 31 % are culture negative [99]. Of the gram-positive organisms, coagulase-negative Staphylococci are most common. A significant worldwide variation in the microbiology of peritonitis and in the frequency of culture-negative infections was also evident in the IPPR analysis (Fig. 11.5).

11.5.1.4 Treatment

Empiric antibiotic treatment should be initiated as soon as the diagnosis of peritonitis is considered and an effluent sample is obtained for culture and Gram's stain using a standardized technique [57]. The antibiotic regimen used should provide coverage for both gram-positive and gram-negative organisms and should be given by the intraperitoneal route to ensure immediate bioavailability. The recently published pediatric peritonitis treatment guidelines propose empiric monotherapy with the fourth-generation cephalosporin cefepime where available, and in the absence of a history of methicillin-resistant *S. aureus* (Fig. 11.6). An alternative ap-

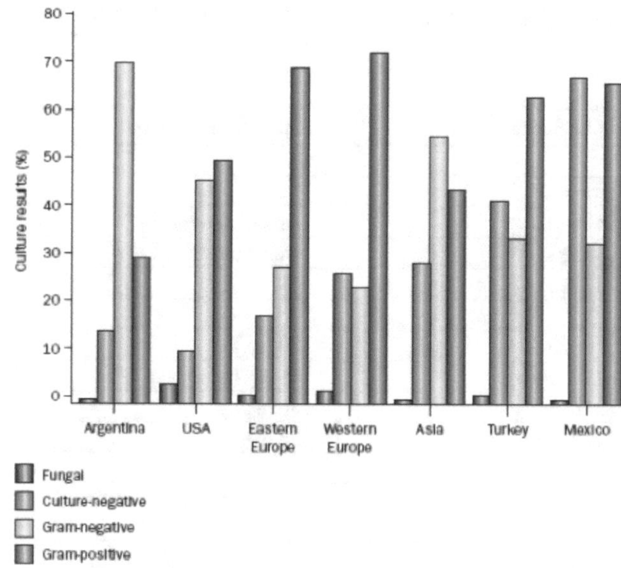

Fig. 11.5 Distribution of peritonitis culture results according to geographical regions. (Source: Used with permission from Schaefer [125])

proach consists of the use of a first-generation cephalosporin or a glycopeptide (e.g., vancomycin) combined with ceftazidime or an aminoglycoside. In all cases, empiric therapy should be guided by the center-specific susceptibility pattern, and maintenance antibiotic therapy should be instituted once the antibiotic susceptibilities of the cultured organism have been determined (Table 11.5). In the IPPR analysis, 89 % of the episodes were followed by full functional recovery, with only an 8.1 % incidence of technique failure and <1 % mortality rate [99].

11.5.1.5 Exit-Site and Tunnel Infection

Exit-site and tunnel infections are significant causes of peritonitis and catheter failure [100]. Early efforts to reduce the incidence of these infections include the provision of intravenous prophylactic antibiotics (usually a first-generation cephalosporin) within 60 min *prior* to the incision for PD catheter placement, immobilization of the catheter without a suture following catheter placement to decrease the risk for exit-site trauma, and limited postoperative dressing changes [57, 101]. Subsequent measures should include delayed onset of dialysis (if possible) to decrease the risk of dialysate leakage, regular cleansing of the exit site with an antiseptic solution followed by the application of a topical antibiotic, proper hand hygiene, and regular exit-site and tunnel monitoring using a standardized scoring system to permit early detection of infection [57, 101, 102]. The combined use of topical mupirocin and sodium hypochlorite solution for exit-site care has been associated with reduced rates of catheter-related infections and prolonged catheter survival in children [103].

The diagnosis of an exit-site infection does not require a positive culture, as long as there is purulent discharge from the sinus tract or marked pericatheter swelling, redness, or tenderness. However, *S. aureus* does account for the major-

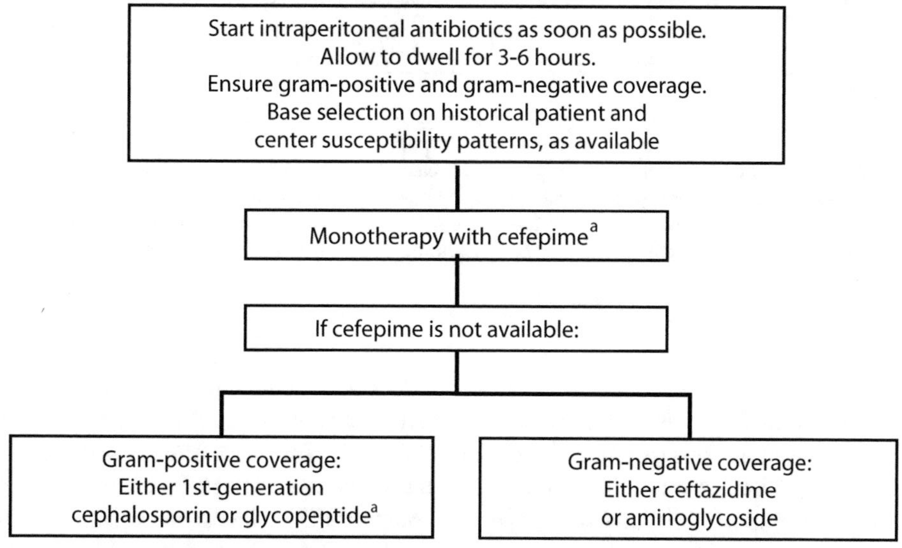

a. *If the center's rate of methicillin-resistant Staphylococcus aureus (MRSA) exceeds 10%, or if the patient has history of MRSA infection of colonization, glycopeptide (vancomycin or teicoplanin) should be added to cefepime or should replace the first-generative cephalosporin for gram-positive coverage.*

Glycopeptide use can also be considered if the patient has a history of severe allergy to penicillins and cephalosporins.

Fig. 11.6 Empiric therapy of peritonitis. (Source: Used with permission from Warady [57]

Table 11.5 Antibiotic dosing recommendations for the treatment of peritonitis [57]. (Source: Used with permission from Warady [57])

	Therapy type		
	Continuous[a]		
Antibiotic type	Loading dose	Maintenance dose	Intermittent therapy[a]
Aminoglycosides (IP)[b]			
Gentamicin	8 mg/L	4 mg/L	
Netilmycin	8 mg/L	4 mg/L	Anuric: 0.6 mg/kg
Tobramycin	8 mg/L	4 mg/L	Non-anuric: 0.75 mg/kg
Amikacin	25 mg/L	12 mg/L	
Cephalosporins (IP)			
Cefazolin	500 mg/L	125 mg/L	20 mg/kg
Cefepime	500 mg/L	125 mg/L	15 mg/kg
Cefotaxime	500 mg/L	250 mg/L	30 mg/kg
Ceftazidime	500 mg/L	125 mg/L	20 mg/kg
Glycopeptides (IP)[c]			
Vancomycin	1000 mg/L	25 mg/L	30 mg/kg: repeat dosing: 15 mg/kg every 3–5 days
Teicoplanin[d]	400 mg/L	20 mg/L	15 mg/kg every 5–7 days
Penicillins (IP)[b]			
Ampicillin	–	125 mg/L	–
Quinolones (IP)			
Ciprofloxacin	50 mg/L	25 mg/L	–
Others			
Aztreonam (IP)	1000 mg/L	250 mg/L	–
Clindamycin (IP)	300 mg/L	150 mg/L	–
Imipenem-cilastin (IP)	250 mg/L	50 mg/L	–
Linezolid (PO)	<5 Years: 30 mg/kg daily, divided into 3 doses 5–11 Years: 20 mg/kg daily, divided into 2 doses ≥12 Years: 600 mg/dose, twice daily		
Metronidazole (PO)	30 mg/kg daily, divided into 3 doses (maximum: 1.2 g daily)		
Rifampin (PO)	10–20 mg/kg daily, divided into 2 doses (maximum: 600 mg daily)		
Antifungals			
Fluconazole (IP, IV, or PO)	6–12 mg/kg every 24–48 h (maximum: 400 mg/daily)		
Caspofungin (IV only)	70 mg/m^2 on day 1 (maximum: 70 mg daily)	50 mg/m^2 daily (maximum: 50 mg daily)	

IP intraperitoneal, *PO* oral, *IV* intravenously

[a]For continuous therapy, the exchange with the loading dose should dwell for 3–6 h; all subsequent exchanges during the treatment course should contain the maintenance dose. For intermittent therapy, the dose should be applied once daily in the long-dwell, unless otherwise specified

[b]Aminoglycosides and penicillins should not be mixed in dialysis fluid because of the potential for inactivation

[c]In patients with residual renal function, glycopeptide elimination may be accelerated. If intermittent therapy is used in such a setting, the second dose should be time-based on a blood level obtained 2–4 days after the initial dose. Re-dosing should occur when the blood level is < 15 mg/L for vancomycin, or < 8 mg/L for teicoplanin. Intermittent therapy is not recommended for patients with residual renal function unless serum levels of the drug can be monitored in a timely manner

[d]Teicoplanin is not currently available in the United States

ity of infections, followed by *Enterococci*, *Pseudomonas*, *E. coli,* and *Klebsiella*. Antibiotic therapy is typically given by the oral route, should be based on the susceptibilities of the cultured organism and should be 2–4 weeks in duration and at least 7 days following resolution of the infection [57].

11.6 Noninfectious Complications of Peritoneal Dialysis

11.6.1 Sclerosing Encapsulating Peritonitis

Sclerosing encapsulating peritonitis (SEP) is a rare and extremely serious complication of PD characterized by the presence of continuous, intermittent, or recurrent bowel obstruction associated with gross thickening of the peritoneum [104,105]. The cause of the disorder is likely multifactorial, but virtually all affected patients have received a prolonged course of PD, and most have evidence of high peritoneal permeability. The incidence in children has been documented to be 6.6 % and 22 % in those patients receiving PD for > 5 years and > 10 years, respectively[106]. The diagnosis is typically suspected based on clinical findings and confirmed by computed tomography (CT) or ultrasound. Treatment consists of cessation of PD and aggressive nutritional management in all, along with immunosuppressive therapy and surgery as deemed necessary [104, 107].

11.6.2 Hernia

The incidence of hernias in children receiving PD (8–57%) is inversely proportional to the patient's age, with the highest percentage noted in children <1 year of age [108]. The most common presentation is a painless swelling and 75% requires surgical correction followed by no/low volume dialysis for several days.

11.6.3 Hydrothorax

Hydrothorax, or the accumulation of dialysis fluid within the pleural space, occurs in 1.6–10% of patients. Contributing factors include increased IPP, a pleura-peritoneal pressure gradient, and congenital diaphragmatic defects. Whereas a presenting feature may consist of shortness of breath following the initiation of PD, the diagnosis may also be made when the displaced dialysate is evident on routine chest X-ray (usually right sided). Diagnostic techniques include scintigraphy or thoracentesis, with the detection of pleural fluid with a high dextrose concentration (>300 mg/dL) characteristic of dialysate consistent with the diagnosis. CT or magnetic resonance imaging (MRI) may be used to investigate a site of communication. Common approaches to management include permanent or temporary cessation of PD, decreased exchange volume, obliteration of the pleural space, or surgical repair of a diaphragmatic defect [109, 110].

11.7 Nutritional Management of Children on Peritoneal Dialysis

Malnutrition is a common complication in children who receive dialysis as a result of anorexia and poor intestinal absorption of nutrients [111]. Moreover, the protein needs of children with ESRD are increased when taking into account the protein losses that occur via the peritoneum. The KDOQI pediatric nutrition guidelines suggest following parameters of nutritional status and growth including dietary intake, length or height, height velocity, estimated dry weight, BMI, and head circumference based upon the child's age for PD patients [112]. Children on PD should receive at least 100% of the estimated energy requirements for normal age-dependent needs, with additional intake as need to address growth requirements [112]. The KDOQI guidelines also suggest that children on PD should receive a dietary protein intake of 100% of the daily recommended intake for ideal body weight, as well as additional protein intake to address protein losses via dialysis. Current recommendations for daily dietary protein intake are shown in Table 11.6.

Table 11.6 Recommended daily protein intake (DPI) [112]. (Source: Used with permission from [112])

Age (months)	DPI (g/kg/day)
0–6	1.8
7–12	1.5
1–3	1.3
4–13	1.1
14–18	1.0

DPI daily protein intake

Special attention must also be directed to the dietary management of sodium, potassium, and phosphorus. Infants, especially those with obstructive uropathy and poor renal tubular function, can have significant sodium losses via the dialysate and the native kidneys. Therefore, some infants require sodium supplementation to maintain total body sodium levels. A lack of supplementation can result in hyponatremia, severe central nervous system (CNS) manifestations, and poor growth [113]. Aggressive use of potassium-binding agents in infant formula can result in hypokalemia, a potential risk factor for peritonitis [114]. Finally, some infants on PD experience hypophosphatemia due to the use of low phosphorous infant formulas [115]. In those pediatric PD patients who experience hyperphosphatemia, management of dietary phosphorous intake is of critical importance because of the impact phosphorous has on bone turnover and linear growth, in addition to cardiovascular health.

11.8 Technique and Patient Survival

The need to terminate PD for reasons other than transplantation is most commonly the result of infectious complications. A NAPRTCS study found that 20% of patients transitioned from PD to HD over a 6-year period, the result of infection in 43% of the cases, followed by UF failure, patient/family choice and access failure as the most frequent reasons [116]. More recent data from the IPPN registry demonstrated similar findings with the following reasons for discontinuation of PD: kidney transplantation (60%), technique failure and switch to HD (20%), death (7%), and partial recovery of renal function (2%) [7].

Compared with adults, patient survival is excellent in children on PD, and there has been a steady improvement in mortality rates over the last 20 years, particularly in the youngest patients. Recent data from the USRDS based on children undergoing either chronic PD or HD have revealed mortality rates of 112.2 and 83.4 per 1000 person-years in those initiating dialysis in 1990–1994 and 2005–2010, respectively [117]. The highest mortality rates are seen in those patients who receive PD during the first year of life [118, 119]. Data from the Australia and New Zealand Dialysis and Transplant (ANZDATA) registry and the Italian dialysis registry are similar, but with more pronounced differences between various age groups [120, 121]. In addition to young age itself, an important predictor of mortality is the presence of nonrenal disease [122]. Data from the

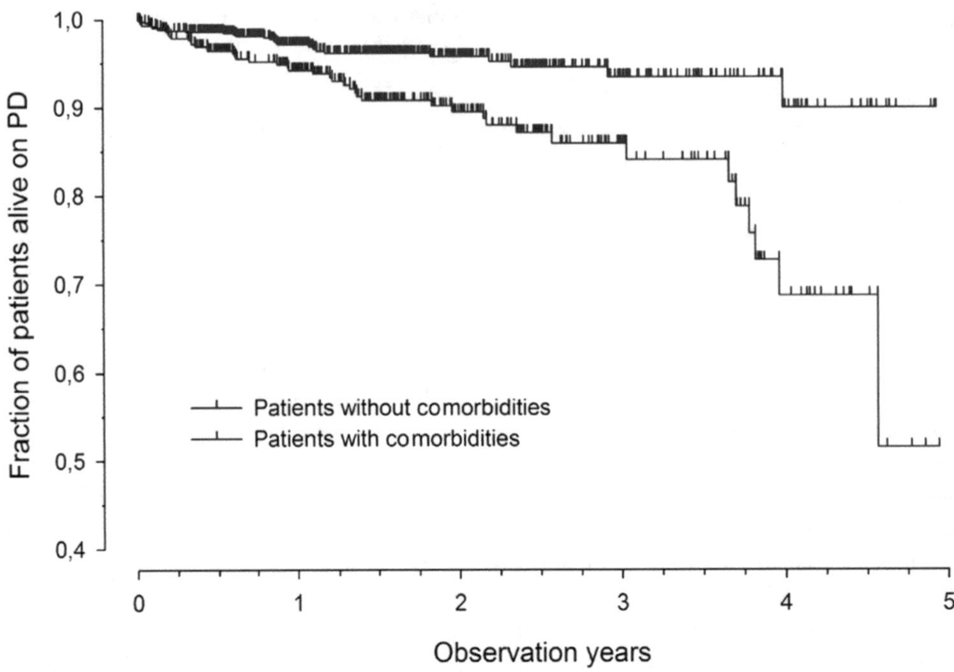

Fig. 11.7 Cumulative survival of pediatric peritoneal dialysis *(PD)* patients by absence or presence of at least one comorbidity. (Source: Used with permission from Neu [123]

IPPN have demonstrated that pediatric patients on chronic PD with a comorbidity (i.e., neurocognitive impairment or congenital heart disease) had a significantly lower survival rate compared with patients not having a comorbidity [123] (Fig. 11.7).

References

1. Blackfan K, Maxcy K. The intraperitoneal injection of saline solution. Am J Dis Child. 1918;15:19.
2. Bloxsum A, Powell N. The treatment of acute temporary dysfunction of the kidneys by peritoneal irrigation. Pediatrics. 1948;1:52–7.
3. Swan H, Gordon HH. Peritoneal lavage in the treatment of anuria in children. Pediatrics. 1949;4(5):586–95. (PubMed PMID: 15391042. Epub 1949/11/01).
4. Tenckhoff H, Schechter H. A bacteriologically safe peritoneal access device. Transac—Am Soc Artif Intern Organs. 1968;14:181–7. (PubMed PMID: 5701529. Epub 1968/01/01).
5. Popovich R, Moncrief J, Decherd J, et al. The definition of a novel portable/wearable equilibrium dialysis technique. Transac—Am Soc Artif Intern Organs. 1976;5.
6. Price CG, Suki WN. Newer modifications of peritoneal dialysis: options in the treatment of patients with renal failure. Am J Nephrol. 1981;1(2):97–104. (PubMed PMID: 7349048. Epub 1981/01/01).
7. Schaefer F, Borzych-Duzalka D, Azocar M, Munarriz RL, Sever L, Aksu N, et al. Impact of global economic disparities on practices and outcomes of chronic peritoneal dialysis in children: insights from the International Pediatric Peritoneal Dialysis Network Registry. Perit Dial Int. 2012;32(4):399–409. (PubMed PMID: 22859840. Pubmed Central PMCID: PMC3524840. Epub 2012/08/04).
8. U.S. Renal Data System, USRDS. Annual data report: atlas of chronic kidney disease and end-stage renal disease in the United States. Bethesda: National Institutes of Health, National Institute of Diabetes and Digestive and Kidney Diseases; 2013.
9. Putiloff P. Materials for the study of the laws of growth of the human body in relation to the surface areas of different systems: the trial on Russian subjects of planigraphic anatomy as a means for exact anthropometry; one of the problems of anthropology. Report of Dr. P. Putiloff at the meeting of the Siberian Branch of the Russian Geographic Society; 1884.
10. Esperanca M, Collins D. Peritoneal dialysis efficiency in relation to body weight. J Pediatr Surg. 1966;1:162–9.
11. Gruskin A, Lerner G, Fleischmann L. Developmental aspects of peritoneal dialysis kinetics. In: Fine R, editor. Chronic ambulatory peritoneal dialysis and chronic cycling peritoneal dialysis in children topics in renal medicine. Vol. 4. Boston: Martinus Nijhoff Publishing; 1987. pp. 33–45.
12. Fischbach M, Warady BA. Peritoneal dialysis prescription in children: bedside principles for optimal practice. Pediatr Nephrol (Berlin, Germany). 2009;24(9):1633–42. (quiz 40, 42. PubMed PMID: 18807074. Pubmed Central PMCID: PMC2719743. Epub 2008/09/23).
13. Nolph KD. Peritoneal anatomy and transport physiology. In: Drukker W, Parson FM, Maher JF, editors. Replacement of renal function by dialysis. Second edition. Boston. Martinus Nijhoff Publishing; 1983. p. 440.
14. Warady BA, Alexander SR, Hossli S, Vonesh E, Geary D, Watkins S, et al. Peritoneal membrane transport function in children receiving long-term dialysis. J Am Soc Nephrol. 1996;7(11):2385–91. (PubMed PMID: 8959629. Epub 1996/11/01).
15. Leypoldt JK. Solute transport across the peritoneal membrane. J Am Soc Nephrol. 2002;13(Suppl 1):S84–91. (PubMed PMID: 11792767. Epub 2002/01/17).
16. Waniewski J. Mathematical models for peritoneal transport characteristics. Perit Dial Int. 1999;19(Suppl 2):S193–201. (PubMed PMID: 10406518. Epub 1999/07/16).
17. Pyle W. Mass transfer in peritoneal dialysis. Austin: Univertisy of Texas; 1987.

18. Goldstein SL. Adequacy of dialysis in children: does small solute clearance really matter? Pediatr Nephrol (Berlin, Germany). 2004;19(1):1–5. (PubMed PMID: 14673636. Epub 2003/12/16).
19. Balfe J, Hanning R, Vigneus A. A comparison of peritoneal water and solute movement in younger and older children on CAPD. In: Fine R, Schaefer F, Mehls O, editors. CAPD in children. New York: Springer-Verlag; 1985. pp. 14–9.
20. Kohaut EC, Waldo FB, Benfield MR. The effect of changes in dialysate volume on glucose and urea equilibration. Perit Dial Int. 1994;14(3):236–9. (PubMed PMID: 7948234. Epub 1994/01/01).
21. Schroder CH, Reddingius RE, van Dreumel JA, Theeuwes AG, Monnens LA. Transcapillary ultrafiltration and lymphatic absorption during childhood continuous ambulatory peritoneal dialysis. Nephrol Dial Transplant. 1991;6(8):571–3. (PubMed PMID: 1956557. Epub 1991/01/01).
22. de Boer AW, van Schaijk TC, Willems HL, de Haan AF, Monnens LA, Schroder CH. Follow-up study of peritoneal fluid kinetics in infants and children on peritoneal dialysis. Perit Dial Int. 1999;19(6):572–7. (PubMed PMID: 10641778. Epub 2000/01/21).
23. Schaefer F, Fischbach M, Heckert KH et al. Hydrostatic intraperitoneal pressure in children on peritoneal dialysis. Perit Dial Int. 1996;16(S2):S79.
24. Phadke KD, Dinakar C. The challenges of treating children with renal failure in a developing country. Perit Dial Int. 2001;21(Suppl 3):S326–9. (PubMed PMID: 11887846. Epub 2002/03/13).
25. Bunchman TE, McBryde KD, Mottes TE, Gardner JJ, Maxvold NJ, Brophy PD. Pediatric acute renal failure: outcome by modality and disease. Pediatr Nephrol (Berlin, Germany). 2001;16(12):1067–71. (PubMed PMID: 11793102. Epub 2002/01/17).
26. Arikan AA, Zappitelli M, Goldstein SL, Naipaul A, Jefferson LS, Loftis LL. Fluid overload is associated with impaired oxygenation and morbidity in critically ill children. Pediatr Crit Care Med. 2011;13(3):253–8. (PubMed PMID: 21760565).
27. Goldstein SL. Overview of pediatric renal replacement therapy in acute kidney injury. Semi Dial. 2009;22(2):180–4. (PubMed PMID: 19426425. Epub 2009/05/12).
28. Goldstein SL, Devarajan P. Pediatrics: acute kidney injury leads to pediatric patient mortality. Nat Rev Nephrol. 2012;6(7):393–4. (PubMed PMID: 20585319).
29. Sutherland SM, Zappitelli M, Alexander SR, Chua AN, Brophy PD, Bunchman TE, et al. Fluid overload and mortality in children receiving continuous renal replacement therapy: the prospective pediatric continuous renal replacement therapy registry. Am J Kidney Dis. 2011;55(2):316–25. (PubMed PMID: 20042260).
30. Payen D, de Pont AC, Sakr Y, Spies C, Reinhart K, Vincent JL. A positive fluid balance is associated with a worse outcome in patients with acute renal failure. Crit Care (London. England). 2008;12(3):R74. (PubMed PMID: 18533029).
31. Bunchman TE. Acute peritoneal dialysis access in infant renal failure. Perit Dial Int. 1996;16(Suppl 1):S509–11. (PubMed PMID: 8728258).
32. Auron A, Warady BA, Simon S, Blowey DL, Srivastava T, Musharaf G, et al. Use of the multipurpose drainage catheter for the provision of acute peritoneal dialysis in infants and children. Am J Kidney Dis. 2007;49(5):650–5. (PubMed PMID: 17472847).
33. Chadha V, Warady BA, Blowey DL, Simckes AM, Alon US. Tenckhoff catheters prove superior to cook catheters in pediatric acute peritoneal dialysis. Am J Kidney Dis. 2000;35(6):1111–6. (PubMed PMID: 10845825).
34. Cullis B, Abdelraheem M, Abrahams G, Balbi A, Cruz DN, Frishberg Y, et al. Peritoneal dialysis for acute kidney injury. Perit Dial Int. 2014 (7–8);34(5):494–517. (PubMed PMID: 25074995. Pubmed Central PMCID: PMC4114667. Epub 2014/07/31).
35. Rusthoven E, van de Kar NA, Monnens LA, Schroder CH. Fibrin glue used successfully in peritoneal dialysis catheter leakage in children. Perit Dial Int. 2004;24(3):287–9. (PubMed PMID: 15185778. Epub 2004/06/10).
36. Sojo ET, Grosman MD, Monteverde ML, Bailez MM, Delgado N. Fibrin glue is useful in preventing early dialysate leakage in children on chronic peritoneal dialysis. Perit Dial Int. 2004;24(2):186–90. (PubMed PMID: 15119641. Epub 2004/05/04).
37. Rusthoven E, Krediet RT, Willems HL, Monnens LA, Schroder CH. Sodium sieving in children. Perit Dial Int. 2005;25(Suppl 3):S141–2. (PubMed PMID: 16048281. Epub 2005/07/29).
38. North American Pediatric Renal Trials and Collaborative Studies (NAPRTCS). Annual dialysis report. Rockville: Emmes Corporation; 2011.
39. Warady BA, Alexander SR, Watkins S, Kohaut E, Harmon WE. Optimal care of the pediatric end-stage renal disease patient on dialysis. Am J Kidney Dis. 1999;33(3):567–83. (PubMed PMID: 10070923. Epub 1999/03/10).
40. Alexander SR, Salusky IB, Warady BA, Watkins SL. Peritoneal dialysis workshop: pediatrics recommendations. Perit Dial Int. 1997;17(Suppl 3):S25–7. (PubMed PMID: 9304653. Epub 1997/01/01).
41. Salusky IB, Holloway M. Selection of peritoneal dialysis for pediatric patients. Perit Dial Int. 1997;17(Suppl 3):S35–7. (PubMed PMID: 9304656. Epub 1997/01/01).
42. Warady B, Schaefer F, Alexander S, Firanek C, Mujais S. Care of the pediatric patient on peritoneal dialysis. Clinical process for optimal outcomes. McGaw Park: Baxter Healthcare; 2004. p. 89.
43. Al-Hermi BE, Al-Saran K, Secker D, Geary DF. Hemodialysis for end-stage renal disease in children weighing less than 10 kg. Pediatr Nephrol (Berlin, Germany). 1999;13(5):401–3. (PubMed PMID: 10412860. Epub 1999/07/21).
44. Kovalski Y, Cleper R, Krause I, Davidovits M. Hemodialysis in children weighing less than 15 kg: a single-center experience. Pediatr Nephrol (Berlin, Germany). 2007;22(12):2105–10. (PubMed PMID: 17940806. Epub 2007/10/18).
45. Eisenstein I, Tarabeih M, Magen D, Pollack S, Kassis I, Ofer A, et al. Low infection rates and prolonged survival times of hemodialysis catheters in infants and children. Clin J Am Soc Nephrol: CJASN. 2011;6(4):793–8. (PubMed PMID: 21127138. Pubmed Central PMCID: PMC3069371. Epub 2010/12/04).
46. Dolan NM, Borzych-Duzalka D, Suarez A, Principi I, Hernandez O, Al-Akash S, et al. Ventriculoperitoneal shunts in children on peritoneal dialysis: a survey of the International Pediatric Peritoneal Dialysis Network. Pediatr Nephrol (Berlin, Germany). 2013;28(2):315–9. (PubMed PMID: 22972407. Epub 2012/09/14).
47. Watson AR, Hayes WN, Vondrak K, Ariceta G, Schmitt CP, Ekim M, et al. Factors influencing choice of renal replacement therapy in European paediatric nephrology units. Pediatr Nephrol (Berlin, Germany). 2013;28(12):2361–8. (PubMed PMID: 23843162. Epub 2013/07/12).
48. Strazdins V, Watson AR, Harvey B. Renal replacement therapy for acute renal failure in children: European guidelines. Pediatr Nephrol (Berlin, Germany). 2004;19(2):199–207. (PubMed PMID: 14685840. Pubmed Central PMCID: PMC1766478. Epub 2003/12/20).
49. Verrina E, Cappelli V, Perfumo F. Selection of modalities, prescription, and technical issues in children on peritoneal dialysis. Pediatr Nephrol (Berlin, Germany). 2009;24(8):1453–64. (PubMed PMID: 18521632. Pubmed Central PMCID: PMC2697927. Epub 2008/06/04).
50. Collins AJ, Foley RN, Herzog C, Chavers B, Gilbertson D, Herzog C, et al. US Renal Data System 2012 Annual Data Report. Am J Kidney Dis. 2013;61(1 Suppl 1):A7, e1–476. (PubMed PMID: 23253259. Epub 2013/01/04).

51. Warady BA, Bohl V, Alon U, Hellerstein S. Symptomatic peritoneal calcification in a child: treatment with tidal peritoneal dialysis. Perit Dial Int. 1994;14(1):26–9. (PubMed PMID: 8312409. Epub 1994/01/01).
52. Watson AR, Gartland C. Guidelines by an Ad, Hoc European Committee for elective chronic peritoneal dialysis in pediatric patients. Perit Dial Int. 2001;21(3):240–4. (PubMed PMID: 11475338. Epub 2001/07/28).
53. NKF-K/DOQI. Clinical practice guidelines for vascular access update 2000. Am J Kidney Dis. 2001;37(1 Suppl 1):S137–81. (PubMed PMID: 11229969).
54. Borzych-Dazalka D, Patel H, Flynn J, White C, Hooman N, Brophy P, et al. Peritoneal dialysis access revision, management and outcome—findings from the International Pediatric Peritoneal Dialysis Network (IPPN). Perit Dial Int. 2014 2014;Abstracts from the Annual Dialysis Conference:S18.
55. Zappitelli M, Goldstein S, Symons J, Somers M, Baum M, Brophy P, et al. Protein and calorie prescription for children and young adults receiving continuous renal replacement therapy: a report from the prospective pediatric continuous renal replacement therapy registry group. Crit Care Med. 2008;36(12):3239–45.
56. Chadha V, Jones LL, Ramirez ZD, Warady BA. Chest wall peritoneal dialysis catheter placement in infants with a colostomy. Adv Perit Dial. 2000;16:318–20. (PubMed PMID: 11045319. Epub 2000/10/25).
57. Warady BA, Bakkaloglu S, Newland J, Cantwell M, Verrina E, Neu A, et al. Consensus guidelines for the prevention and treatment of catheter-related infections and peritonitis in pediatric patients receiving peritoneal dialysis: 2012 update. Perit Dial Int. 2012;32(Suppl 2):S32–86. (PubMed PMID: 22851742. Pubmed Central PMCID: PMC3524923. Epub 2012/08/08).
58. Washburn KK, Currier H, Salter KJ, Brandt ML. Surgical technique for peritoneal dialysis catheter placement in the pediatric patient: a North American survey. Adv Perit Dial. 2004;20:218–21. (PubMed PMID: 15384830. Epub 2004/09/24).
59. White CT, Gowrishankar M, Feber J, Yiu V. Clinical practice guidelines for pediatric peritoneal dialysis. Pediatric nephrology (Berlin, Germany). 2006;21(8):1059–66. (PubMed PMID: 16819641. Epub 2006/07/05).
60. Nicholson ML, Burton PR, Donnelly PK, Veitch PS, Walls J. The role of omentectomy in continuous ambulatory peritoneal dialysis. Perit Dial Int. 1991;11(4):330–2. (PubMed PMID: 1751599).
61. Cribbs RK, Greenbaum LA, Heiss KF. Risk factors for early peritoneal dialysis catheter failure in children. J Pediatr Surg. 2010;45(3):585–9. (PubMed PMID: 20223324. Epub 2010/03/13).
62. Rinaldi S, Sera F, Verrina E, Edefonti A, Gianoglio B, Perfumo F, et al. Chronic peritoneal dialysis catheters in children: a fifteen-year experience of the Italian Registry of Pediatric Chronic Peritoneal Dialysis. Perit Dial Int. 2004;24(5):481–6. (PubMed PMID: 15490990. Epub 2004/10/20).
63. Conlin MJ, Tank ES. Minimizing surgical problems of peritoneal dialysis in children. J Urol. 1995;154(2 Pt 2):917–9. (PubMed PMID: 7609212. Epub 1995/08/01).
64. Phan J, Stanford S, Zaritsky JJ, DeUgarte DA. Risk factors for morbidity and mortality in pediatric patients with peritoneal dialysis catheters. J Pediatr Surg. 2013;48(1):197–202. (PubMed PMID: 23331815. Epub 2013/01/22).
65. Rees L, Brandt ML. Tube feeding in children with chronic kidney disease: technical and practical issues. Pediatr Nephrol (Berlin, Germany). 2010;25(4):699–704. (PubMed PMID: 19949817).
66. von Schnakenburg C, Feneberg R, Plank C, Zimmering M, Arbeiter K, Bald M, et al. Percutaneous endoscopic gastrostomy in children on peritoneal dialysis. Perit Dial Int. 2006;26(1):69–77. (PubMed PMID: 16538878. Epub 2006/03/17).
67. Ledermann SE, Spitz L, Moloney J, Rees L, Trompeter RS. Gastrostomy feeding in infants and children on peritoneal dialysis. Pediatr Nephrol (Berlin, Germany). 2002;17(4):246–50. (PubMed PMID: 11956875).
68. Ramage IJ, Harvey E, Geary DF, Hebert D, Balfe JA, Balfe JW. Complications of gastrostomy feeding in children receiving peritoneal dialysis. Pediatr Nephrol (Berlin, Germany). 1999;13(3):249–52. (PubMed PMID: 10353416).
69. Warady BA, Bashir M, Donaldson LA. Fungal peritonitis in children receiving peritoneal dialysis: a report of the NAPRTCS. Kidney Int. 2000;58(1):384–9. (PubMed PMID: 10886585. Epub 2000/07/08).
70. Neu AM, Miller MR, Stuart J, Lawlor J, Richardson T, Martz K, et al. Design of the standardizing care to improve outcomes in pediatric end stage renal disease collaborative. Pediatr Nephrol (Berlin, Germany). 2014;29(9):1477–84. (PubMed PMID: 25055994. Epub 2014/07/25).
71. Schaefer B, Macher-Goeppinger S, Testa S, Holland-Cunz S, Querfeld U, Schaefer F, et al. An International Peritoneal Dialysis Biopsy Study in Children on peritoneal dialysis and healthy controls. Perit Dial Int. 2013;33(Suppl 1).
72. Canepa A, Verrina E, Perfumo F. Use of new peritoneal dialysis solutions in children. Kidney Int Suppl. 2008;(108):S137–44. (PubMed PMID: 18379537. Epub 2008/05/03).
73. Schroder CH. Optimal peritoneal dialysis: choice of volume and solution. Nephrol Dial Transplant. 2004;19(4):782–4. (PubMed PMID: 15031330. Epub 2004/03/20).
74. Rusthoven E, Krediet RT, Willems HL, Monnens LAH, Schröder CH. Peritoneal transport characteristics with glucose polymer-based dialysis fluid in children. J Am Soc Nephrol. 2004;15(11):2940–7.
75. Dart A, Feber J, Wong H, Filler G. Icodextrin re-absorption varies with age in children on automated peritoneal dialysis. Pediatr Nephrol (Berlin, Germany). 2005;20(5):683–5. (PubMed PMID: 15719251. Epub 2005/02/19).
76. McIntyre CW. Update on peritoneal dialysis solutions. Kidney Int. 2007;71(6):486–90. (PubMed PMID: 17299524. Epub 2007/02/15).
77. Durand PY. Optimization of fill volumes in automated peritoneal dialysis. Perit Dial Int. 2000;20(6):601–2. (PubMed PMID: 11216546. Epub 2001/02/24).
78. Fischbach M, Terzic J, Menouer S, Haraldsson B. Optimal volume prescription for children on peritoneal dialysis. Perit Dial Int. 2000;20(6):603–6. (PubMed PMID: 11216547. Epub 2001/02/24).
79. Schaefer F, Warady BA. Peritoneal dialysis in children with end-stage renal disease. Nat Rev Nephrol. 2011;7(11):659–68. (PubMed PMID: 21947118. Epub 2011/09/29).
80. Fischbach M, Terzic J, Laugel V, Escande B, Dangelser C, Helmstetter A. Measurement of hydrostatic intraperitoneal pressure: a useful tool for the improvement of dialysis dose prescription. Pediatr Nephrol (Berlin, Germany). 2003;18(10):976–80. (PubMed PMID: 12898379. Epub 2003/08/05).
81. KDOQI. Clinical practice guidelines and clinical practice recommendations for updates. Hemodialysis adequacy, peritoneal dialysis adequacy and vascular access. Am J Kidney Dis. 2006;28(Sup pl 1):S1.
82. Twardowski ZJ, Nolph KD, Khanna R. Limitations of the peritoneal equilibration test. Nephrol Dial Transplant. 1995;10(11):2160–1. (PubMed PMID: 8643196. Epub 1995/11/01).
83. Johnson D, Mudge D, Blizzard S, Arndt M, O'Shea A, Watt R, et al. A comparison of peritoneal equilibration tests performed 1 and 4 weeks after PD commencement. Perit Dial Int. 2004;24(5):460–5.
84. Rocco MV, Jordan JR, Burkart JM. Changes in peritoneal transport during the first month of peritoneal dialysis. Perit Dial Int. 1995;15(1):12–7. (PubMed PMID: 7734554. Epub 1995/01/01).

85. Schaefer F, Klaus G, Mehls O. Peritoneal transport properties and dialysis dose affect growth and nutritional status in children on chronic peritoneal dialysis. Mid-European Pediatric Peritoneal Dialysis Study Group. J Am Soc Nephrol. 1999;10(8):1786–92. (PubMed PMID: 10446947. Epub 1999/08/14).
86. Verrina E, Amici G, Perfumo F, Trivelli A, Canepa A, Gusmano R, The use of the PD Adequest mathematical model in pediatric patients on chronic peritoneal dialysis. Perit Dial Int. 1998;18(3):322–8. (PubMed PMID: 9663898. Epub 1998/07/15).
87. Warady BA, Jennings J. The short PET in pediatrics. Perit Dial Int. 2007;27(4):441–5. (PubMed PMID: 17602153. Epub 2007/07/03).
88. Cano F, Sanchez L, Rebori A, Quiroz L, Delucchi A, Delgado I, et al. The short peritoneal equilibration test in pediatric peritoneal dialysis. Pediatr Nephrol (Berlin, Germany). 2010;25(10):2159–64. (PubMed PMID: 20574772. Epub 2010/06/25).
89. Fadrowski JJ, Frankenfield D, Amaral S, Brady T, Gorman GH, Warady B, et al. Children on long-term dialysis in the United States: findings from the 2005 ESRD clinical performance measures project. Am J Kidney Dis. 2007;50(6):958–66. (PubMed PMID: 18037097. Epub 2007/11/27).
90. Paniagua R, Amato D, Correa-Rotter R, Ramos A, Vonesh EF, Mujais SK. Correlation between peritoneal equilibration test and dialysis adequacy and transport test, for peritoneal transport type characterization. Mexican Nephrology Collaborative Study Group. Perit Dial Int. 2000;20(1):53–9. (PubMed PMID: 10716584. Epub 2000/03/15).
91. Lo WK, Lui SL, Chan TM, Li FK, Lam MF, Tse KC, et al. Minimal and optimal peritoneal Kt/V targets: results of an anuric peritoneal dialysis patient's survival analysis. Kidney Int. 2005;67(5):2032–8. (PubMed PMID: 15840054. Epub 2005/04/21).
92. Morgenstern BZ, Mahoney DW, Warady BA. Estimating total body water in children on the basis of height and weight: a reevaluation of the formulas of Mellits and Cheek. J Am Soc Nephrol. 2002;13(7):1884–8. (PubMed PMID: 12089384. Epub 2002/06/29).
93. Bakkaloglu SA, Borzych D, Soo Ha I, Serdaroglu E, Buscher R, Salas P, et al. Cardiac geometry in children receiving chronic peritoneal dialysis: findings from the International Pediatric Peritoneal Dialysis Network (IPPN) registry. Clini J Am Soc Nephrol: CJASN. 2011;6(8):1926–33. (PubMed PMID: 21737855. Pubmed Central PMCID: PMC3359542. Epub 2011/07/09).
94. Mitsnefes MM, Daniels SR, Schwartz SM, Meyer RA, Khoury P, Strife CF. Severe left ventricular hypertrophy in pediatric dialysis: prevalence and predictors. Pediatr Nephrol (Berlin, Germany). 2000;14(10–11):898–902. (PubMed PMID: 10975295. Epub 2000/09/07).
95. Mitsnefes M, Stablein D. Hypertension in pediatric patients on long-term dialysis: a report of the North American Pediatric Renal Transplant Cooperative Study (NAPRTCS). Am J Kidney Dis. 2005;45(2):309–15. (PubMed PMID: 15685509. Epub 2005/02/03).
96. Warady BA, Ellis EN, Fivush BA, Lum GM, Alexander SR, Brewer ED, et al. "Flush before fill" in children receiving automated peritoneal dialysis. Perit Dial Int. 2003;23(5):493–8. (PubMed PMID: 14604204. Epub 2003/11/08).
97. Strippoli GF, Tong A, Johnson D, Schena FP, Craig JC. Catheter-related interventions to prevent peritonitis in peritoneal dialysis: a systematic review of randomized, controlled trials. J Am Soc Nephrol. 2004;15(10):2735–46. (PubMed PMID: 15466279. Epub 2004/10/07).
98. Bakkaloglu SA. Prevention of peritonitis in children: emerging concepts. Perit Dial Int. 2009;29(Suppl 2):S186–9. (PubMed PMID: 19270214. Epub 2009/05/16).
99. Warady BA, Feneberg R, Verrina E, Flynn JT, Muller-Wiefel DE, Besbas N, et al. Peritonitis in children who receive long-term peritoneal dialysis: a prospective evaluation of therapeutic guidelines. J Am Soc Nephrol. 2007;18(7):2172–9. (PubMed PMID: 17582162. Epub 2007/06/22).
100. Chadha V, Schaefer F, Warady B. Peritonitis and exit-site infections. In: Warady B, Schaefer F, Alexander S, editors. Pediatric sialysis. New York: Springer; 2012. pp. 231–56.
101. Warady BA, Neu AM, Schaefer F. Optimal care of the infant, child, and adolescent on dialysis: 2014 update. Am J Kidney Dis. 2014;64(1):128–42. (PubMed PMID: 24717681. Epub 2014/04/11).
102. Bernardini J, Price V, Figueiredo A. Peritoneal dialysis patient training, 2006. Perit Dial Int. 2006;26(6):625–32. (PubMed PMID: 17047225. Epub 2006/10/19).
103. Chua AN, Goldstein SL, Bell D, Brewer ED. Topical mupirocin/sodium hypochlorite reduces peritonitis and exit-site infection rates in children. Clin J Am Soc Nephrol: CJASN. 2009;4(12):1939–43. (PubMed PMID: 19820132. Pubmed Central PMCID: PMC2798867. Epub 2009/10/13).
104. Honda M, Warady BA. Long-term peritoneal dialysis and encapsulating peritoneal sclerosis in children. Pediatr Nephrol (Berlin, Germany). 2010;25(1):75–81. (PubMed PMID: 21476232. Pubmed Central PMCID: PMC2778779. Epub 2010/01/01Eng).
105. Vidal E, Edefonti A, Puteo F, Chimenz R, Gianoglio B, Lavoratti G, et al. Encapsulating peritoneal sclerosis in paediatric peritoneal dialysis patients: the experience of the Italian Registry of Pediatric Chronic Dialysis. Nephrol Dial Transplant. 2013;28(6):1603–9. (PubMed PMID: 23585587. Epub 2013/04/16).
106. Hoshii S, Honda M. High incidence of encapsulating peritoneal sclerosis in pediatric patients on peritoneal dialysis longer than 10 years. Perit Dial Int. 2002;22(6):730–1. (PubMed PMID: 12556080. Epub 2003/01/31).
107. Kawaguchi Y, Saito A, Kawanishi H, Nakayama M, Miyazaki M, Nakamoto H, et al. Recommendations on the management of encapsulating peritoneal sclerosis in Japan, 2005: diagnosis, predictive markers, treatment, and preventive measures. Perit Dial Int. 2005;25(Suppl 4):S83–95. (PubMed PMID: 16300277. Epub 2005/11/23).
108. Bakkaloglu A. Non-infectious compolications of peritoneal dialysis in children. In: Warady BASF, Alexander S, editors. Pediatric dialysis. 2nd ed. New York: Springer; 2012. pp. 257–71.
109. Bakkaloglu SA, Ekim M, Tumer N, Gungor A, Yilmaz S. Pleurodesis treatment with tetracycline in peritoneal dialysis-complicated hydrothorax. Pediatr Nephrol (Berlin, Germany). 1999;13(7):637–8. (PubMed PMID: 10507835. Epub 1999/10/03).
110. Szeto CC, Chow KM. Pathogenesis and management of hydrothorax complicating peritoneal dialysis. Current Opin Pulm Med. 2004;10(4):315–9. (PubMed PMID: 15220759. Epub 2004/06/29).
111. Canpolat N, Caliskan S, Sever L, Tasdemir M, Ekmekci OB, Pehlivan G, et al. Malnutrition and its association with inflammation and vascular disease in children on maintenance dialysis. Pediatr Nephrol (Berlin, Germany). 2013;28(11):2149–56. (PubMed PMID: 23765444. Epub 2013/06/15).
112. KDOQI. Clinical practice guideline for nutrition in children with CKD. Am J Kidney Dis. 2009;53(Suppl 2):S1.
113. Paulson WD, Bock GH, Nelson AP, Moxey-Mims MM, Crim LM. Hyponatremia in the very young chronic peritoneal dialysis patient. Am J Kidney Dis. 1989;14(3):196–9. (PubMed PMID: 2773922. Epub 1989/09/01).
114. Chuang Y-W, Shu K-H, Yu T-M, Cheng C-H, Chen C-H. Hypokalaemia: an independent risk factor of enterobacteriaceae peritonitis in CAPD patients. Nephrol Dial Transplant. 2009;24(5):1603–8.
115. Roodhooft AM, Van Hoeck KJ, Van Acker KJ. Hypophosphatemia in infants on continuous ambulatory peritoneal dialysis. Clin Nephrol. 1990;34(3):131–5. (PubMed PMID: 2225564. Epub 1990/09/01Eng).

116. Leonard MB, Donaldson LA, Ho M, Geary DF. A prospective cohort study of incident maintenance dialysis in children: a NAPRTCS study. Kidney Int. 2003;63(2):744–55. (PubMed PMID: 12631143. Epub 2003/03/13).
117. Mitsnefes MM, Laskin BL, Dahhou M, Zhang X, Foster BJ. Mortality risk among children initially treated with dialysis for end-stage kidney disease, 1990–2010. JAMA. 2013;309(18):1921–9. (PubMed PMID: 23645144. Pubmed Central PMCID: PMC3712648. Epub 2013/05/07).
118. Coulthard MG, Crosier J. Outcome of reaching end stage renal failure in children under 2 years of age. Arch Dis Child. 2002;87(6):511–7. (PubMed PMID: 12456551Eng).
119. Shroff R, Rees L, Trompeter R, Hutchinson C, Ledermann S. Long-term outcome of chronic dialysis in children. Pediatr Nephrol (Berlin, Germany). 2006;21(2):257–64. (PubMed PMID: 16270221Eng).
120. McDonald SP, Craig JC. Long-term survival of children with end-stage renal disease. N Engl J Med. 2004;350(26):2654–62. (PubMed PMID: 15215481. Epub 2004/06/25).
121. Verrina E, Edefonti A, Gianoglio B, Rinaldi S, Sorino P, Zacchello G, et al. A multicenter experience on patient and technique survival in children on chronic dialysis. Pediatric Nephrol (Berlin, Germany). 2004;19(1):82–90. (PubMed PMID: 14648343).
122. Wood EG, Hand M, Briscoe DM, Donaldson LA, Yiu V, Harley FL, et al. Risk factors for mortality in infants and young children on dialysis. Am J Kidney Dis. 2001;37(3):573–9. (PubMed PMID: 11228182Eng).
123. Neu AM, Sander A, Borzych-Duzalka D, Watson AR, Valles PG, Ha IS, et al. Comorbidities in chronic pediatric peritoneal dialysis patients: a report of the International Pediatric Peritoneal Dialysis Network. Perit Dial Int. 2012;32(4):410–8. (PubMed PMID: 22859841. Pubmed Central PMCID: PMC3524853. Epub 2012/08/04. Eng).
124. Warady BA. Peritoneal dialysis. In: Silverstein DM, Symons JM, Alon US, editors Pediatric nephrology: a handbook for training healthcare providers. Singapore: World Scientific Publishing (In Press.). pp. 551–84.
125. Schaefer F, Feneberg R, Aksu N, Donmez O, Sadikoglu B, Alexander SR, et al. Worldwide variation of dialysis-associated peritonitis in children. Kidney Int. 2007;72(11):1374–9.

12 Special Problems in Caring for Patients on Peritoneal Dialysis

Olof Heimbürger

12.1 Changes in Water and Solute Transport with Time on Peritoneal Dialysis (PD)

12.1.1 The Peritoneal Transport Process

The capillary wall is considered to be the main transport barrier for diffusion and convection through the peritoneal barrier (although it is likely that the interstitium may be a significant transport barrier in pathological conditions with thickening and fibrosis of the peritoneal membrane). The peritoneal capillaries behave functionally as having a heteroporous structure, with a large number of "ultra-small" water pores (radius 4–6 Å), a large number of "small pores" (radius 40–65 Å), and a small number of large pores (radius 200–400 Å) through which macromolecules are filtered due to convective flow [1–3]. The anatomical correlates of the water channels are aquaporin-1, of the small pores are the inter-endothelial clefts, and of the large pores are likely larger inter-endothelial clefts on the venules, but this is less established. Only water may pass through the aquaporins, whereas the small pores do not restrict the passage of small solutes but are impermeable for macromolecules larger than albumin [1–3]. In addition to the transcapillary exchange between plasma and dialysate, there is a peritoneal absorptive flow of fluid and solutes, comprising two different pathways [1–3]: (1) direct lymphatic absorption (about 0.3 ml/min) and (2) fluid absorption into interstitial tissues (about 1.2 ml/min) where it is absorbed into the capillaries due to the Starling forces.

O. Heimbürger (✉)
Department of Renal Medicine, Department of Clinical Science, Intervention and Technology, Karolinska University Hospital, Karolinska Institutet, Stockholm, Sweden
e-mail: olof.heimburger@ki.se

12.1.2 How to Evaluate the Peritoneal Transport Rate

There are several tests available for the assessment of peritoneal transport characteristics, but in the clinical setting, mainly the peritoneal equilibration test (PET) [4] and the personal dialysis capacity (PDC) test are used [5]. Commercial computer programs have been developed based on these tests and the three-pore model and make it possible to assess basic peritoneal transport parameters and to predict effects of various treatment schedules on peritoneal small solute clearances and, to some extent, on ultrafiltration [5–7]. However, the results will be closely dependent on the quality of data put into the computer. The lab methods are also important; for example, when creatinine in dialysate is measured by the Jaffé method, it must be corrected for the interference by the high glucose concentrations in dialysate [8].

12.1.3 The PET

The PET is by far the most widely used test for evaluation of the peritoneal transport characteristics in individual patients. Briefly, in the most commonly used version of the PET, 2 l of 2.27% glucose dialysis fluid are infused, after drain of the overnight dialysate. Usually, dialysate samples are taken after infusion, at 2 and 4 h when the dialysate is drained and the volume is recorded. A blood sample is drawn at 2 h dwell time. The net ultrafiltration, the dialysate to plasma concentration (D/P) for creatinine, and the dialysate concentration/initial dialysate concentration (D/D_0) for glucose are compared to standard values. The patients are usually classified according to D/P creatinine at 4 h into fast transporters (above mean + 1 SD), fast average transporters (between mean and mean + 1 SD), slow average transporters (between mean and mean − 1 SD), and slow transporters (below mean − 1 SD) [4, 8], Table 12.1. Twardowski categorized the patients into high, high-average, low-average, and low transport groups. However, fast and slow transport should be a better terminol-

A. K. Singh et al. (eds.), *Core Concepts in Dialysis and Continuous Therapies,* DOI 10.1007/978-1-4899-7657-4_12

Table 12.1 Peritoneal transport groups classified according to D/P creatinine at 4 h from the PET using Twardowski's initial classification. [4]

Transport group	D/P creatinine	Ao/Δx (cm/1.73 BSA)	Ultrafiltration capacity
Fast	> 0.81	> 30,000	–
Fast average	0.65–0.81	23,600–30,000	+
Slow average	0.50–0.65	17,200–23,600	++
Slow	< 0.50	< 17,200	+++

ogy compared to high and low transport, as the net removal of very small solutes, for example, urea, is often low in "high" transporters due to the poor ultrafiltration and lower drained volume. Fast and fast-average transporters have more rapid equilibration of creatinine and poorer net ultrafiltration due to more rapid glucose absorption, whereas slow-average and slow transporters have slower solute transport, resulting in slow glucose absorption and high net ultrafiltration but low peritoneal clearances for creatinine and larger solutes [8]. As most studies show an average creatinine D/P equilibration rate slightly faster than in the study of Twardowski [1, 4], most patients will fall into the fast-average category.

It has been suggested to use 3.86% instead of 2.27% glucose solution for the PET, as the higher glucose concentration will result in better ultrafiltration and consequently a better estimate of ultrafiltration capacity (UFC). In addition, it also makes it possible to use the decrease in dialysate sodium as an additional parameter to identify patients with poor ultrafiltration [9]. With a normal UFC, there is a marked dip in dialysate sodium concentration after 1–2 h of a dwell with hypertonic solution due to sieving of sodium as about half of the ultrafiltered fluid will pass through the aquaporins (which are impermeable for sodium).

12.1.4 Changes in Peritoneal Transport After the Initiation of PD

After the initiation of PD, there are often changes in the peritoneal transport rate during the first 3–6 months with an increase in D/P creatinine but rather stable ultrafiltration rates [1]. Although the peritoneal transport rate seems to be relatively stable during the initial years of PD, there is a tendency toward faster peritoneal transport rates (and increasing D/P creatinine) with time on PD. This increased diffusion rate, likely due to increased peritoneal capillary surface area, also results in a more rapid absorption of glucose, resulting in a more rapid decline in dialysate glucose concentration and shorter duration of the osmotic gradient between plasma and dialysate resulting in decreased net ultrafiltration. This is usually a gradual process which in parallel to the loss of residual renal function with time may result in fluid overload, hypertension, and cardiovascular complications.

The tendency toward increasing small solute transport (as assessed by D/P creatinine) and decreasing ultrafiltration is evident in almost all prospective studies, whereas macromolecule transport (as assessed by protein clearances) seems to be stable or even decreases with time on PD [1]. The reason behind this discrepancy is not completely understood, but likely related to the remodeling of the peritoneal membrane with epithelial-to-mesenchymal transition of mesothelial cells and submesothelial expansion with fibrosis of the interstitial matrix, and angiogenesis [1]. The expanded interstitium will separate the peritoneal microvasculature from the dialysis fluid and make transperitoneal transport less efficient and will markedly decrease the osmotic pressure close to the capillary. However, the increased surface area due to neoangiogenesis will compensate for the larger diffusion distance and result in a more rapid transport of small solutes, such as creatinine (and a more rapid absorption of glucose at the capillary), whereas proteins may be retarded in the expanded fibrotic interstitium resulting in unchanged net protein transport. The net result will be increased small solute transport, decreased ultrafiltration, and unchanged protein transport.

12.2 Loss of Ultrafiltration Capacity

With time, the changes in the peritoneal transport may progress, resulting in loss of UFC. Using the standard lactate-based solutions, the risk of developing loss of UFC (using a clinical definition) increases markedly after 4 years of PD, being 9% after 4 years and 35% after 6 years of PD [10]. Today, UFC is usually defined as less than 400 ml of ultrafiltration during a PET with 2 l of 3.86% glucose solution. The transport pattern is not similar in all patients with loss of UFC (Table 12.2). The most common pattern observed is an increased transport of small solutes with rapid glucose absorption [10, 11], resulting in rapid loss of the osmotic driving force and, consequently, a rapid decline in ultrafiltration rate. However, detailed kinetic analyses of patients with UFC due to rapid diffusive transport show that this is most commonly associated with a decreased osmotic conductance, that is, the remaining osmotic gradient cannot induce water flow as effectively as in patients with normal UFC [12]. This is associated with a decreased dip in dialysate sodium concentration that is usually seen after 1–2 h of an exchange with hypertonic glucose solution.

Table 12.2 Different patterns in patients with reduced ultrafiltration capacity [1, 10, 11]. Note that combinations are common

Observation	Mechanism of reduced ultrafiltration	Frequency
Increased D/P creatinine and low D/D0 glucose	Loss of the osmotic driving force	Common
Less ultrafiltration than expected from the osmotic gradient, low sodium dip	Decreased osmotic conductance for glucose	Common in combination with 1 in long-term PD
Low D/P creatinine and high D/D0 glucose	"Hypopermeable" peritoneum due to fibrosis and multiple adhesions and fibrosis	Extremely rare
Low ultrafiltration and normal D/P creatinine, D/D0 glucose and sodium dip	Increased peritoneal fluid absorption. Dialysate leak	Rare

Loss of peritoneal surface area with slow solute transport due to loss of peritoneal surface area, fibrosis, and formation of adhesions has been reported during the late stage of encapsulating peritoneal sclerosis (EPS, previously called sclerosing encapsulating peritonitis) in a few cases. However, detailed studies in patients developing EPS showed increasing peritoneal solute transport rate in almost all of them [1], suggesting that loss of UFC associated with increased solute transport in these patients was an early sign that preceded the development of more overt signs of EPS. However, slow solute transport is extremely rare and very few cases have been reported.

Increased peritoneal fluid absorption has also been reported as the cause of UFC loss [10, 11]. This has often been attributed to increased lymphatic absorption, but detailed kinetic studies show no increase in lymphatic absorption, but increased fluid absorption into the peritoneal interstitial tissue, that may be due to changes in the interstitial tissue fluid hydraulic conductivity [1]. However, a subcutaneous or retroperitoneal leakage of the dialysate must be excluded, for example, by using computed tomography with contrast in the dialysate.

The pathophysiological mechanisms behind the structural and functional alterations in the peritoneal membrane are not clear, but it is generally believed that uremia per se, bioincompatibility of the conventional PD solutions, and the effect of local peritoneal inflammation due to bioincompatibility of the solutions and peritonitis are the contributing factors [13].

12.2.1 Treatment Options

There are no known specific treatments to stop the changes in the structure and function of the peritoneal membrane in long-term PD patients. It has been suggested that use of modern, more biocompatible, neutral pH PD solutions with low content of reactive glucose degradation products (GDP) will result in less changes in the peritoneal membrane [14]. This has some support from the BalANZ study, which is so far the largest randomized controlled trial of biocompatible PD solution [15]. In this study, 185 new PD patients were randomized to neutral, low-GDP PD solution or standard solution. The patients randomized to the biocompatible PD solution had higher initial D/P creatinine and lower initial ultrafiltration than the control group, but during the 2-year study period, D/P creatinine was stable and ultrafiltration increased in the biocompatible PD solution group over the 2-year study period. The patients in the control group had increasing D/P and decreasing ultrafiltration with time. This may be interpreted that the biocompatible solution has rapid effects on the initial transport pattern, perhaps due to vasodilation and increased surface area, whereas the control solution exerts its effect by neoangiogenesis. If this speculation is correct, the long-term effect of the biocompatible solutions would be clearly beneficial, but it is too early to make any definitive conclusions regarding this.

With regard to treatment options for patients with decreasing UFC due to increased glucose absorption, these patients are very well suited for use of icodextrin solution, which usually causes excellent ultrafiltration in these patients [8]. These patients are also excellently suited for automated peritoneal dialysis (APD), where shorter cycles will result in both high clearances and adequate ultrafiltration [8].

12.3 Malnutrition

In this chapter, the term "protein-energy wasting (PEW)" will be used as recommended by the International Society of Renal Nutrition and Metabolism [16] as it is a more specific term than malnutrition for the syndrome of loss of body protein mass and fuel reserves. The further suggested criteria for the diagnosis of PEW are given in Table 12.3. It is in general important to differentiate between PEW caused by low nutritional intake only and when it is more frequently associated with chronic inflammation, increased catabolism, and metabolic disturbances, in addition to low nutritional intake [16].

12.3.1 PEW in PD Versus HD

PEW is common in dialysis patients and a strong predictor of poor outcome. Surveys using classical methods to assess nutritional status suggest that, in general, about 50% of dialysis patients show signs of wasting [16]. In general, there

Table 12.3 Criteria to define PEW in dialysis patients from the International Society of Renal Nutrition and Metabolism. [16]

Abnormal serum chemistry	S-albumin < 38 g/l
	S-prealbumin < 300 mg/l
	S-cholesterol < 2.6 mmol/l (100 mg/dl)
Low body mass	BMI < 23
	Unintentional weight loss > 5 % in 3 months
	Total fat mass < 10 %
Reduced muscle mass	> 5 % reduction in 3 months
	> 10 % reduced mid-arm muscle circumference area compared to 50th percentile of the normal
	Reduced creatinine appearance
Unintentionally low dietary intake	Protein intake (< 0.8 g/kg body weight for 2 months)
	Energy intake (< 25 kcal/kg body weight for 2 months)

At least three of the four categories (and at least one test in each category) are needed for the diagnosis of renal PEW

seems to be little difference in nutritional status between PD and hemodialysis (HD) patients, but it has previously been suggested that PD patients in general tend to have more fat mass and less muscles. However, recently, a large European multicenter study of 491 pairs of HD and PD patients (matched for country, gender, age and dialysis vintage) was performed using bioimpedance spectroscopy for assessment of body composition [17]. In this study, lean tissue index (representing muscle mass) was slightly better preserved in PD patients, whereas fat mass was increased in both HD and PD, but not different between the groups.

12.3.2 Factors Contributing to PEW in PD Patients

There are multiple causes of PEW in patients on dialysis, but there are clear differences in the dialysis process of HD and PD, which may affect the nutritional status. In particular, PD is a continuous dialysis process with a stable metabolic situation, but on the other hand, PD patients are constantly exposed to glucose absorption from the dialysis fluid as well as losses of protein and amino acids into the dialysate. As PEW is a strong predictor of poor outcome, it is important to be aware of the multiple factors contributing to PEW as well to have a treatment strategy based on the multifactorial pathogenetic mechanisms [18].

Factors contributing to PEW among PD patients are summarized in Table 12.4. Anorexia and poor nutritional intake (particularly of protein) are common factors and have multiple causes, including impaired olfactory and taste functions, depression, elevated cytokine levels due to chronic inflammation, inadequate dialysis, as well as glucose absorption from the dialysate. Further factors contributing to

Table 12.4 Important factors contributing to malnutrition in PD patients

Inadequate dietary intake	
Anorexia due to	Inadequate dialysis
	Inflammation
	Gastrointestinal problems
	Multiple medications
	Comorbidity
	Glucose absorption from the dialysate
	Impaired olfactory function
	Depression
Altered metabolism	Increased energy consumption
	Increased protein catabolism
	Changes in organ-dependent amino acid metabolism
	Insulin resistance
	Hypogonadism, testosterone deficiency
	High myostatin
	Low growth hormone and IGF-1
Effects of the PD procedure	Loss of amino acids and protein into the dialysate (5–15 g)
	Glucose absorption from the dialysis fluid (100–200 g/day)
Inadequate dialysis	Loss of residual renal function
	Metabolic acidosis
Inflammation	Chronic inflammation, often due to comorbidity
	Acute inflammatory episodes, in particular peritonitis
	Other infective episodes

PEW include inadequate dialysis, acidosis, comorbidity, and chronic inflammation, as well as endocrine abnormalities. Many patients have increased energy consumption and increased protein catabolism, often due to inflammation, acidosis, as well as losses of protein and amino acids into the dialysate (5–15 g/24 h).

Chronic inflammation, with elevated plasma levels of several proinflammatory cytokines (e.g., TNF-α, IL-1, and IL-6), is very common among PD patients and contributes to several negative effects including anorexia, insulin resistance, increased energy expenditure, and increased protein catabolism due to activation of the ubiquitin proteasome pathway. Acute inflammatory bursts due to infections (in particular peritonitis) and other acute illnesses will further aggravate these alterations.

12.3.3 Treatment of PEW in PD Patients

The treatment and prevention of PEW in PD patients must be individualized based on the patients' individual situation and special needs [18]. In particular, adequate treatments of comorbidities and dental problems are crucial parts of the management of PEW. As chronic inflammation is very common in PD patients, and may contribute to PEW in multiple ways, it is most important to assess signs of inflammation by measuring C-reactive protein and to seek for the cause(s) of inflammation. Adequate treatment of comorbidities is of course essential.

It is important to supply adequate amounts of protein and energy, where current recommendations suggest a protein intake of at least 1.0 g/kg body weight and an energy intake of 30–35 kcal/kg in patients with a normal body mass index (BMI) (including glucose absorption form the dialysate, usually about 100–200 g/24 h). The glucose absorption can easily be calculated from measurement of glucose in a 24-h collection of dialysate and the used bag volumes and glucose concentrations in the bags. (Record the weight of the unused bags as most bags are overfilled.) In patients with a low or high BMI, these recommendations should be recalculated to a normal BMI for the individual patient's height. In patients with low nutritional intake, a systematic review of enteral multinutrient support in dialysis patients found evidence that this significantly increases serum albumin concentrations and improves total dietary intake [19]. An alternative way to provide protein supplementation is to use amino acid-based PD solution. One 2-l bag provides 22 g of amino acids (of which about 70 % is absorbed) without potassium and phosphate and may compensate for the daily losses of protein and amino acids into the dialysate [20]. Amino acid-based dialysis solutions have been shown to improve nitrogen balance in a short-term study [21] and to be well tolerated during long-term use [22]. However, the results have been relatively modest and amino acid solutions should be seen as a way to secure protein intake in patients where it is low.

Studies have reported that nutritional intake improves if an inadequate dialysis dose is increased [23]. However, an increase in the dialysis dose in patients with a Kt/V above the present target of a weekly Kt/V of 1.7 does not always improve the nutritional intake [23]. Acidosis may contribute to increase protein catabolism by stimulation of the ubiquitin-proteasome pathway and, even though acidosis is less of a problem in PD compared to HD patients, it is important to treat acidosis in PD patients. Bicarbonate supplementation has been shown to improve nutritional status in a randomized controlled trial [24]. Physical exercise is a very important part of treatment and prevention of PEW and should be strongly encouraged [25]. Appetite stimulants, anabolic hormones, and anti-inflammatory therapy are potential future treatments that need further validation. Of these, in particular hypogonadism and testosterone deficiency are common in male PD patients and could be assessed by a simple blood test. Among deficient patients, testosterone supplementation could be tested, though there are no good randomized trials in dialysis patients.

12.4 PD in Patients with Diabetes

There is a worldwide epidemic of obesity and diabetes and today diabetes is the most common cause of chronic kidney disease (CKD). In the USA, as much as 44 % of new dialysis patients have CKD due to diabetes [26].

12.4.1 Choice of Dialysis Therapy in Patients with Diabetes

It has been debated for several years if the outcome of diabetic patients is worse in PD compared to HD, due to worse outcome of elderly female diabetic patients on PD in an analysis from the United States Renal Data System (USRDS) data from the 1990s [27]. However, the outcome of PD has improved markedly in the USA during recent years and studies from other countries have in general showed similar outcome of diabetic patients on PD, compared to HD. A recent systematic review (searching MEDLINE, EMBASE, and CENTRAL databases until February 2014) included 25 observational studies [28]. Patient survival results were inconsistent and varied across study designs, follow-up period, and subgroups. In summary, there was no evidence that selecting HD or PD as the first treatment for diabetic patients with CKD would affect the outcome. They concluded that modality selection should be governed by patient preference, after unbiased patient information.

12.4.2 Hemoglobin A1c and Glycemic Control

Hemoglobin A1c (HbA1c) is presently the most common standard used for glycemic monitoring in patients with diabetes [29]. The International Federation of Clinical Chemistry (IFCC) developed a reference measurement system for HbA1c that reports HbA1c as mmol HbA1c/mol hemoglobin instead of percentage. This change in units avoids any confusion between IFCC results and previous results that in general were not only higher due to unspecific methods but also varied due to the method used. It is possible to convert older units to this new standard [29]. For example, the HbA1c from the National Glycohemoglobin Standardization Program (NGSP) can be converted to the IFCC using the so-called master equation: $NGSP = [0.09148 \times IFCC] + 2.152$, making the results comparable to each other. However, the use of HbA1c has some specific problems in patients with CKD. In particular, HbA1c may be decreased in patients with CKD due to reduced life span of erythrocytes, use of erythropoesis stimulating agents, iron therapy, and the uremic environment itself [29]. Some older methods for determination of HbA1c are also unspecific and may result in overestimation of HbA1c due to interaction with carbamylated hemoglobin. It may not also reflect the long-term glycemic control, even in patients without CKD, and the association between glycemic control and outcome may be different in patients with CKD [29].

However, alternative methods to assess glycemic control in diabetic patients with CKD (fructosamine, glycated albumin, 1,5-anhydroglucitol) have so far not been shown to have a superiority in patients with CKD. The better documentation, low price, and easy availability still make HbA1c the present standard for glycemic monitoring in patients with CKD [29].

Continuous glucose monitoring is likely the best method for evaluation for the glycemic control in patients on PD. It is unaffected by erythrocyte life span but it is a little more cumbersome to use and it has so far only been used sparsely in PD patients. It may represent a major improvement in the care for diabetic patients on PD, but it will need further evaluation if adjustment in diabetic treatment from this method will result in improved clinical outcome.

12.4.3 Importance of Glycemic Control

In spite of the large number of diabetic PD patients, and the general belief in glycemic control, very few studies have assessed the impact of glycemic control on survival in these patients. Recently, Duong et al. reported on the analysis of the relationship between HbA1c and outcome in 2798 diabetic PD patients from the DaVita dialysis clinics in the USA in the period 2001–2006 and found the benefit of moderate metabolic control [30]. In this study, a time-averaged HbA1c of 64 mmol/mol (8%) or a glucose of 16.7 mmol/l (300 mg/dl) was associated with higher all-cause mortality, and this association was particularly robust in patients with a hemoglobin above 110 g/l [30]. A subgroup analysis suggested a lower threshold for HbA1c of 53 mmol/mol (7%) in Caucasians, men, and patients with serum albumin 38 g/l. A recent study of 3157 dialysis patients (HD and PD) from the UK renal registry reported on an increased mortality in younger patients (age <60 years) with HbA1c 69 mmol/mol (8.5%) with a hazard ratio of 1.5 (1.2–1.9) [31]. However, no association was found between HbA1c and death in patients with age ≥60 years. These findings suggest that moderate hyperglycemia may not be a mortality risk factor among PD patients. This is also supported by the results of the ACCORD study [32] in patients without CKD but with long duration of diabetes. In this study, intensive therapy targeting HbA1c 42 mmol/mol (6%) in type 2 diabetics with cardiovascular disease (CVD) or additional cardiovascular risk factors resulted in an increased 5-year mortality. Thus, the complications of diabetes may be too severe, and the risk of hypoglycemic complications too high, to justify intense glucose control in diabetic patients on PD.

Higher HbA1c at start of PD has also been found to be associated with increased risk of exit-site infections and poor technique survival after peritonitis, but not with the risk of peritonitis [33].

12.4.4 Use of Insulin and Oral Hypoglycemic Drugs

As most oral glucose-lowering drugs have been considered contraindicated in severe CKD, insulin therapy has been the cornerstone to control blood glucose levels. In PD patients, intraperitoneal injection into the dialysis fluid was frequently used in early days of PD. It was regarded as more physiological, with lower peripheral insulin levels and equal or better glycemic control. However, intraperitoneal insulin is rarely used today, as it was demonstrated to be associated with increased risk of peritonitis and hepatic subcapsular steatosis. With the increased use of multiple subcutaneous injections, it is often possible to achieve a reasonable glucose control. The insulin requirements increase slightly at start of continuous ambulatory peritoneal dialysis (CAPD), but the dosage of insulin must be adjusted due to the glucose concentration used. Particularly, when PD patients are prescribed hypertonic glucose solution, the insulin dose needs to be increased [34], and when using non-glucose-based PD solutions, the insulin dosage may be reduced. APD is a special challenge due to the glucose absorption during the night, which needs to be taken into account when dosing insulin.

Most oral hypoglycemic drugs are considered to be contraindicated in patients on dialysis [35]. There are very limited data available, but there are some drugs that, in principle, should be possible to use in dialysis patients, and there is some clinical documentation for at least glipizide, pioglitazone, and some of the DPP-4 inhibitors (sitagliptin, saxagliptin, and alogliptin) in dialysis patients (excellently reviewed in [35]). Although metformin has been considered to be contraindicated even in CKD 3, there is presently a discussion that it may be used in patients with CKD 3–4 if the dose is adjusted, and the medication stopped in situations of dehydration, use contrast agents, etc. [35]. There is even one study using metformin in PD patients [36], but this usage cannot be recommended until there are further data, particularly related to safety.

12.4.5 Dialysis Prescription in Diabetic Patients on PD

The dialysis prescription in diabetic patients should, to a large extent, be similar to that in nondiabetic patients. Regarding the weekly Kt/V target of ≥1.7, there is no reason to believe that it should be different in diabetic patients. In the ADEMEX trial, in which 965 PD patients were randomized to standard or increased dose of PD, almost half of the patients were diabetic ($n=418$) and the results were similar in diabetic and nondiabetic patients [37].

Glucose-sparing PD prescriptions using alternative osmotic agents, either of one exchange of icodextrin-based solution or one exchange of icodextrin-based and one of amino acid-based PD solutions, have been shown to improve the glycemic control in diabetic PD patients using continuous glucose monitoring [38]. In addition, a randomized control trial of 59 diabetic PD patients (with fast or fast-average transport rate) randomized to one exchange of icodextrin solution, or to glucose-based solutions only, demonstrated better ultrafiltration, lower blood pressure, less glucose load and insulin need, better glycemic control, and triglyceride (TG) levels in the icodextrin group [39]. In the combined IMPENDIA and EDEN trials, a total of 251 diabetic PD patients were randomized to a glucose-sparing regimen with one exchange of amino acid-based solution and one of icodextrin-based solution compared to a glucose-based solution only [40]. The results showed significantly improved HbA1c of 5 mmol/mol (0.5 %) in the intervention group. However, death and serious adverse events related to fluid expansion increased in the intervention group and close monitoring of fluid status is important.

When using icodextrin-based solution, it is extremely important to be aware of the false elevation of blood glucose levels when measured with glucose dehydrogenase pyrroloquinoline quinone (GDH-PQQ)-based glucose self-monitoring systems [41]. The GDH-PQQ method is not specific to glucose and reacts to the increased plasma levels of icodextrin metabolites, in particular maltose and maltotriose. This is potentially dangerous as the elevated maltose levels may be misinterpreted as hyperglycemia with the risk of subsequent overinjection of insulin. Therefore, glucose self-monitoring systems based on the GDH-PQQ method should not be used in PD patients [41].

12.4.6 Management of Comorbidities

When caring for diabetic PD patients, it is mandatory not to forget about the standard care and follow-up of diabetic patients with other diabetic complications in particular retinopathy, CVD, peripheral vascular disease, neuropathy, foot status, etc. It is important that the patient has a standardized follow-up of this, which could be done at the PD clinic or at a diabetes clinic depending on the local organization. Finally, physical exercise should always be encouraged though there are no large randomized trials on this issue.

12.5 Obesity and Weight Gain

In the past three decades, the prevalence of obesity has risen dramatically and the World Health Organization acknowledges obesity as one of the top 10 global health problems. It is considered as a major threat to health due to its association with several complications including type 2 diabetes mellitus, hypertension, hyperlipidemia, coronary artery disease, sleep apnea, gallbladder disease, and premature death [42]. For PD patients, obesity is a special challenge due to the absorption of glucose from the peritoneal cavity.

12.5.1 Peritoneal Dialysis and Obesity

Obesity represents a significant problem among PD patients and several studies report on weight gain and accumulation of fat tissue during the first year of PD [43–45]. In the early 2000s, weight gain and increased fat mass were reported to be common in PD patients, particularly in diabetics, females, patients with obesity at the start of treatment, and patients with a fast peritoneal transport rate [44–46]. Excessive weight gain (10 kg in 2 years on PD) was reported in 7 % of the patients in one cohort [46]. However, excessive weight gain seems to be less of a problem today, likely because of the increased use of icodextrin-based solution in PD patients with fast peritoneal transport rate.

12.5.2 Why Do PD Patients Tend to Increase Body Fat Mass

The energy requirements are dependent on the level of physical activity. In PD patients, an energy intake of 30–35 kcal/kg body weight/day is recommended for individuals not performing heavy physical exercise. (In underweight and overweight patients, the normal intake should be scaled to a normal body weight for height). In obese patients, the energy intake is recommended to be lower.

However, the glucose absorption from the dialysate should be taken into account and due to this the energy intake may still be too high in many PD patients.

It is generally assumed that the accumulation of adipose tissue in patients starting PD is related to the glucose absorption from the dialysate. For standard CAPD with glucose-based solutions, about 100–200 g of glucose are absorbed during 24 h and this represents a significant portion of the total energy intake [47]. However, in most studies, there is no clear relation between the gains in weight as there are marked variations between patients [48, 49].

Genetic factors may contribute to about 70 % of the variations in BMI in nonrenal patient groups [50] and genetic factors are important also in PD patients. Obviously, there is no way to accumulate excess adipose tissue without disequilibrium between the intake and expenditure of calories. One reason for decreased energy expenditure appears to entail a decreased thermogenesis in adipose tissue. A key element in adipose tissue is the unique expression of a mitochondrial inner membrane protein called uncoupling protein (UCP), which is a transporter of free fatty acid anions, allowing free fatty acids to function as proton carriers. UCP2 has a wide tissue distribution and it has been speculated that UCP2 may play a role in fat tissue accumulation [48] and the deletion/deletion UCP2 genotype has been demonstrated to be associated with fat accumulation during the first year of PD treatment [48].

12.5.3 Consequences of Obesity in PD Patients

In patients without CKD, obesity and, in particular, accumulation of abdominal fat, are an important risk factor for CVD. Therefore, it is a concern that patients starting PD have been reported to develop an increase in intra-abdominal fat [51] similar to what is seen in the metabolic syndrome, as well as an atherogenic lipid profile. In HD patients, obesity has been associated with better survival, the so-called reverse epidemiology phenomenon, that is, the well-known association between established risk factors in the general population, such as hypercholesterolemia, and obesity appear to be reversed in patients with advanced CKD [52]. However, in contrast to HD patients, this phenomenon is not evident in PD patients as regards obesity [53, 54].

12.5.4 Special Problems in Patients with Obesity

PD catheter placement needs special attention in obese patients and an experienced operator is important. Obese PD patients have a higher risk of catheter loss due to infection [55] and the placement of the exit site is important for good exit-site care. Sometimes, it is impossible to implant a standard catheter due to obesity and presternal exit catheters, and two-piece extended catheters are available where the exit could be placed at a remote site [56].

Regarding the adequacy of PD, obesity has often been an overestimated issue. It is usually possible to achieve an adequate Kt/V, but it should be noted that the Watson formula overestimates total body water in the obese patients [57] and, therefore, underestimates the achieved Kt/V. On the other hand, obesity has been reported to be associated with a slightly more rapid decline of the residual renal function [58].

Table 12.5 Treatment of obesity in peritoneal dialysis patients

Reduced energy intake in diet	Important, but the peritoneal glucose absorption is a problem
Physical exercise	Likely very important, but difficult in some patients due to fatigue, comorbidity, etc.
Behavioral therapy	Motivation needed
Reduce glucose absorption from dialysate	Reduce the needed glucose concentration in the dialysis fluid by restriction of water and in particular sodium
	Use icodextrin solution during the long dwell
Pharmacological treatment	No efficient therapy available
	Not established in PD patients
Surgery	Anecdotal reports of success in PD patients, but no systematic study has been performed

12.5.5 Treatment of Obesity

Although the treatment of obesity in PD patients should be based on the same principles as the treatment in nonrenal patients (Table 12.5), it may be even more difficult as many PD patients have comorbidity and fatigue that make physical exercise difficult. Also, diet therapy is hampered due to the glucose absorption from the dialysate, usually about 100–200 g glucose/24 h corresponding to 300–800 kcal/24 h [47]. Thus, reduction of the peritoneal caloric load is important. To be able to reduce the peritoneal glucose load, the patients need to have a diet that (in addition to energy restriction) is restricted in fluid and particularly sodium intake to reduce the need of ultrafiltration. Also, the replacement of glucose-based dialysis solution by icodextrin-based dialysis solution for the long dwell may, particularly in high transporters, result in a markedly reduced glucose absorption. Icodextrin-based solution may be beneficial in several ways. First, the replacement of glucose solution during the long dwell will result in a reduced absorption of carbohydrates. Use of icodextrin during an 8-h dwell reduces the caloric load of more than 100 kcal compared to a 4.25 % glucose solution [59]. Furthermore, the absorbed icodextrin will not be completely metabolized and a significant fraction will be dialyzed away in the form of maltose and maltotriose resulting in an even lower caloric load. Finally, the increased ultrafiltration and more efficient sodium removal during the icodextrin dwell will result in a lower need for ultrafiltration during the other exchanges. Two randomized controlled double-blind trials of icodextrin compared to 2.5 % glucose solution reported on a stable body weight in patients randomized to icodextrin compared to an increase in body weight in control patients [60, 61].

No studies have reported the use of pharmacological therapy for obesity in PD patients, and there are no good alternatives. Orlistat (Xenical^{TM}) prevents the gut from digesting and absorbing fat by blocking lipases in the gut. This results in fat malabsorption and a reduction in body weight.

However, the effect of orlistat is often insufficient. Orlistat may likely be used in PD patients, but its effect is in general modest and it is associated with significant side effects.

12.6 Hyperlipidemia

12.6.1 Lipid Disorders in PD Patients

Patients with CKD have a high prevalence of CVD to which both traditional risk factors (such as diabetes, smoking, hypertension, and hyperlipidemia) and nontraditional risk factors (such as inflammation, oxidative stress, endothelial dysfunction, hyperphosphatemia, and vascular calcification) are considered to contribute.

12.6.2 Dyslipidemia in PD Patients

Hyperlipidemia is common in patients with CKD in general, and PD patients usually have an even more atherogenic lipid profile [62, 63] (Table 12.6). Compared to nondialyzed patients with CKD stage 5 and HD patients, PD patients usually have higher low-density lipoprotein (LDL) cholesterol, apolipoprotein B levels, and markedly increased TG and lipoprotein(a) levels. It may be advisable to measure apolipoprotein B level in PD patients as the LDL cholesterol level cannot always be calculated using the Fridewald equation because of marked hypertriglyceridemia in some patients. There are also reports that PD patients have increased levels of particularly atherogenic small dense LDL particles [62]. The high-density lipoprotein (HDL) cholesterol and apolipoprotein A1 levels are usually low in PD patients. In addition, HDL maturation and function is impaired as in other patients with CKD.

The pathogenetic mechanisms behind the lipid disturbances in PD patients are not well understood, but both the peritoneal protein loss (about 5–10 g/day) and the resulting slight hypoalbuminemia are considered to stimulate increased hepatic synthesis of cholesterol-enriched lipoproteins, resulting in increased levels of LDL cholesterol and lipoprotein(a) similar to in the nephrotic syndrome [62, 63]. The hypertriglyceridemia is a result of increased hepatic production of very-low-density lipoprotein (VLDL) and lipoprotein lipase deficiency. In addition, the glucose absorption from the dialysate and the resulting hyperinsulinemia may contribute to the lipid disturbances, in general, and to the elevated TG and lipoprotein(a) levels, in particular [62–64]. The low HDL cholesterol may, at least partly, be due to the loss of HDL in the dialysate.

Table 12.6 Typical pattern of dyslipidemia in patients with CKD 5

	Nondialyzed patients	HD patients	PD patients
LDL cholesterol	=	=	↑
HDL cholesterol	↓	↓	↓
Triglycerides	↑	↑	↑↑
Lipoprotein (a)	↑	↑	↑↑
Apolipoprotein B	= or ↑	= or ↑	↑↑
Apolipoprotein A1	↓	↓	↓
Oxidized LDL	↑	↑	↑ or ↑↑

12.6.3 Hyperlipidemia and Outcome in PD Patients

The association between lipid disturbances and cardiovascular outcome in patients with CKD is complicated by the so-called reverse epidemiology phenomenon: that is, the well-known association between established risk factors in the general population, such as hypercholesterolemia, and obesity appears to be reversed in patients with advanced CKD [52]. Part of the explanation for this is likely that there are different time profiles for different risk factors in the different populations, as premature deaths in CKD patients preclude the impact of complications, which are more important for long-term mortality [52]. Furthermore, persistent inflammation and/or PEW, both of which are common in advanced CKD (and both associated with low cholesterol as well as with increased mortality), seems to a large extent account for the seemingly paradoxical association between hypercholesterolemia and improved cardiovascular outcome among these patients [52, 65]. In summary, in spite of the reverse epidemiology between lipid levels and clinical outcome in patients with advanced CKD, hyperlipidemia is still considered to be harmful and to contribute to atherosclerosis and CVD in the longer perspective.

12.6.4 Use of Statins to Treat Lipid Disorders in PD Patients

In the population without renal disease, there is strong evidence that hydroxymethylglutaryl-coenzyme A reductase inhibitors, more commonly known as statins, reduce the progression of coronary atherosclerosis and reduces mortality from CVD. Statins are equally effective in reducing LDL cholesterol and apolipoprotein B levels in dialysis patients (in both PD and HD), and are usually well tolerated in dialysis patients [62, 63, 66–70].

Three relatively large, randomized controlled trials have been published concerning the effect of statins in dialysis patients: the 4D [67, 68], the AURORA [69], and the SHARP studies [70], of which only the SHARP study included PD patients (Table 12.7).

The 4D-study [67], in which 1255 prevalent diabetic HD patients were randomized to 20 mg atorvastatin or placebo,

Table 12.7 Randomized placebo-controlled trials of statin therapy in dialysis patients

Study	Number of patients	Therapy used	Decrease in LDL cholesterol	Median follow up	Result
4D [67, 68]	1255 HD	Atorvastatin (20 mg)	42 %	4 years	No significant difference in the composite primary end point (subgroup analysis suggests effect in patients with LDL cholesterol in the highest quartile)
AURORA [69]	2773 HD	Rosuvastatin (10 mg)	43 %	3.8 years	No significant difference in the composite primary end point
SHARP [70]	9270 (6247 CKD, 2527 HD, 496 PD)	Simvastatin (20 mg) + ezetimibe (10 mg)	39 %	4.9 years	17 % reduction in the primary end point. (No significant effect in subgroup analysis of the dialysis patients)

showed no effect of statin treatment on the composite primary end point (cardiovascular death, nonfatal myocardial infarction, and stroke). However, in the atorvastatin group, there was a positive effect on all cardiac events combined (a secondary end point) [67], and a post hoc analysis [68] found that high LDL cholesterol levels tended to increase the risks and atorvastatin significantly reduced the rates of adverse outcomes in patients in the highest quartile of LDL cholesterol (3.76 mmol/l, 145 mg/dl), whereas no effects were seen in the three other quartiles. Similarly, in the AURORA study [69], in which 2773 HD patients were randomized to 10-mg rosuvastatin versus placebo, no effect was found on the primary end point (death from cardiovascular causes, nonfatal myocardial infarction, or nonfatal stroke) or on the individual components of the primary end point.

The SHARP study was the only study in the group to include PD patients ($N=496$ PD patients) and randomized 9270 CKD patients to placebo or 20-mg simvastatin in combination with 10-mg ezetimibe (which blocks the absorption of cholesterol in the small intestine) with a median follow-up of 4.9 years [70]. It showed a significant 17 % decrease in the primary end point of major atherosclerotic events (11.3 vs. 13.4 %, $p=0.0021$). There "was no good evidence that the proportional effect on major atherosclerotic events differed from the summary rate ration [sic] in any subgroup examined" including in dialysis patients [70]. However, there was no significant effect in dialysis patients (event rates were 15 and 16.5 % in patients with active treatment and placebo, respectively), but the study was not powered for dialysis patients. In PD patients, the risk ratio (treatment/placebo) was more beneficial (0.70) compared to HD patients (0.95), but the 95 % confidence intervals were wide (0.46–1.08 in PD patients). It is likely that the treatment had better effect in PD patients due to the more atherogenic lipid profile in PD patients, but this study was not powered for this analysis [70].

There is further support for a positive effect of statins in PD patients from observational studies. In a retrospective analysis of the effect of lipid-lowering therapy on clinical outcome in 1053 incident PD patients from the USRDS prospective dialysis morbidity and mortality Wave 2 study, use of lipid-lowering therapy (mainly statins) was associated with significantly decreased cardiovascular mortality (hazard ratio 0.67; 95 % confidence interval 0.47–0.95) of similar magnitude as in the SHARP study, as well as reduced all-cause mortality (hazard ratio 0.74; 95 % confidence interval 0.56–0.95) [71]. Similarly, in a recent retrospective cohort study including 1024 incident PD patients from Korea, using a propensity score-matched comparison to reduce potential confounding, statin use (in 38 % of the patients) was found to be associated with a 41 % lower risk for death ($p=0.002$) [72]. In summary, these data suggest that statin therapy is indicated in PD patients with hyperlipidemia, at least in patients with elevated LDL cholesterol and a high cardiovascular risk. However, it is not possible to define a clear treatment target for the LDL cholesterol level in PD patients. Guidelines for the general population may be used for guidance, but their relevance for PD patients is not well documented.

Furthermore, there are theoretical and experimental support that statins may have beneficial effects on the peritoneal membrane remodeling mediated by their pleiotropic effects, independent of the lipid-lowering effect [73].

12.6.5 Additional Therapeutic Strategies

Other lipid-lowering strategies have no evidence with regard to clinical outcome in PD patients, although several drugs have a demonstrated lipid-lowering effect in this patient population. Fibrates are not recommended due to their renal elimination and the risk of rhabdomyolysis.

Low-glucose PD regimens using alternative osmotic agents (icodextrin- and amino acid-based PD solutions) may also improve the lipid profile, although the effects are not dramatic. However, the use of icodextrin in PD patients with poor ultrafiltration and a high glucose load may dramatically reduce glucose absorption resulting in less weight gain and reduced TG levels [39]. In a 6-month prospective open-label controlled trial, 251 diabetic PD patients were randomized to a low-glucose PD regimen (one exchange of icodextrin-based solution and one exchange of amino acid-based solution) or to glucose-based PD solutions only. The low-glucose PD regimen significantly improved the atherogenic lipoprotein profile with lower TG, VLDL cholesterol, and apolipoprotein B [74].

However, for the majority of PD patients with marked lipid disturbances, statin therapy is the therapy of choice as it is generally well tolerated, effective to reduce LDL cholesterol levels, and has the best documented effect in PD patients.

In summary, PD patients have a more atherogenic lipid profile compared to HD patients and nondialyzed CKD 5 patients. Several studies suggest that lipid-lowering therapy has beneficial effects in PD patients, though no large randomized outcome study has been performed on this patient group. Use of low-glucose PD regimens also has beneficial effects on the lipid levels. In addition, the role of exercise, dietary interventions, and other pharmacological therapy need to be better evaluated in PD patients.

12.7 PD in Patients with Ostomies and Gastronomy Tubes

Colostomies and ileostomies are usually regarded as contraindications to PD. There is a high risk for adhesions in the peritoneal cavity and malfunction of the dialysis due to mechanical problems. However, there are occasional case reports of successful cases, but no systematic report or case series have been published.

There are several reports on the use of gastrostomy tubes in children treated with PD to allow adequate enteral nutrition. There was a recent report of 17 children, in 15 of whom gastrostomy tubes were inserted after the start of PD. PD was in these cases usually stopped for 24 h (range 0–72 h) and prophylactic antibiotics were given [75]. The results were generally good, even though two early episodes of bacterial peritonitis occurred. None of the patients experienced an episode of fungal peritonitis. In adults, the results are less encouraging. A recent review of published case reports of percutaneous endoscopic gastrostomy (PEG) tubes suggested that the insertion of a PD catheter in a patient with a preexistent and well-healed PEG may be safe, but the insertion of PEG tubes in adults receiving PD is associated with major adverse events including leaks and fatal or nonfatal peritonitis [76]. They considered placement of PEG tubes in adult PD patients to be contraindicated. However, occasional successful cases have been reported [77], but it may be needed to temporarily switch to HD to let the PEG heal, though this is not always successful [76].

References

1. Heimbürger O. Peritoneal physiology. In: Pereira BJG, Sayegh MH, Blake P, editors. Chronic kidney disease, dialysis and transplantation: a companion to brenner and rector's the kidney. ed 2. Philadelphia: Elsevier Saunders; 2005. p. 491–513.
2. Rippe B, Rosengren BI, Venturoli D. The peritoneal microcirculation in peritoneal dialysis. Microcirculation. 2001;8:303–20.
3. Flessner MF. Peritoneal transport physiology: insights from basic research. J Am Soc Nephrol. 1991;2:122–35.
4. Twardowski ZJ, Nolph KD, Khanna R, Prowant BF, Ryan LP, Moore HL, Nielsen MP. Peritonealequilibration test. Perit Dial Bull. 1987;7:138–47.
5. Haraldsson B. Assessing the peritoneal dialysis capacities of individual patients. Kidney Int. 1995;47:1187–98.
6. Vonesh EP, Lysaght MJ, Moran J, Farrell P. Kinetic modeling as a prescription aid in peritoneal dialysis. Blood Purif. 1991;9:246–70.
7. Vonesh EF, Rippe B. Net fluid absorption under membrane transport models of peritoneal dialysis. Blood Purif. 1992;10:209–26.
8. van Biesen W, Heimburger O, Krediet R, Rippe B, Lamilia V, Covic A, Vanholder R, ERBP working group on peritoneal dialysis. Evaluation of peritoneal membrane characteristics: a clinical advice for prescription management by the ERBP working group. Nephrol Dial Transplant. 2010;25:2052–62.
9. Mujais S, Nolph KD, Gokal R, Blake P, Burkhart J, Coles G, Kawaguchi Y, Kawanishi H, Korbet S, Krediet RT, Lindholm B, Oreopoulos DG, Rippe B, Selgas R. International society of peritoneal dialysis ad hoc committee on ultrafiltration management in peritoneal dialysis: evaluation and management of ultrafiltration problems in peritoneal dialysis. Perit Dial Int. 2000;20(Suppl 4):S5–21.
10. Heimbürger O, Waniewski J, Werynski A, Tranaeus A, Lindholm B. Peritoneal transport in CAPD patients with permanent loss of ultrafiltration capacity. Kidney Int. 1990;38:495–506.
11. Ho-dac-Pannekeet MM, Atasever B, Struijk DG, Krediet RT. Analysis of ultrafiltration failure in peritoneal dialysis patients by means of standard peritoneal permeability analysis. Perit Dial Int. 1997;17:144–50.
12. Waniewski J, Heimbürger O, Werynski A, Lindholm B. Osmotic conductance of the peritoneum in CAPD patients with permanent loss of ultrafiltration capacity. Perit Dial Int. 1996;16:488–96.
13. Devuyst O, Margetts PJ, Topley N. The pathophysiology of the peritoneal membrane. J Am Soc Nephrol. 2010;21:1077–85.
14. Cho Y, Johnson DW, Badve SV, Craig JC, Strippoli GF, Wiggins KJ. The impact of neutral-pH peritoneal dialysates with reduced glucose degradation products on clinical outcomes in peritoneal dialysis patients. Kidney Int. 2013;84:969–79.
15. Johnson DW, Brown FG, Clarke M, Boudville N, Elias TJ, Foo MWY, Jones B, Kulkarni H, Langham R, Ranganathan D, Schollum J, Suranyi MG, Tan SH, Voss D, balANZ Trial Investigators. The effect of low glucose degradation product, neutral pH vs. standard peritoneal dialysis solutions on peritoneal membrane function: the balANZ trial. Nephrol Dial Transplant. 2012;27:4445–53.
16. Fouque D, Kalantar-Zadeh K, Kopple J, Cano N, Chauveau P, Cuppari L, Franch H, Guarnieri G, Ikizler TA, Kaysen G, Lindholm B, Massy Z, Mitch W, Pineda E, Stenvinkel P, Treviño-Becerra A, Wanner C. A proposed nomenclature and diagnostic criteria for protein-energy wasting in acute and chronic kidney disease. Kidney Int. 2008;73:391–8.
17. van Biesen W, Claes K, Covic A, Fan S, Lichodziejewska-Niemierko M, Schoder V, Verger C, Wabel P. A multicentric, international matched pair analysis of body composition in peritoneal dialysis versus haemodialysis patients. Nephrol Dial Transplant. 2013;28:2620–8.
18. Carrero JJ, Heimbürger O, Chan M, Axelsson J, Sternvinkel P, Lindholm B. Protein-energy malnutrition/wasting during peritoneal dialysis (Chapter 12). In: Khanna R, Krediet RT, editors. Nolph and Gokal's textbook of peritoneal dialysis. 3rd ed. New York: Springer; 2009.
19. Stratton RJ, Bircher G, Fouque D, Stenvinkel P, de Mutsert R, Engfer M, Elia M. Multinutrient oral supplements and tube feeding in maintenance dialysis: a systematic review and meta-analysis. Am J Kidney Dis. 2005;46:387–405.

20. Jones MR, Gehr TW, Burkart JM, Hamburger RJ, Kraus AP Jr, Piraino BM, Hagen T, Ogrinc FG, Wolfson M. Replacement of amino acid and protein losses with 1.1% amino acid peritoneal dialysis solution. Perit Dial Int. 1998;18:210–6.
21. Kopple JD, Bernard D, Messana J, Swartz R, Bergström J, Lindholm B, Lim V, Brunori G, Leiserowitz M, Bier DM, et al. Treatment of malnourished CAPD patients with an amino acid based dialysate. Kidney Int. 1995;47:1148–57.
22. Li FK, Chan LY, Woo JC, Ho SK, Lo WK, Lai KN, Chan TM. A 3-year, prospective, randomized, controlled study on amino acid dialysate in patients on CAPD. Am J Kidney Dis. 2003;42:173–83.
23. Szeto CC, Wong TY, Chow KM, Leung CB, Wang AY, Lui SF, Li PK. The impact of increasing the daytime dialysis exchange frequency on peritoneal dialysis adequacy and nutritional status of Chinese anuric patients. Perit Dial Int. 2002;22:197–203.
24. Szeto CC, Wong TY, Chow KM, Leung CB, Li PK. Oral sodium bicarbonate for the treatment of metabolic acidosis in peritoneal dialysis patients: a randomized placebo-control trial. J Am Soc Nephrol 2003;14:2119–26.
25. Ikizler TA, Cano NJ, Franch H, Fouque D, Himmelfarb J, Kalantar-Zadeh K, Kuhlmann MK, Stenvinkel P, TerWee P, Teta D, Wang AY, Wanner C, International Society of Renal Nutrition and Metabolism. Prevention and treatment of protein energy wasting in chronic kidney disease patients: a consensus statement by the international society of renal nutrition and metabolism. Kidney Int. 2013;84:1096–107.
26. UNITED STATES RENAL DATA SYSTEM Annual Data Report. 2014. www.usrds.org.
27. Collins AJ, Hao W, Xia H, Ebben JP, Everson SE, Constantini EG, Ma JZ. Mortality risks of peritoneal dialysis and hemodialysis. Am J Kidney Dis. 1999;34:1065–74.
28. Couchoud C, Bolignano D, Nistor I, Jager KJ, Heaf J, Heimburger O. Van Biesen W, European Renal Best Practice (ERBP) Diabetes Guideline Development Group. Dialysis modality choice in diabetic patients with end-stage kidney disease: a systematic review of the available evidence. Nephrol Dial Transplant. 2014;30(2):310–20. pii: gfu293. [Epub ahead of print].
29. Speeckaert M, Van Biesen W, Delanghe J, Slingerland R, Wiecek A, Heaf J, Drechsler C, Lacatus R, Vanholder R, Nistor I, European Renal Best Practice Guideline Development Group on Diabetes in Advanced CKD. Are there better alternatives than haemoglobin A1c to estimate glycaemic control in the chronic kidney disease population? Nephrol Dial Transplant. 2014;29:2167–77.
30. Duong U, Mehrotra R, Molnar MZ, Noori N, Kovesdy CP, Nissenson AR, Kalantar-Zadeh K. Glycemic control and survival in peritoneal dialysis patients with diabetes mellitus. Clin J Am Soc Nephrol. 2011;6:1041–8.
31. Adler A, Casula A, Steenkamp R, Fogarty D, Wilkie M, Tomlinson L, Nitsch D, Roderick P, Tomson CR. Association between glycemia and mortality in diabetic individuals on renal replacement therapy in the U.K. Diabetes Care. 2014;37:1304–11.
32. ACCORD Study Group, Gerstein HC, Miller ME, Genuth S, Ismail-Beigi F, Buse JB, Goff DC Jr, Probstfield JL, Cushman WC, Ginsberg HN, Bigger JT, Grimm RH Jr, Byington RP, Rosenberg YD, Friedewald WT. Long-term effects of intensive glucose lowering on cardiovascular outcomes. N Engl J Med. 2011;364:818–28.
33. Rodríguez-Carmona A, Pérez-Fontán M, López-Muñiz A, Ferreiro-Hermida T, García-Falcón T. Correlation between glycemic control and the incidence of peritoneal and catheter tunnel and exit-site infections in diabetic patients undergoing peritoneal dialysis. Perit Dial Int. 2014;34:618–26.
34. Szeto CC, Chow KM, Leung CB, Kwan BC, Chung KY, Law MC, Li PK. Increased subcutaneous insulin requirements in diabetic patients recently commenced on peritoneal dialysis. Nephrol Dial Transplant. 2007;22:1697–702.
35. Arnouts P, Bolignano D, Nistor I, Bilo H, Gnudi L, Heaf J, van Biesen W. Glucose-lowering drugs in patients with chronic kidney disease: a narrative review on pharmacokinetic properties. Nephrol Dial Transplant. 2014;29:1284–300.
36. Al-Hwiesh AK, Abdul-Rahman IS, El-Deen MA, Larbi E, Divino-Filho JC, Al-Mohanna FA, Gupta KL. Metformin in peritoneal dialysis: a pilot experience. Perit Dial Int. 2014;34:368–75.
37. Paniagua R, Amato D, Vonesh E, Correa-Rotter R, Ramos A, Moran J, Mujais S, Mexican Nephrology Collaborative Study Group. Effects of increased peritoneal clearances on mortality rates in peritoneal dialysis: ADEMEX, a prospective, randomized, controlled trial. J Am Soc Nephrol. 2002;13(5):1307–20.
38. Marshall J, Jennings P, Scott A, Fluck RJ, McIntyre CW. Glycemic control in diabetic CAPD patients assessed by continuous glucose monitoring system (CGMS). Kidney Int. 2003;64:1480–6.
39. Paniagua R, Ventura MD, Avila-Díaz M, Cisneros A, Vicenté-Martínez M, Furlong MD, García-González Z, Villanueva D, Orihuela O, Prado-Uribe MD, Alcántara G, Amato D. Icodextrin improves metabolic and fluid management in high and high-average transport diabetic patients. Perit Dial Int. 2009;29:422–32.
40. Li PK, Culleton BF, Ariza A, Do JY, Johnson DW, Sanabria M, Shockley TR, Story K, Vatazin A, Verrelli M, Yu AW, Bargman JM, IMPENDIA and EDEN Study Groups. Randomized, controlled trial of glucose-sparing peritoneal dialysis in diabetic patients. J Am Soc Nephrol. 2013;24:1889–900.
41. Tsai CY, Lee SC, Hung CC, Lee JJ, Kuo MC, Hwang SJ, Chen HC. False elevation of blood glucose levels measured by GDH-PQQ-based glucometers occurs during all daily dwells in peritoneal dialysis patients using icodextrin. Perit Dial Int. 2010;30:329–35.
42. Wolf C, Tanner M. Obesity. West J Med. 2002;176:23–8.
43. Heimbürger O, Lönnqvist F, Danielsson A, Nordenström J, Stenvinkel P. Serum-immunoreactive leptin concentration and its relation to body fat content in chronic renal failure. J Am Soc Nephrol. 1997;8:1423–30.
44. Jager KJ, Merkus MP, Huisman RM, Boeschoten EW, Dekker FW, Korevaar JC, Tijssen JGP, Krediet RT, NECOSAD Study Group. Nutritional status over time in haemodialysis and peritoneal dialysis. J Am Soc Nephrol. 2001;12:1272–9.
45. Stenvinkel P, Lindholm B, Lönnqvist F, Katzarski K, Heimbürger O. Increases in serum leptin during peritoneal dialysis are associated with inflammation and a decrease in lean body mass. J Am Soc Nephrol. 2000;11:1303–9.
46. Jolly S, Chatatalsingh C, Bargman J, Vas S, Chu M, Oreopoulos DG. Excessive weight gain during peritoneal dialysis. Int J Artif Organs. 2001;24:197–202.
47. Heimbürger O, Waniewski J, Werynski A, Lindholm B. A quantitative description of solute and fluid transport during peritoneal dialysis. Kidney Int. 1992;41:1320–32.
48. Nordfors L, Heimbürger O, Lönnqvist F, Lindholm B, Helmrich J, Schalling M, Stenvinkel P. Fat tissue accumulation during peritoneal dialysis is associated with a polymorphism in uncoupling protein 2. Kidney Int. 2000;57:1713–9.
49. Davies SJ, Russell L, Bryan J, Phillips L, Russell GI. Impact of peritoneal absorption of glucose on appetite, protein catabolism and survival in CAPD patients. Clin Nephrol. 1996;45:194–8.
50. Yanowski JA, Yanowski SZ. Recent advances in basic obesity research. JAMA. 1999;282:1504–6.
51. Fernström A, Hylander B, Å M, Jacobsson H, Rössner S. Increase of intra-abdominal fat in patients treated with continuous ambulatory peritoneal dialysis. Perit Dial Int. 1998;18:166–71.
52. Kalantar-Zadeh K, Block G, Humphreys MH, Kopple JD. Reverse epidemiology of cardiovascular risk factors in maintenance dialysis patients. Kidney Int. 2003;63:793–808.
53. Abbott KC, Glanton CW, Trespalacios FC, Oliver DK, Ortiz MI, Agodoa LY, Cruess DF, Kimmel PL. Body mass index, dialysis modality, and survival: analysis of the United States renal data system dialysis morbidity and mortality wave II study. Kidney Int. 2004;65:597–605.

54. McDonald SP, Collins JF, Johnson DW. Obesity is associated with worse peritoneal dialysis outcomes in the Australia and New Zealand patient populations. J Am Soc Nephrol. 2003;14:2894–901.
55. Piraino B, Bernardini J, Centa PK, Johnston JR, Sorkin M. The effect of body weight on CAPD related infections and catheter loss. Perit Dial Int. 1991;11:64–8.
56. Crabtree JH, Burchette RJ. Comparative analysis of two-piece extended peritoneal dialysis catheters with remote exit-site locations and conventional abdominal catheters. Perit Dial Int. 2010;30:46–55.
57. Johansson AC, Samuelsson O, Attman PO, Bosaeus I, Haraldsson B. Limitations in anthropometric calculations of total body water in patients on peritoneal dialysis. J Am Soc Nephrol. 2001;12:568–73.
58. Johnson DW, Mudge DW, Sturtevant JM, Hawley CM, Campbell SB, Isbel NM, Hollett P. Predictors of decline of residual renal function in new peritoneal dialysis patients. Perit Dial Int. 2003;23:276–83.
59. Gokal R, Moberly J, Lindholm B, Mujais S. Metabolic and laboratory effects of icodextrin. Kidney Int. 2002;62 Suppl 81:62–71.
60. Wolfson M, Piraino B, Hamburger RJ, Morton AR, Icodextrin Study Group. A randomized controlled trial to evaluate the efficacy and safety of icodextrin in peritoneal dialysis. Am J Kidney Dis. 2002;40:1055–65.
61. Davies SJ, Woodrow G, Donovan K, Plum J, Williams P, Johansson AC, Bosselmann HP, Heimbürger O, Simonsen O, Davenport A, Tranaeus A, Divino Filho JC. Icodextrin improves the fluid status of peritoneal dialysis patients: results of a double-blind randomized controlled trial. J Am Soc Nephrol. 2003;14:2338–44.
62. Prichard SS. Management of hyperlipidemia in patients on peritoneal dialysis: current approaches. Kidney Int 2006(suppl 103):S115–7.
63. Epstein M, Vaziri ND. Statins in the management of dyslipidemia associated with chronic kidney disease. Nat Rev Nephrol. 2012;8:214–23.
64. Heimbürger O, Stenvinkel P, Berglund L, Tranoeus A, Lindholm B. Increased plasma lipoprotein(a) in continuous ambulatory peritoneal dialysis is related to peritoneal transport of proteins and glucose. Nephron. 1996;72:135–44.
65. Liu Y, Coresh J, Eustace JA, Longnecker JC, Jaar B, Fink NE, Tracy RP, Powe NR, Klag MJ. Association between cholesterol level and mortality in dialysis patients. Role of inflammation and malnutrition. JAMA. 2004;291:451–9.
66. Navaneethan SD, Nigwekar SU, Perkovic V, Johnson DW, Craig JC, Strippoli GF. HMG CoA reductase inhibitors (statins) for dialysis patients. Cochrane Database Syst Rev. 2009;15(2):CD004289.
67. Wanner C, Krane V, März W, Olschewski M, Mann J, Ruf G, Ritz E. German diabetes and dialysis study investigators: atorvastatin in patients with type 2 diabetes mellitus undergoing hemodialysis. N Engl J Med. 2005;353:238–48.
68. März W, Genser B, Drechsler C, Krane V, Grammer TB, Ritz E, Stojakovic T, Scharnagl H, Winkler K, Holme I, Holdaas H, Wanner C, German Diabetes and Dialysis Study Investigators. Atorvastatin and low-density lipoprotein cholesterol in type 2 diabetes mellitus patients on hemodialysis. Clin J Am Soc Nephrol. 2011;6:1316–25.
69. Fellström BC, Jardine AG, Schmieder RE, Holdaas H, Bannister K, Beutler J, Chae DW, Chevaile A, Cobbe SM, Grönhagen-Riska C, De Lima JJ, Lins R, Mayer G, McMahon AW, Parving HH, Remuzzi G, Samuelsson O, Sonkodi S, Sci D, Süleymanlar G, Tsakiris D, Tesar V, Todorov V, Wiecek A, Wüthrich RP, Gottlow M, Johnsson E, Zannad F, AURORA Study Group. Rosuvastatin and cardiovascular events in patients undergoing hemodialysis. N Engl J Med. 2009;360:1395–407.
70. Baigent C, Landray MJ, Reith C, Emberson J, Wheeler DC, Tomson C, Wanner C, Krane V, Cass A, Craig J, Neal B, Jiang L, Hooi LS, Levin A, Agodoa L, Gaziano M, Kasiske B, Walker R, Massy ZA, Feldt-Rasmussen B, Krairittichai U, Ophascharoensuk V, Fellström B, Holdaas H, Tesar V, Wiecek A, Grobbee D, de Zeeuw D, Grönhagen-Riska C, Dasgupta T, Lewis D, Herrington W, Mafham M, Majoni W, Wallendszus K, Grimm R, Pedersen T, Tobert J, Armitage J, Baxter A, Bray C, Chen Y, Chen Z, Hill M, Knott C, Parish S, Simpson D, Sleight P, Young A, Collins R, SHARP Investigators. The effects of lowering LDL cholesterol with simvastatin plus ezetimibe in patients with chronic kidney disease (Study of Heart and Renal Protection): a randomised placebo-controlled trial. Lancet. 2011;377:2181–92.
71. Goldfarb-Rumyantzev AS, Habib AN, Baird BC, Barenbaum LL, Cheung AK. The association of lipid-modifying medications with mortality in patients on long-term peritoneal dialysis. Am J Kidney Dis. 2007;50:791–802.
72. Lee JE, Oh K-H, Choi KH, Kim SB, Kim Y-S, Do J-Y, Kim Y-L, Kim DJ. Statin therapy is associated with improved survival in incident peritoneal dialysis patients: propensity-matched comparison. Nephrol Dial Transplant. 2011;26:4090–4.
73. Heimburger O. Lipid disorders, statins and the peritoneal membrane. Contrib Nephrol. 2009;163:177–82.
74. Sniderman AD, Sloand JA, Li PK, Story K, Bargman JM. Influence of low-glucose peritoneal dialysis on serum lipids and apolipoproteins in the IMPENDIA/EDEN trials. J Clin Lipidol. 2014;8:441–7.
75. Prestidge C, Ronaldson J, Wong W, Stack M, Kara T. Infectious outcomes following gastrostomy in children receiving peritoneal dialysis. Pediatr Nephrol. 2015;30:849–54. [Epub ahead of print].
76. Dahlan R, Biyani M, McCormick BB. High mortality following gastrostomy tube insertion in adult peritoneal dialysis patients: case report and literature review. Endoscopy. 2013;45(Suppl 2) UCTN:E313–4.
77. Paudel K, Fan SL. Successful use of continuous ambulatory peritoneal dialysis in 2 adults with a gastrostomy. Am J Kidney Dis. 2014;64:316–7.

Home Hemodialysis

13

Joel D. Glickman and Rebecca Kurnik Seshasai

13.1 Introduction

Home hemodialysis (HHD), though novel and maybe even intimidating for many nephrologists, is not a new option for renal replacement therapy (RRT). First utilized in Japan in 1963 [1], HHD was the predominate dialysis modality until after the 1972 amendment to the Medicare Social Security Act created the financial impetus to develop in-center hemodialysis (HD). Though a significant number of patients remained on HHD, fewer and fewer patients utilized this treatment until a rejuvenated interest at the beginning of this millennium stimulated new growth. The driving force was the efforts of a few nephrologists who were determined to improve outcomes in HD patients by increasing time and frequency of dialysis treatments. Short daily hemodialysis (SDHD) was initially described in 1969, but was not financially viable and was abandoned until revived in the 1990s [2]. More frequent home nocturnal hemodialysis (NHD) was first introduced by Dr. Uldall in 1994 after obtaining a grant from the Ministry of Health, Province of Ontario [3]. Improvement in dialysis equipment and a decrease in cost of supplies made "daily" dialysis more financially attractive, yet still more expensive than thrice-weekly dialysis. However, the major cost-saving was performing dialysis at home with a patient functioning as a nonpaid dialysis technician. Finally, for HHD to be attractive for patients, novel dialysis equipment had to be developed that was unobtrusive in the home (small), simple to use, financially sound, and, ideally, portable. Industry has responded to these needs and we can expect even more innovative dialysis platforms in the future. Thus, more frequent HD at home evolved and was suddenly a very attractive option for many patients.

In this chapter, we review the benefits of HHD acknowledging that, as is true for most clinical subjects in nephrology, rigorous and scientifically sound data is limited. However, we need to recognize that the patients we treat today cannot afford to wait 5 or 10 years for the possibility that more studies will be done. Potential complications of HHD as well as solutions to manage the complications are outlined. We also describe appropriate dialysis prescriptions using traditional and more novel dialysis platforms. Finally, we review strategies to build a successful HHD program that includes an approach for discussion of modality selection options with patients.

13.2 Clinical Outcomes

Over the past decade, many observational studies and a few randomized control trials (RCTs) have been published examining a range of clinical outcomes for HHD patients. Although the studies encompass a variety of study designs, evaluate a number of outcomes, and are not all consistent with each other, the overwhelming take-away message from this growing body of literature is that more frequent dialysis (typically performed in the home) offers favorable clinical outcomes for patients. However, it is important to realize that this is largely observational data and thus we must interpret with caution. In addition, it is important to note that the general term "home hemodialysis" includes both SDHD and NHD. For the purpose of this chapter, "home hemodialysis" refers to "more frequent" or "daily" HD options performed at home. Both modalities offer overall more time on dialysis per week and are typically performed in the home, but are different from each other in prescription and should not be lumped together when discussing clinical outcomes. In this section, we will discuss the major clinical outcomes described in the literature and end with some special cases in which HHD may be a particularly attractive modality.

J. D. Glickman (✉)
Hospital of the University of Pennsylvania, One Founders, 3400 Spruce Street, Philadelphia, PA 19104, USA
e-mail: joel.glickman@uphs.upenn.edu

R. K. Seshasai
Drexel University College of Medicine, 245 North 15th Street Suite 6144 NCB, Philadelphia, PA 19102, USA

A. K. Singh et al. (eds.), *Core Concepts in Dialysis and Continuous Therapies*, DOI 10.1007/978-1-4899-7657-4_13

13.2.1 Randomized Control Trials

There are two key RCTs that evaluate clinical outcomes in HHD. The Frequent Hemodialysis Network (FHN) trial was a multicenter RCT with both an SDHD arm (6 days per week) [4], which included 245 subjects, and an NHD arm (6 nights per week) [5], which included 87 subjects, compared with conventional in-center thrice-weekly dialysis (CHD). The primary composite outcomes at 12 months were (1) death or 1-year change from baseline in left ventricular (LV) mass, and (2) death or 1-year change in physical health based on a RAND health survey. There were a number of secondary outcomes that were evaluated and many ancillary studies have been subsequently performed. The SDHD trial showed statistically significant improvement in both co-primary outcomes ($p<0.001$, $p=0.007$, respectively) although the NHD trial showed no difference in primary outcomes from the conventional arm. The FHN trial had a number of limitations, including, notably, the low enrollment in the NHD trial and the fact that many of the controls in the NHD trial were actually doing traditional thrice-weekly HD at home instead of in-center, but it is one of only a few RCTs we have to evaluate HHD and so it is important to review.

The other RCT, by Culleton et al., randomized 52 subjects to 6 days per week NHD versus CHD and subjects were followed for 6 months [6]. The primary endpoint was change in LV mass, as measured by cardiovascular magnetic resonance imaging (MRI), and prespecified secondary outcomes included self-reported quality of life, blood pressure, mineral metabolism, and medication usage. In this study, frequent NHD significantly improved LV mass ($p=0.04$) and had favorable impact on systolic blood pressure (SBP) control, mineral metabolism, and some measures of quality of life.

13.2.2 Quality of Life

Performing dialysis at home, either as SDHD or NHD, affords the patient significantly more flexibility and freedom to tailor treatments around their daily lives. It allows patients to remain employed, spend more time with family and friends, and gain more freedom to do what they choose. In addition, patients generally report fewer intradialytic symptoms and shorter recovery time post-dialysis. The increased time on dialysis overall allows for smaller quantities of fluid removal and less extreme solute fluctuations in a given time period. In the Following Rehabilitation, Economics and Everyday-Dialysis Outcome Measurements (FREEDOM) study, a prospective cohort study of SDHD patients, improvement in quality of life was demonstrated using the SF-36 survey at initiation of SDHD and then subsequently at 4 months and 12 months [7]. The percentage of patients with depressive symptoms, using the Beck Depression Scale, significantly decreased during 12 months of follow-up as well [8]. Furthermore, there was a significant drop in post-dialysis recovery time at 12 months from 8 h in the thrice-weekly HD patients to only 1 h in the SDHD patients. Lockridge described his experience with NHD patients in Lynchburg, Virginia, and using patients as their own controls, he showed that the hospital admission rate dropped by 42 % and the number of hospital days by 60 % following initiation of NHD [9]. In addition, he found that his patients had statistically significant improvement in both the physical and mental components of the SF-36 scores after transitioning to NHD. Finally, in a cohort of 12 patients converted from CHD to NHD, Jassel demonstrated improvement in cognitive functioning on a battery of neuropsychiatric tests performed at baseline and after 6 months on NHD. The most impressive improvement was in attention and working memory, which improved by 32 %. Patients' own perception of their cognitive function also improved significantly [10].

13.2.3 Phosphorous Control

Improvement in the control of phosphorous levels has been shown in many studies with HHD. Phosphorous removal entails a two-phase model, with early phosphorous removal from the extracellular compartment related to the concentration gradient from the blood to the dialysate. The second phase of phosphorous removal requires much more time, to allow for mobilization of phosphorous from the intracellular compartment. This two-phase removal process is why NHD, with its relatively longer treatments, has more profound effects on phosphorous removal than SDHD [11]. Patients using NHD often require few, if any, phosphorous binders and can follow a much more liberal diet which includes phosphorous-containing foods.

A number of studies have evaluated phosphorous control in SDHD patients and showed overall a modest improvement in phosphorous levels and some reduction in phosphate binder use [11, 12]. However clinically, NHD provides better control of phosphorous. In the RCT by Culleton et al., 19 of 26 NHD patients decreased or discontinued phosphorous binders compared with only 3 of 25 in the conventional arm [6]. Similarly, 40 patients followed longitudinally by Lockridge required no phosphorous binders after initiating NHD [9]. Kim et al. described the case of a patient with extraosseous tumoral calcification which resolved after daily NHD. The calcium–phosphorous product dropped from 85 mg^2/dL^2 to <55 mg^2/dL^2 [13]. Finally, in the NHD FHN trial, not only did 73 % of the 87 patients not require any phosphorous binders, 42 % required supplemental phosphorous in the dialysate to maintain normal phosphorous levels [5].

In addition to the improvement in control of phosphorous, frequent dialysis has been shown to improve overall nutritional status. In a study of eight patients on SDHD, Galland demonstrated improvement in serum albumin, protein intake, and lean body mass [14]. Similarly, improvement in appetite, protein intake, and energy were seen in a study of 14 NHD patients. However, they cautioned that fat intake also increased and put patients at increased risk of becoming overweight [15].

13.2.4 Cardiovascular

End-stage renal disease (ESRD) patients in the USA have an annual mortality rate of approximately 20 % [16], and cause of death is overwhelmingly related to cardiovascular events. Patients using conventional dialysis have long 2–3-day interdialytic intervals in which they become relatively volume-expanded and have more hypertension. Patients using frequent dialysis have overall more stable blood pressure and volume status. In addition, they do not have large volumes of fluid removed over short intervals of time (lower ultrafiltration rate) and therefore have fewer episodes of myocardial stunning and regional wall motion abnormalities [17].

SDHD has been shown to lower blood pressure and reduce the number of anti-hypertensive medications that are required. Fagugli studied 12 patients who transitioned from conventional to SDHD and observed that average SBP dropped 20 mm Hg, use of anti-hypertensive medications decreased, and left ventricular mass index (LVMI), which has been independently associated with increased mortality in the ESRD population, decreased significantly [18]. In the SDHD FHN trial, patients on frequent dialysis had an average of 10 mm Hg decrease in SBP and significant reduction in the mean LV mass as well, compared with the CHD control arm [4].

Similar improvements in blood pressure control and cardiovascular outcomes are demonstrated in a number of studies of NHD. In the RCT of NHD patients by Culleton, there was a significant reduction in LV mass in the NHD group after 6 months of follow-up [6]. In addition, 16 of 26 patients on NHD stopped or reduced the number of blood pressure meds they were taking and concurrently the SBP in the NHD group dropped on average by 7 mm Hg. Chan et al. observed 28 patients who switched from CHD to NHD and found a reduction in SBP of more than 20 mm Hg, a reduction in the average number of blood pressure meds per person from 1.8 to 0.3, as well as a significant reduction in LVMI [19]. There was no change in extracellular volume concurrently, which suggests that more frequent dialysis improves blood pressure control not only because of improved volume control but also by decreasing peripheral vascular resistance. Indeed, endothelial dependent and independent vasodilation improved in NHD patients. Norepinephrine levels were also noted to be lower [19, 20]. NHD has also been shown to improve the cardiac ejection fraction and reduce the frequency of apneic episodes in patients with sleep apnea [21, 22].

13.2.5 Survival

Many, but not all, of the studies addressing survival in frequent dialysis suggest at least a modest mortality benefit for patients. Blagg et al. found that 117 SDHD patients had 61 % better survival than comparable CHD patients [23]. The largest observational study of SDHD to evaluate survival investigated 1873 SDHD patients matched 1:5 with a group of CHD from the United States Renal Data System (USRDS) and showed a modest improvement in survival among patients using SDHD [24]. Similarly, studies comparing NHD show improved survival as well [25, 26]. Nesrallah et al. compared an international group of 338 patients receiving intensive home dialysis treatments (average of 4.8 times per week, 7.4 h per session) with matched CHD controls from the Dialysis Outcomes and Practice Patterns Study (DOPPS) and found a 13 % mortality in the intense dialysis group versus 21 % mortality in the CHD group, during median follow-up of 1.8 years. Finally, patients using NHD have been shown to have comparable survival to recipients of deceased donor kidney transplants [27].

13.2.6 Anemia

The effect of SDHD or NHD on anemia management is less clear. There have been a number of observational studies suggesting improved hemoglobin and reduction in dose required of erythropoietin-stimulating agents (ESA) as well as many studies which show no difference [28, 29]. The FHN trial, both SDHD and NHD arms, shows no difference in hemoglobin or ESA dose [30] nor does the RCT in NHD by Culleton et al. [6].

13.2.7 Special Uses of Home Hemodialysis

13.2.7.1 Pregnancy

Young women on dialysis are typically less fertile, often with impaired ovulation and even amenorrhea, and thus rates of pregnancy are lower than in the general population. For women who do conceive, pregnancy complications include intrauterine fetal death, preterm delivery, and more intrauterine growth restriction [31]. There have been a number of small studies suggesting that more frequent and intensive dialysis, delivered as NHD, is associated with improved fertility and better maternal and fetal outcomes [32, 33]. Gangji et al. described a 31-year-old woman on CHD who began menstruating 8 months after transitioning to NHD and had a successful full-term pregnancy 2 years after using NHD. During her pregnancy, she received 7.5 h of dialysis seven nights per week [34].

13.2.7.2 Ascites

Patients with ascites, from any cause, can particularly benefit from NHD. Pauly et al. described two patients with ascites who did poorly on CHD with no improvement in ascites because of intradialytic hypotension, cramping, and difficulty removing fluid. Once each patient was transferred to NHD, they experienced resolution of the ascites [35].

13.2.8 Ventilators

Dialysis patients who require continuous or intermittent mechanical ventilation may have difficulty finding a dialysis unit which can accommodate them for in-center treatments. Sometimes, these chronically ill patients cannot sit upright in a chair and would require a bed for dialysis treatments. Oftentimes, the clinical staff at the dialysis unit is not trained and comfortable in handling routine or emergency ventilator care. Finally, it may simply be more cumbersome to transport a patient who requires a ventilator to dialysis thrice weekly. For all of these reasons, mechanically ventilated patients may benefit from HHD if they have the necessary space and someone who can help with their home treatments (personal experience).

13.2.9 Summary

In summary, the overwhelming evidence available suggests that HHD offers an array of improved clinical outcomes for patients, including improved quality of life metrics, improved blood pressure control and reduction in LV hypertrophy, improved phosphorous control, and likely improved survival. In addition to providing all patients with more flexibility and ownership over their own dialysis treatments, NHD in particular can be particularly favorable for certain patient populations such as pregnant women or patients with ascites or who like to have free time during the day to work or pursue other pleasures in life.

13.3 Complications of Home Hemodialysis

With proper training, HD can be performed safely in the home. When patients are selected to be appropriate candidates for this modality, spend weeks training with a nurse before dialyzing independently, receive retraining at specified intervals, and follow specified safety precautions consistently, the rate of complications is very low. One large HHD program in Canada reviewed their HHD population and performed a quality assurance (QA) analysis. From 2001 to 2012, the HHD programs in Edmonton and Ottawa, Canada, trained 190 patients. In total, they estimate 500 patient-years and 117,000 HHD treatments of experience. Over those 11 years, they had only one death (from exsanguination) and six life-threatening procedure-related adverse events, or an event rate of 0.06 per 1000 dialysis treatments. Five events were definitely and two events were possibly attributed to human error and failure to follow specified protocols [36]. Some programs have instituted home-monitoring for patients dialyzing at night. While this provides some patients with reassurance, data have not shown that this practice improves outcomes or reduces complications. The London Daily/Nocturnal Study suggested that home monitoring may be helpful for a period of 3 months, until the patient is completely comfortable with performing dialysis at home [37]. Out of 4096 patient treatments, there were 5351 alarms, 322 calls to patients' home because of slow or nonresponse, and zero calls to emergency medical services. At this time, most practices do not utilize continuous home-monitoring.

There are several preventable, though potentially dangerous, complications of HHD including major hemorrhage, vascular access complications, cardiovascular events during dialysis, equipment malfunction, and psychosocial stress. It is imperative to instruct patients regarding these potential complications during training to underscore the importance of careful attention to procedures and technique. Some patients and health-care providers are concerned about safety of dialyzing alone at home without a partner. Though most programs recommend a partner, there are no data examining this subject, and many physicians have confidence in the experience of their home dialysis team and allow patients to dialyze at home alone. For example, we have a very safe and successful 7-year experience with patients who perform nocturnal HHD alone.

Perhaps the most concerning potential complication of HHD is major hemorrhage. In order to prevent this major complication, patients are taught to meticulously secure the needles with tape and then pull on the tubing to make sure needles do not move. In addition, they are instructed to use blood leak sensors (enuresis alarms) wrapped around the access site and placed strategically on the floor around the machine, which sound an alarm if blood or leaking dialysate is detected.

HHD patients appear to have increased risk of vascular access complications but there is no difference seen in access loss. This result was seen in a number of studies, including both arms of the FHN trials [38]. There is debate in the literature about the best cannulation technique for patients with arteriovenous fistulas—the "rope ladder technique" versus "buttonhole." The rope ladder technique is most commonly used in-center and uses sharp needles and rotating access cannulation sites. The buttonhole uses a blunt needle and uses the same track with each cannulation. Some literature suggests increased access survival, reduced complications, reduced aneurysms, pain, and infiltrations with the buttonhole technique. However, there is a suggestion of increased risk of staphylococcus infection with buttonholes because of the track that forms [38–41]. Recent experience suggests that the increasing use of topical mupirocin seems to reduce buttonhole-related infection rate. Furthermore, there may be opportunity to decrease vascular access infection in the home by developing "best demonstrated practices" for home dialysis access use. When patients and nurses were surveyed regarding vascular access cannulation, not a single patient or nurse reported performing all steps in accordance with general accepted practice for access cannulation [42]. This study suggests there is tremendous opportunity to improve home cannulation technique and training.

Intradialytic hypotension and dialysis-related symptoms are less common in HHD [43]. There are also reports of a decrease in episodes of myocardial stunning. Myocardial stunning can lead to a decrease in ejection fraction and ventricular arrhythmias during dialysis [17]. Improvement in the aforementioned parameters is probably related to decreased ultrafiltration rates that occur with more frequent sessions and increased overall dialysis time.

Patients who use conventional dialysis equipment need to rigorously follow water treatment and testing guidelines to avoid problems with water quality. It is quite safe to use water in the home for HHD with the portable reverse osmosis machines and carbon filter as long as the patient is meticulous and appropriate water testing and cultures are done at regular intervals. For patients who use NxStage therapy, the NxStage PureFlow system makes ultrapure water from tap water which is mixed with sterile dialysate concentrate. This process is automated and thus is less likely to lead to complications in water treatment.

Finally, HHD can have major psychosocial benefits as well as complications for patients. For the motivated patient with social support, HHD can offer increased independence to tailor treatments around other activities. Many patients report improved physical and mental functioning. However, "burnout" is a major issue, with the discontinuation rate within 1 year of starting HHD in the 25–30% range [8, 24, 44]. HHD requires significant commitment, time, and energy, and can be difficult for patients as well as their families to maintain. Decreased compliance with treatment frequency can also become a problem in these cases [44].

13.4 Prescription Management

13.4.1 Introduction

There are three components of a home dialysis prescription: solute removal, fluid removal, and quality of life. Solute removal encompasses more than just urea and the physician needs to consider, for example, other small solutes and electrolytes, phosphate and middle molecules. Fluid removal is more complicated than just achieving dry weight because we have to adjust fluid removal to a patient's inherent "refill rate" of the intravascular space to avoid myocardial stunning and the increase in mortality rate-associated high ultrafiltration rates. Finally, if the prescription does not match the patient's lifestyle and will be difficult to adhere to, it will lead to patient dissatisfaction, burnout, and possible dropout from the home program.

There are several different options for HHD including SDHD, NHD, traditional thrice-weekly HD, and even a hybrid plan that enables patients to do different types of treatments according to their schedule. We have patients who do several NHD treatments intermixed with SDHD in a week that varies according to their work and travel schedule with the caveat that changes to prescriptions can be done only with the physician's approval. In order to prescribe HHD correctly, make appropriate changes when target solute and fluid removal is not met, and to develop novel prescriptions to meet the personal needs of the home patient, the physician needs to understand the theory and nuances of each dialysis platform. Though currently there are only two dialysis platforms approved for use in the home, Fresenius 2008K@home (Fresenius) machine and NxStage System One (NxStage), there are new machines in clinical trial and development that will utilize other technologies (e.g., sorbent technology) that will require the physician to learn even more. Typical dialysis prescriptions for current dialysis machines and different HHD modalities are summarized in Table 13.1.

Table 13.1 Hemodialysis prescriptions

	Conventional HD equipment			NxStage	
	HD	SDHD	NHD	SDHD	NHD
Treatments/week	3	5–6	5–6	5–6	5–6
Treatment time (h)*	4	2	6–8	2–3.5	6–8
Q_b (mL/min)	400–450	400–450	200–300	400–450	200–300
Q_d (mL/min)	600–800	600–800	300	100–300	60–100

* we recommend a minimum weekly treatment time of 12 hours

HD hemodialysis, *SDHD* short daily hemodialysis, *NHD* nocturnal hemodialysis

13.4.2 Kt/V

Appropriate solute clearance is difficult to define because we have few tools to measure solute removal and even fewer tools to define what optimal removal is. Kt/V_{Urea} (Kt/V) has become the standard for adjusting dialysis dose for thrice-weekly conventional HD treatments. Dialysis modalities with different levels of continuousness have different degrees of efficiency and therefore cannot be compared by spKt/V. Take, for example, peritoneal dialysis (PD) and continuous RRT modalities, in which the serum blood urea nitrogen (BUN) level does not vary significantly during the day, yet over the course of 24 hours, urea removal is significant. To address this and to have a tool to compare dialysis treatments with different frequencies and duration, the (weekly) standard Kt/V (stdKt/V) model was developed. This model expresses dialysis dose for each modality as an equivalent, normalized (theoretical) continuous clearance [45]. The stdKt/V is the same for all modalities that produce the same mid-week pre-dialysis BUN. Though this model has never been clinically validated as a predictor of clinical outcomes, Kidney Disease Outcomes Quality Initiative (KDOQI) guidelines suggest a stdKt/V of 2.1.

The formula for stdKt/V is quite complex:

$$\text{stdKt}/\text{V} = 168*\left[1-\exp\left(-\text{eKt}/\text{V}\right)\right]/\text{t}/\left[\left(1-\exp\left(-\text{eKt}/\text{V}\right)\right)/\text{eKt}/\text{V}+168/\text{N}/\text{t}-1\right] \quad [45]$$

Where: "eKt/V" is equilibrated Kt/V per treatment, "N" is treatments per week and "t" is time per treatment in hours. This formula can be used to generate a nomogram (Fig. 13.1) to estimate, for a given frequency of dialysis, the target per treatment spKt/V to achieve a stdKt/V of 2.0. For example, if a patient performs HD 5 days per week, then target per treatment spKt/V is about 0.6. Note that for thrice-weekly, 4 h HD treatments, a spKt/V of 1.2 is equivalent to a stdKt/V of 2.0.

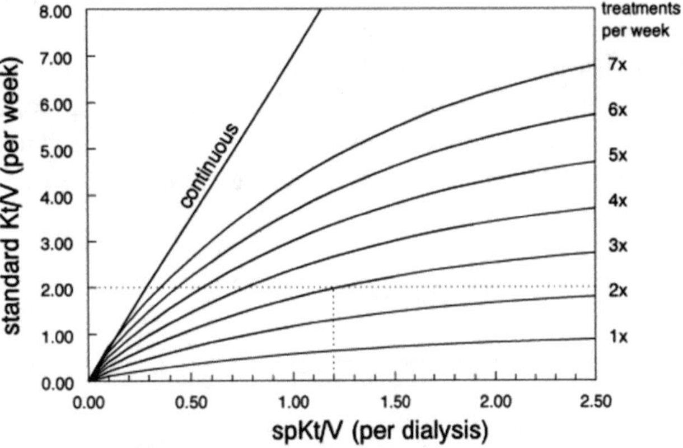

Fig. 13.1 Graph represents relationship between *spKt/V* and *stdKt/V* according to frequency of hemodialysis treatment [45]

The two dialysis machines approved for use in the home, Fresenius and NxStage, use different approaches to achieve target urea clearance and maintain electrolyte levels in the normal range.

13.4.3 Fresenius

Fresenius is a traditional dialysis machine that requires electrical and plumbing modification to the home to accommodate the dialysis machine and water treatment equipment (typically reverse osmosis). Prescription changes are fundamentally the same as using traditional dialysis equipment for in-center HD. SDHD is typically a 2 h treatment, at typical blood flow rates (Q_b) of 400–450 mL/min and typical dialysate flow rates (Q_d). If target spKt/V is not achieved then treatment duration, Q_b and Q_d can be adjusted in the same manner as in-center HD. Electrolyte content of dialysate is prescribed and altered according to blood tests. Ultrafiltration rates should be kept below 10–13 mL/Kg/h as is done for in-center HD patients [46]. For NHD, given the long duration of therapy, lower rates are used. Given lower Q_d rates overall, dialysate volumes are about the same and therefore dialysate electrolyte content is nearly the same as traditional HD. However, longer treatments will result in lower phosphate binder use and therefore, depending on the binder used, serum calcium levels may be lower resulting in higher parathyroid hormone (PTH) levels. In that situation, calcium supplementation or higher dialysate calcium may be required [47]. Occasional patients become hypophosphatemic and phosphate (0.7 mmol/L) is added to the dialysate [48].

13.4.4 NxStage

Patients prefer a simple, easy-to-use dialysis machine that requires minimal storage space, is energy and water efficient, and requires no significant electrical modification to the home. A low dialysate volume approach, though theoretically applicable to any dialysis machine, is a requirement for the NxStage. The hallmark of this machine is adjusting the relationship between Q_d and Q_b to maximize saturation of lower amounts of dialysate. In-center dialysis centers produce relatively large volumes of dialysate. At higher Q_d, urea clearance increases but relatively inefficiently, as noted by a plateau in clearance (Fig. 13.2). However, at low Q_d and relatively high Q_b, dialysate is highly saturated and therefore dialysate is used efficiently. The term "Flow fraction" (FF) is defined as Q_d/Q_b. When the FF is low, dialysate saturation is high (Fig. 13.3).

Part of the prescription for NxStage is selecting a maximum FF that is programmed into the machine. Setting a maximum FF sets minimum dialysate saturation. By fixing

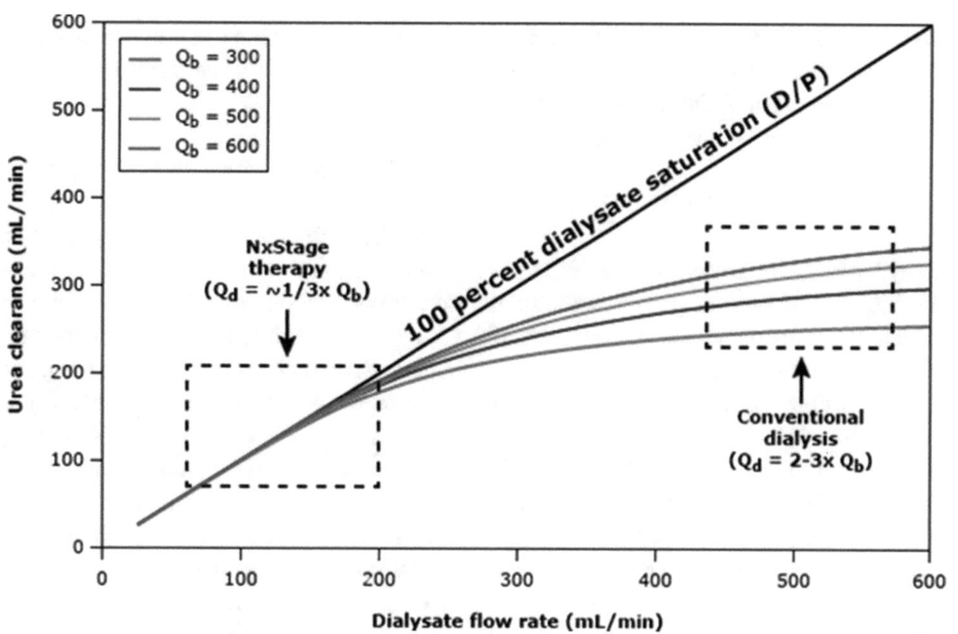

Fig. 13.2 Urea clearance is depicted as a function of dialysate flow rates (Q_d) at different blood flow rates (Q_b). At slower Q_d, dialysate is nearly 100 % saturated with urea. NxStage therapy uses low Q_d to maximize dialysate saturation whereas conventional dialysis uses higher Q_d with lower dialysate saturation. (Data reproduced with permission from NxStage Medical, Inc. Copyright © 2012)

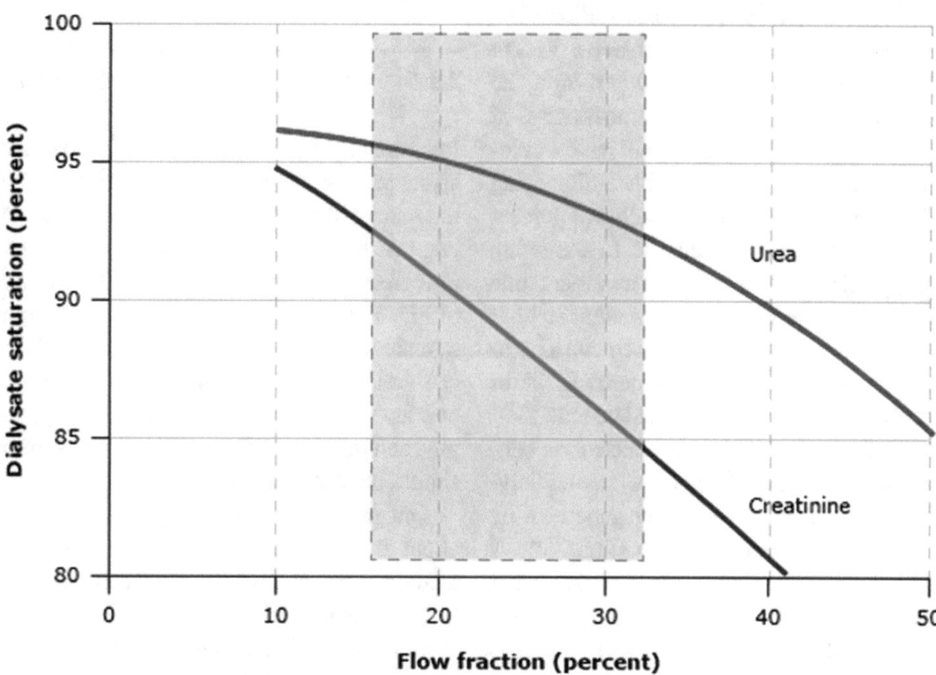

Fig. 13.3 Graphs represent dialysate saturation in relationship to flow fraction (FF). At lower FF, dialysate saturation is higher. (Data reproduced with permission from NxStage Medical, Inc. Copyright © 2012)

the minimum saturation (saturation can be higher but not lower during a treatment), the patient will receive their target Kt/V as long as they complete their treatment with the prescribed amount of fluid. The methodology to measure stdKt/V is exactly the same as any HD treatment; a urea reduction ratio (URR) is obtained and converted to a spKt/V which is converted to a stdKt/V as previously described in this chapter.

However, to appropriately adjust the prescription to achieve target Kt/V, it is useful to conceptually consider Kt/V for HD just as we do for PD. In PD, the volume of PD dialysate drained multiplied by D/P urea (percent saturation of PD fluid relative to plasma) will equal the amount of drained dialysate that is completely (100 %) saturated (Kt). Then Kt is divided by an estimate of V. This is represented by the formula:

$$Kt / V = (D / P_{Urea})(\text{Dialysate drain volume}) / V.$$

For NxStage, therapy (D/P_{Urea}), or percent saturation, is determined by the FF (Q_d/Q_b). To increase percent saturation, we decrease FF, which invariably means Q_d will be lower. If Q_d is lower, it will take longer to process the fixed amount of dialysate and treatment time will be longer. Similarly, if the prescribed dialysate volume is increased, at the same FF (same Q_d), the treatment will be longer. Finally, because Kt is equal to the product of percent saturation and dialysate volume, one could generously increase dialysate volume and modestly decrease percent saturation and still achieve a higher Kt/V.

For example, if we have a 76 kg patient who wants to do 5-day-per-week SDHD, we will need to target a per treatment spKt/V of about 0.6 (Fig. 13.1). Assuming his V is about 38 L, he will need a Kt of about 23 L (0.6 multiplied by 38 L). If we decided to use 25 L of fluid, it will need to be 92 % saturated to yield 23 L of 100 % saturated fluid. We can estimate the patient needs a flow fraction of about 0.3 to achieve a percent saturation of 92 (Fig. 13.3). Assuming Q_b is 400 mL/min, the Q_d will be about 120 mL/min. If we have to process 25 L of dialysate at a rate of 120 mL/min, the patient will have a treatment time of nearly 210 min. If we redo the calculation using 30 L of dialysate, we could use a FF of 0.5, achieve percent saturation of 85 %, and Kt will be more than 25 L. Assuming Q_b of 400 mL/min, Q_d will be 200 mL/min and treatment time will be about 150 min. We are able to save the patient an hour of treatment time, improve quality of life, and achieve a higher Kt/V! Remember, regardless of our estimate of Kt/V for a given prescription, we measure URR to calculate stdKt/V.

There are limited options for altering the electrolyte content of the dialysate when using the NxStage system. Dialysate is available in pre-packaged 5 L bags, or generated by a self-contained dialysate generating system (PureFlow™ SL). PureFlow™ SL makes ultrapure water from tap water and then adds it to sterile dialysate concentrate to produce dialysate in 40, 50, or 60 L batches. The dialysate buffer is lactate which is metabolized in the liver to bicarbonate in a 1:1 ratio. The composition of dialysate currently available is:

- Lactate—40 or 45 mEq/L
- Potassium—1.0 mEq/L and for 2.0 for some of the batches
- Sodium—140 mEq/L
- Calcium—3.0 mEq/L
- Magnesium—1.0 mEq/L
- Chloride—105 mEq/L
- Glucose—100 mg/dL

Note that hypokalemia and hypercalcemia are unusual because of the relatively low volume of dialysate used [49].

13.4.5 Blood Pressure Management

Regardless of dialysis equipment used at home, most HHD patients require significantly less blood pressure medication. Blood pressure may fall even within days of beginning therapy and therefore it is very important to reduce the anti-hypertensive regimen *prior* to beginning SDHD or NHD by as much as 50 % and monitor blood pressure closely to avoid hypotensive events. Initially, most patients will be able to achieve a lower estimated dry weight once they are dialyzing more frequently, and blood pressure medications often need to be reduced or discontinued as the dry weight is reduced. With time, many patients may gain body weight, blood pressures tend to decrease again, and dry weights need to be increased. Patients need education regarding the risk of hypotension at home and to report low blood pressures promptly to the HHD nurse. Eventually, if the prescription and dry weight are correct, most patients require no or just one anti-hypertensive medication.

13.5 Developing a Home Dialysis Program

Intentionally, we describe how to build a successful home dialysis program as opposed to just an HHD program because the many similarities between HHD and PD essentially dictate that these two programs live under one roof. Strategies to increase utilization of HHD will also increase utilization of PD. Teaching methods to improve training and retraining of patients are similar for HHD and PD. Programs to develop QA and continuous quality improvement (CQI) initiatives overlap for these two modalities. Finally, the goals, philosophy, and mission of PD and HHD programs are the same and should be clearly stated and practiced.

Our program's philosophy keeps it very simple: "It's all about the patient." That is, we practice "patient-centric" medicine and try to incorporate the patient's vantage point in every aspect of the program. For example: we typically present patients with options for prescription changes to make sure it is compatible with their lifestyle, and we organize comprehensive, multidisciplinary monthly clinic visits to minimize patient visits and allow us to address all of their needs at one time. Every project, miscue, and opportunity for improvement in the process of setting up a home program will turn into a success if the entire home dialysis team focuses on the patient's needs (and not necessarily ours).

There are three major components of a home dialysis program: the people, the physical infrastructure, and the policies and procedures that operate the clinic. For certain, the peo-

Table 13.2 The medical team

At least one person needs to be the program champion
Nurses
Physician
Social worker
Dietician
Administrator
Biomedical engineer
Administrative assistant
Patient care technician
Interventional radiologist
Surgeon (vascular and laparoscopic for PD)

PD peritoneal dialysis

Table 13.3 Sources and strategies to recruit patients

In-center hemodialysis
"Lobby days"
Chairside machine demonstrations
"Try it you will like it" programs
Patient support groups
CKD patients
CKD education
One-on-one meetings with home dialysis nurse
Acute start patients
In-hospital modality education
Maintain contact with patients interested but not ready to commit
Transplant patients
Develop relationships with transplant program

CKD chronic kidney disease

ple are most important and patients are paramount because without patients there is no program (Table 13.2). A home dialysis facility needs to project census prior to developing space and hiring staff. It is shortsighted to build a space that will be too small within a year or two or have to mothball because of inadequate utilization. Set a goal for projected census growth. Though there is limited literature, realistically, 5–10 % of dialysis patients will embrace HHD. PD literature is much better defined. Given the opportunity to choose a dialysis modality, 35–40 % of incident patients select PD [50]. Of course, there will be some variation according to demographics and some practices will have higher utilization. However, a beautiful home and a college education is not a requirement. We have single mothers with barely high school education succeeding tremendously on HHD and similarly we have octogenarians and functionally illiterate patients thriving while on PD.

All patients deserve the opportunity to learn about options for RRT without bias or prejudice of health-care providers. Our paradigm for presentation of options is straightforward. Patients who are interested in transplant are referred for transplant evaluation, and patients who may not benefit or are not interested in RRT are counseled on options for appropriate medical care. Patients who are interested in RRT are told they can have dialysis treatments done in the comfort of their own home or they come to a dialysis clinic 3 days per week. We then review home options (PD vs. HHD), as well as benefits and disadvantages of each modality. In-center thrice-weekly HD as well as NHD is also offered. After this relatively brief outline is presented, we refer every patient to one of our home dialysis nurse educators for a more detailed one-on-one meeting. During these meetings, patients have the opportunity to see home dialysis equipment and receive all the information they need to make an educated decision regarding RRT. Finally, prospective patients frequently speak directly with current home dialysis patients to get a different and insightful perspective.

There are several sources of patients. Robust chronic kidney disease (CKD) education programs for both outpatients and inpatients will help attract patients. For HHD, the largest source of patients is probably transfers from in-center HD. To recruit patients from your in-center program, consider "lobby days" where patients can receive educational materials and see HHD machines. For those patients who are great candidates, do an up-close machine demonstration while they receive in-patient HD. And for the patient who is highly motivated but not 100 % confident, consider investing in a trial of SDHD training. If the patient likes it, they can complete training. If they don't feel any better (unlikely), they will return in-center. Finally, a relatively high proportion of our home dialysis patients have failed kidney transplants or developed renal failure as a consequence of chronic immunosuppression for other solid organ transplants. Develop programs to attract these patients (Table 13.3).

The medical staff needs at least one "leader" or "champion" and preferably two from different disciplines (e.g., physician and nurse), but everyone on the team needs to understand the special needs of the home patient. The physician needs to be the point person for patient recruitment but, along with the nurse champion, develop staff education programs, policies and procedures, program development, and QA and CQI projects. The day-to-day operation of the program rests on the shoulders of the nurse. Having a great nurse is the key to success so make sure to recruit the right nurses and invest in their education. Dietary restrictions for patients improve but do not disappear with home dialysis, so a dietician knowledgeable about home therapies is essential. The social worker is the key to provide support to patients and families, and identify potential changes in the home that may lead to patient burnout or dropout from the program.

The physical infrastructure includes the clinic space and layout as well as dialysis equipment. In keeping with the theme of "it's all about the patient," we strongly believe that the space needs to be beautiful, comfortable, warm, and appealing (Fig. 13.4 and 13.5). It is often difficult to retrofit existing space for home dialysis in most dialysis facilities because a storage closet converted to a multiuse training and exam room is rarely attractive and does not allow for growth.

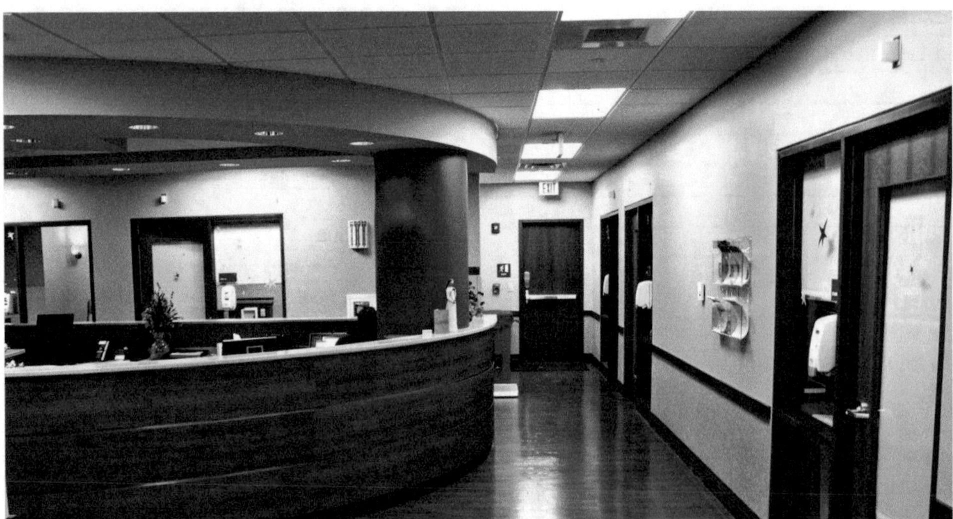

Fig. 13.4 Home dialysis unit with a central nursing work area surrounded by training and exam rooms

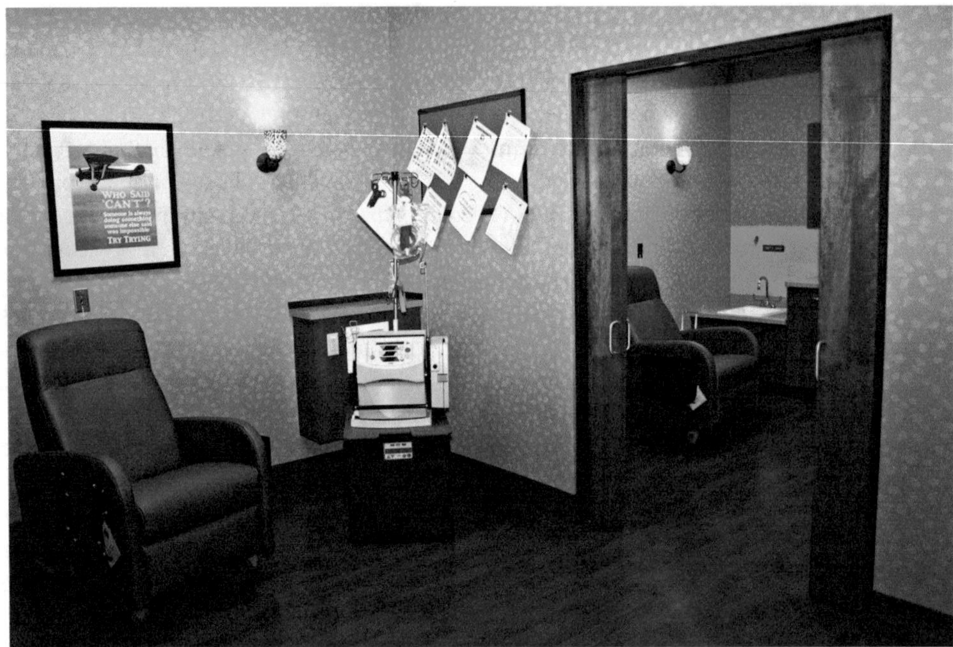

Fig. 13.5 Two home hemodialysis rooms separated by a sliding pocket door allow a nurse to monitor two patients at once yet provide privacy when needed

A new program will focus primarily on training patients but eventually the nursing staff will spend a significant portion of their time with monthly, routine, and urgent clinic visits. A space that focuses only on training rooms and not the workflow of the staff during clinic visits will fall short of needs and will lead to tremendous inefficiencies and frustrations for the nurses. As an example, we elected to have a central nursing station with work spaces and rooms surrounding the nursing station. The nurses also have laptops with a wireless connection so they can document and enter orders easily in every room. We also like having two training rooms connected by sliding pocket doors so they can be used to take care of two patients at once during training yet also provide privacy when needed. We have designated clinic rooms that are not used for training but the training rooms can be used for clinic visits during those very busy days. The training rooms should obviously have appropriate drains for used dialysate, and if you plan to use the Fresenius 2008K@Home machine, make sure there is appropriate water and electric connections. The NxStage machine does not require special plumbing and runs on standard electric outlets. It's size, simplicity, and portability makes it the machine of choice for almost all of our patients.

Developing policies and procedures is beyond the scope of this limited article. Suffice to say some policies are universal and apply to both in-center HD and HHD. But there need to be home dialysis-specific policies, procedures, and protocols. As previously noted, we believe in the multidisciplinary model of home dialysis care and schedule monthly patient visits at the home dialysis center with the nurse, physician, social worker, and dietitian all present. Some programs have a separate nursing visit at the facility and a physician visit at the physician's office or at the facility on another day. But we mandate that physicians participate in the multidisciplinary visit because we find that we are much more effective and thorough when the entire team sees the patient at the same time.

Finally, QA and CQI projects are especially important not only in the early, developmental phase of the program but also as the program matures. Identify quality indicators other than the usual Kt/V, anemia, and albumin for example, which the medical team feel are important and specific to the program such as dropout, blood pressure control, and adherence to treatments. If outcomes fall short of predetermined goals, develop projects and teams to fix them. The quality of the program helps increase the census of the program because dropout rates will be lower. But having a larger program will not guarantee better outcomes if the right staff, facility, and procedures are not developed. QA and CQI projects are a win-win situation: they improve patient care and the professional satisfaction of the whole dialysis team.

13.6 Conclusions

There are many options for RRT, and it is important for the nephrologist and patient to work together to figure out what the best dialysis modality is for the individual patient at a given time. Both the literature and the experience of established home dialysis programs suggest improved clinical outcomes and patient satisfaction with HHD. However, it is important that the patient and nephrologist are comfortable with managing a dialysis patient at home to reduce the risk of complications. The development of new technology has already made and will likely continue to make performing dialysis at home simpler and safer. It is our belief and hope that with proper education and training of patients and physicians, the prevalence of HHD use in the USA can grow, allowing us to provide dialysis care tailored to our ESRD patients.

References

1. Blagg CR. A brief history of home hemodialysis. Advances Ren Replace Ther. 1996;3(2):99–105. Epub 1996/04/01.
2. DePalma JR, Pecker EA, Maxwell MH. A new automatic coil dialyzer system for 'daily' dialysis. Hemodial Int. 2004;8(1):19–23. Epub 2004/01/01.
3. Uldall P, Francoeur R, Ouwendyk M. Simplified nocturnal home hemodialysis (SNHHD): a new approach to renal replacement therapy. J Am Soc Nephrol. 1994;5:428.
4. Chertow GM, Levin NW, Beck GJ, Depner TA, Eggers PW, Gassman JJ, et al. In-center hemodialysis six times per week versus three times per week. N Engl J Med. 2010;363(24):2287–300. Epub 2010/11/26.
5. Rocco MV, Lockridge RS Jr, Beck GJ, Eggers PW, Gassman JJ, Greene T, et al. The effects of frequent nocturnal home hemodialysis: the frequent hemodialysis network nocturnal trial. Kidney Int. 2011;80(10):1080–91. Epub 2011/07/22.
6. Culleton BF, Walsh M, Klarenbach SW, Mortis G, Scott-Douglas N, Quinn RR, et al. Effect of frequent nocturnal hemodialysis vs conventional hemodialysis on left ventricular mass and quality of life: a randomized controlled trial. JAMA. 2007;298(11):1291–9.
7. Finkelstein FO, Schiller B, Daoui R, Gehr TW, Kraus MA, Lea J, et al. At-home short daily hemodialysis improves the long-term health-related quality of life. Kidney Int. 2012;82(5):561–9. Epub 2012/05/25.
8. Jaber BL, Lee Y, Collins AJ, Hull AR, Kraus MA, McCarthy J, et al. Effect of daily hemodialysis on depressive symptoms and postdialysis recovery time: interim report from the FREEDOM (following rehabilitation, economics and everyday-dialysis outcome measurements) study. Am J Kidney Dis. 2010;56(3):531–9. Epub 2010/08/03.
9. Lockridge RS Jr, Spencer M, Craft V, Pipkin M, Campbell D, McPhatter L, et al. Nightly home hemodialysis: five and one-half years of experience in Lynchburg, Virginia. Hemodial Int. 2004;8(1):61–9. Epub 2004/01/01.
10. Jassal SV, Devins GM, Chan CT, Bozanovic R, Rourke S. Improvements in cognition in patients converting from thrice weekly hemodialysis to nocturnal hemodialysis: a longitudinal pilot study. Kidney Int. 2006;70(5):956–62. Epub 2006/07/14.
11. Achinger SG, Ayus JC. The role of daily dialysis in the control of hyperphosphatemia. Kidney Int Suppl. 2005;95:28–32. Epub 2005/05/11.
12. Daugirdas JT, Chertow GM, Larive B, Pierratos A, Greene T, Ayus JC, et al. Effects of frequent hemodialysis on measures of CKD mineral and bone disorder. J Am Soc Nephrol. 2012;23(4):727–38. Epub 2012/03/01.
13. Kim SJ, Goldstein M, Szabo T, Pierratos A. Resolution of massive uremic tumoral calcinosis with daily nocturnal home hemodialysis. Am J Kidney Dis. 2003;41(3):E12. Epub 2003/03/04.
14. Galland R, Traeger J, Arkouche W, Cleaud C, Delawari E, Fouque D. Short daily hemodialysis rapidly improves nutritional status in hemodialysis patients. Kidney Int. 2001;60(4):1555–60. Epub 2001/09/29.
15. Sikkes ME, Kooistra MP, Weijs PJ. Improved nutrition after conversion to nocturnal home hemodialysis. J Ren Nutr. 2009;19(6):494–9. Epub 2009/07/21.
16. U.S. Renal Data System, USRDS. Annual data report: atlas of end-stage renal disease in the United States. Bethesda: National Institutes of Health, National Institute of Diabetes and Digestive and Kidney Diseases; 2012. [Database on the Internet].
17. Jefferies HJ, Virk B, Schiller B, Moran J, McIntyre CW. Frequent hemodialysis schedules are associated with reduced levels of dialysis-induced cardiac injury (myocardial stunning). Clin J Am Soc Nephrol (CJASN). 2011;6(6):1326–32. Epub 2011/05/21.

18. Fagugli RM, Reboldi G, Quintaliani G, Pasini P, Ciao G, Cicconi B, et al. Short daily hemodialysis: blood pressure control and left ventricular mass reduction in hypertensive hemodialysis patients. Am J Kidney Dis. 2001;38(2):371–6. Epub 2001/08/02.
19. Chan CT, Floras JS, Miller JA, Richardson RM, Pierratos A. Regression of left ventricular hypertrophy after conversion to nocturnal hemodialysis. Kidney Int. 2002;61(6):2235–9. Epub 2002/05/25.
20. Chan CT, Harvey PJ, Picton P, Pierratos A, Miller JA, Floras JS. Short-term blood pressure, noradrenergic, and vascular effects of nocturnal home hemodialysis. Hypertension. 2003;42(5):925–31. Epub 2003/10/15.
21. Chan C, Floras JS, Miller JA, Pierratos A. Improvement in ejection fraction by nocturnal haemodialysis in end-stage renal failure patients with coexisting heart failure. Nephrol Dial Transpl. 2002;17(8):1518–21. Epub 2002/07/31.
22. Hanly PJ, Pierratos A. Improvement of sleep apnea in patients with chronic renal failure who undergo nocturnal hemodialysis. N Engl J Med. 2001;344(2):102–7. Epub 2001/01/11.
23. Blagg CR, Kjellstrand CM, Ting GO, Young BA. Comparison of survival between short-daily hemodialysis and conventional hemodialysis using the standardized mortality ratio. Hemodial Int. 2006;10(4):371–4. Epub 2006/10/04.
24. Weinhandl ED, Liu J, Gilbertson DT, Arneson TJ, Collins AJ. Survival in daily home hemodialysis and matched thrice-weekly in-center hemodialysis patients. J Am Soc Nephrol. 2012;23(5):895–904. Epub 2012/03/01.
25. Johansen KL, Zhang R, Huang Y, Chen SC, Blagg CR, Goldfarb-Rumyantzev AS, et al. Survival and hospitalization among patients using nocturnal and short daily compared to conventional hemodialysis: a USRDS study. Kidney Int. 2009;76(9):984–90. Epub 2009/08/21.
26. Nesrallah GE, Lindsay RM, Cuerden MS, Garg AX, Port F, Austin PC, et al. Intensive hemodialysis associates with improved survival compared with conventional hemodialysis. J Am Soc Nephrol. 2012;23(4):696–705. Epub 2012/03/01.
27. Pauly RP, Gill JS, Rose CL, Asad RA, Chery A, Pierratos A, et al. Survival among nocturnal home haemodialysis patients compared to kidney transplant recipients. Nephrol Dial Transpl. 2009;24(9):2915–9. Epub 2009/07/09.
28. Woods JD, Port FK, Orzol S, Buoncristiani U, Young E, Wolfe RA, et al. Clinical and biochemical correlates of starting "daily" hemodialysis. Kidney Int. 1999;55(6):2467–76. Epub 1999/06/03.
29. Ting GO, Kjellstrand C, Freitas T, Carrie BJ, Zarghamee S. Long-term study of high-comorbidity ESRD patients converted from conventional to short daily hemodialysis. Am J Kidney Dis. 2003;42(5):1020–35. Epub 2003/10/29.
30. Ornt DB, Larive B, Rastogi A, Rashid M, Daugirdas JT, Hernandez A, et al. Impact of frequent hemodialysis on anemia management: results from the frequent hemodialysis network (FHN) trials. Nephrol Dial Transpl. 2013;28(7):1888–98. Epub 2013/01/30.
31. Chao AS, Huang JY, Lien R, Kung FT, Chen PJ, Hsieh PC. Pregnancy in women who undergo long-term hemodialysis. Am J Obstet Gynecol. 2002;187(1):152–6. Epub 2002/07/13.
32. Asamiya Y, Otsubo S, Matsuda Y, Kimata N, Kikuchi K, Miwa N, et al. The importance of low blood urea nitrogen levels in pregnant patients undergoing hemodialysis to optimize birth weight and gestational age. Kidney Int. 2009;75(11):1217–22. Epub 2009/02/27.
33. Barua M, Hladunewich M, Keunen J, Pierratos A, McFarlane P, Sood M, et al. Successful pregnancies on nocturnal home hemodialysis. Clin J Am Soc Nephrol (CJASN). 2008;3(2):392–6. Epub 2008/03/01.
34. Gangji AS, Windrim R, Gandhi S, Silverman JA, Chan CT. Successful pregnancy with nocturnal hemodialysis. Am J Kidney Dis. 2004;44(5):912–6. Epub 2004/10/20.
35. Pauly RP, Sood MM, Chan CT. Management of refractory ascites using nocturnal home hemodialysis. Semin Dial. 2008;21(4):367–70. Epub 2008/06/25.
36. Wong B, Zimmerman D, Reintjes F, Courtney M, Klarenbach S, Dowling G, et al. Procedure-related serious adverse events among home hemodialysis patients: a quality assurance perspective. Am J Kidney Dis. 2014;63(2):251–8. Epub 2013/09/03.
37. Heidenheim AP, Leitch R, Kortas C, Lindsay RM, London Daily/Nocturnal Hemodialysis Study. Patient monitoring in the London daily/nocturnal hemodialysis study. Am J Kidney Dis. 2003;42(Suppl 1):61–5. Epub 2003/06/28.
38. Suri RS, Larive B, Sherer S, Eggers P, Gassman J, James SH, et al. Risk of vascular access complications with frequent hemodialysis. J Am Soc Nephrol. 2013;24(3):498–505. Epub 2013/02/09.
39. van Loon MM, Goovaerts T, Kessels AG, van der Sande FM, Tordoir JH. Buttonhole needling of haemodialysis arteriovenous fistulae results in less complications and interventions compared to the rope-ladder technique. Nephrol Dial Transpl. 2010;25(1):225–30. Epub 2009/09/01.
40. Muir CA, Kotwal SS, Hawley CM, Polkinghorne K, Gallagher MP, Snelling P, et al. Buttonhole cannulation and clinical outcomes in a home hemodialysis cohort and systematic review. Clin J Am Soc Nephrol (CJASN). 2014;9(1):110–9. Epub 2013/12/29.
41. Macrae JM, Ahmed SB, Hemmelgarn BR, Alberta Kidney Disease Network. Arteriovenous fistula survival and needling technique: long-term results from a randomized buttonhole trial. Am J Kidney Dis. 2014;63(4):636–42. Epub 2013/11/19.
42. Spry L, Burkart JM, Holcroft C, Mortier L, Glickman JD. Anonymous survey among home hemodialysis patients and nursing staff regarding vascular access site use and care. Hemodial Int. 2014 (In press).
43. Pierratos A. Nocturnal home haemodialysis: an update on a 5-year experience. Nephrol Dial Transpl. 1999;14(12):2835–40. Epub 1999/11/26.
44. Hawley CM, Jeffries J, Nearhos J, Van Eps C. Complications of home hemodialysis. Hemodial Int. 2008;12(Suppl 1):21–5. Epub 2008/07/22.
45. Gotch FA. The current place of urea kinetic modelling with respect to different dialysis modalities. Nephrol Dial Transpl. 1998;13(Suppl 6):10–4. Epub 1998/08/27.
46. Flythe JE, Kimmel SE, Brunelli SM. Rapid fluid removal during dialysis is associated with cardiovascular morbidity and mortality. Kidney Int. 2011;79(2):250–7. Epub 2010/10/12.
47. Al-Hejaili F, Kortas C, Leitch R, Heidenheim AP, Clement L, Nesrallah G, et al. Nocturnal but not short hours quotidian hemodialysis requires an elevated dialysate calcium concentration. J Am Soc Nephrol. 14(9):2322–8. Epub 2003/08/26.
48. Lindsay RM, Alhejaili F, Nesrallah G, Leitch R, Clement L, Heidenheim AP, et al. Calcium and phosphate balance with quotidian hemodialysis. Am J Kidney Dis. 2003;42(Suppl 1):24–9. Epub 2003/06/28.
49. King RS, Glickman JD. Electrolyte management in frequent home hemodialysis. Semin Dial. 2010;23(6):571–4. Epub 2010/12/21.
50. Golper T. Patient education: can it maximize the success of therapy? Nephrol Dial Transpl. 2001;16(Suppl 7):20–4. Epub 2001/10/09.

Wearable Dialysis Devices

14

Andrew Davenport

14.1 Introduction

Cellular metabolism leads to the production of nitrogenous waste products which are transported out of cells through active or passive transport systems. These compounds may then circulate freely in plasma water, or bound to proteins and lipids. Although intermittent haemodialysis may effectively clear small water-soluble solutes from plasma water, the clearance of many of the nitrogenous waste products of metabolism is dependent on the rate of passage of solutes from intracellular compartment to extracellular compartment and the dynamic equilibrium between binding to proteins and lipids and the free plasma concentration. As such, a continuous dialysis modality would potentially prove to be a more effective treatment in clearing the waste products of cellular metabolism (Fig. 14.1). In addition, a continuous treatment modality would permit a slower ultrafiltration rate allowing patients to better tolerate fluid removal, so reducing the risk of treatment-associated hypotension and the potentially adverse effects of hypoperfusion on the heart and brain.

14.2 Historical Developments in Designing a Wearable Dialysis Device

Haemodialysis was originally restricted to patients with acute kidney injury due to the technical problems of obtaining vascular access, the limited availability of haemodialysis machines, clotting within the extracorporeal circuit and providing reliable quality dialysate. It was only when these hurdles were overcome in the mid-to-late 1960s that regular haemodialysis for patients with chronic kidney disease started to become an established treatment. However, it was soon appreciated that life-saving regular thrice-weekly therapy imposed numerous restrictions on patients' lifestyles, not only in terms of limiting dietary and fluid intake but also limiting the distance that a patient could live from a dialysis centre. As such, the concept of a wearable dialysis device is not new and dates back to the 1970s [1], but the technology at that time did not permit a solution.

The first step in developing a wearable device was to invent a portable haemodialysis machine, which could then allow patients to travel beyond their dialysis centre [2]. The first commercially available device, which could be transported in an automobile, was powered by rechargeable batteries and used a 20-L batch of fresh dialysate, which was then regenerated by passing the spent dialysate through a charcoal module [3]. These early pioneers reported successful treatment outcomes for a small number of patients treated with short daily treatment sessions of less than 2 h. However, the device weighed some 17 kg mainly due to the weight of the large rechargeable batteries and the blood and dialysate pumps, and then with the dialysate weighed around 40 kg [4]. After an initial wave of enthusiasm, the design team abandoned their project as they were unable to significantly reduce the weight and size of the haemodialysis machine [5].

The next major technological advance in the design for a wearable dialysis device followed advances in sorbent technology. Sorbents potentially allowed the regeneration of spent dialysate, so permitting effective dialysis without the constant need for a ready supply of fresh dialysate. Charcoal, although an effective adsorbent for many of the compounds which are retained in patients with chronic kidney disease, including β2 microglobulin, bilirubin, indoxyl sulphate, p-aminohippurate and 3-carboxy-4-methyl-5-propyl-2 furanpropionic acid, does not effectively bind urea. Thus alternative strategies were required to clear urea. One approach was to enzymatically degrade urea using urease which cleaves urea to produce ammonia and carbon dioxide. As ammonia is potentially toxic, any ammonia produced has to be removed before it can circulate back to the patient. This then led to the development of a layered sorbent system, as

A. Davenport (✉)
Royal Free Hospital, University College Medical School, Pew Street, London NW3 2QG, UK
e-mail: adavenport@nhs.org

A. K. Singh et al. (eds.), *Core Concepts in Dialysis and Continuous Therapies*, DOI 10.1007/978-1-4899-7657-4_14

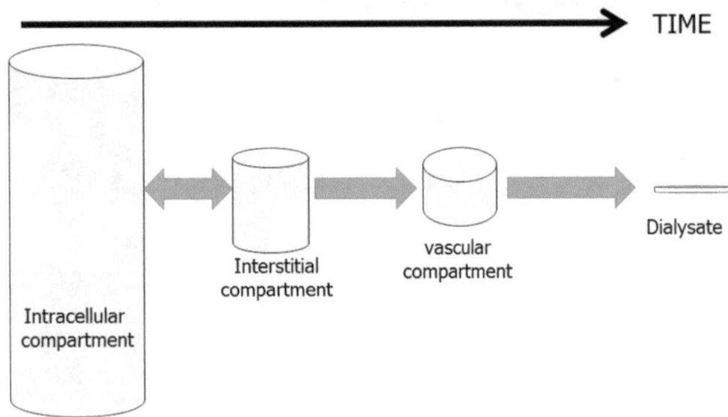

Fig. 14.1 The products of intracellular metabolism pass from the *intracellular compartment* into the extracellular space and into the plasma. Cartoon depicting the relative volume of distribution of azotaemic solutes, which would be more effectively cleared by continuous forms of dialysis

although activated carbon adsorbs compounds, other sorbents are essentially ionic exchangers, adsorbing some compounds but releasing others in exchange (Fig. 14.2). The Redy® system using this layered sorbent technology was commercially introduced into North America and Western Europe, and so permitted haemodialysis patients greater freedom to travel and dialyse away from home and dialysis centres [6].

The next wave of enthusiasm for developing wearable haemodialysis devices came following the introduction of haemofiltration. Improvements in dialyzer design and biomaterials now permitted patients to be treated by continuous ultrafiltration [7]. These early pioneering devices used the patient's native arterial pulse pressure to provide the hydrostatic pressure required for ultrafiltration, using either a Scribner shunt at the wrist (radial artery) or a Thomas shunt in the groin (femoral artery), with ultrafiltration simply controlled by manually adjusting a gate clamp. These simple experimental devices had many hurdles to overcome not only regulation of blood flow and ultrafiltration rates but also patient safety and as such were never commercially developed [7]. Although these wearable haemofiltration devices could successfully control fluid balance they could not satisfactorily control uraemia, as large volumes of ultrafiltrate were needed to obtain sufficient uraemic solute clearance, and this would then require the reinfusion of a corresponding amount of fresh replacement fluid to prevent volume depletion. Some designers tried to overcome this problem by recycling the spent ultrafiltrate through a sorbent cartridge and then returning the regenerated fluid back to the patient [8]. However, these designs then increased device complexity by adding a number of pumps, as blood flow had to be regulated to provide a controlled ultrafiltrate flow through the sorbents, and a continuous heparin infusion was required to prevent clotting in the extracorporeal circuit [8]. Although described as a wearable haemofiltration device by the inventors, this prototype was only used to treat two hospital inpatients. The sorbent cartridges based on the sorbent system used by the Redy® system quickly became saturated and had to be changed up to three or four times each day [9]. As such, this device was never commercially developed.

Newer dialysis machine developments based on a batch dialysate system either made from domestic water or using sterile bags of dialysate have been recently designed for the home haemodialysis market, such as the NxStage System 1 (NxStage Medical Inc, Lawrence, Massachusetts, USA)

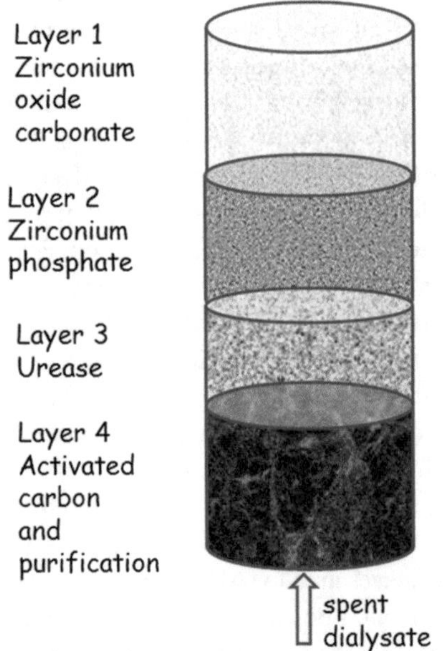

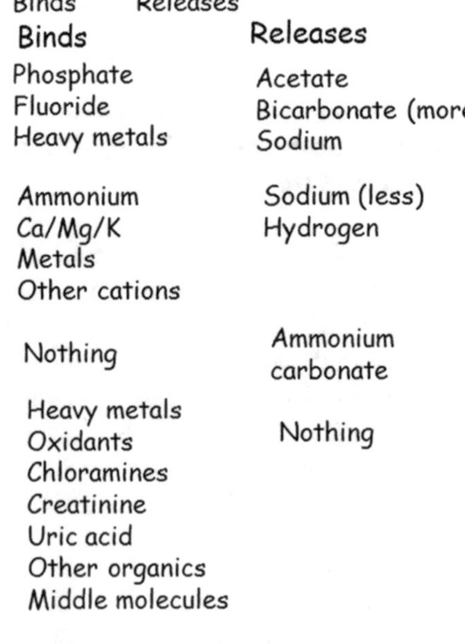

Binds Releases
Binds
Releases
Phosphate
Fluoride
Heavy metals
Acetate
Bicarbonate (more)
Sodium
Ammonium
Ca/Mg/K
Metals
Other cations
Sodium (less)
Hydrogen
Nothing
Ammonium carbonate
Heavy metals
Oxidants
Chloramines
Creatinine
Uric acid
Other organics
Middle molecules
Nothing

Fig. 14.2 Schematic representation of a sorbent cartridge depicting a specific sequence of sorbents

[10]. These machines allow patients to travel and dialyse in hotels and houses, but again patients essentially still require an automobile to pack the dialysis machine and bags of sterile dialysate.

Due to the technological challenges in developing a truly wearable hemodialysis device, there has been little progress until recently.

14.3 Current Approaches to Developing a Wearable Dialysis Device

14.3.1 Continuous Wearable Peritoneal Dialysis Devices

It could be argued that peritoneal dialysis (PD) is both a wearable and portable dialysis therapy. However, continuous ambulatory peritoneal dialysis (CAPD) typically requires three or four exchanges with fresh dialysate each day, and although automated cycler peritoneal dialysis (APD) typically allows the patient daytime freedom, the patient has to be connected to the machine overnight, and treatment requires the use and storage of relatively large volumes of fresh dialysate and then the disposal of spent dialysate and used consumables. As such, a number of designs have been proposed to develop a wearable PD system based on sorbent technology to regenerate spent dialysate effluent to limit additional fresh dialysate fluid exchanges.

The Vicenza group proposed a wearable artificial kidney (ViWAK) [11] which utilised a novel dual lumen peritoneal catheter so allowing a continuous flow of peritoneal dialysate into and out of the peritoneum driven by a small light weight battery powered mini-pump. The ViWAK was a relatively simple device, as it required the patient to start the day by instilling a fresh standard glucose-based dialysate, which was then left to dwell for 2 h. Thereafter the dialysate pump would start and peritoneal dialysate then continuously recycled with spent dialysate pumped first through a filter to remove proteins and prevent them coating the sorbents, and then a series of sorbent cartridges containing a mixture of microporous activated carbon and polystyrene resin. Then in the evening, the spent dialysate was to be drained out and a fresh 7.5 % icodextrin dialysate instilled for overnight dialysis. The system relied on residual renal function and the icodextrin exchange to achieve volume control. The inventors proposed that the device could potentially be modified to include a small pouch of glucose, which could then be added to the recycled dialysate to improve ultrafiltration [11]. As such, the proposed ViWAK required two standard CAPD exchanges each day compared to the conventional four.

Currently, the ViWAK has only been tested in short-term in vitro experiments and awaits animal and human clinical trials to determine the adsorptive capacity of the sorbents.

An alternative design based on peritoneal dialysis is the automated wearable artificial kidney (AWAK) which differs from the ViWAK in having a traditional single lumen peritoneal dialysis catheter. As dialysate flow is discontinuous with the AWAK, a reservoir is required to store regenerated dialysate before it is pumped back into the patient [12] (Fig. 14.3 and 14.4). In contrast to the ViWAK, the AWAK device is designed to continuously regenerate dialysate from a single standard glucose containing peritoneal dialysate for

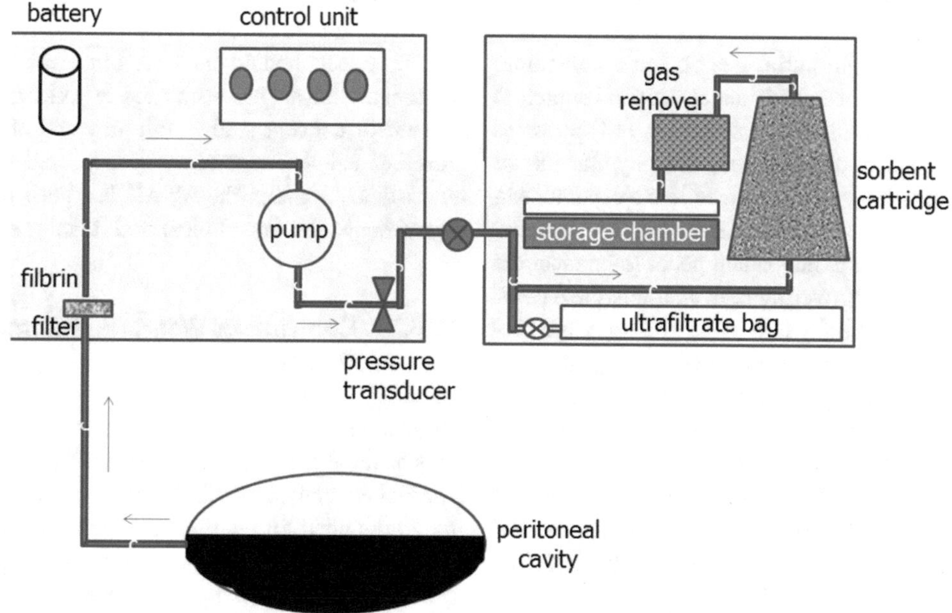

Fig. 14.3 Outflow circuit of the automated wearable artificial kidney (AWAK) peritoneal dialysis device

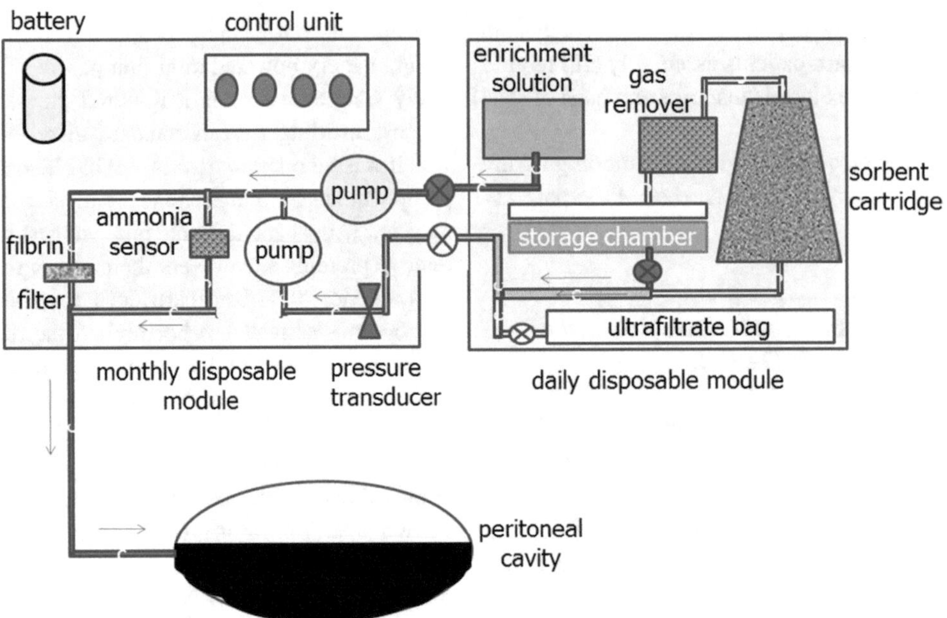

Fig. 14.4 Inflow circuit of the automated wearable artificial kidney (AWAK) peritoneal dialysis device

up to 1 month. As such the dialysate not only has to be recycled through a series of sorbents but also refreshed by adding glucose, bicarbonate and other electrolytes. Thus, the design is more complex than the ViWAK requiring an additional chamber containing electrolytes, lactate and glucose to refresh the regenerated dialysate. The sorbents contain urease to enzymatically degrade urea, then as ammoniais released the device requires a sensor to check that no ammonia is returned to the patient, and alarm to inform the patient that the sorbents have become saturated and need changing.

The AWAK differs from conventional peritoneal dialysis in that it is designed around a high-flow tidal peritoneal dialysis prescription, with an initial fresh glucose containing peritoneal dialysate fill of approximately 750 ml which is then recirculated in a tidal manner at 4.0 L/h [13] powered by a rechargeable battery driven pump, with any ultrafiltrate generated over an 8–10-h period drained into a separate bag attached to the daily exchangeable module (Fig. 14.3). As the battery requires recharging, the patient needs to connect the device to mains electricity overnight. In addition, the AWAK is designed to have both daily and monthly disposable sections, designed for ease of replacement (Fig. 14.4), with the daily replacement section containing the sorbents, reservoir, degassing unit and refreshing electrolyte/bicarbonate/glucose pouch. To change this section the patient would have to perform a standard drain out and then once re-inserted, start again instilling a fresh glucose-based dialysate. As such, if the sorbents had to be replaced twice or three times a day, then not only would there be the financial costs of replacing items, but in essence the patient would be performing three manual daytime exchanges and then overnight recharging the battery using mains electricity.

To put this into context, a healthy 70 kg dialysis patient would be expected to generate around 9–10 g of urea nitrogen daily when eating a recommended dietary protein intake of 1 g/kg [14]. Although urease and 250 g of zirconium can readily catalyze 2 g urea/h and adsorb ammonia released, this projected urea clearance would exhaust the sorbent combination within a day. As such, this would require either more sorbent with an increased weight, or more than one daily cartridge exchange. Thus the AWAK has been designed with two sorbent cartridges of different size: the smaller one designed to extract 3.5 g urea nitrogen and the larger one to remove 10 g urea nitrogen [15].

The concept behind the AWAK in terms of high-flow tidal peritoneal dialysis has been tried in patients for up to 5 h as a proof of concept study, with an extrapolated weekly Kt/Vurea of 3.4–4.5 depending upon patient transporter characteristics. Although the AWAK has been trialed in animal experiments, the first clinical trial remains awaited.

14.3.2 Continuous Wearable Haemodialysis Devices

The challenges to design and manufacture a wearable continuous haemodialysis device are somewhat similar to those for a peritoneal dialysis device but have two more complications due to the need for continuous blood access and prevention of clotting in the extracorporeal circuit. In the intensive care setting, continuous renal replacement therapy (CRRT) using slower blood and dialysate flows than standard intermittent haemodialysis can deliver both significantly higher small and middle molecular weight solute clearances.

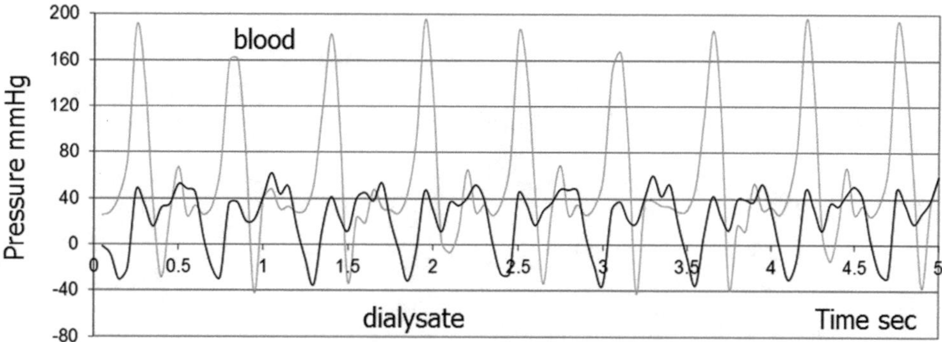

Fig. 14.5 Pressure wave profiles generated by the bellows mini-pump that powers blood and dialysate flow in the wearable artificial kidney (WAK) device

Two different approaches are currently at the design stage and undergoing trials. Firstly, a European consortium based in Holland using a simple modification of the CRRT circuit in which the ultrafiltrate is passed through a nanoporous biopolymer made from clay designed to absorb albumin bound toxins, and the 'cleaned' ultrafiltrate is then returned to the patient after a further mini-filter to ensure no sorbent microparticles pass back into the patient [16]. Potentially, some of the ultrafiltrate can be discarded to regulate hydration status. So far, this device has been used in a goat model of uraemia with short-term experimental results reporting a urea removal 10–15 mmol/h, creatinine 0.6 mmol/h, potassium 2.0 mmol/h and phosphate 0.75 mmol/h. Although effective, these preliminary data should be interpreted with caution, as removal rates are dependent upon serum concentrations, and protein caking of the dialyzer capillary fibres, and may also fall with time as sorbents become saturated. However, as this design has no dialysate and there is no replacement solution containing electrolytes or bicarbonate, then patients treated by such a device will most likely require additional bicarbonate supplementation to correct the metabolic acidosis of chronic kidney disease, and in addition may develop electrolyte imbalances due to differences in adsorption and release of cations by the sorbents. The current prototype does not have any separate ultrafiltration module, although this is anticipated in later designs. As yet this device has had limited testing in an animal model as a proof of concept trial, and will require additional animal model testing and require the addition of safety control features prior to human trials.

The other device, termed as wearable artificial kidney (WAK), was developed in Los Angeles and differred in a number of key issues. First, it employs a small, lightweight battery-powered pump that contains two chambers, so that when one is full the other is empty. This changes the pressure either side of the capillary fibre (Fig. 14.5), whereas with the conventional haemodialysis machine, roller blood pump design pressure is constant, and as such this novel pump design reduces protein deposition on the capillary surface so maintaining solute clearances over time [17]. Second, as the risk of clotting in the extracorporeal circuit is increased at blood–air interfaces, the arterial and venous reservoir and air-detector have been removed from the circuit and replaced by water impermeable but gas permeable plastic tubing to allow for the removal of carbon dioxide microbubbles, formed by the reversible reaction between bicarbonate and hydrogen ions and water and carbon dioxide, with the reaction equilibrium depending upon the pressure and temperature within the extracorporeal circuit. Similarly as urease is also used in the sorbent system, gas permeable plastic tubing is also used in the dialysate circuit again to remove carbon dioxide microbubbles. As the dialysate needs to be regenerated, then after passage through a series of sorbents the small volume of recirculating dialysate is 'refreshed' by the infusion of bicarbonate and electrolytes to correct metabolic acidosis and maintain electrolyte balance due to ion exchange with the sorbents (Fig. 14.6).

This device has been tested in the laboratory and in both animal experiments of acute kidney injury and also in dialysis dependent chronic kidney disease patients for up to 8 h [18]. These studies have shown that the small solute, urea and creatinine clearances were similar to those achieved by CRRT; however, the relative clearance of phosphate and beta 2 microglobulin were higher than anticipated, most likely due to the action of the pulsatile pump reducing protein deposition of the capillary dialyzer membrane [19]. Safety studies did not show any significant haemolysis with the novel blood/dialysate pump design. Similarly, the sorbents were not exhausted after 72 h in animals and after 8 h in humans. Unfractionated heparin was used to anticoagulated the WAK circuit and provided the systemic activated partial thromboplastin time was maintained > 60 s, no extracorporeal clotting was observed. However, it must be recognised that these are preliminary studies, and these encouraging results need to be confirmed in further longer duration clinical trials to determine the life expectancy of the sorbents and the frequency of sorbent exchange. In the long-term oral anticoagulants, either factor Xa or thrombin inhibitors may well be a better option than heparin, due to the individual

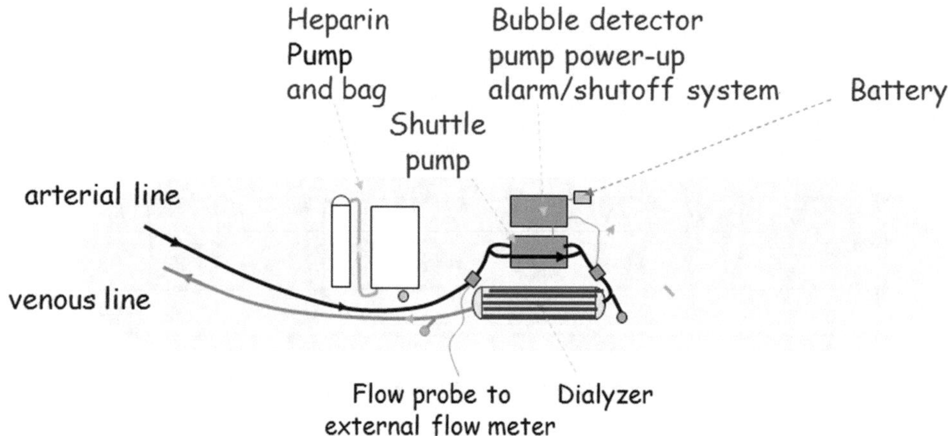

Fig. 14.6 Blood circuit diagram of wearable artificial kidney (WAK) showing micro-shuttle pump, refreshing electrolyte solution, heparin pump and ultrafiltration pump

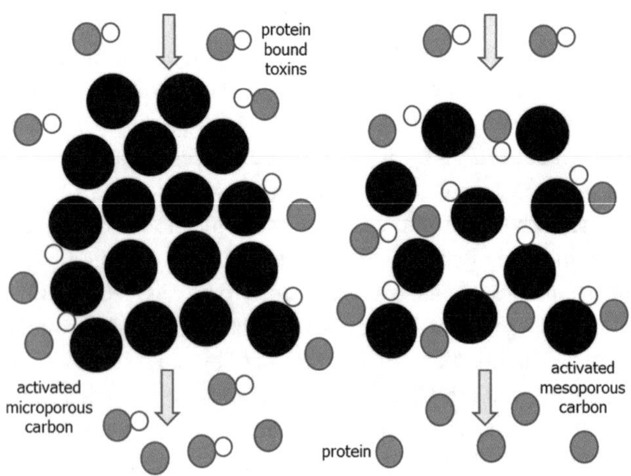

Fig. 14.7 Cartoon depicting the difference between micoporous activate carbon and mesoporous carbon in adsorbing protein bound toxins

sensitivity to unfractionated heparin and the potential side effects of long-term heparin exposure including osteoporosis and heparin induced thrombocytopaenia.

One problem with sorbents for wearable devices is balancing the amount and weight of sorbent against the duration of activity. More recently activated mesoporous carbon has been introduced as a sorbent. This differs from the traditional activated microporous carbon in that the pores are larger, and as such this allows proteins including albumin to permeate through the structure which not only increases the effective absorptive capacity by increasing relative surface area but also increases removal of protein bound azotaemic toxins (Fig. 14.7). Due to the rekindling of interest in sorbents [20], this has led to the design and creation of sorbents specifically targeting different solutes (Table 14.1). Traditional sorbents do not clear urea, and as such many devices have used enzymatic clearance. Although activated microporous carbons do not bind urea, some of the newer mesoporous carbons can bind urea, although this may be due to the mixer agents used to create the three-dimensional structure of the mesocarbon monoliths. Other approaches to remove urea include electro-oxidisation using carbon electrodes, although this process releases both carbon dioxide and chlorine, so requiring not only a degassing unit to remove carbon dioxide but also an additional carbon filter to remove chlorine.

Table 14.1 Specific sorbents designed to remove a target compound

Target for absorption	Sorbent composition
Phosphate	Ferric hydroxide-coated polymer
	Magnesium Ferrous hydrocalcite
Potassium	Sodium bentonite
Urea	Starch
	Ureases

14.4 Alternative Strategies to Wearable Dialysis Devices—Implantable Devices

14.4.1 The Implantable Artificial Kidney

A totally different approach is to try and design an artificial dialysis device based on the normal human kidney, with a filtration unit and then a tubular unit to process the ultrafiltrate. If such a device could be implanted inside a patient then potentially it could operate without the patient having to change sorbent cartridges, juggle with anticoagulant dosing and manage connection and disconnection problems and avoid the potential infection risks associated with central venous access catheters used by the external wearable haemodialysis devices and changing modules. Such a device could also be offered to a wider spectrum of patients than the wearable devices. However, to be successful not only has the device to provide adequate solute clearances and allow regulation of hydration status but also the lifespan of any such implantable artificial kidney device anastomosed to the iliac vessels and connected to the bladder would have to be of sufficient duration to overcome the disadvantages of replacement or subsequent removal of the whole system or parts of the device.

As an implantable device would use the patient's arterial pulse pressure to drive ultrafiltration, it requires no external pump or electrical supply. However, designing the vascular access then becomes the first hurdle in developing any implantable device. Whereas, synthetic arterial grafts have been a major clinical advance, both synthetic and vein grafts used for arterio-venous vascular access have had limited success in dialysis patients, due to venous stenoses and thrombosis. Preliminary in vivo animal studies using synthetic silicon darts inserted into pig femoral veins for vascular access darts led to the development of mural thrombi and adherent clot. However, this could be reduced by modifying the silicon surface of the dart with polyethylene glycol [21]. However, further extensive work is required before these vascular access devices could be used on humans.

The traditional dialyzer design would not be able to provide the ultrafiltration volume required to be an effective artificial glomerulus. As such the proposed artificial glomerulus has been designed with a nanotechnology produced silicon-based parallel multi-slit membrane, similar to street storm drain designed to remove flood water (Fig. 14.8) [22]. Nanotechnology manufacturing can reliably produce flat-sheet silicon wafer membranes with elongated 5–10 nm slit-shaped pores that in vitro and in vivo testing have matched predicted hydraulic permeability and steric and electrostatic hindrances [23].

However, this design, although very efficient at removing ultrafiltrate, poses the problem of haemoconcentration and deposition of plasma proteins at the dialyzer membrane surface, as such increasing protein deposition. Protein fouling of a biomaterial is a complex sequence of events resulting in soluble proteins being irreversibly deposited on the dialyzer membrane [24]. Although short-term in vitro studies have shown that modification of the silicon membrane with polyethylene glycol retained hydraulic permeability and sieving curves over 4 days, additional longer animal studies are required before this technology could be tried on humans, and it may well be that a different approach is required to achieve the longevity required of an implantable device.

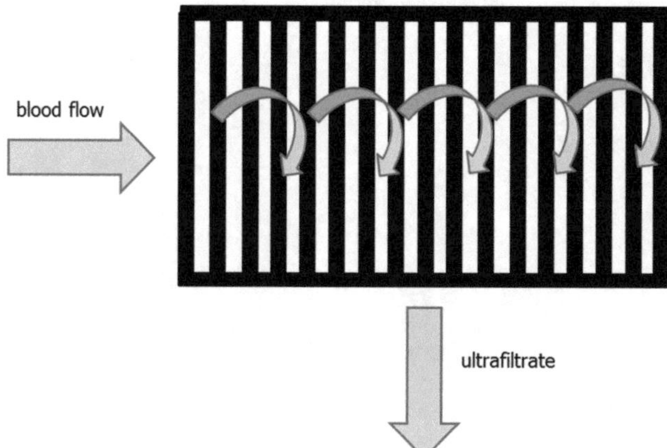

Fig. 14.8 Cartoon depicting the slit pore nanotechnology produced membranes that have designed for the artificial glomerulus for implantable dialysis devices

The normal kidney produces an ultrafiltrate of around 140 l/day, and as such any implantable artificial 'glomerular' device has to be linked to a 'tubule' device designed to reabsorb large volumes of ultrafiltrate, so that patients only pass 1–2 L of urine per day, yet excrete sufficient waste products to remain healthy. The reverse osmosis membrane used in conventional haemodialysis is designed to treat large volumes of fluid, and produce a much smaller volume or purified water. As such an artificial tubule could potentially be developed based on this design of a coiled membrane. However compared to the native renal tubule the key to any artificial device is whether it could differentiate between which solutes to reabsorb and which to excrete. Unfortunately such a design remains to be created. Another possibility for the future would be to design a renal tubule cell bioreactor, but this is some years away, as current devices are somewhat large and bulky and could not be implanted as yet [25]. As such a renal tubular-based bioreactor linked to a synthetic 'glomerular' membrane could potentially provide both the reabsorptive capacity for the ultrafiltrate as well as providing some additional tubular metabolic control.

14.5 Summary

Although haemodialysis has moved from an experimental treatment restricted to patients with acute kidney injury to one providing routine outpatient treatments to more than 2 million patients worldwide, the mortality of patients with chronic kidney disease remains unacceptably high. Daily and continuous dialysis treatments allow the potential for greater solute removal and better control of hydration and as such would be expected to provide not only improved patient survival but also better quality of life by allowing more liberal fluid and dietary intake.

The advent of nanotechnology manufacturing has allowed the development of wearable artificial kidney prototypes for the treatment of patients with CKD5d, with a number of devices based on current haemodialysis and peritoneal dialysis paradigms, and three devices currently planning clinical trials. Success of these devices will depend not only upon solute removal but also their ability to control electrolyte, acid–base and volume status on one hand, but equally important success will be judged on patient acceptance and in the current financial climate the cost per treatment. These newer treatment paradigms may well not be suitable for all chronic kidney disease patients, but could potentially offer more patients the advantage of both more frequent and longer dialysis treatments than current in-centre or satellite dialysis centre-based haemodialysis programs. On the other hand, looking further into the future implantable devices could potentially offer a treatment solution for the majority, and over the next few years, proof-of-concept experiments need to be performed to show the feasibility of such innovative renal replacement devices mirroring the native kidney.

As such, we are potentially at the start of a new era in the treatment of chronic kidney disease patients with new treatment paradigms on the horizon based on wearable and implantable devices that could not only potentially improve patient survival but also quality of life.

References

1. Lande AJ, Roberts M, Pecker EA (1977) In search of a 24 hours per day artificial kidney. J Dialysis. 1:805–23.
2. Jacobsen SC, Stephen RL, Bulloch EC, Luntz RD, Kolf WJ (1975) A wearable artificial kidney: functional description of hardware and clinical results. Proc Clin Dial Transplant Forum. 5:65–71.
3. Stephens RL, Jacobsen SC, Atkin-Thor E, Kolf WJ (1976) A portable wearable artificial kidney (WAK): initial evaluation. Proc Euro Dial Transplant Assoc. 12:511–18.
4. Kolff WJ, Jacobsen S, Stephen RL, Rose D (1976) Towards a wearable artificial kidney. Kidney Int. 7(suppl):S300–4.
5. Stephen RL, Kablitz C, Jacobsen S, Kolff WJ (1978) Combined technological clinical approach to wearable dialysis. Kidney Int suppl. 8:S125–32.
6. Blumenkrantz MJ, Gordon A, Roberts M, Lewin AJ, Pecker EA, Moran JK, Coburn JW, Maxwell MH (1979) Applications of the Redy sorbent system to hemodialysis and peritoneal dialysis. Artif Organs. 3(3):230–6.
7. Shaldon S, Beau MC, Deschodt G, Lysaght MJ, Ramperez P, Mion C (1980) Continuous ambulatory hemofiltration. Trans Am Soc Artif Intern Organs. 26:210–23.
8. Murisasco A, Baz M, Boobes Y, Bertocchio P, el Mehdi M, Durand C, Reynier JP, Ragon A (1986) A continuous hemofiltration system, using sorbents for hemofiltrate regeneration. Clin Nephrol. 26(Suppl. 1):S53–7.
9. Murisasco A, Reynier JP, Ragon A, Boobes Y, Baz M, Durand C, Bertocchio P, Agenet C, el Mehdi M (1986) Continuous arterio-venous hemofiltration in a wearable device to treat end-stage renal disease. Trans Am Soc Artif Intern Organs. 32:567–71.
10. Takahashi S (2012) Future home hemodialysis—advantages of the NxStage system one. Contrib Nephrol. 177:117–26.
11. Ronco C, Fecondini L (2007) The Vicenza wearable artificial kidney for peritoneal dialysis (ViWAK PD). Blood Purif. 25:383–8.
12. Roberts M, Ash SR, Lee DB (1999) Innovative peritoneal dialysis: flow-thru and dialysate regeneration. ASAIO J. 45(5):372–8.
13. Lee DBN, Roberts M (2008) A peritoneal based automated wearable artificial kidney. Clin Exper Nephrol. 12:171–80.
14. Maroni BJ, Steinman TI, Mitch WE (1985) A method for estimating nitrogen intake of patients with chronic renal failure. Kidney Int. 27:58–65.
15. Roberts M, Lee DBN (2006) Wearable artificial kidneys. A peritoneal dialysis approach. Dial Transplant. 36:780–2.
16. Wester M, Simonis F, Gerritsen KG, Boer WH, Wodzig WK, Kooman JP, Joles JA (2013) A regenerable potassium and phosphate sorbent system to enhance dialysis efficacy and device portability: an in vitro study. Nephrol Dial Transplant. 28(9):2364–71.
17. Gura V, Davenport A, Beizai M, Ezon C, Ronco C (2009) Beta 2-microglobulin and phosphate clearances using a wearable artificial kidney: a pilot study. Am J Kidney Dis. 54:104–11.
18. Davenport A, Gura V, Ronco C, Beizai M, Ezon C, Rambod E (2007) A wearable hemodialysis device for patients with end-stage renal failure: a pilot study. Lancet. 370:2005–10.
19. Gura V, Macy AS, Beizai M, Ezon C, Golper TA (2009) Technical breakthroughs in the wearable artificial kidney (WAK). Clin J Am Soc Nephrol. 4(9):1441–8.
20. Ash SR (2008) The Allient dialysis system. Semin Dial. 17:164–6.
21. Melvin ME, Fissell WH, Roy S, Brown DL (2010) Silicon induces minimal thrombo-inflammatory response during 28-Day intravascular implant testing. ASAIO J. 56:344–8.
22. Hofmann CL, Fissell WH (2010) Middle-molecule clearance at 20 and 35 ml/kg/h in continuous veno-venous haemodiafiltration. Blood Purif. 29:259–63.
23. Fissell WH, Dubnisheva A, Eldridge AN, Fleischman AJ, Zydney AL, Roy S (2009) High-performance silicon nanopore hemofiltration membranes. J Memb Sci. 326:58–63.
24. Holland NB, Qiu Y, Ruegsegger M, Marchant RE (1998) Biomimetic engineering of non-adhesive glycocalyx-like surfaces using oligosaccharide surfactant polymers. Nature. 392:799–801.
25. Fissell WH, Kimball J, MacKay SM, Funke A, Humes HD (2001) The role of a bioengineered artificial kidney in renal failure. Annals New York Acad Sci. 944:284–95.

Part III
Continuous Therapies

Continuous Renal Replacement Therapies (CRRT) Overview

15

Manoj Bhattarai, Ridhmi Rajapakase and Paul M. Palevsky

15.1 Introduction

Severe acute kidney injury (AKI) occurs in more than 5% of the critically ill patients and has been associated with mortality rates ranging from approximately 40% to more than 70% [1–6]. In the absence of specific pharmacologic interventions, the management of AKI is primarily supportive including optimization of volume status, treatment of electrolyte and acid–base disturbances, nutritional support, and adjustment in medication dosing. Renal replacement therapy (RRT) is often required as an adjunctive therapy, particularly when more conservative management is unable to prevent progressive volume overload and normalize electrolyte and acid–base disturbances or when AKI is prolonged and progressive azotemia or uremic manifestations supervene. Multiple modalities of RRT may be used in the management of critically ill patients with AKI including conventional intermittent hemodialysis (IHD), prolonged intermittent renal replacement therapy (PIRRT; also known as extended duration dialysis, EDD or sustained low-efficiency dialysis, SLED), peritoneal dialysis, and various modalities of continuous renal replacement therapy (CRRT). The modalities of CRRT provide extracorporeal blood purification with an intent to deliver uninterrupted therapy for 24 h a day. CRRT facilitates slow fluid removal and provides greater ability to maintain fluid balance in patients who require large daily fluid intake and provides more stable control of electrolyte and other solutes as compared to conventional IHD.

P. M. Palevsky (✉)
VA Pittsburgh Healthcare System, Mail Stop 111F-U, University Drive, Pittsburgh, PA 15240, USA
e-mail: palevsky@pitt.edu

M. Bhattarai · R. Rajapakase
University of Pittsburgh, A-915 Scaife Hall, 3550 Terrace Street, Pittsburgh, PA 15213, USA

15.2 History

Peter Kramer and colleagues published the initial description of continuous arteriovenous hemofiltration (CAVH) for the management of patients with oliguric AKI and volume overload in 1977 [7]. Their technique utilized an extracorporeal circuit with a hemofilter interposed between the femoral artery and vein to provide ultrafiltration (UF) and maintain biochemical balance [7–9]. Subsequently, Paganini and colleagues described a similar method for the performance of slow continuous ultrafiltration (SCUF) for the management of volume overload in oliguric patients [10]. Further description of clinical experience and operational characteristics by others including Luer et al. in 1983 [11], Kaplan et al. in 1984 [12], and Golper in 1985 [13] heralded wider adoption of CAVH. Relatively low rates of solute clearance, particularly in patients with high catabolic states, was a major limitation to CAVH and led to the use of counter-current dialysate flow to augment the clearance of urea and other small solutes in continuous arteriovenous hemodialysis (CAVHD) and continuous arteriovenous hemodiafiltration (CAVHDF) [14, 15]. However, these techniques could not overcome the disadvantages inherent to an arteriovenous (AV) circuit including dependence of blood flow on the pressure gradient between mean arterial pressure and central venous pressure, which limited flow, particularly in hypotensive and hemodynamically unstable patients, and complications related to prolonged arterial cannulation, including bleeding, thromboembolism, and infection. These inherent problems with the AV circuit led to the development of pumped venovenous (VV) systems [16–18]. The use of a VV circuit, however, sacrificed the technical simplicity of the AV system, necessitating the addition of air detectors and pressure monitors. While early VV circuits were cobbled together from individual components, progressive improvement in technology has yielded sophisticated machines with integrated blood and fluid pumps, pressure monitoring alarms, blood leak detectors, and UF controls to assure accurate fluid balance. With progressive advances in technology, CRRT has advanced

A. K. Singh et al. (eds.), *Core Concepts in Dialysis and Continuous Therapies,* DOI 10.1007/978-1-4899-7657-4_15

from a treatment used by a small number of innovators for the most desperately ill patients to a mainstream therapy that is widely used for the management of critically ill patients with AKI,

15.3 Modalities of Continuous Renal Replacement Therapy

CRRT is defined as any extracorporeal blood purification-technique intended to substitute for impaired kidney function that is designed to be utilized on a continuous (i.e., 24 h per day) basis. These modalities may be provided using either an AV or a VV extracorporeal circuit. In AV therapies, blood enters the extracorporeal circuit through a cannula in an artery, flows through the hemofilter/hemodialyzer driven by the pressure gradient between mean arterial pressure and central venous pressure, and is returned though a catheter in the femoral or central veins. In the VV therapies, vascular access is provided by a double-lumen catheter in the femoral or central veins, with pump-driven blood flow through the extracorporeal circuit. While the use of VV modalities require greater technical complexity, including blood pumps, pressure monitors, and return-line air detectors, the ability to provide higher blood flow rates independent of mean arterial blood pressure and avoidance of prolonged arterial cannulation has led to predominant use of these modalities [19].

Beginning in the mid-1990s, a standard terminology was developed to describe the multiple modalities of CRRT (Table 15.1) [20–22]. SCUF provides UF for the management of volume overload (Fig. 15.1). Since the UF rate does not exceed the refilling of the intravascular compartment from the interstitium, intravenous replacement fluids are not required. Although SCUF is effective for the management of volume overload, for example, in patients with decompensated heart failure, solute clearance rates are negligible and it is not suitable for the management of azotemia or the acid-base and electrolyte disturbances associated with kidney failure. In continuous hemofiltration (continuous arteriovenous hemofiltration, CAVH; continuous venovenous hemofiltration, CVVH), high-volume UF is performed at rates exceeding those needed for volume management and the excess ultrafiltrate is replaced intravenously with a balanced electrolyte solution (Fig. 15.2). Solute removal is primarily convective, with clearance rates of urea and other

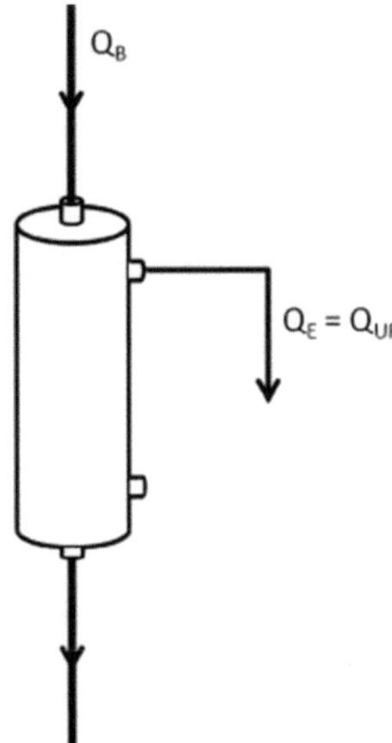

Fig. 15.1 Slow continuous ultrafiltration. Schematic diagram illustrating slow continuous ultrafiltration. Blood is shown flowing through a hollow-fiber hemofilter. An ultrafiltrate is generated at a rate equal to the rate of desired fluid loss and is discarded as effluent (Q_B blood flow, Q_E effluent flow, Q_{UF} ultrafiltrate flow)

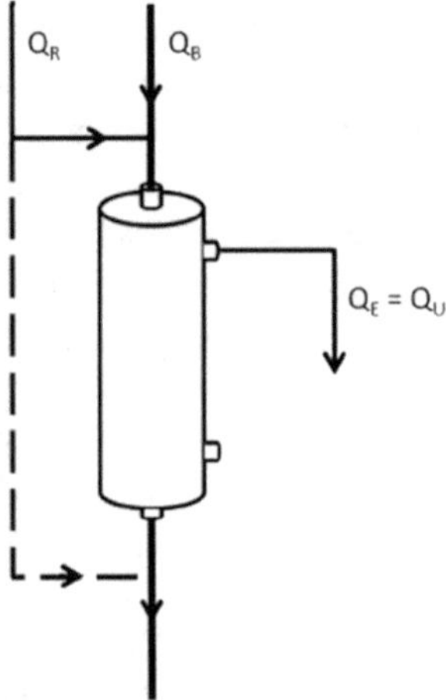

Fig. 15.2 Continuous hemofiltration. Schematic diagram illustrating continuous hemofiltration. Blood is shown flowing through a hollow-fiber hemofilter. An ultrafiltrate is generated at a rate which exceeds the desired rate of net fluid loss. Intravenous fluid is administered either prior to the hemofilter *(solid line)* or after the hemofilter *(dashed line)* to replace the volume of ultrafiltrate that exceeds the desired net fluid loss. The effluent volume is equal to the ultrafiltration rate (Q_B blood flow, Q_E effluent flow, Q_{UF} ultrafiltrate flow, Q_R replacement fluid)

Table 15.1 Modalities of continuous renal replacement therapy

Modality	Volume management	Solute clearance	Replacement fluids	Dialysate
Slow continuous ultrafiltration (SCUF)	Yes	Minimal	No	No
Continuous hemofiltration (CAVH, CVVH)	Yes	Yes	Yes	No
Continuous hemodialysis (CAVHD, CVVHD)	Yes	Yes	No	Yes
Continuous hemodiafiltration (CAVHDF, CVVHDF)	Yes	Yes	Yes	Yes

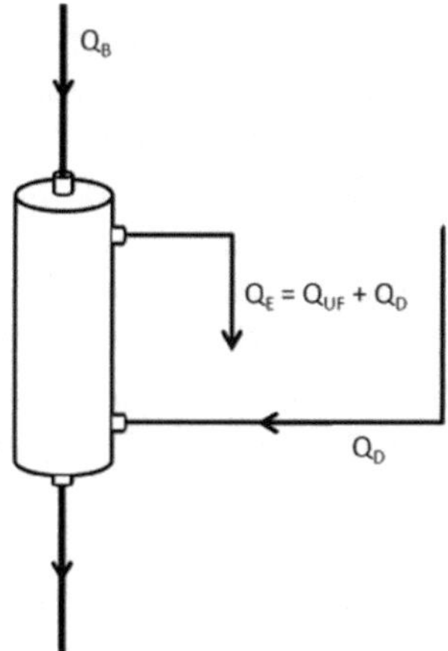

Fig. 15.3 Continuous hemodialysis. Schematic diagram illustrating continuous hemofiltration. Blood is shown flowing through a hollow-fiber hemodialyzer. Dialysate is perfused through the ultrafiltrate compartment countercurrent to the direction of flood flow. Ultrafiltration occurs at the rate desired for net negative fluid balance. The effluent volume is equal to the rate of dialysate flow plus the ultrafiltration rate (Q_B blood flow, Q_E effluent flow, Q_{UF} ultrafiltrate flow, Q_D dialysate)

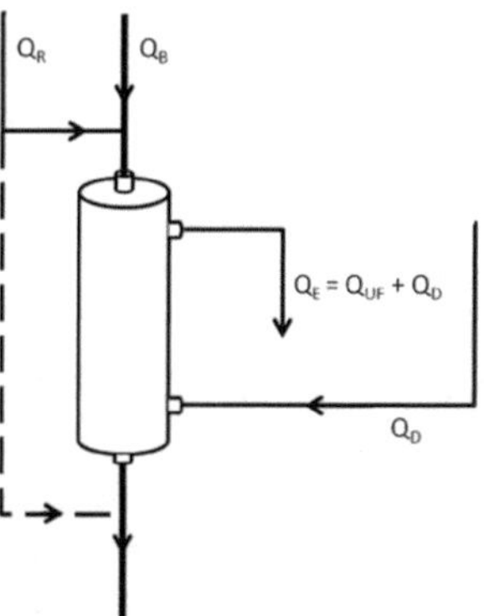

Fig. 15.4 Continuous hemodiafiltration. Schematic diagram illustrating continuous hemodiafiltration. Blood is shown flowing through a hollow-fiber hemodiafilter. Dialysate is perfused through the ultrafiltrate compartment countercurrent to the direction of flood flow. An ultrafiltrate is generated at a rate which exceeds the desired rate of net fluid loss. Intravenous fluid is administered either prior to the hemofilter *(solid line)* or after the hemofilter *(dashed line)* to replace the volume of ultrafiltrate that exceeds the desired net fluid loss. The effluent volume is equal to the rate of dialysate flow plus the ultrafiltration rate (Q_B blood flow, Q_E effluent flow, Q_{UF} ultrafiltrate flow, Q_R replacement fluid, Q_D dialysate)

small solutes proportional to the total UF rate. In continuous hemodialysis (continuous arteriovenous hemodialysis, CAVHD; continuous venovenous hemodialysis, CVVHD), dialysate is perfused across the opposite side of the membrane from the blood and solutes are removed primarily by diffusion down a concentration gradient (Fig. 15.3). As in SCUF, UF is limited to the rate necessary for the optimization of volume status and intravenous replacement fluids are not required. Continuous hemodiafiltration (continuous arteriovenous hemodiafiltration, CAVHDF; continuous venovenous hemodiafiltration, CVVHDF) combines the convective solute removal of continuous hemofiltration with the diffusive solute removal of continuous hemodialysis (Fig. 15.4). Dialysate is perfused through the hemodiafilter on the opposite side of the membrane from the blood, permitting diffusion of low-molecular-weight solutes while high-volume UF is performed to provide convective solute removal, with the ultrafiltrate volume exceeding the desired rate of volume removal replaced intravenously with a balanced electrolyte solution.

15.4 Mechanisms of Solute Removal During CRRT

RRT involves the transfer of fluid and solutes across a semipermeable membrane. Although fluid and solute flux is predominantly from the blood into the dialysate/ultrafiltrate compartment, diffusion and backfiltration from the dialysate/ultrafiltrate compartment may occur. In the modalities of CRRT, UF of fluid is driven by hydrostatic pressure across the hemodialysis/hemofilter membrane and solute removal occurs via diffusion, convection, or a combination.

15.4.1 Ultrafiltration

Ultrafiltration (UF) describes the removal of plasma water across a semipermeable membrane driven by a transmembrane pressure gradient (TMP). The ultrafiltration rate (Q_{UF}) is determined by the product of the hydraulic permeability of the membrane (K_M), the membrane surface area (A), and the transmembrane pressure gradient (TMP).

$$Q_{UF} = K_M \times A \times TMP.$$

The transmembrane pressure is the difference between the driving effect of hydrostatic pressure (ΔP) and restraining effect from the oncotic pressure (Π) generated by plasma proteins (since the ultrafiltrate is essentially protein free, the oncotic pressure of the ultrafiltrate is considered to be zero).

$$TMP = \Delta P - \Pi$$

In the AV modalities of CRRT, blood flow rates and the transmembrane hydrostatic pressure were relatively low. As UF occurred over the length of the hemofilter, the oncotic pressure in the blood compartment increased, providing a significant restraining effect on UF, occasionally to the point where $\Pi \approx \Delta P$ and further UF ceased. In the pump-driven VV modalities of CRRT, the blood flow rate and ΔP are sufficiently high that oncotic pressure is of little consequence as a determinant of UF.

15.4.2 Diffusion

Diffusion is the movement of solutes in solution from a region of higher concentration to a region of lower concentration. During dialytic therapies, diffusive clearance occurs when there is a concentration gradient between the blood and dialysate across the semipermeable dialysis membrane. The diffusive flux of a given solute (J_D) is a function of membrane characteristics including surface area (A) and thickness (Δx), the diffusion coefficient of solute (K_D), and the solute concentration between the blood and dialysate compartments (ΔC), and can be expressed as:

$$J_D = K_D \times A \times \left(\frac{\Delta C}{\Delta x}\right).$$

In order to maximize the concentration gradient between the blood and dialysate compartments, dialysate is commonly run countercurrent to the direction of blood flow on the opposite side of the membrane. As solutes diffuse from blood into dialysate, the solute concentration in the blood decreases while the corresponding concentration in the dialysate increases. By maintaining countercurrent flow, the concentration gradient is maximized along the length of the dialysis membrane. The diffusivity of a given solute is inversely related to its molecular weight. Thus, diffusive therapies, such as continuous hemodialysis (CHD), are more efficient in clearing low-molecular-weight solutes (<500 Da), such as urea and creatinine, as compared to higher molecular weight solutes (>1500 Da), such as β_2-microglobulin and cytokines.

15.4.3 Convection

Convection is the bulk flow of solute across a semipermeable membrane as the result of solvent flux across the membrane. During UF, solutes are entrained in the flow of plasma water across the dialysis membrane, a process referred to as "solvent drag." Solute flux is therefore dependent upon the net flux of solvent across the membrane (ultrafiltration rate, Q_{UF}) and is independent of the concentration gradient across the membrane. The ability of a given solute to cross a semipermeable membrane by convection is a function of the charge and molecular radius of the solute and the structure of the pores in the membrane. Thus, in contrast to diffusion, the relative clearance of lower- and higher molecular weight solutes are similar; with restriction in convective flux only as the solute's molecular radius approaches the effective size of the pores in the membrane.

The ability of a solute to cross a membrane by convection is quantified by the membrane reflection coefficient, σ, with values ranging from 0, for solutes that are not restricted by the membrane, to 1, for solutes that are unable to cross the membrane. In clinical practice, however, it is more common to express the ability of solutes to cross the membrane by convection in terms of the sieving coefficient (S), which is equal to $1-\sigma$ and can be readily calculated from the ratio of solute concentration in the ultrafiltrate (C_{UF}) and blood (C_B):

$$S = \frac{C_{UF}}{C_B}.$$

The membrane's sieving coefficient for a specific solute may decline over the duration of treatment. Plasma proteins, which are too large to cross the membrane, accumulate along the membrane surface, a phenomenon known as protein concentration polarization. This accumulation of proteins along the membrane surface may restrict access to membrane pores and alter the charge characteristics of the membrane surface [23].

The convective flux (J_C) of a solute is expressed as the product of the ultrafiltration rate (Q_{UF}), the concentration of the solute in the blood (C_B) and the membrane's sieving coefficient for the solute (S):

$$J_C = Q_{UF} \times C_B \times S.$$

Since convective clearance (K_C) is equal to convective solute flux divided by the solute concentration in blood (J_C/C_B), convective clearance of a solute can be expressed as the product of the UF rate and the sieving coefficient:

$$K_C = Q_{UF} \times S.$$

For low-molecular-weight solutes such as urea, S is approximately unity. Thus, convective clearance for these solutes approximates the UF rate.

Theoretically, the biophysical mechanisms of solute transport in each of the different modalities of CRRT should result in different solute clearance profiles. Continuous hemofiltration, a predominantly convective therapy, should provide more efficient removal of higher molecular weight species than continuous hemodialysis, a predominantly diffusive therapy. The clinical relevance of this is, however, uncertain, as clinical outcomes with hemofiltration and hemodialysis are similar [24]. Filtration and backfiltration occurring over the length of the dialysis membrane during continuous hemodialysis, particularly when very high-flux membranes are used, can result in significant unmeasured convection within the hemodialyzer, augmenting the amount of convective clearance during the predominantly diffusive therapy [25] .

15.5 Calculation of Solute Clearance

Solute clearance during extracorporeal RRT can be calculated based on either the disappearance of solute from the blood or from its appearance in the effluent. Since during continuous hemodialysis, the dialysate flow rate is usually substantially less than the blood flow rate and during hemofiltration the solute concentration in the ultrafiltrate is similar to that in plasma water, the change in solute concentration over the length of the hemodialyzer/hemofilter tends to be small. As a result, solute clearance (K) during CRRT is most commonly calculated based on solute appearance in the hemofilter/hemodialyzer effluent [26], expressed as:

$$K = \frac{[(Q_E \times C_E) - (Q_D \times C_D)]}{C_B},$$

where Q_E and Q_D are the effluent outflow and dialysate inflow rates, respectively, and C_E, C_D, and C_B are the solute concentrations in effluent, dialysate, and blood, respectively. Since the ultrafiltration rate (Q_{UF}) is equal to the difference between the effluent outflow rate and dialysate inflow rate ($Q_{UF} = Q_E - Q_D$), the calculation of solute clearance may be rewritten as:

$$K = \frac{Q_{UF} \times C_E}{C_B} + \frac{Q_D \times (C_E - C_D)}{C_B}.$$

Since, when there is no dialysate flow, $Q_E = Q_{UF}$ and C_E/C_B is equal to the sieving coefficient (S), the first term of this equation may be rewritten as $Q_{UF} \times S$, which represents the convective component of solute clearance (K_C). The second term of the equation, $Q_D \times (C_E - C_D)/C_B$, represents the solute clearance that would occur in the absence of UF and can be considered to represent the diffusive component of clearance (neglecting any convective flux resulting from filtration/backfiltration over the length of the hemofilter/hemodialyzer). For solutes that are not present in dialysate ($C_D = 0$), this term simplifies to $Q_D \times C_E/C_B$, where C_E/C_B represents the degree of solute equilibration between blood and dialysate. Thus, similar to convective clearance, diffusive clearance can be considered to be approximated by the product of the dialysate flow rate times and fractional equilibration of solute between blood and dialysate

15.5.1 Determinants of Convective Clearance

As previously discussed, solute clearance in continuous hemofiltration is equal to the product of the UF rate and sieving coefficient. For solutes with relatively low molecular weights, such as urea, sieving coefficients are approximately unity and solute clearance is equal to the UF or effluent flow rate [27, 28]. For higher molecular weight solutes, a more complex relationship may be observed. For example, the sieving coefficient for β-2 microglobulin is less than one but increases with increasing UF rate, resulting in a nonlinear increase in clearance with increasing effluent flow [27, 28]. The mechanism for this phenomenon is incompletely understood. Higher transmembrane pressure required to augment UF rates may result in recruitment of additional pores and/or changes in pore geometry allowing for the increase in sieving coefficient. Solute concentration polarization may also contribute to the augmentation of convective flux.

Blood flow rate and membrane surface area are of secondary importance in determining convective clearance. Increasing UF at a constant blood flow rate increases the fraction of plasma water removed, resulting in hemoconcentration of cells and plasma proteins, increasing the viscosity of the blood exiting the hemofilter. This filtration fraction (FF) can be calculated as the ratio of UF rate to plasma water, expressed as:

$$FF = \frac{Q_{UF}}{[Q_B \times (1 - Hct)]},$$

where Q_{UF} is the ultrafiltration rate, Q_B is the blood flow rate, and Hct is the patient's hematocrit. Optimally, the FF should be maintained <0.2; values exceeding 0.3 are associated with decreased hemofilter longevity [29]. FF may be minimized by increasing blood flow rate or by administering replacement fluid prior to the hemofilter. This latter strategy, while minimizing FF, decreases the concentration of solutes entering the hemofilter resulting in a lower solute concentration in the ultrafiltrate. The effective clearance (K_{eff}) is thus reduced by the ratio of the blood flow rate to the sum of the blood flow rate and prefilter replacement fluid (Q_R):

$$K_{eff} = Q_{UF} \times S \times \left[\frac{Q_B}{(Q_B + Q_R)}\right].$$

The characteristics of the hemofilter membrane determine the sieving coefficient for a given solute. Increasing the membrane surface area for a given membrane increases the hydraulic permeability and, hence, the maximal achievable UF rate. Thus, increasing membrane size allows for increased UF and increased clearance; however, if blood flow remains constant, this is at the expense of an increased UF rate. If UF is held constant, increasing the hemofilter surface area will have no effect on convective clearance.

15.5.2 Determinants of Diffusive Clearance

In conventional IHD, the dialysate flow rate usually exceeds blood flow rate and diffusive equilibration of solute between blood and dialysate is therefore incomplete. In contrast, during continuous hemodialysis, the blood flow rates utilized generally exceed dialysate flow allowing for near equilibration between blood and dialysate ($C_D/C_B \sim 1$) for low-molecular-weight solutes (<500−1500 Da) such as urea [27]. If blood flow rate is held constant, as dialysate flow rate increases the degree of equilibration between blood and dialysate tends to fall [27]. For example, at a blood flow rate of 150 mL/min and a dialysate flow of 16.7 mL/min (1 L/h) equilibration of both urea and uric acid was essentially complete; when dialysate flow was increased to 41.7 mL/min (2.5 L/h) the fractional equilibration of urea decreased to 0.96 and fractional equilibration of uric acid decreased to 0.76 [27]. Despite this decline in equilibration between blood and dialysate, dialysate flow is the major determinant of low-molecular-weight solute clearance. Higher molecular weight solutes, such as β-2 microglobulin, are poorly cleared by diffusion and exhibit minimal dependence of dialysate flow [27]. It is likely that the clearance of these higher molecular weight solutes during continuous hemodialysis is the result of convective flux provided by unmeasured filtration/backfiltration within the hemodialyzer [25, 30]. This conjecture is supported by the observed lack of augmentation of clearance when diffusive therapy is added to convection in CVVHDF [28].

Unlike conventional IHD, under the operational conditions used during continuous hemodialysis and hemodiafiltration, diffusive clearance exhibits only minimal dependence on blood flow, so long as the blood flow rate is more than 3–5 times the dialysate flow rate [26, 31]. If solute equilibration between blood and dialysate is complete, increasing the surface area of the dialysis membrane will not augment clearance; however, if equilibration is incomplete, increasing the membrane surface may permit more complete equilibration and higher clearance rates.

15.5.3 Interaction Between Diffusive and Convective Clearance

Although in the discussion above, diffusion and convection were treated as independent processes, the overall clearance during hemodiafiltration may be less than the arithmetic sum of the clearances when dialysis (diffusive clearance) and hemofiltration (convective clearance) are performed separately [32, 33]. The magnitude of this interaction is related to the UF rate. When there is low convective flux minimal interaction is observed [26]; however, when higher UF rates are employed observed clearances during hemodiafiltration are less than predicted from the individual components of therapy [27, 30].

15.6 CRRT Extracorporeal Circuit

At a minimum, the extracorporeal circuit for CRRT consists of a vascular access which permits sufficient blood flow from and back to the patient, the hemofilter/hemodialyzer, and pumps to regulate the UF rate, replacement fluid administration and/or dialysate inflow. In the AV therapies, the driving force for flow through the circuit is the pressure gradient between the mean arterial pressure and central venous pressure. In order to maximize flow, the resistance of the circuit needs to be minimized. The caliber of the catheters used for arterial and venous access need to be as large as the cannulated vessels will permit, their lengths should be relatively short to minimize resistance to flow and the overall extracorporeal circuit length should be kept as short as possible. Since the hemofilter/hemodialyzer represents the major site of resistance in the AV circuit, hemofilter/hemodialyzer configuration has a major effect on circuit function. Optimization of flow is provided by using hollow-fiber hemofilters/hemodialyzers with a large cross-sectional area and short axial length [34]. Increasing the diameter of the individual fibers decreases resistance, although at the expense of diminished effective surface area per unit volume of blood [34]. It has been suggested that the use of parallel plate hemodialyzers enhances diffusive clearance in CAVHD as compared to hollow-fiber dialyzers of equivalent surface area [35]. In the absence of a blood pump, pressure monitors and air detectors are generally not used in AV circuits.

Many of the considerations for optimization of AV circuits do not pertain to VV CRRT circuits. While the overall length of the VV CRRT circuit should not be excessive, there is not the same critical need for minimization and the tubing length should be sufficient to position the CRRT equipment without hindering patient access. Similarly, the need to minimize resistance to flow within the hemofilter/hemodialyzer does not pertain, and standard hemodialyzer configurations can be used. However, the use of a blood pump mandates the presence of an air detector with an integrated blood pump shutoff on the return line to minimize the risk of air embolization. The use of a pumped system also requires the use of pressure monitors to assess circuit patency, at a minimum on the inflow line, between the catheter and the blood pump, and on the return line, between the hemofilter/hemodialyzer and the catheter. Given the higher UF rates that can be achieved with pumped VV therapies, most VV therapies are now provided using dedicated equipment with fluid balancing capability to match dialysate and/or replacement fluid flow rates to effluent flow, thereby providing control of net fluid balance [36] .

15.6.1 Vascular Access

Wide-bore arterial and venous catheters are the most common vascular access for AV CRRT [37]. Historically, AV (Scribner) shunts were also used; however, catheters generally provided higher blood flow rates, especially in the setting of hypotension [38]. Since it is readily cannulated and provides high blood flow rates, the femoral artery is the most common site for arterial access; however, the brachial and axillary arteries in the upper limb and more distal vessels in both the upper and lower limbs may also be used. In order to optimize flow, the arterial catheter should be non-tapered with a single end-hole and should be of the largest diameter that the vessel can accommodate, preferably no smaller than 8 French [37]. Venous return can be through the femoral, subclavian, or internal jugular veins. The venous catheter should be relatively short, non-tapered with as large an internal diameter as feasible in order to minimize resistance to flow. The use of AV access, primarily the need for prolonged arterial cannulation with a large-bore catheter, is associated with more frequent and serious complications than seen with the VV therapies [39]. The major complications include bleeding, thromboembolism with distal limb ischemia, arterial aneurysms, or AV fistulas at the site of cannulation and infection. Caution must be used, particularly in patients with underlying peripheral vascular disease, to ensure that the arterial catheter does not compromise distal circulation. The catheter site and distal extremity must be monitored closely for evidence of infection or vascular injury while the catheter remains in place. The arterial catheter should be removed as soon as possible once treatment can be terminated. Anticoagulation should be reversed prior to removing the catheter and prolonged pressure applied after removal in order to assure adequate hemostasis.

Access for VV therapies may be obtained by placement of two separate single-lumen venous catheters, or more commonly, by the use of a standard double-lumen dialysis catheter. The KDIGO Clinical Practice Guideline for Acute Kidney Injury recommend the right jugular vein as the most optimal site for catheter placement, followed by the femoral veins, left internal jugular vein, and lastly the subclavian veins, with preference for placement on the dominant side [40]. The preference for the right internal jugular vein is based on lower rates of catheter dysfunction based on venous anatomy as compared to the left internal jugular vein [41]. There is a general preference for catheters above the waist as compared to catheters in the femoral veins due to increased risk of infection; however, in a randomized trial of 750 patients requiring dialysis for AKI the incidence of catheter-related blood stream infection was not higher in patients with femoral catheters [42]. Although subclavian catheters are associated with the lowest rate of infectious complications [43], they may result in the development of central venous stenosis which may complicate long-term vascular access in patients who do not recover kidney function and remain dialysis dependent [40, 44].

Ultrasound guidance during catheter insertion is recommended, particularly for insertion of catheters into the jugular veins [40, 45, 46]. A chest radiograph should be obtained to confirm position of internal jugular and subclavian catheters prior to initial use [40]. Catheter position is important for optimization of catheter function. Depending on the specific catheter used, the catheter tip should either be at the junction of the superior vena cava and the right atrium or in the right atrium. When catheters are placed in the femoral position, the longest available catheter should be used so that the tip of the catheter is in the inferior vena cava. Aseptic techniques should be used during catheter insertion and during catheter care so as to minimize the risk of infection and use of the catheter should be restricted to dialytic therapies. Tunneled dialysis catheters can be used for CRRT, but are not recommended as the initial vascular access for most patients with AKI given an average duration of RRT of less than 2 weeks [40]. In patients with end-stage renal disease who require CRRT in the setting of critical illness, it is generally not recommended to use an existing AV fistula or graft for CRRT access given the risks of dislodgement or infiltration of rigid fistula needles during the course of care during prolonged therapy [47].

15.6.2 Hemofilter/Hemodialyzer

The membranes used for continuous hemofiltration must have a high hydraulic permeability in order to permit sufficient UF without necessitating excessive transmembrane pressure. This is in contrast to the membrane characteristics required for continuous hemodialysis, in which high UF rates are not required. The critical characteristic of a membrane used for continuous hemodialysis is its coefficient of diffusion, which is related to its composition, thickness, and surface area. While commercially available membranes are generally suitable for both hemofiltration and hemodialysis, some membranes that are optimized for convective therapy may provide inadequate diffusive clearance [31]. Although there has been controversy in the past regarding the effect of membrane biocompatibility on recovery of kidney function in AKI [48–53], the clinical relevance of this controversy is relatively limited given the wide availability of biocompatible synthetic membranes. The KDIGO Clinical Practice Guideline for Acute Kidney Injury recommends the use of biocompatible synthetic membranes over cellulosic membranes for CRRT and other modalities of extracorporeal RRT in patients with AKI [40].

15.6.3 Pumps and Safety Monitors

Initial descriptions of pumped VV CRRT generally used a combination of a peristaltic blood pump to provide blood flow and volumetric infusion pumps to regulate flow of dialysate, replacement fluid, and effluent. Oftentimes, pressure monitors were not used and the only safety monitor was an air detector on the venous return line. In addition, UF control was relatively poor as the linear peristaltic pumps used to regulate fluids and UF were not designed to operate against significant pressure gradients and were often prone to errors [54]. These improvised systems have been supplanted by integrated machines specifically designed for the performance of CRRT that are equipped with fluid-balancing technology to ensure delivery of the prescribed fluid management and integrated safety alarms, including air detectors and pressure monitors [36]. The equipment varies by manufacturer, with some machines capable of all modalities of VV CRRT while other machines can only provide continuous hemodialysis or hemodiafiltration but cannot provide hemodiafiltration.

15.7 Dialysate and Replacement Fluids

The use of dialysate and/or intravenous replacement solutions will depend on the modality of CRRT employed. In continuous hemofiltration, intravenous replacement fluids are administered to replace ultrafiltrate losses that exceed desired net fluid loss. In continuous hemodialysis, dialysate is perfused through the dialysate compartment of the hemodialyzer as in conventional IHD to provide diffusive clearance. In continuous hemodiafiltration, both dialysate and replacement fluids are utilized.

The compositions of dialysate and replacement fluid are similar; both should have an electrolyte composition similar to that of plasma, although often with lower potassium and higher buffer concentrations to permit correction of hyperkalemia and metabolic acidosis. The glucose concentration can vary; although some treatment protocols call for glucose-free solutions, most regimens use physiologic concentrations of approximately 100 mg/dL. Use of supraphysiologic glucose concentrations will result in glucose loading and may contribute to hyperglycemia. The concentration of calcium and magnesium are usually at physiologic to slightly supraphysiologic levels, with the exception that low or calcium-free solutions are often used in conjunction with citrate anticoagulation (see below). Most CRRT fluids contain no phosphate; although there is the potential for calcium phosphate deposition when phosphate is added to solutions containing calcium, stability has been demonstrated with phosphate concentrations of up to 1.2 mmol/L [55]. The addition of phosphate can prevent the development of hypophosphatemia and obviate the need for intravenous phosphate supplementation.

Various buffers have been used in fluids for CRRT including lactate, acetate, and bicarbonate. In the past, bicarbonate-buffered solutions could not be stored for prolonged periods of time and bicarbonate-buffered solutions for CRRT not were commercially available. The available solutions were buffered with either sodium lactate or sodium acetate, both of which are rapidly metabolized to bicarbonate. When lactate-buffered solutions were used as dialysate or replacement fluid during CRRT, infusion rates could exceed metabolic clearance and modest elevations in blood lactate levels were common, although marked elevations were generally seen only in patients with underlying lactic acidosis or impaired hepatic metabolism [56–58]. Whether or not the modest elevations in lactate levels seen in most patients were associated with increased morbidity is not clear. Elevations in blood lactate and alterations in the pyruvate:lactate ratio are associated with increased protein catabolism and may contribute to myocardial depression. Several studies suggested that lactate-buffered fluids were less effective for controlling metabolic acidosis and were associated with increased hemodynamic instability as compared to bicarbonate-buffered fluids [59–61]. The KDIGO Clinical Practice Guideline for Acute Kidney Injury suggests that bicarbonate-buffered fluids be used rather than lactate-buffered solutions [40]. With the current ready availability of commercially prepared bicarbonate buffered fluids, these have generally replaced the use of acetate- and lactate-buffered CRRT solutions.

Replacement fluid must be sterile and pyrogen free; dialysate does not need to meet the same stringency of bacteriologic purity, as is also true for dialysate for conventional IHD, although commercially available dialysate for CRRT is both sterile and endotoxin free. Prior to the availability of commercially prepared fluids for CRRT, dialysate and replacement fluids were often compounded locally by pharmacy or by bedside nursing staff. Unfortunately, local preparation of solutions and the use of "custom" CRRT fluids has been associated with catastrophic compounding errors and should be discouraged [62, 63]. If fluids are compounded locally, they should be assayed prior to use to ensure that the electrolyte composition is correct.

15.8 Anticoagulation

Clotting of the extracorporeal circuit is the most common complication of CRRT and results in interruption of treatment and reduction in the delivered dose of therapy [64]. Multiple anticoagulation regimens have been used for prevention of clotting [65]. The optimal anticoagulation strategy will prevent clotting in the extracorporeal circuit while minimizing the risks of systemic bleeding; a particular concern in critically ill patients who often are in the immediate postoperative period or who have thrombocytopenia or underlying coagulopathy. Agents that have been utilized include unfractionated heparin, low-molecular-weight heparins, danaparoid, direct thrombin inhibitors such as hirudin and argatroban, nafamostat, and citrate [65].

The KDIGO Clinical Practice Guideline for Acute Kidney Injury recommends using anticoagulation during CRRT in patients who do not have increased bleeding risk or impaired coagulation and are not already receiving systemic anticoagulation [40]. Data from clinical trials suggest that 40–60% of patients undergoing CRRT receive therapy without anticoagulation [5, 6], the majority of whom are thrombocytopenic or coagulopathic. System patency in the absence of anticoagulation is optimized by maximizing the blood flow rate, ensuring that the FF is less than 30%, and minimizing interruptions in blood flow because of machine alarms or catheter malfunction. Restricted inflow of blood or increased resistance to blood return as the result of catheter malfunction is among the most common reasons for machine alarms and transient interruptions of treatment. Catheter malfunction may result from it being too short, malposition, kinking, or development of a fibrin sheath outside or an intraluminal clot within. If catheter malfunction is present, initiation or intensification of anticoagulation will provide minimal benefit and the catheter should be repositioned or replaced.

15.8.1 Heparin

Unfractionated heparin is the most commonly used anticoagulant for CRRT [5, 6, 66]. Heparin is infused into the afferent limb (pre-filter) of the extracorporeal circuit as close to the vascular access as possible. Heparin acts by potentiating the action of antithrombin III, resulting in inhibition of factors IIa (thrombin) and Xa. Inhibition of factor IIa prolongs the activated partial thromboplastin time (aPTT) allowing ready monitoring of heparin dosing. Multiple regimens for heparin infusion have been proposed. In general, an initial bolus of 10–30 IU/kg is given followed by an infusion of 5–10 IU/kg/h, with a target aPTT of 1.5–2.0 times the upper limit of normal. Regional anticoagulation with protamine reversal has been used in patients at high risk for bleeding [67, 68]. This approach is technically cumbersome and difficult to standardize, and the use of protamine may be associated with complications including hypotension, anaphylaxis, and thrombocytopenia [69]. Low–molecular-weight heparins have also been used for anticoagulation of extracorporeal dialysis circuits, primarily in the chronic IHD setting [70, 71]. Specific data in CRRT are limited; however, from several small trials low-molecular-weight heparins appear to be at least as efficacious and unfractionated heparin with similar profiles for bleeding risk [72, 73]. Because low-molecular-weight heparins predominantly inhibit factor Xa, they do not prolong at aPTT and specific monitoring of anti-Xa activity is required (this may not be easily available). One limitation of low-molecular-weight heparins is that they accumulate in renal failure. The use of heparin is contraindicated in patients with heparin-induced thrombocytopenia and anticoagulation with argatroban (a direct thrombin inhibitor) or factor Xa inhibitors is recommended [40].

15.8.2 Citrate

Calcium is an obligate cofactor for coagulation; citrate chelates ionized calcium, thereby inhibiting the coagulation cascade. In regional citrate anticoagulation, citrate is infused into the afferent limb of the extracorporeal CRRT circuit as close to the vascular access as possible (ideally just where the afferent blood exits the catheter). Optimal anticoagulation is achieved when the ionized calcium level in the extracorporeal circuit is $\leq$0.35 mmol/L, measured post filter. Since the calcium–citrate complex is a small molecule, it will be readily cleared by either hemofiltration or hemodialysis. The remaining calcium–citrate complex that is returned to the body will be rapidly metabolized by the liver and skeletal muscle, generating three molecules of bicarbonate for each citrate molecule metabolized and releasing the bound calcium back into the circulation. In order to maintain calcium balance and prevent the development of systemic hypocalcemia, the calcium lost across the hemofilter/hemodialyzer membrane must be replaced with a systemic calcium infusion [65, 74]. The use of regional citrate anticoagulation requires close monitoring of the ionized calcium concentration in the return line of the extracorporeal circuit and systemically to ensure both adequate extracorporeal calcium chelation and maintenance of normal systemic ionized calcium concentration. Since citrate is metabolized to bicarbonate, acid-base status needs to be closely monitored to ensure that metabolic alkalosis does not develop. Depending on the specific citrate solution used, the buffer content of dialysate and/or replacement fluids may need to be reduced. In addition, many of the available citrate solutions have a high sodium content and can cause hypernatremia; if a hypernatric solution is used, the serum sodium concentration needs to be closely monitored and the sodium concentration of dialysate and/or replacement fluids decreased. Citrate accumulation may occur in patients with impaired citrate metabolism, such as patients with severe liver failure or lactic acidosis. In these patients, the use of citrate as an anticoagulant may be contraindicated as it may lead to citrate toxicity with severe systemic hypocalcemia [74–76]. Shock liver—which may coexist with ischemic AKI—is not of itself a contraindication to use of citrate. Multiple randomized trials have compared regional citrate anticoagulation to anticoagulation with either unfractionated or low-molecular-weight heparin in CRRT, finding increased circuit life and fewer bleeding events associated with citrate, with no increase in metabolic complications [77–84]. In one study, citrate anticoagulation was associated with improved renal recovery and hospital survival, although in this study, citrate anticoagulation was not associated with improved circuit patency [81]. Based on these data, the KDIGO Clinical Practice Guideline for Acute Kidney Injury suggests preferential use of citrate anticoagulation over heparin for CRRT in patients who do not have a contraindication to citrate administration [40]. However, no citrate formulation is currently approved for use in anticoagulation of CRRT by the US Food and Drug Administration.

15.9 Comparison of Modalities of CRRT

The advantages of VV CRRT as compared to AV therapies have been previously discussed. The higher clearance of higher molecular weight solutes, including pro-inflammatory cytokines, has led to the hypothesis that continuous hemofiltration would have greater benefit, as compared to continuous hemodialysis, particularly in patients with sepsis-associated AKI [85, 86]. However, this hypothesis has not been borne out by clinical data. In a randomized controlled trial comparing high-volume to standard-volume CVVH in patients with sepsis-associated AKI, more intensive convective therapy was not associated with improved outcomes [87]. In a meta-analysis of 19 clinical trials, 16 of which utilized CRRT, no benefit was observed with convective therapies as compared to diffusive therapy [24]. Thus, based on current data, the modalities of CRRT should be considered equivalent and no recommendation can be made regarding use of continuous hemofiltration, hemodialysis, or hemodiafiltration.

15.10 Dosing of CRRT

As previously discussed, the clearance of urea and other low-molecular-weight molecules during CRRT is approximately equal to the total effluent flow rate, usually normalized to body weight. Several single-center randomized controlled trials suggested that CRRT delivered at effluent flow rates greater than 20 mL/kg/h were associated with improved patient outcomes as compared to CRRT at lower effluent flow rates [88, 89]; however, these results were not consistent across all trials [90, 91]. In two large, multicenter randomized controlled trials, higher doses of CRRT were not associated with improved clinical outcomes [5, 6]. In the Acute Renal Failure Trial Network (ATN) study, patients who received CVVHDF at an effluent flow rate of 35 mL/kg/h did not have improved survival at 60 days or recovery of kidney function as compared with patients who received CVVHDF at an effluent flow rate of 20 mL/kg/h [5]. Similarly, in the Randomized Evaluation of Normal versus Augmented Level (RENAL) Replacement Therapy study, which randomized 1508 patients to CVVHDF at an effluent flow of either 25 mL/kg/h or 40 mL/kg/h there was no difference in mortality at 90 days, ICU or hospital survival, or recovery of kidney function between groups [6]. Based on these results, the KDIGO Clinical Practice Guideline for Acute Kidney Injury recommends delivering an effluent volume of 20–25 mL/kg/h for CRRT in AKI [40]. Based on the observation that delivered therapy is often less than prescribed due to interruptions of therapy (leaving the ICU for imaging studies or therapeutic procedures or clotting of the extracorporeal circuit [64, 92]), the guideline suggests that this will usually require prescription of a higher effluent volume in order to achieve the target delivered dose [40]. Dosing of therapy must also take into account the individual patient's clinical status and the need to achieve adequate control of azotemia and electrolyte, acid-base, and volume status. In particular, higher doses of therapy may be needed in hypercatabolic patients in order to control hyperkalemia, metabolic acidosis, and azotemia.

15.11 Comparison of CRRT with Other Modalities of RRT

There has been substantial debate regarding the relative benefits of CRRT as compared to other modalities of RRT in patients with AKI. Individual randomized controlled trials comparing CRRT to conventional IHD have not demonstrated superiority of either modality of therapy [93–98]. Three meta-analyses pooling these data confirmed the absence of superiority for either intermittent or continuous therapy with regard to patient survival [99–101]. Observational studies have suggested that CRRT may be associated with improved recovery of kidney function as compared to conventional IHD. In a meta-analysis of 16 observational studies, conventional IHD was associated with an almost twofold increased risk of persistent dialysis dependence as compared to CRRT [102]. However, this benefit was not present in a pooled analysis of data from seven randomized controlled trials [102]. The reason for difference in the apparent benefit between the observational and randomized studies is most likely related to differences in the patients treated with intermittent as compared to continuous therapy in the observational trials, as evidenced by higher mortality rates in the CRRT cohorts in these studies. CRRT has been shown to be associated with a greater ability to achieve negative fluid balance than conventional IHD [103]. Given the absence of clear benefit of either modality, the KDIGO Clinical Practice Guideline for Acute Kidney Injury proposes that the modalities be considered complementary therapies in AKI patients and that the specific modality should be chosen based on patient characteristics as well as on available expertise and resources [40]. The guidelines do suggest, however, that CRRT be used preferentially over conventional intermittent therapy in hemodynamically unstable patients [40]. Data also suggest that CRRT may minimize the risk of compromised cerebral perfusion in patients with acute brain injury or other causes of increased intracranial pressure or cerebral edema [40, 104, 105]. There are only limited data comparing

CRRT to prolonged intermittent RRT; however, these data suggest similar metabolic and clinical outcomes [106, 107].

References

1. Brivet FG, Kleinknecht DJ, Loirat P, Landais PJ. Acute renal failure in intensive care units—causes, outcome, and prognostic factors of hospital mortality; a prospective, multicenter study. French study group on acute renal failure. Crit Care Med. 1996;24(2):192–8.
2. Star RA. Treatment of acute renal failure. Kidney Int. 1998;54(6):1817–31.
3. Uchino S, Kellum JA, Bellomo R, Doig GS, Morimatsu H, Morgera S, et al. Acute renal failure in critically ill patients: a multinational, multicenter study. JAMA. 2005;294(7):813–8.
4. Uchino S. The epidemiology of acute renal failure in the world. Curr Opin Crit Care. 2006;12(6):538–43.
5. Palevsky PM, Zhang JH, O'Connor TZ, Chertow GM, Crowley ST, Choudhury D, et al. Intensity of renal support in critically ill patients with acute kidney injury. N Engl J Med. 2008;359(1):7–20.
6. Bellomo R, Cass A, Cole L, Finfer S, Gallagher M, Lo S, et al. Intensity of continuous renal-replacement therapy in critically ill patients. N Engl J Med. 2009;361(17):1627–38.
7. Kramer P, Wigger W, Rieger J, Matthaei D, Scheler F. Arteriovenous haemofiltration: a new and simple method for treatment of over-hydrated patients resistant to diuretics. Klin Wochenschr. 1977;55(22):1121–2.
8. Kramer P, Kaufhold G, Grone HJ, Wigger W, Rieger J, Matthaei D, et al. Management of anuric intensive-care patients with arteriovenous hemofiltration. Int J Artif Organs. 1980;3(4):225–30.
9. Kramer P, Schrader J, Bohnsack W, Grieben G, Grone HJ, Scheler F. Continuous arteriovenous haemofiltration. A new kidney replacement therapy. Proc Eur Dial Transpl Assoc. 1981;18:743–9.
10. Paganini EP, Nakamoto S. Continuous slow ultrafiltration in oliguric acute renal failure. Trans Am Soc Artif Intern Organs. 1980;26:201–4.
11. Lauer A, Saccaggi A, Ronco C, Belledonne M, Glabman S, Bosch JP. Continuous arteriovenous hemofiltration in the critically ill patient. Clinical use and operational characteristics. Ann Intern Med. 1983;99(4):455–60.
12. Kaplan AA, Longnecker RE, Folkert VW. Continuous arteriovenous hemofiltration. A report of six months' experience. Ann Intern Med. 1984;100(3):358–67.
13. Golper TA. Continuous arteriovenous hemofiltration in acute renal failure. Am J Kidney Dis. 1985;6(6):373–86.
14. Geronemus R, Schneider N. Continuous arteriovenous hemodialysis: a new modality for treatment of acute renal failure. Trans Am Soc Artif Intern Organs. 1984;30:610–3.
15. Ronco C. Arterio-venous hemodiafiltration (A-V HDF): a possible way to increase urea removal during C.A.V.H. Int J Artif Organs. 1985;8(1):61–2.
16. Ing TS, Purandare VV, Daugirdas JT, Hano JE, Battersby DG, Gandhi VC. Slow continuous hemodialysis. Int J Artif Organs. 1984;7(1):53.
17. Wendon J, Smithies M, Sheppard M, Bullen K, Tinker J, Bihari D. Continuous high volume venous-venous haemofiltration in acute renal failure. Intensive Care Med. 1989;15(6):358–63.
18. Storck M, Hartl WH, Inthorn D. Pump-driven haemofiltration. Lancet. 1991 Jun 8;337(8754):1415.
19. Palevsky PM, Bunchman T, Tetta C. The acute dialysis quality initiative—part V: operational characteristics of CRRT. Adv Ren Replace Ther. 2002;9(4):268–72.
20. Bellomo R, Ronco C, Mehta RL. Nomenclature for continuous renal replacement therapies. Am J Kidney Dis. 1996;28(Suppl 3):S2–S7.
21. Ronco C, Bellomo R. Continuous renal replacement therapy: evolution in technology and current nomenclature. Kidney Int Suppl. 1998;66:S160–4.
22. Gibney RT, Kimmel PL, Lazarus M. The acute dialysis quality initiative—part I: definitions and reporting of CRRT techniques. Adv Ren Replace Ther. 2002;9(4):252–4.
23. Clark WR, Ronco C. Continuous renal replacement techniques. Contrib Nephrol. 2004;144:264–77.
24. Friedrich JO, Wald R, Bagshaw SM, Burns KE, Adhikari NK. Hemofiltration compared to hemodialysis for acute kidney injury: systematic review and meta-analysis. Crit Care. 2012;16(4):R146.
25. Ronco C, Bellomo R. Continuous high-flux dialysis: an efficient renal replacement. In: Vincent JL, editor. Yearbook of intensive care and emergency medicine. Heidelberg: Springer; 1996. pp. 690–6.
26. Sigler MH, Teehan BP. Solute transport in continuous hemodialysis: a new treatment for acute renal failure. Kidney Int. 1987;32(4):562–71.
27. Brunet S, Leblanc M, Geadah D, Parent D, Courteau S, Cardinal J. Diffusive and convective solute clearances during continuous renal replacement therapy at various dialysate and ultrafiltration flow rates. Am J Kidney Dis. 199;34(3):486–92.
28. Troyanov S, Cardinal J, Geadah D, Parent D, Courteau S, Caron S, et al. Solute clearances during continuous venovenous haemofiltration at various ultrafiltration flow rates using Multiflow-100 and HF1000 filters. Nephrol Dial Transpl. 2003;18(5):961–6.
29. Clark WR, Turk JE, Kraus MA, Gao D. Dose determinants in continuous renal replacement therapy. Artif Organs. 2003;27(9):815–20.
30. Golper TA, Cigarran-Guldris S, Jenkins RD, Brier ME. The role of convection during simulated continuous arteriovenous hemodialysis. Contrib Nephrol. 1991;93:146–8.
31. Relton S, Greenberg A, Palevsky PM. Dialysate and blood flow dependence of diffusive solute clearance during CVVHD. ASAIO J. 1992;38(3):691–6.
32. Jaffrin MY, Gupta BB, Malbrancq JM. A one-dimensional model of simultaneous hemodialysis and ultrafiltration with highly permeable membranes. J Biomech Eng. 1981;103(4):261–6.
33. Husted FC, Nolph KD, Vitale FC, Maher JF. Detrimental effects of ultrafiltration on diffusion in coils. J Lab Clin Med. 1976;87(3):435–42.
34. Ronco C. Continuous renal replacement therapies in the treatment of acute renal failure in intensive care patients. Part 1. Theoretical aspects and techniques. Nephrol Dial Transpl. 1994;9(Suppl 4):191–200.
35. Yohay DA, Butterly DW, Schwab SJ, Quarles LD. Continuous arteriovenous hemodialysis: effect of dialyzer geometry. Kidney Int. 1992;42(2):448–51.
36. Ronco C, Bellomo R, Kellum JA. Continuous renal replacement therapy: opinions and evidence. Adv Ren Replace Ther. 2002;9(4):229–44.
37. Uldall R. Vascular access for continuous renal replacement therapy. Semin Diaolysis. 1996;9(2):93–7.
38. Olbricht CJ, Haubitz M, Habel U, Frei U, Koch KM. Continuous arteriovenous hemofiltration: in vivo functional characteristics and its dependence on vascular access and filter design. Nephron. 1990;55(1):49–57.
39. Bellomo R, Parkin G, Love J, Boyce N. A prospective comparative study of continuous arteriovenous hemodiafiltration and continuous venovenous hemodiafiltration in critically ill patients. Am J Kidney Dis. 1993;21(4):400–4.
40. Disease K. Improving global outcomes (KDIGO) acute kidney injury work group. KDIGO clinical practice guideline for acute kidney injury. Kidney Int Suppl. 2012;2:1–138.
41. Oliver MJ, Edwards LJ, Treleaven DJ, Lambert K, Margetts PJ. Randomized study of temporary hemodialysis catheters. Int J Artif Organs. 2002;25(1):40–4.

42. Parienti JJ, Thirion M, Megarbane B, Souweine B, Ouchikhe A, Polito A, et al. Femoral vs jugular venous catheterization and risk of nosocomial events in adults requiring acute renal replacement therapy: a randomized controlled trial. JAMA. 2008;299(20):2413–22.
43. O'Grady NP, Alexander M, Dellinger EP, Gerberding JL, Heard SO, Maki DG, et al. Guidelines for the prevention of intravascular catheter-related infections. (Centers for disease control and prevention. MMWR Recommendations and reports: Morbidity and mortality weekly report Recommendations and reports/Centers for Disease Control). Infect Control Hosp Epidemiol. 2002;23(12):759–69.
44. Vascular Access Work Group. Clinical practice guidelines for vascular access. Am J Kidney Dis. 2006;48(Suppl 1):S176–S247.
45. Karakitsos D, Labropoulos N, De Groot E, Patrianakos AP, Kouraklis G, Poularas J, et al. Real-time ultrasound-guided catheterisation of the internal jugular vein: a prospective comparison with the landmark technique in critical care patients. Crit Care. 2006;10(6):R162.
46. Leung J, Duffy M, Finckh A. Real-time ultrasonographically-guided internal jugular vein catheterization in the emergency department increases success rates and reduces complications: a randomized, prospective study. Ann Emerg Med. 2006;48(5):540–7.
47. Vijayan A. Vascular access for continuous renal replacement therapy. Semin Dial. 2009;22(2):133–6.
48. Schiffl H, Lang SM, Konig A, Strasser T, Haider MC, Held E. Biocompatible membranes in acute renal failure: prospective case-controlled study. The Lancet. 1994;344(8922):570–2.
49. Hakim RM, Wingard RL, Parker RA. Effect of the dialysis membrane in the treatment of patients with acute renal failure. N Engl J Med. 1994;331(20):1338–42.
50. Himmelfarb J, Tolkoff Rubin N, Chandran P, Parker RA, Wingard RL, Hakim R. A multicenter comparison of dialysis membranes in the treatment of acute renal failure requiring dialysis. J Am Soc Nephrol. 1998;9(2):257–66.
51. Subramanian S, Venkataraman R, Kellum JA. Influence of dialysis membranes on outcomes in acute renal failure: a meta-analysis. Kidney Int. 2002;62(5):1819–23.
52. Jaber BL, Lau J, Schmid CH, Karsou SA, Levey AS, Pereira BJ. Effect of biocompatibility of hemodialysis membranes on mortality in acute renal failure: a meta-analysis. Clin Nephrol. 2002;57(4):274–82.
53. Alonso A, Lau J, Jaber BL. Biocompatible hemodialysis membranes for acute renal failure. Cochrane Database Syst Rev. 2008;1:CD005283.
54. Roberts M, Winney RJ. Errors in fluid balance with pump control of continuous hemodialysis. Int J Artif Organs. 1992;15(2):99–102.
55. Troyanov S, Geadah D, Ghannoum M, Cardinal J, Leblanc M. Phosphate addition to hemodiafiltration solutions during continuous renal replacement therapy. Intensive Care Med. 2004;30(8):1662–5.
56. Davenport A, Will EJ, Davison AM. Hyperlactataemia and metabolic acidosis during haemofiltration using lactate-buffered fluids. Nephron. 1991;59(3):461–5.
57. Clasen M, Bohm R, Riehl J, Gladziwa U, Dakshinamurty KV, Schacht B, et al. Lactate or bicarbonate for intermittent hemofiltration? Contrib Nephrol. 1991;93:152–5.
58. Hilton PJ, Taylor J, Forni LG, Treacher DF. Bicarbonate-based haemofiltration in the management of acute renal failure with lactic acidosis. QJM. 1998;91(4):279–83.
59. Barenbrock M, Hausberg M, Matzkies F, de la Motte S, Schaefer RM. Effects of bicarbonate- and lactate-buffered replacement fluids on cardiovascular outcome in CVVH patients. Kidney Int. 2000;58(4):1751–7.
60. McLean AG, Davenport A, Cox D, Sweny P. Effects of lactate-buffered and lactate-free dialysate in CAVHD patients with and without liver dysfunction. Kidney Int. 2000;58(4):1765–72.
61. Barenbrock M, Schaefer RM. Cardiovascular outcome in critically ill patients treated with continuous haemofiltration—beneficial effects of bicarbonate-buffered replacement fluids. Edtna Erca J. 2002;2:4–6.
62. Johnston RV, Boiteau P, Charlebois K, Long S, David U. Responding to tragic error: lessons from Foothills Medical Centre. CMAJ. 2004;170(11):1659–60.
63. Culley CM, Bernardo JF, Gross PR, Guttendorf S, Whiteman KA, Kowiatek JG, et al. Implementing a standardized safety procedure for continuous renal replacement therapy solutions. Am J Health Syst Pharm. 2006;63(8):756–63.
64. Venkataraman R, Kellum JA, Palevsky P. Dosing patterns for continuous renal replacement therapy at a large academic medical center in the United States. J Crit Care. 2002;17(4):246–50.
65. Tolwani AJ, Wille KM. Anticoagulation for continuous renal replacement therapy. Semin Dial. 2009;22(2):141–5.
66. Davenport A, Mehta S. The Acute Dialysis Quality Initiative—part VI: access and anticoagulation in CRRT. Adv Ren Replace Ther. 2002 Oct;9(4):273–81.
67. Morabito S, Guzzo I, Solazzo A, Muzi L, Luciani R, Pierucci A. Continuous renal replacement therapies: anticoagulation in the critically ill at high risk of bleeding. J Nephrol. 2003;16(4):566–71.
68. van der Voort PH, Gerritsen RT, Kuiper MA, Egbers PH, Kingma WP, Boerma EC. Filter run time in CVVH: pre- versus post-dilution and nadroparin versus regional heparin-protamine anticoagulation. Blood Purif. 2005;23(3):175–80.
69. Horrow JC. Protamine: a review of its toxicity. Anesth Analg. 1985;64(3):348–61.
70. Lim W, Cook DJ, Crowther MA. Safety and efficacy of low-molecular-weight heparins for hemodialysis in patients with end-stage renal failure: a meta-analysis of randomized trials. J Am Soc Nephrol. 2004;15(12):3192–206.
71. Section V. Chronic intermittent haemodialysis and prevention of clotting in the extracorporal system. Nephrol Dial Transpl. 2002;17(Suppl 7):63–71.
72. Joannidis M, Kountchev J, Rauchenzauner M, Schusterschitz N, Ulmer H, Mayr A, et al. Enoxaparin vs. unfractionated heparin for anticoagulation during continuous veno-venous hemofiltration: a randomized controlled crossover study. Intensive Care Med. 2007;33(9):1571–9.
73. Reeves JH, Cumming AR, Gallagher L, O'Brien JL, Santamaria JD. A controlled trial of low-molecular-weight heparin (dalteparin) versus unfractionated heparin as anticoagulant during continuous venovenous hemodialysis with filtration. Crit Care Med. 1999;27(10):2224–8.
74. Tolwani A, Wille KM. Advances in continuous renal replacement therapy: citrate anticoagulation update. Blood Purif. 2012;34(2):88–93.
75. Kramer L, Bauer E, Joukhadar C, Strobl W, Gendo A, Madl C, et al. Citrate pharmacokinetics and metabolism in cirrhotic and noncirrhotic critically ill patients. Crit Care Med. 2003;31(10):2450–5.
76. Bakker AJ, Boerma EC, Keidel H, Kingma P, van der Voort PH. Detection of citrate overdose in critically ill patients on citrate-anticoagulated venovenous haemofiltration: use of ionised and total/ionised calcium. Clin Chem Lab Med. 2006;44(8):962–6.
77. Monchi M, Berghmans D, Ledoux D, Canivet JL, Dubois B, Damas P. Citrate vs. heparin for anticoagulation in continuous venovenous hemofiltration: a prospective randomized study. Intensive Care Med. 2004;30(2):260–5.
78. Kutsogiannis DJ, Gibney RT, Stollery D, Gao J. Regional citrate versus systemic heparin anticoagulation for continuous renal replacement in critically ill patients. Kidney Int. 2005;67(6):2361–7.
79. Betjes MG, van Oosterom D, van Agteren M, van de Wetering J. Regional citrate versus heparin anticoagulation during venovenous hemofiltration in patients at low risk for bleeding: similar hemofilter survival but significantly less bleeding. J Nephrol. 2007;20(5):602–8.
80. Fealy N, Baldwin I, Johnstone M, Egi M, Bellomo R. A pilot randomized controlled crossover study comparing regional hepa-

rinization to regional citrate anticoagulation for continuous venovenous hemofiltration. Int J Artif Organs. 2007;30(4):301–7.
81. Oudemans-van Straaten HM, Bosman RJ, Koopmans M, van der Voort PH, Wester JP, van der Spoel JI, et al. Citrate anticoagulation for continuous venovenous hemofiltration. Crit Care Med. 2009;37(2):545–52.
82. Hetzel GR, Schmitz M, Wissing H, Ries W, Schott G, Heering PJ, et al. Regional citrate versus systemic heparin for anticoagulation in critically ill patients on continuous venovenous haemofiltration: a prospective randomized multicentre trial. Nephrol Dial Transpl. 2011;26(1):232–9.
83. Park JS, Kim GH, Kang CM, Lee CH. Regional anticoagulation with citrate is superior to systemic anticoagulation with heparin in critically ill patients undergoing continuous venovenous hemodiafiltration. Korean J Intern Med. 2011;26(1):68–75.
84. Wu MY, Hsu YH, Bai CH, Lin YF, Wu CH, Tam KW. Regional citrate versus heparin anticoagulation for continuous renal replacement therapy: a meta-analysis of randomized controlled trials. Am J Kidney Dis. 2012;59(6):810–8.
85. Ronco C, Tetta C, Mariano F, Wratten ML, Bonello M, Bordoni V, et al. Interpreting the mechanisms of continuous renal replacement therapy in sepsis: the peak concentration hypothesis. Artif Organs. 2003;27(9):792–801.
86. Ronco C, Bonello M, Bordoni V, Ricci Z, D'Intini V, Bellomo R, et al. Extracorporeal therapies in non-renal disease: treatment of sepsis and the peak concentration hypothesis. Blood Purif. 2004;22(1):164–74.
87. Joannes-Boyau O, Honore PM, Perez P, Bagshaw SM, Grand H, Canivet JL, et al. High-volume versus standard-volume haemofiltration for septic shock patients with acute kidney injury (IVOIRE study): a multicentre randomized controlled trial. Intensive Care Med. 2013;39(9):1535–46.
88. Ronco C, Bellomo R, Homel P, Brendolan A, Dan M, Piccinni P, et al. Effects of different doses in continuous veno-venous haemofiltration on outcomes of acute renal failure: a prospective randomised trial. Lancet. 2000;356(9223):26–30.
89. Saudan P, Niederberger M, De Seigneux S, Romand J, Pugin J, Perneger T, et al. Adding a dialysis dose to continuous hemofiltration increases survival in patients with acute renal failure. Kidney Int. 2006;70(7):1312–7.
90. Bouman CS, Oudemans-Van Straaten HM, Tijssen JG, Zandstra DF, Kesecioglu J. Effects of early high-volume continuous venovenous hemofiltration on survival and recovery of renal function in intensive care patients with acute renal failure: a prospective, randomized trial. Crit Care Med. 2002;30(10):2205–11.
91. Tolwani AJ, Campbell RC, Stofan BS, Lai KR, Oster RA, Wille KM. Standard versus high-dose CVVHDF for ICU-related acute renal failure. J Am Soc Nephrol. 2008;19(6):1233–8.
92. Vesconi S, Cruz DN, Fumagalli R, Kindgen-Milles D, Monti G, Marinho A, et al. Delivered dose of renal replacement therapy and mortality in critically ill patients with acute kidney injury. Crit Care. 2009;13(2):R57.
93. Mehta RL, McDonald B, Gabbai FB, Pahl M, Pascual MT, Farkas A, et al. A randomized clinical trial of continuous versus intermittent dialysis for acute renal failure. Kidney Int. 2001;60(3):1154–63.
94. Augustine JJ, Sandy D, Seifert TH, Paganini EP. A randomized controlled trial comparing intermittent with continuous dialysis in patients with ARF. Am J Kidney Dis. 2004;44(6):1000–7.
95. Uehlinger DE, Jakob SM, Ferrari P, Eichelberger M, Huynh-Do U, Marti HP, et al. Comparison of continuous and intermittent renal replacement therapy for acute renal failure. Nephrol Dial Transpl. 2005;20(8):1630–7.
96. Vinsonneau C, Camus C, Combes A, Costa de Beauregard MA, Klouche K, Boulain T, et al. Continuous venovenous haemodiafiltration versus intermittent haemodialysis for acute renal failure in patients with multiple-organ dysfunction syndrome: a multicentre randomised trial. Lancet. 2006;368(9533):379–85.
97. Lins RL, Elseviers MM, Van der Niepen P, Hoste E, Malbrain ML, Damas P, et al. Intermittent versus continuous renal replacement therapy for acute kidney injury patients admitted to the intensive care unit: results of a randomized clinical trial. Nephrol Dial Transpl. 2009;24(2):512–8.
98. Schefold JC, Haehling S, Pschowski R, Bender T, Berkmann C, Briegel S, et al. The effect of continuous versus intermittent renal replacement therapy on the outcome of critically ill patients with acute renal failure (CONVINT): a prospective randomized controlled trial. Crit Care. 2014;18(1):R11.
99. Rabindranath K, Adams J, Macleod AM, Muirhead N. Intermittent versus continuous renal replacement therapy for acute renal failure in adults. Cochrane Database Syst Rev. 2007(3):CD003773.
100. Bagshaw SM, Berthiaume LR, Delaney A, Bellomo R. Continuous versus intermittent renal replacement therapy for critically ill patients with acute kidney injury: a meta-analysis. Crit Care Med. 2008;36(2):610–7.
101. Pannu N, Klarenbach S, Wiebe N, Manns B, Tonelli M. Renal replacement therapy in patients with acute renal failure: a systematic review. JAMA. 2008;299(7):793–805.
102. Schneider AG, Bellomo R, Bagshaw SM, Glassford NJ, Lo S, Jun M, et al. Choice of renal replacement therapy modality and dialysis dependence after acute kidney injury: a systematic review and meta-analysis. Intensive Care Med. 2013;39(6):987–97.
103. Bouchard J, Soroko SB, Chertow GM, Himmelfarb J, Ikizler TA, Paganini EP, et al. Fluid accumulation, survival and recovery of kidney function in critically ill patients with acute kidney injury. Kidney Int. 2009;76(4):422–7.
104. Davenport A. Continuous renal replacement therapies in patients with acute neurological injury. Semin Dial. 2009;22(2):165–8.
105. Davenport A. Continuous renal replacement therapies in patients with liver disease. Semin Dial. 2009;22(2):169–72.
106. Kielstein JT, Kretschmer U, Ernst T, Hafer C, Bahr MJ, Haller H, et al. Efficacy and cardiovascular tolerability of extended dialysis in critically ill patients: a randomized controlled study. Am J Kidney Dis. 2004;43(2):342–9.
107. Schwenger V, Weigand MA, Hoffmann O, Dikow R, Kihm LP, Seckinger J, et al. Sustained low efficiency dialysis using a single-pass batch system in acute kidney injury—a randomized interventional trial: the renal replacement therapy study in intensive care unit patients. Crit Care. 2012;16(4):R140.

Continuous Renal Replacement Therapy Technology

16

Federico Nalesso and Claudio Ronco

16.1 Introduction to CRRT Thechnology

Continuous renal replacement therapies (CRRTs) are a group of continuous therapies used in the intensive care unit (ICU) setting. In the past, CRRTs were seen reductively as therapies directed to the replacement of renal function only. In recent years, thanks to improvements in hardware and software technology and the introduction of more specific filters, the role of CRRTs has expanded beyond the replacement of renal function in the setting of severe acute kidney injury (AKI). For example, CRRTs are now used in the setting of less severe AKI associated with liver failure, heart failure, or sepsis.

In order to achieve optimum results with CRRT, it is necessary to have close cooperation between nephrologists and intensivists, as described in "Vicenza Model" [1]. In this model, the critically ill patient is followed in partnership by the nephrologist and intensivist so that they can prescribe and deliver *in a timely fashion* the best type of CRRT for the single patient's clinical condition.

16.2 CRRT in Renal Replacement Therapies

Extracorporeal blood purification (EBP) is a treatment in which a patient's blood is passed through a device where solute, toxins, and fluid are removed. EBP is primarily used in patients with renal failure but more than 20 years ago, it was suggested that EBP could remove inflammatory mediators from the plasma of patients with sepsis and improve pulmonary function [2]. Subsequently, surrogate clinical improvements with hemofiltration have been reported in animal and human studies, and cytokine removal from the circulation of animals and humans with sepsis has been demonstrated [3]. Shortly after, a survival benefit associated with higher dosages of continuous hemofiltration was reported [4]. With these advances, CRRT as a treatment for human septic shock was born. Since that time, many technological advances have occurred along with substantial changes in our basic understanding of sepsis and the inflammatory response. Newer filter and machine technologies now allow removal of inflammatory mediators via convection, diffusion, or adsorption. Of course, these inflammatory mediators are removed only from the plasma; the effects of CRRT on local tissue concentrations are less well understood. There are other ways by which CRRT may improve outcomes in sepsis: better acid–base control, better fluid balance and temperature control, cardiac support, protective lung support, brain protection with preservation of cerebral perfusion, bone marrow protection, and blood detoxification and liver support. Cardiac support can be achieved by the optimization of fluid balance, the reduction of organ edema, and the restoration of desirable levels of preload and afterload. By optimizing the patient's volume state and offering the ability to remove interstitial fluid, CRRT may provide additional support to the failing lung [5]. Blood purification may improve the encephalopathy of sepsis by removing uremic toxins and amino acid derivatives and correcting acidemia. Continuous therapies also offer the advantages of minimizing both osmotic shifts and hemodynamic insults that threaten cerebral perfusion pressure [6]. Through the removal of uremic toxins, blood purification also reverses immunoparalysis [7] and may improve bone marrow function such as erythropoiesis [8]. Thus, CRRT is increasingly recognized to be a multiple organ support therapy (MOST) .

16.3 Definition and Settings of CRRT

CRRT uses three processes for blood purification: convection (hemofiltration), diffusion (dialysis), and adsorption (onto the blood surface of the fibers of the filter). All may be combined in the one treatment. Improvements in filter and

F. Nalesso (✉) · C. Ronco
Department of Nephrology, Dialysis, Transplant, San Bortolo Hospital, Vicenza, Italy
e-mail: nalesso.federico@gmail.com

A. K. Singh et al. (eds.), *Core Concepts in Dialysis and Continuous Therapies,* DOI 10.1007/978-1-4899-7657-4_16

Table 16.1 Definitions and characteristic of the different continuous renal replacement therapy (CRRT) types

Treatment	Abbreviation	Type of process	Molecules target	Note
Dialysis	CVVHD	Diffusion	Low molecular weight If high cutoff membrane is used this treatment can remove high molecular weight molecules; it is important to be aware of possible albumin loss	According to the filter, cutoff is possible to enhance the removal of middle and high molecular weight molecules
Hemofiltration	CVVH	Convection	Middle/high molecules	According to the exchange of plasma water and the type of filter is possible to extend the molecules removal to the high molecular weight molecules (e.g., cytokines)
Hemodiafiltration	CVVHDF	Diffusion and convection	Middle molecules	This treatment is the combination of CVVHD and CVVH (the reinfusion can be done in pre- or post-dilution or both according to the software and hardware available)
Highflux dialysis	CVVHFD	Diffusion and convection (back filtration)	Middle molecules	This treatment is a subtype of CVVHDF. The convection is due to the filter characteristic of high flux that determines an ultrafiltration of plasma water in the first part of the filter and back filtration of the dialysate (reinfusion) in the second part of the filter
Pulse high volume	pHVHF	24 h cycles of HVHF followed by CVVH	High molecular weight molecules	Sequential treatment (HVHF followed by CVVH, this treatment in 24 h provides high dialytic dose in convection)

CRRT machine technology now allow great flexibility in adjusting the convection/diffusion/adsorption prescription for a given patient. For example, high cutoff filters are now available which allow removal (by diffusion) of molecules with a molecular weight just below that of albumin. Other high-flow filters permit plasma water exchanges of about 6–9 L per hour. High-adsorption membranes can increase removal of high molecular weight inflammatory molecules not otherwise removed by convection or diffusion.

Adequate vascular access is very important in facilitating the blood flow (Q_B) needed to deliver an appropriate dose and filtration fraction (FF). Arterial access for CRRT is very rarely used today. Hence, we have used a "veno-venous" classification of current CRRT therapies, as below (see also Table 16.1):

- CVVHD: Continuous veno-venous hemodialysis (diffusion)
- CVVHFD: Continuous veno-venous high flux hemodialysis (diffusion and convection due to back filtration thanks to the high flux filter used)
- CVVHDF: Continuous veno-venous hemodiafiltration (diffusion and convection)
- CVVH: Continuous veno-venous hemofiltration (convection)
- pHVHF: Pulse high volume hemofiltration (a combination of HVHF followed by CVVH, convection)

In all of the above treatments, it is possible to enhance blood purification by increasing the adsorption characteristics of the filter used. For example, it is possible to use a filter with the ability to filter out endotoxin.

pHVHF is a subtype of CRRT. In this type of treatment, used to treat patients with severe sepsis or septic shock, it is possible to provide a high diffusive dose during the day by the HVHF (Q_R: 4–9 L/h)—this facilitates removal of inflammatory cytokines. The HVHF is followed by CVVH (Q_R: 3–4 L/h) to maintain the clinical results during the night.

All these types of CRRT can be used in critically ill patients according to the target of molecules to be removed—allowing optimal treatment of critically ill patient with multiple organs dysfunction syndrome/multiple organs failure syndrome (MODS/MOFS).

Typical CRRT prescriptions are summarized in Table 16.2. These prescriptions are only guidelines and they can vary according to the local policy, the available software and hardware, and the experience and availability of nurses. For example, pHVHF treatment is not feasible if adequate staff time is not available to change the large number of bags required. The important point is to prescribe *on a daily basis* the best locally available form of CRRT for an individual patient.

The main options for anticoagulation are heparin, citrate, or none. Anticoagulation is discussed in detail in Chap. 15, where clotting of the extracorporeal circuit is a concern (e.g., when no anticoagulation is used). A number of strategies

Table 16.2 Renal and septic dose suggested in continuous renal replacement therapy (CRRT)

Treatment	Abbreviation	Type of process	Renal dose $Q_{B\ ml/min}/Q_{D\ L/min}/Q_{R\ L/min}$ Provide at least 25–30 ml/kg/h[a]	Septic dose[b] $Q_{B\ ml/min}/Q_{D\ L/min}/Q_{R\ L/min}$ Provide at least 35–40 ml/kg/h More than 40 ml/kg/h in septic shock[a]
Dialysis	CVVHD	Diffusion	150–200/2–3/–	150–200/6/–
Hemofiltration	CVVH	Convection	150–200/0/2[c]	150–200/0/3–4[c]
Hemodiafiltration	CVVHDF	Diffusion and convection	150–200/2–3/1[d]	150–200/6/2[d]
Highflux dialysis	CVVHFD	Diffusion and convection (back filtration)	150–200/2–3/0	150–200/6/0
Pulse high volume	pHVHF	24 h cycles of HVHF followed by CVVH	–	HVHF: 150–200/–/4–6 CVVH: 1 50–200/–/3–4[c]

[a] The dose must to be corrected depending on the percentage of infusion in pre-dilution that decreases the efficiency of diffusion and convection (post-dilution) due to the blood dilution pre-filter

[b] During treatments in sepsis or septic shock, it is recommended to use high flux filters or high cutoff membrane in order to enhance the removal of high molecular weight molecules such as cytokines. According to the membrane cutoff, the treatment can be switched to CVVHD in order to avoid albumin losses that occur during convection

[c] It is suggested to use a percentage between 100 and 60 % in pre-dilution according to: Q_B (Filtration fraction must to be below 15–20 %), possibility to provide anticoagulation (decreasing FF), monitor type, clinical conditions

[d] Pre or post-dilution according to the filtration fraction (FF). Pre-dilution if FF is more than 20 %

can be used: increasing the blood flow to maintain the FF below 15–20 %, increasing the pre-dilution of replacement fluid in CVVH to 80–100 % and in CVVHD mode, using dialysis more than filtration.

16.4 Indications to Start CRRT

Currently, the use of renal replacement therapy (RRT) in patients with AKI is extremely variable and is based primarily on experience, habits, and local resources. Indications to start CRRT in isolated AKI are "classical indications" and are summarized in Table 16.3. In practice, patients with AKI in the ICU setting often have MODS/MOFS—earlier initiation of CRRT may be beneficial in such patients. There is increasing evidence that fluid overload associated with AKI contributes significantly to morbidity and mortality and this concern may prompt "early" initiation of CVVH, especially in children or in patients after cardiac surgery. There is ongoing interest in developing biomarkers of early AKI (such as kidney injury molecule-1 (KIM-1) and neutrophil gelatinase associated lipocalin (NGAL))—such biomarkers might facilitate appropriate earlier initiation of CRRT in certain patients.

Initiation of CRRT results in a considerable escalation in both the complexity and cost of care. While CRRT is extensively used in clinical practice, there remains uncertainty about the ideal circumstances of when to initiate RRT and for what indications. The process of deciding when to initiate RRT in critically ill patients is complex and is influenced by numerous factors, including patient-specific and

Table 16.3 Classical indications to start continuous renal replacement therapy (CRRT) in isolated acute kidney injury (AKI)

Indications	Characteristics	Absolute (A)/relative (R)
Metabolic abnormality	BUN > 76 mg/dl	R
	BUN > 100 mg/dl	A
	K > 6 mEq/L	R
	K > 6 mEq/L with ECG abnormalities	A
	Dysnatremia	R
	Mg > 8 mEq/L	R
	Mg > 8 mEq/L with anuria and absent deep tendon reflexes	A
Acidosis	pH > 7.15	R
	pH < 7.15	A
	Lactic acidosis related to metformin use	A
Anuria/oliguria	RIFLE class R	R
	RIFLE class I	R
	RIFLE class F	R
Fluid overload	Diuretic sensitive	R
	Diuretic resistant	A

clinician-specific factors and those related to local organizational/logistical issues (Fig. 16.1). Studies have shown marked variation between clinicians, and across institutions and countries. As a consequence, analysis of ideal circumstances under which to initiate RRT is challenging [9]. Early initiation probably improves outcomes. Relative versus absolute indications to start CRRT are more important overall in patients with MODS or MOFS or sepsis. RIFLE (risk, injury, failure, loss, and end-stage kidney staging criteria) class can be used as a surrogate of timing and can be used to follow the clinical trend and trajectory of the patient.

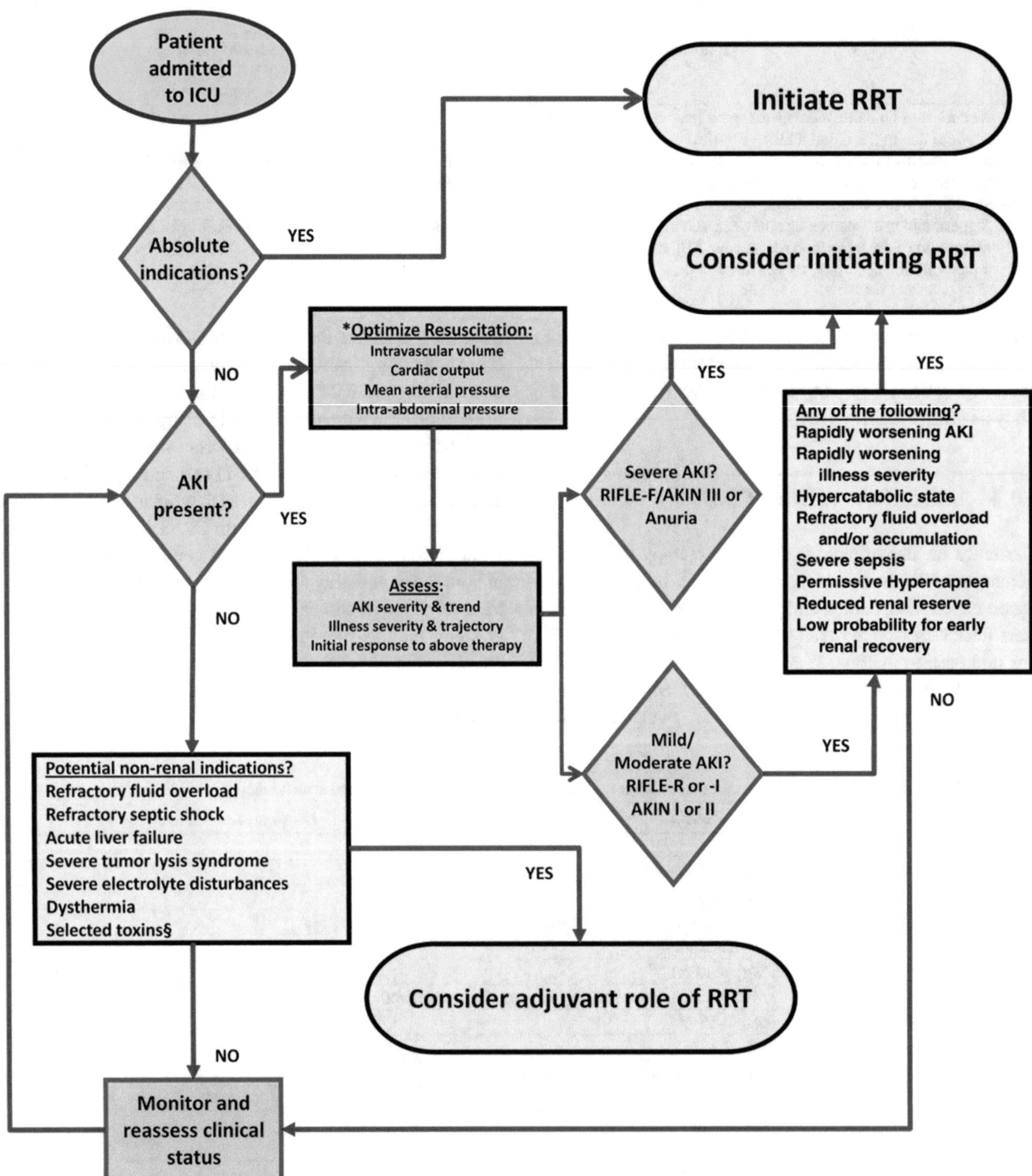

Fig. 16.1 Treatment algorithm. (From: Bagshaw et al. [9])

16.5 Dose of CRRT

It is important to know for every treatment the *real* dose delivered to the patient as opposed to the *prescribed* dose [10]. Often, due to downtime (alarms, problems with vascular access, patient being moved to radiology, etc.), the real dose is significantly lower. Another factor impacting on adequate prescribed and delivered dose of CRRT is underestimation of the patient's weight. This is likely to be a common problem as the majority of ICU patients are in a state of hyperhydration [11] but remain very difficult to weigh.

More CRRT seems to improve outcomes but only until up to a certain point [12]. Optimal dose seems to be between 25 and 35 ml/h/Kg in most patients. Higher doses are sometimes used in septic and hypercatabolic patients. In the case of septic patients, the idea is to remove noxious mediators of inflammation (the benefits of this approach have not yet been well validated in clinical trials). Thus, some have advocated two types of CRRT prescriptions: CRRT at "renal dose" and CRRT at "sepsis dose." Urea kinetics have not been well validated in the AKI setting but in practice measures such as K, Kt, and Kt/V are often used.

16.6 Conclusions

CRRTs are a group of continuous therapies that are now widely used in critical care. Today, thanks to improved hardware and software technology we have a wide spectrum of treatments that can be used during AKI in critically ill patients not only to support and substitute the renal function but also to protect, restore, and maintain the function of other organs. In this paradigm, CRRT has the role of MOST. The process of deciding when to initiate RRT in critically ill patients is complex and is influenced by numerous factors, including patient-specific and clinician-specific factors and those related to local organizational/logistical issues. Relative indications are more important to start CRRT when AKI is a part of a more complex clinical situation of MODS or MOFS. It is important to ensure that the prescribed and delivered (real) dose of CRRT is adequate for a given patient. In order to achieve optimal results with the various forms of CRRT, it is necessary to have close cooperation between nephrologists and intensivists, as described in the "Vicenza Model."

References

1. Ronco C. Critical care nephrology: can we clone the 'Vicenza model'? Int J Artif Organs. 2007;30(3):181–2.
2. Gotloib L, Barzilay E, Shustak A, Lev A. Sequential hemofiltration in nonoliguric high capillary permeability pulmonary edema of severe sepsis: preliminary report. Crit Care Med. 1984;12:997–1000.
3. De Vriese AS, Vanholder RC, Pascual M, et al. Can inflammatory cytokines be removed efficiently by continuous renal replacement therapies? Intensive Care Med. 1999;25:903–10.
4. De Vriese AS, Colardyn FA, Philippe JJ, et al. Cytokine removal during continuous hemofiltration in septic patients. J Am Soc Nephrol. 1999;10:846–53.
5. Huang H, Yao T, Wang W, et al. Continuous ultrafiltration attenuates the pulmonary injury that follows open heart surgery with cardiopulmonary bypass. Ann Thorac Surg. 2003;76:136–40.
6. Davenport A. Renal replacement therapy in the patient with acute brain injury. Am J Kidney Dis. 2001;37:457–66.
7. Yekebas EF, Eisenberger CF, Ohnesorge H, et al. Attenuation of sepsis-related immunoparalysis by continuous veno-venous hemofiltration in experimental porcine pancreatitis. Crit Care Med. 2001;29:1423–30.
8. Righetti M, Ferrario GM, Milani S, et al. A single centre study about the effects of HFR on anemia. G Ital Nefrol. 2004;21(Suppl 30):S168–71.
9. Bagshaw SM, Cruz DN, Gibney RT, Ronco C. A proposed algorithm for initiation of renal replacement therapy in adult critically ill patients. Crit Care. 2009;13(6):317. doi:10.1186/cc8037. (Epub 2009 Nov 11).
10. Vesconi S, Cruz DN, Fumagalli R, Kindgen-Milles D, Monti G, Marinho A, Mariano F, Formica M, Marchesi M, René R, Livigni S, Ronco C, DOse REsponse Multicentre International collaborative Initiative (DO-RE-MI Study Group). Delivered dose of renal replacement therapy and mortality in critically ill patients with acute kidney injury. Crit Care. 2009;13(2):R57. doi:10.1186/cc7784. (Epub 2009 Apr 15).
11. Basso F, Berdin G, Virzì GM, Mason G, Piccinni P, Day S, Cruz DN, Wjewodzka M, Giuliani A, Brendolan A, Ronco C. Fluid management in the intensive care unit: bioelectrical impedance vector analysis as a tool to assess hydration status and optimal fluid balance in critically ill patients. Blood Purif. 2013;36(3–4):192–9.
12. Prowle JR, Schneider A, Bellomo R. Clinical review: optimal dose of continuous renal replacement therapy in acute kidney injury. Crit Care. 2011;15(2):207. doi:10.1186/cc9415. (Epub 2011 Mar 18. Review).

Complications of Continuous Renal Replacement Therapy (CRRT)

17

James Harms, Keith Wille and Ashita Tolwani

17.1 Introduction

Acute kidney injury (AKI) is an increasingly prevalent condition in the intensive care unit (ICU) patient population and is associated with significantly increased mortality. Continuous renal replacement therapy (CRRT) has become the preferred method of renal replacement in these patients because of its perceived benefits of hemodynamic stability, enhanced metabolic control, and more effective volume management. Despite these benefits, CRRT has not been found to have a demonstrable survival benefit when compared to conventional intermittent hemodialysis (IHD). Complications associated with CRRT may partly contribute to its lack of survival advantage. Recognizing the potential complications of CRRT, and thereby preventing them, may improve patient outcomes (see Table 17.1).

17.2 Vascular Access

17.2.1 Catheter Type and Placement

CRRT requires the presence of a vascular access in the form of a large-bore, double-lumen central venous catheter (CVC)—arterial access is very rarely used today. Placement of a CVC is recommended even in chronic hemodialysis patients who need CRRT and already have a functioning fistula or graft. Reasons include the potential risk of fistula or graft damage by the continuous indwelling of the needles and life-threatening hemorrhage from accidental needle dislodgement. Insertion of a CVC is associated with risks of bleeding, pneumothorax, hemothorax, arterial puncture/dilation, venous thrombosis, infection, aneurysm, air embolism, and hematoma [1, 2]. The incidence of complications during catheter insertion varies between 5 and 19 % based on the site selected [3–5]. Standard insertion protocols using sterile technique should be followed and placement performed or supervised by experienced providers to decrease these risks. Ultrasound guidance for internal jugular and subclavian CVCs has been shown to decrease the number of attempts and complications and should be utilized [6, 7]. Although tunneled cuffed catheters have demonstrated significantly increased catheter survival times and less dysfunction as compared to non-tunneled devices, they typically require interventional or surgical expertise for placement and take longer to insert [8]. For these reasons, CRRT is typically initiated via a non-tunneled catheter and later transitioned to a tunneled cuffed catheter if it is anticipated that the patient will need renal replacement therapy for a prolonged duration (>1–3 weeks) [9, 10].

17.2.2 Site

The site of CVC placement can lead to variations in access performance. Despite widespread belief that femoral catheters are more prone to infection, recent trials suggest that infection rates may not be significantly different between femoral and internal jugular-placed catheters [8, 11, 12]. However, catheter malfunction has been found to be the least in right internal jugular position, followed by the femoral position, and finally left internal jugular position [13]. For this reason, Kidney Disease: Improving Global Outcomes (KDIGO) 2012 clinical practice guidelines for AKI suggest that the right internal jugular is the most preferred site for CVC placement (see Table 17.2) [8]. After CVC placement, catheter position should be confirmed by chest radiograph for internal jugular catheters. (An abdominal plain film can be used to confirm the correct position of femoral catheters but is rarely performed.) The radiograph of a properly placed

A. Tolwani (✉) · J. Harms
Division of Nephrology, Department of Medicine, University of Alabama at Birmingham, Birmingham, AL, USA
e-mail: atolwani@uab.edu

K. Wille
Division of Pulmonary, Allergy, and Critical Care Medicine, Department of Medicine, University of Alabama at Birmingham, Birmingham, AL, USA

A. K. Singh et al. (eds.), *Core Concepts in Dialysis and Continuous Therapies,* DOI 10.1007/978-1-4899-7657-4_17

Table 17.1 Complications of continuous renal replacement therapy (CRRT)

Vascular access	Pneumothorax
	Hemothorax
	Arteriovenous fistula formation
	Hematoma
	Catheter-related bacteremia
	Catheter-associated thrombosis
	Recirculation
	Air embolism
	Arrhythmias
Anticoagulation	*Heparin-Related*: Bleeding
	Thrombocytopenia
	Heparin-induced thrombocytopenia
	Citrate Related:
	Metabolic alkalosis
	Metabolic acidosis
	Hypocalcemia
	Hypercalcemia
	Hypernatremia
Hemodynamics	Hypotension
	Hypovolemia
Extracorporeal circuit	Air embolism
	Anaphylaxis
	Hypothermia
	Immunologic activation
	Line disconnection
	Fluid removal errors
Electrolytes and acid-base	Hypophosphatemia
	Hypokalemia
	Hypomagnesemia
	Hyponatremia
	Hypercalcemia
	Hypocalcemia
	Hypernatremia
	Metabolic alkalosis
	Metabolic acidosis
Nutrition	Protein losses
	Vitamin deficiencies
	Mineral deficiencies
Drug administration	Altered drug clearance
	Drug toxicity
	Inadequate dosing

internal jugular catheter should demonstrate the tip ending at the right atrial juncture, while femoral catheters should extend into the inferior vena cava to reduce malfunction and recirculation [14]. Subclavian CVCs are typically avoided because of their propensity for causing venous stenosis and thereby jeopardizing the ipsilateral extremity for future dialysis access [15, 16].

17.2.3 Recirculation and Catheter Malfunction

Recirculation of blood in a CVC can lead to hemoconcentration, reduced solute clearance, and filter clotting [14, 17]. Shorter catheters (15 cm) have more recirculation than longer catheters (24 cm), and femoral catheters tend to have the most recirculation [18, 19]. Optimal catheter length varies depending on the site of placement: 12–15 cm for right internal jugular catheters, 15–20 cm for left internal jugular, and 20–24 cm for femoral catheters (see Table 17.2) [2, 18, 19]. Catheter malfunction can occur when any kinking or manipulation alters laminar blood flow through the catheter, leading to fibrin deposition, reduced delivered dose of dialysis, and shorter catheter and hemofilter lifespan. Signs of CVC malfunction include increased access pressures and poor blood flows [1, 14].

Table 17.2 Central venous catheter site and length for continuous renal replacement therapy (CRRT)[a]

Site	Length of catheter	Characteristics
Right internal jugular vein	12–15 cm	Most preferred site of catheter placement
		Least incidence of catheter malfunction
Femoral vein	20–24 cm	More recirculation
		Concern for greater infectious risks
Left internal jugular vein	15–20 cm	Least preferred side of catheter placement
		Highest incidence of catheter malfunction

[a] Subclavian vein placement not recommended because of propensity to cause central venous stenosis

17.3 Circuit Patency

Clotting of the CRRT circuit prolongs CRRT downtime, reduces treatment efficacy, increases blood loss in the hemofilter, and increases cost. Retrospective studies have shown that patients receive only 68 % of their prescribed dose of CRRT due to circuit downtime [20]. Various technical aspects of the therapy can affect circuit patency and are described below.

17.3.1 Filtration Fraction

Patency of the extracorporeal circuit can be affected by the CRRT technique. Convective CRRT modalities (continuous venovenous hemofiltration, CVVH, and continuous venovenous hemodiafiltration, CVVHDF) using post-filter replacement fluid can increase the risk of hemofilter clotting through an excessive filtration fraction. Filtration fraction is defined as the ratio of ultrafiltration rate to plasma water flow rate and refers to the fraction of plasma that is filtered across the semipermeable membrane (see Table 17.3). Blood flow rate, patient hematocrit, and ultrafiltration rate are important determinants of the filtration fraction. In CRRT, a

Table 17.3 Filtration fraction calculation

FF = Quf/Qp	FF: filtration fraction
	Quf: ultrafiltration rate
	Qp: plasma flow rate
Plasma flow rate is calculated as follows	
Qp = Qb × (1 − Hct/100)	Qp: plasma flow rate
	Qb: blood flow rate
	Hct: hematocrit
Ultrafiltration rate is calculated as follows	
Quf = Qufnet + Qrf	Qufnet: net rate of volume removal
	Qrf: replacement fluid flow rate

filtration fraction above 25% increases the risk of clotting through hemoconcentration and formation of a protein layer within the hemofilter [21]. Increasing the post-filter replacement fluid rate increases the filtration fraction and increases the risk of clotting. The filtration fraction can be decreased by the following: administering the replacement fluid prefilter (thereby decreasing the hematocrit), switching to a dialysate-based CRRT modality (continuous venovenous hemodialysis, CVVHD, or continuous venovenous hemodiafiltration, CVVHDF), or increasing the blood flow rate. The downside of prefilter replacement fluid is that it dilutes the concentration of solutes entering the hemofilter and decreases clearance [22].

17.3.2 Anticoagulation

Although CRRT can be administered without anticoagulation, anticoagulation is generally required to decrease clotting of the circuit. Anticoagulants used for CRRT include systemic unfractionated heparin, regional heparin (in conjunction with protamine sulphate), low molecular weight heparin, regional citrate, thrombin antagonists, and platelet inhibiting agents. Unfractionated heparin (UFH) remains the most widely used form of anticoagulation for CRRT. Studies have demonstrated increased episodes of significant bleeding and increased transfusion requirements in patients receiving heparin anticoagulation, as compared with regional citrate anticoagulation (RCA) [23, 24]. UFH as a systemic anticoagulant has been shown to cause hemorrhagic complications in as many as 50% of patients [25, 26]. Heparin-induced thrombocytopenia (HIT) develops in up to 5% of patients exposed to UFH [27]. HIT can cause devastating consequences including thrombosis and limb ischemia. KDIGO AKI guidelines suggest avoiding the use of heparin in patients who are considered to be high risk for bleeding. High-risk patients are defined as having recent (within 7 days) or active bleeding, recent trauma or surgery, recent stroke, intracranial arteriovenous malformation or aneurysm, retinal hemorrhage, uncontrolled hypertension, or presence of an epidural catheter [8]. Finally, although heparin can be reversed with protamine sulfate, this agent has been associated with hypotension and anaphylaxis [28]. Because of the risks associated with heparin, citrate regional anticoagulation has been gaining greater acceptance.

RCA has been shown to be effective with less bleeding risk than heparin and has become the recommended method of anticoagulation at institutions with well-developed RCA protocols [8]. Citrate is delivered into the blood at the beginning of the CRRT extracorporeal circuit and chelates ionized calcium, effectively removing a key piece of the coagulation cascade and preventing coagulation of the hemofilter. Since a significant amount of the calcium-citrate complex is lost across the hemofilter, calcium infusion to the patient is typically employed to replace extracorporeal loss of calcium. Once the remainder of the calcium-citrate complex enters the systemic circulation, it is rapidly metabolized, primarily in the liver, to bicarbonate, which leads to the release of ionized calcium. By maintaining normal levels of ionized calcium in the systemic circulation, anticoagulation is limited only to the circuit (see Fig. 17.1).

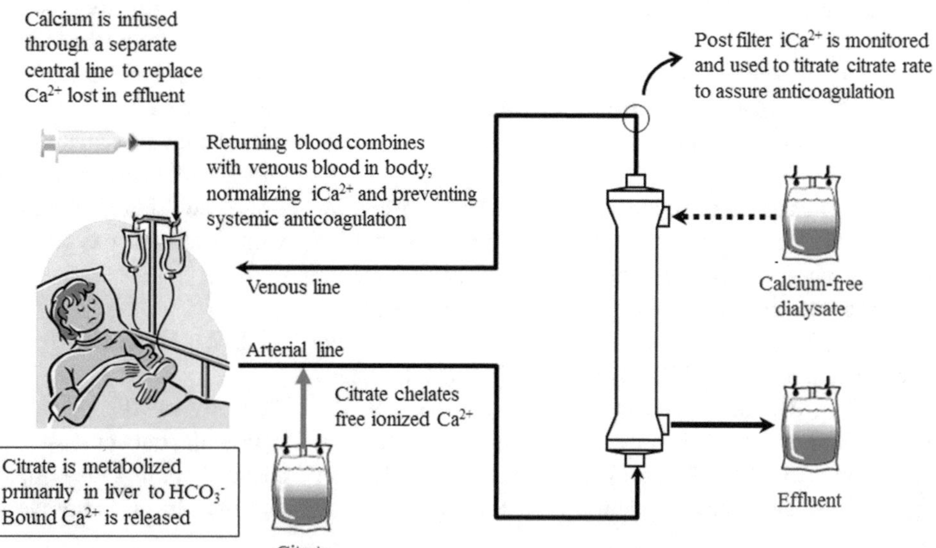
Calcium is infused through a separate central line to replace Ca^{2+} lost in effluent
Post filter iCa^{2+} is monitored and used to titrate citrate rate to assure anticoagulation
Returning blood combines with venous blood in body, normalizing iCa^{2+} and preventing systemic anticoagulation
Venous line
Calcium-free dialysate
Arterial line
Citrate chelates free ionized Ca^{2+}
Citrate is metabolized primarily in liver to HCO_3^- Bound Ca^{2+} is released
Effluent
Citrate

Fig. 17.1 Citrate anticoagulation in continuous renal replacement therapy (CRRT): regional effect in the circuit

Table 17.4 Metabolic complications of regional citrate anticoagulation

Metabolic alkalosis	Citrate overdose
	Excessive bicarbonate load
Metabolic acidosis	Inadequate citrate metabolism in setting of severe liver disease or hypoperfusion
	Inadequate bicarbonate supply
Hypernatremia	Hyperosmolar citrate solutions
Systemic ionized hypercalcemia	Excessive calcium replacement
Systemic ionized hypocalcemia	Inadequate calcium supplementation

Potential complications of RCA include metabolic alkalosis, metabolic acidosis, hypernatremia from the use of commercially available hypertonic citrate solutions (such as 4% trisodium citrate and 2.2% anticoagulant citrate dextrose solution), and hypo- or hypercalcemia (see Table 17.4) [29]. When citrate enters the patient's circulation, each mole of citrate is potentially metabolized in the Krebs cycle to 3 mol of bicarbonate. As a result, metabolic alkalosis can occur with an excessive citrate load. Metabolic acidosis can occur when citrate accumulates in patients who cannot metabolize citrate, such as those with liver failure or severe lactic acidosis, resulting in negative buffer balance. Hallmarks of citrate accumulation include worsening metabolic acidosis, ionized hypocalcemia from unmetabolized calcium-citrate complexes, rising total calcium levels due to a progressively higher calcium infusion rate, and a disproportional rise in total systemic calcium to ionized calcium ratio of greater than 2.5 [30, 31]. Severe ionized hypocalcemia can cause hypotension, arrhythmias, and eventual cardiovascular collapse and death. Protocol driven care with frequent monitoring (every 4–6 h) of acid-base status and other electrolytes, including ionized calcium, total calcium, phosphorous, and magnesium, are necessary for preventing errors. Citrate should be avoided, or used cautiously, in those with severe liver failure. With adequate monitoring and effective protocols, complications associated with RCA are uncommon [32].

17.4 Hemodynamics and Volume Management

CRRT is often utilized in critically ill patients who are considered too hemodynamically unstable to tolerate IHD. In these circumstances, CRRT is generally viewed as being superior to IHD based on studies comparing changes in mean arterial pressure, systemic vascular resistance, and other hemodynamic parameters [33–35]. Despite hypothetical advantages over IHD, CRRT-associated hypotension can still occur. The rate of fluid removal can cause hypotension if it exceeds the rate of interstitial fluid movement into the plasma, leading to intravascular volume depletion [36]. Similarly, osmotic pressure may be decreased by rapid removal of urea, leading to movement of plasma water intracellularly. Strategies for preventing CRRT-related hypotension include beginning therapy with a low blood flow rate (50 ml/min) for the first 5 min, administering a bolus of colloid fluid (200 ml) 1–2 min prior to CRRT initiation, and temporarily increasing vasopressors by 10–15% for 5–10 min prior to initiating therapy [1]. Neonates weighing less than 8–10 kg have an increased risk of hemodynamic instability if more than 10% of their blood volume is in the CRRT circuit and therefore require blood priming to mitigate hypotension [37].

Assessment of intravascular volume status remains a significant challenge to clinicians and can make establishing fluid removal goals with CRRT difficult. Invasive blood pressure monitoring and advanced methods of assessing volume status may be helpful in anticipating and preventing hypotensive events. Static methods of assessing volume status, such as central venous pressure (CVP), pulmonary artery occlusion pressure, and echocardiography, have been shown to be of limited utility. Dynamic measurements are proving to be clinically relevant and increasingly available at the bedside. Dynamic pressure measurement techniques include pulse pressure variation (PPV), stroke volume variation (SVV), esophageal Doppler monitoring, respiratory variation in vena cava diameter, and straight leg raising [38].

17.5 Extracorporeal Circuit Complications

17.5.1 Air Embolism

Negative pressures in the venous intake can allow air entry into the circulation and potentially lead to air emboli. This complication can manifest in the patient as chest pain, dyspnea, hypoxia, tachycardia, cardiopulmonary arrest, and focal signs of end organ damage in cases of arterial embolization [39, 40]. Alarms exist in modern CRRT machines to stop blood flow when air is detected within the circuit, and deaeration chambers are used to extract air prior to blood return to the patient. Patients suspected of having an air embolism should immediately be placed in a left lateral decubitus and Trendelenburg position to optimize pulmonary blood flow. They should subsequently be considered for treatment with hyperbaric oxygen [39, 41].

17.5.2 Hypothermia

As many as 90% of patients on CRRT can experience hypothermia, but some studies have shown that this CRRT-associated cooling may not affect oxygen and energy balance and may in fact improve global hemodynamic parameters

[42, 43]. In certain clinical settings such as cardiac arrest, hypothermia has been shown to decrease neurologic injuries and other end-organ damage [44, 45]. Hypothermia, while theoretically advantageous in some situations, can mask fever, which could potentially lead to delayed response to infection. Clinicians must be vigilant for other signs of infection to help prevent this potential complication. Long-term hypothermia can lead to energy loss (shivering), increased oxygen demand, increased systemic vascular resistance, decreased cardiac output, decreased oxygen delivery, impaired leukocyte function, and coagulation disorders [46, 47]. Undesired hypothermia can be treated with an integrated fluid warmer or blood warmer on equipped CRRT devices. Heating blankets and other external warming devices can also be used.

17.5.3 Immunologic Activation and Anaphylactic Reactions

Prolonged exposure to the hemofilter membrane and artificial surfaces of the extracorporeal circuit can activate immune mediators, which can lead to cytokine production and increased energy expenditure [48]. Anaphylactic reactions have significantly decreased with the advent of the polyacrylonitrile membrane (PAN) [49]. However, there are case reports of anaphylactoid reactions to the CRRT AN69 PAN membrane in patients taking angiotensin converting enzyme inhibitors and rare cases solely from exposure to AN69 membranes [50–52]. Bradykinin activation is thought to be the primary pathophysiologic mechanism and results from blood contact with the negatively charged AN69 membrane [53]. Once a potential anaphylactoid reaction is identified, dialysis should be stopped, the blood in the circuit discarded, and for severe reactions, epinephrine administered. PAN membranes should be avoided in these patients.

In small patients such as children and neonates, blood priming of the circuit with an AN69 membrane can cause profound hypotension at CRRT initiation due to exacerbation of the bradykinin release syndrome from the low pH of the blood prime. Methods for preventing the bradykinin release syndrome include normalizing the pH of the blood prime with bicarbonate, bypassing the hemofilter by giving the blood post filter in conjunction with a saline filter prime, avoiding a blood prime, or using a different membrane than the AN69 [37].

17.5.4 Fluid Balance Errors

Adverse effects due to errors in fluid management can occur from an inadequate prescription, operator error, or inaccuracies in delivery due to machine malfunction or misuse. Given the high ultrafiltration rates often used in CRRT, training in the monitoring and maintenance of desired fluid balance is key to preventing fluid balance errors during therapy [54]. Errors have occurred from inattention to "excess fluid removal" alarms. Some CRRT machines have potential for significant fluid errors if alarms are repeatedly overridden without addressing the underlying problem [55]. Fluid balance errors can be minimized through careful adherence to standardized protocols for the specific CRRT device in use, well-trained personnel, and clearly outlined procedures for device alarms to avoid significant clinical problems.

17.6 Electrolytes and Acid-Base

Phosphate clearance is highly efficient in CRRT, partly because commercially available dialysates and replacement fluids with phosphate are not universally available. As a result, hypophosphatemia is common in CRRT, occurring in as many as 65.1 % of patients treated with this modality [53, 56, 57]. Hypophosphatemia is clinically relevant because it can delay weaning from mechanical ventilation [58]. To prevent complications of ventilator dependence, careful monitoring and repletion of phosphate is recommended. Phosphate may be supplemented by high phosphate-containing enteral feedings as oral supplementation. Several authors have described the safe addition of phosphate to CRRT fluids [59, 60].

Hypokalemia and hypomagnesemia occur less often because commercially available dialysate and replacement fluids contain potassium and magnesium. The frequency of hypokalemia with CRRT has been reported to be between 4 and 24 % and can be mitigated by using dialysate and replacement fluids with potassium concentration of 4 mmol/L [56, 57]. Commercially available CRRT fluids contain magnesium concentration between 2 and 3 mmol/L and have been used successfully without significant hypermagnesemia or hypomagnesemia. Since ionized magnesium is chelated by citrate, intravenous magnesium may be needed in patients treated with citrate anticoagulation.

Both lactate-based and bicarbonate-based solutions are commercially available as CRRT fluids. Although controlled trials have demonstrated similar efficacy of lactate- and bicarbonate-based CRRT solutions in correcting metabolic acidosis, serum lactate levels are typically higher when lactate-based solutions are used and can confound the clinical interpretation of blood lactate levels [61, 62]. Moreover, lactate solutions may worsen metabolic acidosis in patients with liver failure [63]. Studies have shown better control of metabolic acidosis with bicarbonate-based solutions as compared to lactate-based solutions [64]. Bicarbonate is currently the preferred buffer per KDIGO AKI guidelines. Commercially available CRRT fluids contain bicarbonate concentrations in the range of 22–35 mmol/L.

As already mentioned in detail, the use of citrate RCA can predispose to multiple electrolyte and acid-base abnormalities (see Table 17.4). Hypernatremia can develop if hypertonic trisodium citrate solutions are used without adjusting the sodium concentration in the dialysate or replacement fluid. As citrate is metabolized to bicarbonate, metabolic alkalosis can occur with increasing amounts of citrate. Alternatively, metabolic acidosis can occur in patients who are unable to metabolize citrate, as in the setting of hepatic failure. As described previously, citrate functions as an anticoagulant by binding ionized calcium to inhibit the coagulation cascade. Alterations in citrate metabolism can lead to hypo- or hypercalcemia and require frequent monitoring and adjustments in the calcium infusion. A negative calcium balance during RCA can stimulate parathyroid hormone (PTH) release and lead to severe bone reabsorption after prolonged citrate-based CRRT in critically ill patients who are immobilized for extended periods of time. Coexisting secondary hyperparathyroidism (from renal failure) may amplify bone resorption. Immobilization hypercalcemia may be masked by the chelation of calcium during RCA, delaying diagnosis [65].

17.7 Nutrition

Critically ill patients requiring CRRT are generally hypercatabolic leading to mismatch in caloric intake and expenditure and resultant malnutrition. This state of malnutrition can predispose to increased rates of infection, difficulties with wound healing, and muscle wasting [66, 67]. Malnutrition is an independent predictor of mortality in the setting of AKI [68]. CRRT induces additional losses of key nutrients in the effluent, which can contribute to the problem. Amino acid loss in patients on CRRT is estimated between 10 and 20 g/day depending on the amount of effluent [69–71]. CVVH leads to twofold higher total protein losses compared with CVVHDF presumably from increased convective clearance [70]. A protein intake of 2.5 g/kg/day is recommended for optimal nitrogen balance in patients on CRRT, but consultation with a clinical dietitian or nutrition expert is advised. Because of extensive protein and electrolyte losses with CRRT, patients should not be given enteral feeding regimens designed for renal failure (see Table 17.5).

The recommended daily caloric intake for patients on CRRT is 25–35 kcal/kg/day. Optimal glycemic control in critically ill patients can be difficult as hyperglycemia occurs secondary to peripheral insulin resistance and increased hepatic gluconeogenesis [72–74]. Commercially available CRRT solutions typically contain 0–110 mg/dL of glucose. This can account for 40–80 g/day but generally does not cause hyperglycemia [75]. Solutions with supraphysiologic glucose content should be avoided since they can induce hyperglycemia, which is associated with poorer outcomes. CRRT-induced hypoglycemia is limited to circumstances where glucose-free CRRT solutions are used. Close monitoring of blood glucose is necessary in critically ill patients undergoing CRRT.

Table 17.5 Nutrition support recommendations for continuous renal replacement therapy (CRRT) patients

Avoid protein, fluid, and electrolyte restrictions
Protein requirements range from 1.5 to 2.5 g/kg reference weight/day
Energy needs range from 25 to 35 kcal/kg reference weight/day
Water-soluble vitamin supplementation is recommended
Standard vitamin supplements and trace elements are recommended in parenteral nutrition
Hypomagnesemia, hypophosphatemia, and hypokalemia are predictable electrolyte disturbances that should be anticipated and repleted

Water soluble vitamins and trace minerals are freely filtered across the membrane in CRRT and can become quickly depleted [76]. Active vitamin D is readily depleted with CRRT, and if prolonged treatment is expected, vitamin D repletion should be started [14]. Concentrations of thiamine, folic acid, and vitamin C patients are also decreased due to losses through the semipermeable membrane. Vitamin C replacement should not exceed 100–150 mg/day to prevent the development of oxalosis [76]. Additional essential nutrients that are freely filtered include zinc, selenium, copper, manganese, and chromium [77, 78]. The clinical significance of loss of these vitamins and nutrients is unclear at this time. Replacement of selenium 100 µg and thiamine 100 mg daily is recommended by some experts to prevent severe body depletion [76]. Consultation with a clinical dietitian is recommended when prolonged periods of CRRT are anticipated.

17.8 Drug Administration with CRRT

The dosing of drugs with CRRT is an important consideration in critically ill patients and is discussed in detail in Chap. 19. The underdosing of drugs such as antibiotics can lead to inadequate treatment of sepsis, while doses that are too high can lead to drug toxicity. The clearance of drugs on CRRT is complex and highly variable in different situations.

Factors affecting drug dosing include CRRT modality, blood flow rate, effluent rate, location of replacement fluid, and interruptions in CRRT because of filter clotting or need for procedures. CVVHD uses passive diffusion of solutes across a concentration gradient with countercurrent dialysis fluid, and only molecules of small molecular weight (<500 Da) are readily removed with this method. CVVH uses convective clearance, where solutes and plasma water are forced through a membrane by a pressure gradient leading to "solute drag" of particles smaller than the pore size of the membrane. This method can theoretically lead to clearance of middle molecular weight solutes up to the pore size of the membrane (30,000 Da) [21]. In CVVHDF, both methods are used, leading to the clearance of both "small and middle molecular weight solutes." The characteristics of the membrane also affect the clearance of drugs. "High-flux" membranes have larger pore sizes and generally lead to greater drug clearance. The ability of a drug or solute to pass through a membrane is represented by the sieving coefficient (SC). This coefficient is calculated by dividing the concentration of the solute or drug in the effluent by the concentration in the plasma. A SC of 0 indicates no passage through the filter, while a SC of 1 indicates free passage through the filter.

Patient characteristics also lead to alterations in drug clearance on CRRT. Critically ill patients may have altered volumes of distribution from increased or decreased total body water. Drug absorption may be altered by intestinal edema. Drug absorption may increase as volume is removed with CRRT and edema is alleviated. Furthermore, a patient's nutritional and acid-base status may affect protein binding and varying levels of organ dysfunction may alter metabolism. Residual renal function may lead to enhanced drug clearance that will not be accounted for solely with CRRT.

The properties of a drug may also affect its clearance by CRRT. Small molecular weight substances are more likely to be removed by CRRT, while large molecular weight substances are less likely to be removed. Protein bound molecules, particularly when the protein bound complex exceeds 30,000 Da, are unlikely to be removed. Unbound molecules are more likely to be cleared by CRRT. The volume of distribution is affected by the hydrophilic or lipophilic nature of the drug. Hydrophilic molecules generally have a small volume of distribution and are restricted to the vascular space, where they are more readily removed by CRRT. Lipophilic drugs, by contrast, are able to freely cross plasma membranes and have large volumes of distribution, making them less freely cleared by CRRT [21].

All of these characteristics—type of CRRT employed, membrane and patient characteristics, and the pharmacodynamics properties of the drug (concentration dependent vs. time dependent)—must be considered when dosing drugs on CRRT. Therapeutic drug monitoring is recommended when available to ensure adequate dosing, and consultation with a clinical pharmacist is recommended.

References

1. Shingarev R, Wille K, Tolwani A. Management of complications in renal replacement therapy. Semin Dial. 2011;24(2):164–8.
2. Oliver MJ. Acute dialysis catheters. Semin Dial. 2001;14(6):432–5 (Review).
3. Mansfield PF, Hohn DC, Fornage BD, Gregurich MA, Ota DM. Complications and failures of subclavian-vein catheterization. N Engl J Med. 1994;331(26):1735–8 (Clinical Trial Randomized Controlled Trial Research Support, Non-U.S. Gov't).
4. Merrer J, De Jonghe B, Golliot F, Lefrant JY, Raffy B, Barre E, et al. Complications of femoral and subclavian venous catheterization in critically ill patients: a randomized controlled trial. JAMA. 2001;286(6):700–7 (Clinical Trial Comparative Study Multicenter Study Randomized Controlled Trial Research Support, Non-U.S. Gov't).
5. Sznajder JI, Zveibil FR, Bitterman H, Weiner P, Bursztein S. Central vein catheterization. Failure and complication rates by three percutaneous approaches. Arch Intern Med. 1986;146(2):259–61. (Comparative Study).
6. Karakitsos D, Labropoulos N, De Groot E, Patrianakos AP, Kouraklis G, Poularas J, et al. Real-time ultrasound-guided catheterisation of the internal jugular vein: a prospective comparison with the landmark technique in critical care patients. Crit Care. 2006;10(6):R162 (Randomized Controlled Trial).
7. Prabhu MV, Juneja D, Gopal PB, Sathyanarayanan M, Subhramanyam S, Gandhe S, et al. Ultrasound-guided femoral dialysis access placement: a single-center randomized trial. Clin J Am Soc Nephrol. 2010;5(2):235–9 (Randomized Controlled Trial).
8. Disease K, Improving Global Outcomes (KDIGO) Acute Kidney Injury Work Group. KDIGO clinical practice guideline for acute kidney injury. Kidney Inter. 2012;2:1–138.
9. National Kidney Foundation. KDOQI clinical practice guidelines and clinical practice recommendations for 2006 updates: vascular access. Am J Kidney Dis. 2006;48:S176–247.
10. O'Grady NP, Alexander M, Dellinger EP, Gerberding JL, Heard SO, Maki DG, et al. Guidelines for the prevention of intravascular catheter-related infections. Infect Control Hosp Epidemiol. 2002;23(12):759–69 (Guideline Research Support, Non-U.S. Gov't).
11. Gowardman JR, Robertson IK, Parkes S, Rickard CM. Influence of insertion site on central venous catheter colonization and bloodstream infection rates. Intensive Care Med. 2008;34(6):1038–45 (Research Support, Non-U.S. Gov't).
12. Parienti JJ, Thirion M, Megarbane B, Souweine B, Ouchikhe A, Polito A, et al. Femoral vs jugular venous catheterization and risk of nosocomial events in adults requiring acute renal replacement therapy: a randomized controlled trial. JAMA. 2008;299(20):2413–22 (Multicenter Study Randomized Controlled Trial Research Support, Non-U.S. Gov't).
13. Parienti JJ, Megarbane B, Fischer MO, Lautrette A, Gazui N, Marin N, et al. Catheter dysfunction and dialysis performance according to vascular access among 736 critically ill adults requiring renal replacement therapy: a randomized controlled study. Crit Care Med. 2010;38(4):1118–25.
14. Finkel KW, Podoll AS. Complications of continuous renal replacement therapy. Semin Dial. 2009;22(2):155–9 (Review).
15. Cimochowski GE, Worley E, Rutherford WE, Sartain J, Blondin J, Harter H. Superiority of the internal jugular over the subclavian access for temporary dialysis. Nephron. 1990;54(2):154–61 (Comparative Study).
16. Schillinger F, Schillinger D, Montagnac R, Milcent T. Post-catheterization venous stenosis in hemodialysis: comparative angiographic study of 50 subclavian and 50 internal jugular accesses. Nephrologie. 1992;13(3):127–33 (Comparative Study).
17. Tolwani A. Continuous renal-replacement therapy for acute kidney injury. N Engl J Med. 2012;367(26):2505–14 (Review).
18. Leblanc M, Fedak S, Mokris G, Paganini EP. Blood recirculation in temporary central catheters for acute hemodialysis. Clin Nephrol. 1996;45(5):315–9 (Comparative Study).
19. Little MA, Conlon PJ, Walshe JJ. Access recirculation in temporary hemodialysis catheters as measured by the saline dilution technique. Am J Kidney Dis. 2000;36(6):1135–9.

20. Venkataraman R, Kellum JA, Palevsky P. Dosing patterns for continuous renal replacement therapy at a large academic medical center in the United States. J Crit Care. 2002;17(4):246–50 (Comparative Study Review).
21. Zhongping H, Jeffrey JL, Claudo R, William RC. Basic principles of solute transport. In: John AK, Bellomo R, Claudo R, editors. Continuous renal replacement therapy. 1st edition. Oxford: Oxford University Press; 2010. pp. 25–33.
22. Clark WR, Turk JE, Kraus MA, Gao D. Dose determinants in continuous renal replacement therapy. Artif Organs. 2003;27(9):815–20 (Research Support, Non-U.S. Gov't Review).
23. Betjes MG, van Oosterom D, van Agteren M, van de Wetering J. Regional citrate versus heparin anticoagulation during venovenous hemofiltration in patients at low risk for bleeding: similar hemofilter survival but significantly less bleeding. J Nephrol. 2007;20(5):602–8 (Randomized Controlled Trial).
24. Monchi M, Berghmans D, Ledoux D, Canivet JL, Dubois B, Damas P. Citrate vs. heparin for anticoagulation in continuous venovenous hemofiltration: a prospective randomized study. Intensive Care Med. 2004;30(2):260–5 (Clinical Trial Comparative Study Randomized Controlled Trial).
25. Davenport A, Will EJ, Davison AM. Comparison of the use of standard heparin and prostacyclin anticoagulation in spontaneous and pump-driven extracorporeal circuits in patients with combined acute renal and hepatic failure. Nephron. 1994;66(4):431–7 (Clinical Trial Comparative Study Controlled Clinical Trial Research Support, Non-U.S. Gov't).
26. van de Wetering J, Westendorp RG, van der Hoeven JG, Stolk B, Feuth JD, Chang PC. Heparin use in continuous renal replacement procedures: the struggle between filter coagulation and patient hemorrhage. J Am Soc Nephrol. 1996;7(1):145–50.
27. Martel N, Lee J, Wells PS. Risk for heparin-induced thrombocytopenia with unfractionated and low-molecular-weight heparin thromboprophylaxis: a meta-analysis. Blood. 2005;106(8):2710–5 (Meta-Analysis).
28. Horrow JC. Protamine: a review of its toxicity. Anesth Analg. 1985;64(3):348–61 (Review).
29. Tolwani A, Wille KM. Advances in continuous renal replacement therapy: citrate anticoagulation update. Blood Purif. 2012;34(2):88–93.
30. Bakker AJ, Boerma EC, Keidel H, Kingma P, van der Voort PH. Detection of citrate overdose in critically ill patients on citrate-anticoagulated venovenous haemofiltration: use of ionised and total/ionised calcium. Clin Chem Lab Med. 2006;44(8):962–6.
31. Meier-Kriesche HU, Gitomer J, Finkel K, DuBose T. Increased total to ionized calcium ratio during continuous venovenous hemodialysis with regional citrate anticoagulation. Crit Care Med. 2001;29(4):748–52.
32. Tolwani AJ, Prendergast MB, Speer RR, Stofan BS, Wille KM. A practical citrate anticoagulation continuous venovenous hemodiafiltration protocol for metabolic control and high solute clearance. Clin J Am Soc Nephrol. 2006;1(1):79–87.
33. Bellomo R, Farmer M, Wright C, Parkin G, Boyce N. Treatment of sepsis-associated severe acute renal failure with continuous hemodiafiltration: clinical experience and comparison with conventional dialysis. Blood Purif. 1995;13(5):246–54 (Clinical Trial Comparative Study Controlled Clinical Trial).
34. Guerin C, Girard R, Selli JM, Ayzac L. Intermittent versus continuous renal replacement therapy for acute renal failure in intensive care units: results from a multicenter prospective epidemiological survey. Intensive Care Med. 2002;28(10):1411–8 (Multicenter Study Research Support, Non-U.S. Gov't).
35. John S, Griesbach D, Baumgartel M, Weihprecht H, Schmieder RE, Geiger H. Effects of continuous haemofiltration vs intermittent haemodialysis on systemic haemodynamics and splanchnic regional perfusion in septic shock patients: a prospective, randomized clinical trial. Nephrol Dial Transplant. 2001;16(2):320–7 (Clinical Trial Comparative Study Evaluation Studies Randomized Controlled Trial).
36. Gibney N, Cerda J, Davenport A, Ramirez J, Singbartl K, Leblanc M, et al. Volume management by renal replacement therapy in acute kidney injury. Int J Artif Organs. 2008;31(2):145–55 (Case Reports Consensus Development Conference).
37. Goldstein SL. Advances in pediatric renal replacement therapy for acute kidney injury. Semin Dial. 2011;24(2):187–91.
38. Kalantari K, Chang JN, Ronco C, Rosner MH. Assessment of intravascular volume status and volume responsiveness in critically ill patients. Kidney Int. 2013;83(6):1017–28 (Review).
39. Dudney TM, Elliott CG. Pulmonary embolism from amniotic fluid, fat, and air. Prog Cardiovasc Dis. 1994;36(6):447–74 (Review).
40. Heckmann JG, Lang CJ, Kindler K, Huk W, Erbguth FJ, Neundorfer B. Neurologic manifestations of cerebral air embolism as a complication of central venous catheterization. Crit Care Med. 2000;28(5):1621–5 (Case Reports Review).
41. Bateman NT, Leach RM. ABC of oxygen. Acute oxygen therapy. BMJ. 1998;317(7161):798–801 (Review).
42. Jones S. Heat loss and continuous renal replacement therapy. AACN Clin Issues. 2004;15(2):223–30 (Review).
43. Rokyta R Jr, Matejovic M, Krouzecky A, Opatrny K Jr, Ruzicka J, Novak I. Effects of continuous venovenous haemofiltration-induced cooling on global haemodynamics, splanchnic oxygen and energy balance in critically ill patients. Nephrol Dial Transplant. 2004;19(3):623–30 (Clinical Trial Research Support, Non-U.S. Gov't).
44. Aslami H, Juffermans NP. Induction of a hypometabolic state during critical illness—a new concept in the ICU? Neth J Med. 2010;68(5):190–8 (Review).
45. Polderman KH. Induced hypothermia and fever control for prevention and treatment of neurological injuries. Lancet. 2008;371(9628):1955–69 (Review).
46. Manns M, Maurer E, Steinbach B, Evering HG. Thermal energy balance during in vitro continuous veno-venous hemofiltration. ASAIO J. 1998;44(5):M601–5.
47. Yagi N, Leblanc M, Sakai K, Wright EJ, Paganini EP. Cooling effect of continuous renal replacement therapy in critically ill patients. Am J Kidney Dis. 1998;32(6):1023–30.
48. Gutierrez A, Alvestrand A, Wahren J, Bergstrom J. Effect of in vivo contact between blood and dialysis membranes on protein catabolism in humans. Kidney Int. 1990;38(3):487–94 (Clinical Trial Comparative Study Controlled Clinical Trial Research Support, Non-U.S. Gov't).
49. Ebo DG, Bosmans JL, Couttenye MM, Stevens WJ. Haemodialysis-associated anaphylactic and anaphylactoid reactions. Allergy. 2006;61(2):211–20 (Review).
50. Brunet P, Jaber K, Berland Y, Baz M. Anaphylactoid reactions during hemodialysis and hemofiltration: role of associating AN69 membrane and angiotensin I-converting enzyme inhibitors. Am J Kidney Dis. 1992;19(5):444–7.
51. Parnes EL, Shapiro WB. Anaphylactoid reactions in hemodialysis patients treated with the AN69 dialyzer. Kidney Int. 1991;40(6):1148–52 (Case Reports Research Support, Non-U.S. Gov't).
52. Tielemans C, Madhoun P, Lenaers M, Schandene L, Goldman M, Vanherweghem JL. Anaphylactoid reactions during hemodialysis on AN69 membranes in patients receiving ACE inhibitors. Kidney Int. 1990;38(5):982–4 (Case Reports).
53. Schulman G, Hakim R, Arias R, Silverberg M, Kaplan AP, Arbeit L. Bradykinin generation by dialysis membranes: possible role in anaphylactic reaction. J Am Soc Nephrol. 1993;3(9):1563–9 (Research Support, U.S. Gov't, P.H.S.)
54. Baldwin IC. Training, management, and credentialing for CRRT in the ICU. Am J Kidney Dis. 1997;30(5 Suppl 4):S112–6.
55. Ronco C. Fluid balance in CRRT: a call to attention! Int J Artif Organs. 2005;28(8):763–4 (Editorial).

56. Bellomo R, Cass A, Cole L, Finfer S, Gallagher M, Lo S, et al. Intensity of continuous renal-replacement therapy in critically ill patients. N Engl J Med. 2009;361(17):1627–38 (Multicenter Study Randomized Controlled Trial Research Support, Non-U.S. Gov't).
57. Palevsky PM, Zhang JH, O'Connor TZ, Chertow GM, Crowley ST, Choudhury D, et al. Intensity of renal support in critically ill patients with acute kidney injury. N Engl J Med. 2008;359(1):7–20 (Multicenter Study Randomized Controlled Trial Research Support, N.I.H. Extramural Research Support, U.S. Gov't, Non-P.H.S.)
58. Alsumrain MH, Jawad SA, Imran NB, Riar S, DeBari VA, Adelman M. Association of hypophosphatemia with failure-to-wean from mechanical ventilation. Ann Clin Lab Sci. 2010;40(2):144–8.
59. Santiago MJ, Lopez-Herce J, Urbano J, Bellon JM, del Castillo J, Carrillo A. Hypophosphatemia and phosphate supplementation during continuous renal replacement therapy in children. Kidney Int. 2009;75(3):312–6.
60. Troyanov S, Geadah D, Ghannoum M, Cardinal J, Leblanc M. Phosphate addition to hemodiafiltration solutions during continuous renal replacement therapy. Intensive Care Med. 2004;30(8):1662–5.
61. Heering P, Ivens K, Thumer O, Morgera S, Heintzen M, Passlick-Deetjen J, et al. The use of different buffers during continuous hemofiltration in critically ill patients with acute renal failure. Intensive Care Med. 1999;25(11):1244–51.
62. Thomas AN, Guy JM, Kishen R, Geraghty IF, Bowles BJ, Vadgama P. Comparison of lactate and bicarbonate buffered haemofiltration fluids: use in critically ill patients. Nephrol Dial Transplant. 1997;12(6):1212–7.
63. Kierdorf HP, Leue C, Arns S. Lactate- or bicarbonate-buffered solutions in continuous extracorporeal renal replacement therapies. Kidney Int Suppl. 1999;72:S32–6.
64. McLean AG, Davenport A, Cox D, Sweny P. Effects of lactate-buffered and lactate-free dialysate in CAVHD patients with and without liver dysfunction. Kidney Int. 2000;58(4):1765–72.
65. Wang P-L. Bone resorption and "relative" immobilization hypercalcemia with prolonged continuous renal replacement therapy and citrate anticoagulation. Am J Kidney Dis. 2004;44(6):1110–4.
66. Mainous MR, Deitch EA. Nutrition and infection. Surg Clin North Am. 1994;74(3):659–76 (Review).
67. Santos JI. Nutrition, infection, and immunocompetence. Infect Dis Clin North Am. 1994;8(1):243–67 (Review).
68. Obialo CI, Okonofua EC, Nzerue MC, Tayade AS, Riley LJ. Role of hypoalbuminemia and hypocholesterolemia as copredictors of mortality in acute renal failure. Kidney Int. 1999;56(3):1058–63 (Research Support, Non-U.S. Gov't).
69. Hynote ED, McCamish MA, Depner TA, Davis PA. Amino acid losses during hemodialysis: effects of high-solute flux and parenteral nutrition in acute renal failure. JPEN J Parenter Enteral Nutr. 1995;19(1):15–21.
70. Mokrzycki MH, Kaplan AA. Protein losses in continuous renal replacement therapies. J Am Soc Nephrol. 1996;7(10):2259–63.
71. Wooley JA, Btaiche IF, Good KL. Metabolic and nutritional aspects of acute renal failure in critically ill patients requiring continuous renal replacement therapy. Nutr Clin Pract. 2005;20(2):176–91 (Review).
72. Basi S, Pupim LB, Simmons EM, Sezer MT, Shyr Y, Freedman S, et al. Insulin resistance in critically ill patients with acute renal failure. Am J Physiol Renal Physiol. 2005;289(2):F259–64 (Research Support, N.I.H., Extramural Research Support, Non-U.S. Gov't Research Support, U.S. Gov't, P.H.S.)
73. Van den Berghe G, Wilmer A, Hermans G, Meersseman W, Wouters PJ, Milants I, et al. Intensive insulin therapy in the medical ICU. N Engl J Med. 2006;354(5):449–61 (Randomized Controlled Trial Research Support, Non-U.S. Gov't).
74. van den Berghe G, Wouters P, Weekers F, Verwaest C, Bruyninckx F, Schetz M, et al. Intensive insulin therapy in critically ill patients. N Engl J Med. 2001;345(19):1359–67 (Clinical Trial Randomized Controlled Trial Research Support, Non-U.S. Gov't).
75. Bollmann MD, Revelly JP, Tappy L, Berger MM, Schaller MD, Cayeux MC, et al. Effect of bicarbonate and lactate buffer on glucose and lactate metabolism during hemodiafiltration in patients with multiple organ failure. Intensive Care Med. 2004;30(6):1103–10 (Clinical Trial Comparative Study Randomized Controlled Trial).
76. Honore PM, De Waele E, Jacobs R, Mattens S, Rose T, Joannes-Boyau O, et al. Nutritional and metabolic alterations during continuous renal replacement therapy. Blood Purif. 2013;35(4):279–84.
77. Berger MM, Shenkin A. Update on clinical micronutrient supplementation studies in the critically ill. Curr Opin Clin Nutr Metab Care. 2006;9(6):711–6 (Review).
78. Berger MM, Shenkin A, Revelly JP, Roberts E, Cayeux MC, Baines M, et al. Copper, selenium, zinc, and thiamine balances during continuous venovenous hemodiafiltration in critically ill patients. Am J Clin Nutr. 2004;80(2):410–6 (Clinical Trial Randomized Controlled Trial).

Continuous Renal Replacement Therapy in Children

18

Scott M. Sutherland

18.1 Introduction

Over time, continuous renal replacement therapy (CRRT) has become the preferred modality to manage acute kidney injury (AKI) and fluid overload in critically ill children [1, 2]. One reason is that CRRT allows clearance and fluid removal to occur over an extended period of time with remarkable accuracy. This is a boon in unstable patients who are intolerant of abrupt volume and solute concentration changes. Although pediatric CRRT provision is in some ways similar to that in adult populations, there are several considerations that are unique to therapy in children. The goal of this chapter is to describe the principles of pediatric CRRT, highlighting the required adaptations from adult conventions.

18.2 Demographics and Epidemiology

18.2.1 Epidemiology of Pediatric AKI

The majority of children receiving CRRT are critically ill with AKI, so it is important to understand the epidemiology of AKI, especially since it has changed over the past several decades. Single center reports from the 1980s describe hemolytic uremic syndrome and other primary renal diseases, sepsis, and burns as the most common causes of pediatric AKI [3, 4]. Recent studies, however, suggest that most cases of AKI are now occurring due to diseases of other organ systems or as complications of systemic diseases or their treatments. Two large pediatric studies highlight congenital heart disease (and the requisite corrective surgery), acute tubular necrosis (ATN), sepsis, and administration of nephrotoxic medications as the most common causes of pediatric AKI [5, 6]. These findings were corroborated by an analysis of the 2009 Kids' Inpatient Database, a large, all-payer, inpatient care database that contains information included in a typical discharge abstract. This study examined 10,322 hospitalized children with AKI and found that AKI is more commonly associated with systemic or multisystem disease than with primary renal disease [7]. Thus, the majority of children with AKI now commonly have one or more comorbid conditions that are likely to affect their clinical course and outcome. Notably, this shift in AKI epidemiology has occurred primarily in developed countries where the use of CRRT is more prevalent. In developing countries, AKI continues to be caused by primary renal diseases such as hemolytic uremic syndrome, glomerulonephritis, nephrotic syndrome, renal stones, and hypovolemic ATN [8–11]. Additionally, in these situations, many practitioners have found peritoneal dialysis (PD) to be a viable alternative to CRRT in critically ill children [10–13].

18.2.2 Epidemiology of Pediatric CRRT

With regard to CRRT, the most robust pediatric data available come from the prospective pediatric continuous renal replacement therapy (ppCRRT) registry [14]. The registry contains data on children from the 13 US centers with ages ranging from newborn to 25 years and weights ranging from 1.3 to 160 kg [15]. These epidemiologic data highlight the fact that providing CRRT to children requires adaptation and resourcefulness. The underlying diseases seen in this cohort underscore the epidemiologic AKI data described above (Table 18.1). The three most common disease categories were sepsis (23.5 %), stem cell transplantation (16.0 %), and cardiac disease (11.9 %); hepatic disease (8.4 %) was as common as primary renal disease (9.3 %) [15]. A large cohort from Madrid, Spain reported similar findings [16]. Cardiac disease (55 %) and sepsis (20 %) were common; again, primary renal disease was less common, representing the underlying pathophysiology only 12 % of the time (Table 18.1). It is also important to highlight that children receiving CRRT

S. M. Sutherland (✉)
Department of Pediatrics, Lucile Packard Children's Hospital, Stanford University Medical Center, Stanford, CA, USA
e-mail: suthersm@stanford.edu

A. K. Singh et al. (eds.), *Core Concepts in Dialysis and Continuous Therapies*, DOI 10.1007/978-1-4899-7657-4_18

Table 18.1 Underlying diseases among children receiving continuous renal replacement therapy (CRRT)

	Prospective pediatric continuous renal replacement therapy (ppCRRT) registry USA (n=344)		Madrid cohort Spain (n=174)	
	N	%	*N*	%
Sepsis	81	23.5	34	19.5
Stem cell transplant	55	16.0		
Cardiac disease/transplant	41	11.9	97	55.7
Renal disease	32	9.3	21	12.1
Liver disease/transplant	29	8.4		
Malignancy (w/o tumor lysis)	29	8.4		
Ischemia/shock	19	5.5		
Inborn error of metabolism	15	4.4	5	2.9
Drug intoxication	13	3.8	3	1.7
Tumor lysis syndrome	12	3.5	5	2.9
Pulmonary disease/transplant	11	3.2		
Other	7	2.0	9	5.2

ppCRRT prospective pediatric continuous renal replacement therapy

are among the sickest patients in the hospital. The ppCRRT registry reported that at CRRT initiation, 48 % of the patients were receiving diuretics, 74 % were intubated and receiving mechanical ventilation, and 64 % were receiving vasopressor support; nearly 80 % of the patients had multi-organ dysfunction syndrome (MODS) [15]. Thus, it is evident that children requiring CRRT usually have substantial fluid overload with a tendency towards hemodynamic instability.

18.3 Mechanisms of Clearance and CRRT Nomenclature

The majority of CRRT devices can provide diffusive and/or convective clearance (see Chap. 15). The distinction is important since although diffusive and convective clearances are equally effective at small molecule removal, larger molecules move more effectively via convection [17, 18]. CRRT terminology is historically based upon the type of vascular access and the primary method of molecular clearance [17]. Although CRRT was initially developed based on combined arterial and venous access (i.e., continuous arterio-venous hemofiltration, CAVH), the current technique relies upon pump-driven veno-venous access, hence the terms continuous veno-venous hemofiltration (CVVH), continuous veno-venous hemodialysis (CVVHD), and continuous veno-venous hemodiafiltration (CVVHDF). CVVH provides exclusively convective clearance through high ultrafiltration rates. To prevent rapid volume depletion, the majority of the ultrafiltrate is replaced with electrolyte containing fluid. In CVVHD, the majority of clearance is diffusive and occurs via countercurrent infusion of dialysate through the hemofilter. A small amount of convective clearance is provided by the net ultrafiltration used to reduce extracellular fluid volume. CVVHDF employs both diffusive and convective clearance. All these modalities enjoy some degree of popularity, and modality choice is usually center dependent. The ppCRRT registry reported that among the 344 children studied, 21 % of the patients received CVVH, 48 % received CVVHD, and 30 % received CVVHDF [15].

18.4 CRRT and Comparisons to Hemodialysis and Peritoneal Dialysis

CRRT shares many principles with hemodialysis (HD) and PD. One substantial difference between CRRT and HD are the flow rates. CRRT tends to use slower blood and dialysate flow rates (Q_b and Q_d) than HD, resulting in lower clearance rates on an hour-by-hour basis. To compensate for this, CRRT extends the duration of therapy; thus, over a full 24 h period, CRRT can provide solute clearance comparable to that of a 4-h HD session. Additionally, small solute clearance limitations differ between HD and CRRT; different approaches are used to augment molecular removal. HD, given its temporal constraints, employs a dialysate flow rate that far exceeds the blood flow rate, often by a factor of 1.5–3×. Thus, dialytic clearance is limited primarily by the blood flow rate, and increasing the blood flow rate tends to increase solute clearance. CRRT clearance, by comparison, is primarily limited by the dialysate or replacement/effluent rate since these rates can be dwarfed by the blood flow rate; typically, the best way to increase CRRT clearance is to increase the dialysate or replacement/effluent rate. CRRT and the continuous forms of PD commonly used in the critical care setting share their continuous nature. Thus, both CRRT and PD can achieve gradual and continuous solute and fluid removal. However, PD clearance and ultrafiltration rates depend on the quality and characteristics of the peritoneal membrane that can vary from patient to patient; furthermore, ultrafiltration may vary hour to hour. CRRT, on the other hand, allows one to fine tune and stabilize ultrafiltration. Additionally, CRRT allows for much greater daily clearance rates when compared to PD.

While a comprehensive comparison is beyond the scope of this chapter, it is important to understand the general advantages and disadvantages of CRRT therapy. The major advantages are the ability to provide renal replacement therapy (RRT) in a critically ill child while maintaining hemodynamic stability, the ability to remove a large amount of volume over an extended period of time, and the ability to nearly eliminate the need for fluid restriction. This allows optimization of nutritional status and provision of essential medications and blood products. Notably, the continuous nature of CRRT that promotes such hemodynamic stability can also at times be disadvantageous. The ubiquitous presence of the circuit complicates both diagnostic imaging and procedures. Additionally, patients who are neither intubated nor sedated often poorly tolerate the immobility that CRRT requires. Other disadvantages include the potential for hypothermia (addressed with a circuit heating device) and the potential to create electrolyte imbalances (addressed by addition of electrolytes to CRRT fluids and provision of high dose amino acids/protein).

18.5 Technical Aspects of CRRT Provision in Children

CRRT devices often have distinctive features, and variation exists between the machines and circuits made by different manufacturers. However, many technical aspects of pediatric CRRT can be generalized and applied regardless of the device used. Thus, the goal of this section is to describe these generalizable aspects while avoiding machine- or device-specific technicalities. Note that many of these principles are based upon the need for pediatric practitoners to use adult-sized devices on pediatric-sized patients. Recent work towards the creation of a pediatric-specific device [19] is likely to redefine much of pediatric CRRT provision.

18.5.1 Access

Achieving adequate vascular access is essential to the delivery of CRRT and doing so can be especially challenging in children where vessel size is often small. Effective access is governed primarily by Poiseuille's law: Although catheter length is associated with resistance, generally speaking, the internal diameter of the catheter has the greatest effect on flow. One potential caveat is that while longer catheters usually offer greater resistance to flow, there are times where a longer catheter will allow the access to be positioned in a larger blood vessel, resulting in higher blood flow rates despite the increased length; this is especially true for catheters positioned in the femoral vessels. In general, larger diameter catheters allow higher blood flow rates and are associated with greater CRRT circuit survival. This was clearly demonstrated by the ppCRRT data, which showed a stepwise increase in circuit survival as catheter French (Fr) size increased (Fig. 18.1a) [20]. These data highlighted the fact that standard single lumen, 5Fr catheters performed exceedingly poorly; no circuits survived beyond 20 h [20]. While these data led most practitioners to abandon the two single-lumen catheter approach, a group from the University of Alabama, Birmingham (USA) recently published their experience using 3, 4, and 5Fr single lumen cardiac catheterization introducer sheaths with great success [21]. These sheaths are constructed differently than standard dialysis catheters; while the external diameter of the 4Fr sheath is smaller than a 7Fr dialysis catheter, the internal diameter approaches that of a 9 or 10Fr dialysis catheter [21]. While this approach has not been widely adopted and may or may not be feasible

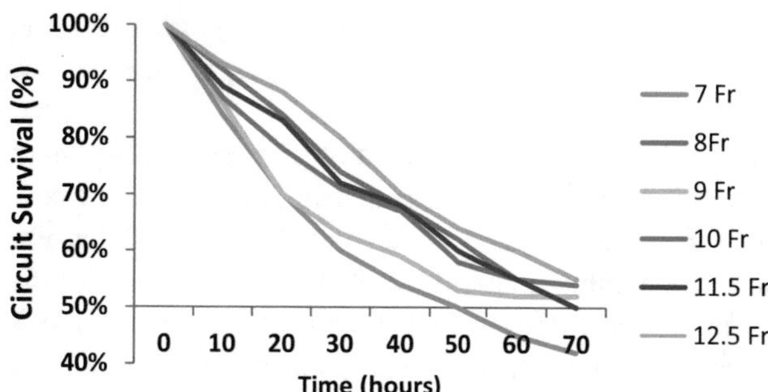

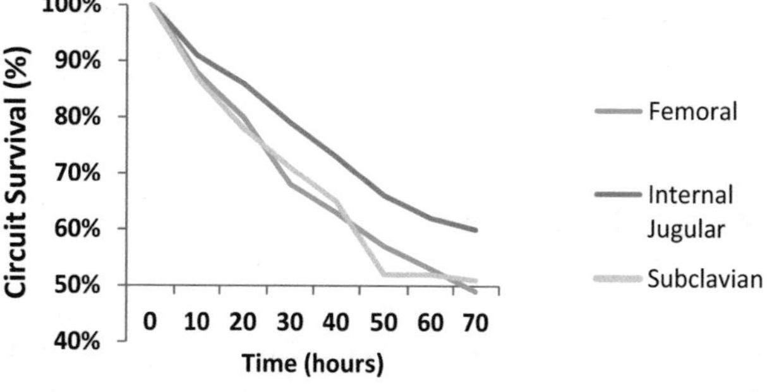

Fig. 18.1 Circuit survival by catheter size (**a**) and insertion location (**b**) [18, 19]. **a** Prospective pediatric continuous renal replacement therapy *(ppCRRT)* data demonstrate that 7 and 8Fr catheters are associated with shorter continuous renal replacement therapy *(CRRT)* circuit survival. Standard single-lumen 5Fr catheters are associated with inadequate circuit survival and their use is not recommended (data not pictured). **b** Catheters placed in the subclavian *(SC)* and femoral veins are associated with similar CRRT circuit survival, however, superior circuit survival is seen with internal jugular *(IJ)* vein catheters

Table 18.2 Temporary catheters for acute continuous renal replacement therapy (CRRT) access

Patient weight/size	Catheter size
Neonate	Dual-lumen 7French
3–6 kg	Dual-lumen 7Fr
6–15 kg	Dual-lumen 8–9Fr
15–30 kg	Dual-lumen 9–10Fr
30 kg	Dual- or triple-lumen 11.5–12.5Fr

Fr French

at certain institutions, it is an impressive example of how CRRT provision in children requires an adaptable approach. Notably, smaller bore catheters such as Broviacs, peripherally inserted central catheters (PICC), and umbilical lines provide insurmountable resistance to flow and cannot be used for CRRT access. At our institution, we have had excellent technical success in neonates using 7Fr catheters placed by the Pediatric Surgery service. Typically, these catheters were inserted into an internal jugular (IJ) vein using a cut-down technique similar to that used for extracorporeal membrane oxygenation (ECMO) cannulation. Suggested catheter sizes based on patient weight are listed in Table 18.2 [17, 22].

Catheter location has an equally substantial effect on circuit survival. Femoral catheters are used for CRRT access more frequently than IJ and subclavian (SC) catheters (69% vs. 16% vs. 8%, respectively); however, IJ catheters are associated with significantly greater circuit survival when compared to femoral or SC catheters (Fig. 18.1b) [20]. Many practitioners prefer femoral catheters due to ease of placement; however, bedside ultrasound devices have become more commonplace and, if available, can facilitate IJ catheter insertions. Additionally, femoral catheters which terminate prior to the inferior vena cava are remarkably sensitive to patient movement and usually require more aggressive patient sedation and, at times, paralysis for successful use. Nephrologists frequently avoid SC catheters since they are associated with stenosis of the SC vein, which is catastrophic from a long-term access standpoint should the patient not regain renal function and require chronic intermittent HD therapy.

18.5.2 Circuit Priming

Prior to connecting the patient to the CRRT circuit, the circuit itself must be primed; this process purges the air contained within the pre-packaged filter and tubing, replacing it with a fluid chosen by the practitioner. Once the circuit is primed in this fashion, the patient can be connected to the circuit and therapy can begin. As blood moves from the patient into the circuit, the priming fluid replaces the volume of the blood which has been displaced into the circuit. Essentially, the circuit expands the intravascular volume of the patient; the impact of this expansion is highly dependent on patient size. For example, a 5 kg neonate has a blood volume of approximately 80 mL/kg, or 400 mL. Often, the priming volume of the CRRT circuit exceeds 150 mL which is nearly 40% of the estimated blood volume; rapidly displacing this amount of blood is likely to have catastrophic hemodynamic effects. Thus, in smaller children, it is imperative to prime large, adult-sized circuits with blood. This approach effectively expands the patient's blood volume to the same degree to which the circuit expands the extracorporeal blood volume and allows initiation of CRRT with a minimum of hemodynamic instability. As a rule of thumb, we tend to prime with blood whenever the extracorporeal volume of the circuit exceeds 10–15% of the patient's estimated blood volume. Several blood priming techniques have been published and used with great success [23–25]. In bigger patients with greater blood volumes, the impact of priming is negligible. Thus, in most large children and adolescents, the circuit can be primed with an isotonic fluid such as normal saline, just as in adults. However, we have found that in some older children who are particularly hemodynamically unstable, a normal saline circuit prime can still result in hypotension which requires intervention. In such situations, we have had great success using 5% albumin to prime the circuit.

18.5.3 Filter/Membrane

Many CRRT hemofilters and membranes have been developed. One of the most commonly used is the AN-69 membrane, which is biocompatible and constructed of polyacrilonitrile. This membrane has been frequently associated with the bradykinin release syndrome (BRS) when used in conjunction with a blood prime. The BRS occurs due to exposure of the blood to the AN-69 membrane which activates prekallikrein and Hageman factor leading to release of bradykinin, which is a powerful vasodilator [17]. This reaction can lead to profound hypotension in infants 5–10 min after initiation of CRRT. Several strategies have been proposed to mitigate or prevent this syndrome including bypassing the CRRT filter during the prime [23] and dialyzing the prime prior to CRRT initiation [24, 25]. However, our center has found that the best option for prevention of the BRS is to avoid the AN-69 membrane altogether. This may not be a feasible strategy at all centers and, if not, the aforementioned BRS avoidance techniques are quite effective. Some practitioners use the AN-69 membranes specifically in patients with sepsis due to their greater cytokine-sieving coefficients when compared to other membranes [26, 27]. However, while studies have indicated that CRRT can remove cytokines and/or mediators of inflammation [27, 28], no studies have been able to confirm that cytokine removal, or implementation of CRRT, have the ability to improve survival in septic patients [29–31]. Notably, our center changed from the AN-69 filter to a polyarylethersulfone (PAES) membrane over 7 years ago; since making that change, the bradykinin release phenomenon is no longer seen. However, PAES membranes are not available on all CRRT devices and they may not be available in pediatric specific sizes. Although we have used an adult-sized PAES membrane successfully even in children less than 10 kg, other polysulfone derivative membranes are available which, when compared with AN-69 membranes, have been associated with lower post-CRRT initiation bradykinin levels [24, 32] .

18.5.4 CRRT Solutions for Dialysate and Replacement Fluid

The introduction of bicarbonate-based solutions has made the delivery of CRRT more feasible and effective. Prior to this, when the solution was buffered with lactate, it was common to see lactic acidosis with resultant cardiac dysfunction and hypotension [33]. Studies comparing these two buffer systems clearly demonstrated the superiority of bicarbonate-based fluids, and now bicarbonate-based dialysate/replacement fluids are considered standard of care in adults and children [34, 35]. It is important to note, however, that many commercially available fluids contain a small, clinically insignificant amount of lactate to improve stability.

CRRT solutions usually contain sodium, potassium, chloride, glucose, phosphate, calcium, and magnesium in various concentrations and combinations. Although many different electrolyte formulations are available from a number of manufacturers, for the sake of simplicity, our institution has tended to stock a single brand in only a few formulations which can then be modified as required. Notably, as the length of CRRT course becomes more prolonged, the composition of the dialysate and replacement fluids tends to determine the electrolyte levels of the patient. A fluid low in potassium, phosphorous, and magnesium may be appropriate at CRRT initiation; however, patients can become markedly deficient in these electrolytes in a surprisingly short period of time. Hypophosphatemia, in particular, is remarkably common without solution supplementation, especially if higher clearance rates are targeted [30, 36]. Supplementation of the CRRT solutions with the necessary electrolytes creates a more physiologic fluid that will result in normalization of the electrolyte levels. If required, the pharmacy can add potassium, *phosphorous,* magnesium, calcium, and additional bicarbonate as required. While we have had great success with this practice, it has the potential for pharmacy errors and may increase costs.

In the majority of situations, if one is using CVVHDF, the replacement and dialysate fluids should have the same composition to reduce staff confusion and the risk for error. One significant exception is when albumin is added to the dialysate fluid. This technique can be used to remove protein-bound medications in the setting of intoxication as well as substances such as bilirubin [37] .

18.5.5 Anticoagulation

Anticoagulation in adults has been discussed in detail in Chap. 15, and the majority of the same principles apply to children. In pediatrics, there is no evidence that heparin or citrate is the superior anticoagulant. The only large observational study in pediatrics demonstrated that heparin and citrate are equally efficacious, but that bleeding complications may be more common with heparin [38]. Most adult studies demonstrate prolonged-circuit life and reduced bleeding with the use of citrate anticoagulation [39, 40]. However, since controlled studies in children are lacking, most centers tend to adopt either heparin or citrate based primarily on local experience and practice; amongst practitioners from the 13 US centers, citrate was used 56 % and heparin 37 % of the time [15]. An additional 7 % of the patients received no anticoagulation, relying on periodic saline flushes of the circuit. While a no-anticoagulation approach might be considered in patients with evidence of existing coagulopathy due to disseminated intravascular coagulation or hepatic failure, this tends to be associated with poor circuit survival [38]. Many of these patients receive periodic fresh frozen plasma and platelet infusions which, without anticoagulation, commonly lead to clotting. Moreover, patients with hepatic failure may have a paradoxical hypercoagulable state. Thus, while either citrate or heparin can provide adequate CRRT anticoagulation, it is clear that avoidance of anticoagulation is associated with markedly inferior circuit life span and a reduced ability to deliver CRRT [38].

18.6 CRRT Prescription and Dosing

18.6.1 Blood Flow Rates

Blood flow (Q_b) is primarily dependent on the access; smaller 7Fr and 9Fr catheters infrequently allow a Q_b greater than 60–80 mL/min. The CRRT device itself can also dictate blood flow rates; for example, while many newer machines have maximal Q_b rates of 450–600 mL/min, some older machines possess lower maximal Q_b rates (150–180 mL/min). However, generally recommended Q_b rates of 3–10 mL/kg/min have been extrapolated from adult data and animal models [41]. Higher Q_b rates (10–12 mL/kg/min) are usually necessary in neonates and small infants for technical reasons when currently available CRRT devices are used. For example, in a 3 kg neonate, a Q_b of 30 mL/min may be necessary to generate access and return pressures adequate to prevent

Table 18.3 Recommended blood flow (Q_b) rates for CRRT

Patient weight/size (kg)	Blood flow rate (mL/min)
0–10	20–60
11–20	50–100
21–50	100–150
>50	150–250

access disconnect alarms. General guidelines for Q_b ranges based on age are shown in Table 18.3. Higher blood flow rates tend to result in longer circuit lifespans due to reduced risk for intrafiber clotting. Again, it is important to remember that a fundamental difference between CRRT and HD is that increasing CRRT Q_b does not necessarily result in greater small solute clearance. Increasing Q_b can, however, facilitate greater clearance by mitigating the reduced efficiency seen with pre-dilution mode CVVH or CVVHDF. Many patients will not tolerate maximal blood flow at the initiation of CRRT and, in general, it is best to advance Q_b to the targeted rate over 20–30 min.

18.6.2 Dialysate Flow Rates (Q_d), Replacement Flow Rates (Q_r), and CRRT Dosing

Although no CRRT dosing studies exist in children, there have been several studies performed in adults (see Chap. 15). As a result, most pediatric practitioners have adopted dosing strategies extrapolated from the available data. Although Ronco and colleagues originally suggested targeting a convective clearance of 35–45 mL/kg/h [42], the Veterans Affairs/National Institutes of Health (VA/NIH) and RENAL studies demonstrated that, in adults, there was no benefit to targeting combined (convective and diffusive) clearances above 20–25 mL/kg/h [30, 31]. While 85–100% of the patients enrolled in these studies received the prescribed dose, successfully delivering the prescribed dose can be difficult in clinical practice. In adults, it has been suggested that critically ill patients may receive 30% less than their prescribed HD dose [43]; this may be even more common in children where smaller diameter catheters and lower blood flow rates encourage circuit malfunction and membrane clotting. Many children require blood priming at CRRT initiation which can substantially delay restarting a failed circuit. Additionally, centers (such as ours) which use pre-dilution CVVH or CVVHDF to reduce the risk of intra-filter hemoconcentration will experience clearances that are reduced by 15–35% [43, 44]. Thus, we typically prescribe a dose of 30–40 ml/kg/h to ensure a sustained dose no lower than 25 mL/kg/h. We, like many centers, tend to divide the dose evenly between dialysate and replacement. Many centers which provide CVVHD will target Q_d of 2000 mL/min/1.73 m^2. One common exception to these dosing strategies are children with inborn errors of metabolism (IEM), which is discussed below.

18.7 Indications for Use of CRRT

For the most part, indications for CRRT are similar in adults and children. Although unique pediatric indications exist, more often than not, CRRT is used in critically ill children with AKI and fluid overload where medical management has failed. The specific triggers for initiation commonly include hyperkalemia and symptomatic uremia (encephalopathy, bleeding, pericarditis) in addition to fluid overload (Table 18.4). The ppCRRT registry data demonstrated that 29% of the children received CRRT to treat isolated fluid overload, 13% to treat isolated electrolyte abnormalities, and 46% to treat both fluid overload and electrolyte abnormalities [15]. Of the remaining patients, 4% received CRRT to treat hyperammonemia associated with an IEM, and 2% received CRRT to treat an intoxication or medication overdose.

18.7.1 CRRT Use and Dose for Inborn Errors of Metabolism

It is worth briefly discussing the use of CRRT in the setting of neonatal hyperammonemia and suspected IEM since this is a uniquely pediatric disease. These patients have acutely elevated ammonia levels, often in excess of 500–1500 mcg/dL and require aggressive management to mitigate the effects of the hyperammonemia. The cornerstones of the most IEM management strategies are aggressive, specific nutritional supplementation and administration of ammonia scavengers, both of which should be initiated as soon as the disease is suspected. However, these interventions often require 24–48 h to be fully effective and RRT is typically used to acutely lower ammonia levels. Similarly, RRT should begin as soon as the diagnosis is suspected. Patients with suspected IEM should receive care at centers with the capacity to deliver either HD or CRRT; ammonia clearance with

Table 18.4 Indications for CRRT in critically ill children with acute kidney injury (AKI)

Indication
Fluid overload
Hyperkalemia
Uremia
Encephalopathy
Refractory bleeding
In preparation for surgery
Pericarditis
Metabolic acidosis
Inability to deliver adequate nutrition
Need to deliver high volumes of medications or blood products
Hyperammonemia/inborn error of metabolism
Intoxication/overdose

PD is inadequate, and this therapy should only be used as a last resort if no other RRT modality is available. While intermittent HD has often been considered the most appropriate therapy due to its ability to achieve high diffusive clearance rates of ammonia, many centers have transitioned to CRRT as the mainstay treatment for IEM associated with hyperammonemia [17, 45]. CRRT can be provided with regional anticoagulation, can be delivered without the need for specialized nursing staff, and avoids the ammonia rebound seen with intermittent HD. If CRRT is used in this situation, it is imperative to deliver higher clearance rates, in the order of 8000 mL/h/1.73 m^2 [17, 26, 45]. Although we have tended to use CVVHD in these babies, CVVH or CVVHDF are likely to be equally efficacious [26]. As previously mentioned, when higher clearance rates are prescribed, it is important to add electrolytes (phosphate, magnesium, and potassium) to the dialysate/replacement fluids to prevent their depletion.

18.7.2 CRRT in Children with Intoxication or Medication Overdose

Children who ingest toxic substances or receive a marked overdose of a medication can experience substantial morbidity. The symptoms and outcomes are highly dependent on the substance ingested or received, the relative size of the dose, and the rapidity with which the intoxication is managed. Although there are no current absolute indications in these settings [46, 47], CRRT has been used successfully in a number of clinical scenarios to manage intoxications. Examples include vancomycin [48], carbamazepine [49], sustained release potassium preparations [50], iron [51], and methotrexate [52]. Typically, in adult patients, HD provides more effective clearance of many toxins/medications, and CRRT is commonly reserved for patients who are hemodynamically unstable or unlikely to tolerate the HD procedure. In smaller children, however, because of the comparatively high dialysate/replacement rates available (relative to an adult sized patient), CRRT can approximate the clearance provided by intermittent HD; use of CRRT in the setting of IEM (above) is an example of this approach [17, 45]. CRRT can also be beneficial in preventing the rebound phenomenon seen following CRRT; in certain situations, CRRT can be initiated immediately following the initial HD session with great success.

18.8 Outcomes in Children Who Receive CRRT

Patients receiving CRRT experience different outcomes depending on the underlying disease state and comorbid conditions, the indication for initiation, and a range of clinical criteria. Adult studies have suggested that mortality in adults with AKI severe enough to require RRT is 50–80% [30, 31, 53]. Factors that have been associated with greater mortality are the need for vasopressor support, use of mechanical ventilation, sepsis, greater severity of illness, muti-organ failure (heart, liver, GI, brain, lungs), and greater positive fluid balance [53–55].

This seems to be the case in children also (Table 18.5). Among patients in the ppCRRT registry, overall mortality was 42%; higher mortality rates were seen in patients with liver failure or liver transplant, pulmonary disease or lung transplant, and stem cell transplant (69, 55, and 55%, respectively) [26, 56]. Smaller children experienced greater morality than bigger children; in children ≤10 kg, survival was 43%, whereas survival was 64% in children >10 kg [57]. Interestingly, when the ≤10 kg cohort was split into ≤5 and 5–10 kg, survival rates were equivalent (44 and 42%, respectively) [57]. Although younger, smaller children had

Table 18.5 Mortality according to underlying diagnosis among pediatric patients receiving continuous renal replacement therapy (CRRT)

	Prospective pediatric continuous renal replacement therapy (ppCRRT) registry USA (n=344)		Madrid cohort Spain (n=174)	
	N	Mortality (%)	*N*	Mortality (%)
Sepsis	33/81	41	15/97	44
Stem cell transplant	30/55	55		
Cardiac disease/transplant	20/41	49	39/97	40
Renal disease	5/32	16	1/21	5
Liver disease/transplant	20/29	69		
Malignancy (w/o tumor lysis)	15/29	52		
Ischemia/shock	6/19	32		
Inborn error of metabolism	4/15	17	2/5	40
Drug intoxication	0/13	0	1/3	33
Tumor lysis syndrome	2/12	17	0/5	0
Pulmonary disease/transplant	6/11	55		
Other	2/7	29	3/3	100

ppCRRT prospective pediatric continuous renal replacement therapy greater mortality, this likely reflects the greater mortality seen in critically ill infants with AKI rather than a CRRT-specific finding.

A retrospective series of 76 pediatric CRRT patients presented similar findings. Across the entire cohort, mortality was 44.7 %; however, mortality was greater in patients with sepsis, MODS, and increased fluid overload [58]. The ppCRRT registry also found a high risk of mortality in the setting of MODS (OR 4.7; 95th CI 2.0–10.7) and cancer (OR 3.2; 95th CI 1.7–6.1) [56]. Another center established that in children requiring CRRT, non-survivors had higher pediatric risk of mortality (PRISM) scores, lower blood pressures, and required more substantial pressor support [59]. Thus, it seems that children with higher disease severity, a greater number of organ systems involved, and hemodynamic instability have a poorer prognosis and worse outcomes.

The relationship between fluid overload and mortality is especially relevant and worthy of further discussion. The ppCRRT registry has demonstrated that greater fluid overload at CRRT initiation is independently associated with greater mortality (Fig. 18.2). After controlling for severity of illness, each 1 % increase in fluid overload was associated with a concomitant 3 % increase in mortality; patients with >20 % fluid overload at CRRT initiation were 8.5 times more likely to die than those with <20 % fluid overload [56]. This association has been seen in adult studies as well. However, adults studies have also been able to demonstrate that outcomes are superior when RRT is initiated earlier in the ICU course [54]. Thus, although the majority of the data remain observational, they certainly suggest that outcomes are likely to be better if CRRT is initiated earlier in the clinical course and at a lesser degree of fluid overload.

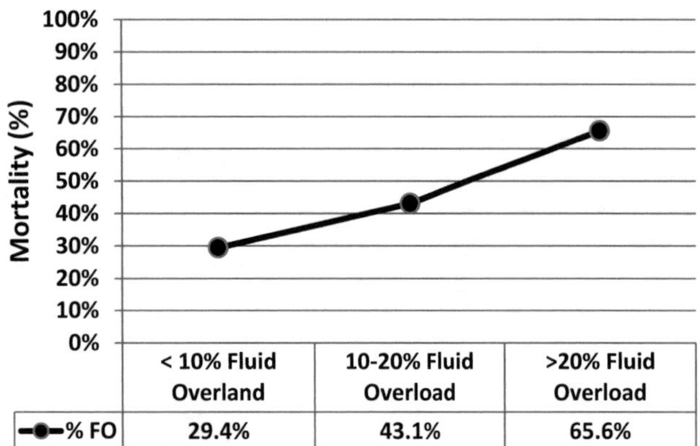

Fig. 18.2 Relationship between fluid overload and mortality in critically ill children receiving continuous renal replacement therapy *(CRRT)* [18, 56]. Prospective pediatric continuous renal replacement therapy *(ppCRRT)* data demonstrate that children with greater fluid overload at CRRT initiation experienced greater mortality

In the pediatric setting, CRRT is often used in combination with ECMO. A large proportion of the patients requiring ECMO develop AKI and oligoanuria. When these patients fail to respond to standard medical interventions, CRRT can be used effectively to treat uremia and fluid overload. We have experienced excellent technical success delivering the therapy directly into the ECMO circuit. The return line can be positioned downstream from the access line and both access points can be placed pre-bladder, pump, and oxygenator, which minimizes the risk of air embolism [17]. Additionally, the heparin-based ECMO anticoagulation is more than adequate anticoagulation for the CRRT circuit, and no additional anticoagulation is required. Although patients receiving ECMO who develop AKI and require CRRT have higher mortality rates, those who do survive have exceptional renal outcomes [60, 61]. In two studies, 93 and 97 % of the ECMO/CRRT therapy patients recovered full renal function [60, 61]. In fact, out of 68 ECMO/CRRT survivors, the only two patients who did not recover renal function had primary renal vasculitis [61]. Thus, although the majority of pediatric AKI survivors develop some degree of chronic kidney disease (CKD) [62, 63], they are quite unlikely to require chronic RRT at the time of hospital discharge.

18.9 Summary

Across the majority of developed countries, CRRT has become the preferred modality to treat AKI and fluid overload in critically ill children; it can provide stable, slow removal of uremic toxins and fluid in patients with hemodynamic instability. CRRT shares some physiologic principles with HD and PD, however, it does have distinct advantages and disadvantages which need to be appreciated in order to deliver high-quality care. Although the technical considerations are similar to those in adults, providing CRRT in children does require an adaptable approach and an understanding of some practical differences and obstacles. Available data suggest that with adequate experience, centers can deliver CRRT to children across the entire spectrum of age and size both safely and effectively [17].

References

1. Belsha CW, Kohaut EC, Warady BA. Dialytic management of childhood acute renal failure: a survey of North American pediatric nephrologists. Pediatr Nephrol. 1995;9(3):361–3.
2. Warady BA, Bunchman T. Dialysis therapy for children with acute renal failure: survey results. Pediatr Nephrol. 2000;15(1–2):11–3.
3. Lattouf OM, Ricketts RR. Peritoneal dialysis in infants and children. Am Surg. 1986;52(2):66–9.
4. Williams D, Sreedhar S, Mickell J, Chan JCM. Acute kidney failure: a pediatric experience over 20 years. Arch Pediatr Adolesc Med. 2002;156(9):893–900.

5. Bunchman TE, McBryde KD, Mottes TE, Gardner JJ, Maxvold NJ, Brophy PD. Pediatric acute renal failure: outcome by modality and disease. Pediatr Nephrol. 2001;16(12):1067–71.
6. Hui Stickle S, Brewer E, Goldstein S. Pediatric ARF epidemiology at a tertiary care center from 1999 to 2001. Am J Kidney Dis. 2005;45(1):96–101.
7. Sutherland SM, Ji J, Sheikhi FH, Widen E, Tian L, Alexander SR, et al. AKI in hospitalized children: epidemiology and clinical associations in a national cohort. Clin J Am Soc Nephrol. 2013;8(10):1661–9.
8. Vachvanichsanong P, Dissaneewate P, Lim A, McNeil E. Childhood acute renal failure: 22-year experience in a University Hospital in Southern Thailand. Pediatrics. 2006;118(3):e786–91.
9. Van Biljon G. Causes, prognostic factors and treatment results of acute renal failure in children treated in a tertiary hospital in South Africa. J Trop Pediatr. 2008;54(4):233–7.
10. Abdelraheem M, Ali ET, Osman R, Ellidir R, Bushara A, Hussein R, et al. Outcome of acute kidney injury in sudanese children—an experience from a Sub-Saharan African unit. Perit Dial Int. 2014;34(5):526–33.
11. Esezobor CI, Ladapo TA, Osinaike B, Lesi FE. Paediatric acute kidney injury in a tertiary hospital in Nigeria: prevalence, causes and mortality rate. PloS One. 2012;7(12):e51229.
12. Bonilla-Félix M. Peritoneal dialysis in the pediatric intensive care unit setting: techniques, quantitations and outcomes. Blood Purif. 2013;35(1–3):77–80.
13. Mishra OP, Gupta AK, Pooniya V, Prasad R, Tiwary NK, Schaefer F. Peritoneal dialysis in children with acute kidney injury: a developing country experience. Perit Dial Int. 2012;32(4):431–6.
14. Goldstein SL, Somers MJG, Brophy PD, Bunchman TE, Baum M, Blowey D, et al. The prospective pediatric continuous renal replacement therapy (ppCRRT) registry: design, development and data assessed. Int J Artif Organs. 2004;27(1):9–14.
15. Symons JM, Chua AN, Somers MJG, Baum MA, Bunchman TE, Benfield MR, et al. Demographic characteristics of pediatric continuous renal replacement therapy: a report of the prospective pediatric continuous renal replacement therapy registry. Clin J Am Soc Nephrol. 2007;2(4):732–8.
16. Santiago M, Lpez-Herce J, Urbano J, Solana M, del Castillo J, Ballestero Y, et al. Clinical course and mortality risk factors in critically ill children requiring continuous renal replacement therapy. Intensive Care Med. 2010;36(5):843–9.
17. Sutherland S, Alexander S. Continuous renal replacement therapy in children. Pediatr Nephrol. 2012;27(11):2007–16.
18. Messer J, Mulcahy B, Fissell WH. Middle-molecule clearance in CRRT: in vitro convection, diffusion and dialyzer area. ASAIO J. 2009;55(3):224–6.
19. Ronco C, Garzotto F, Brendolan A, Zanella M, Bellettato M, Vedovato S, et al. Continuous renal replacement therapy in neonates and small infants: development and first-in-human use of a miniaturised machine (CARPEDIEM). Lancet. 2014;383(9931):1807–13.
20. Hackbarth R, Bunchman TE, Chua AN, Somers MJ, Baum M, Symons JM, et al. The effect of vascular access location and size on circuit survival in pediatric continuous renal replacement therapy: a report from the PPCRRT registry. Int J Artif Organs. 2007;30(12):1116–21.
21. Masri K E, Jackson K, Borasino S, Law M, Askenazi D, Alten J. Successful continuous renal replacement therapy using two single-lumen catheters in neonates and infants with cardiac disease. Pediatr Nephrol. 2013;28(12):2383–7.
22. Goldstein S. Advances in pediatric renal replacement therapy for acute kidney injury. Semin Dial. 2011;24(2):187–91.
23. Brophy PD, Mottes TA, Kudelka TL, McBryde KD, Gardner JJ, Maxvold NJ, et al. AN-69 membrane reactions are pH-dependent and preventable. Am J Kidney Dis. 2001;38(1):173–8.
24. Hackbarth R, Eding D, Gianoli Smith C, Koch A, Sanfilippo D, Bunchman T. Zero balance ultrafiltration (Z-BUF) in blood-primed CRRT circuits achieves electrolyte and acid-base homeostasis prior to patient connection. Pediatr Nephrol. 2005;20(9):1328–33.
25. Pasko D, Mottes T, Mueller B. Pre dialysis of blood prime in continuous hemodialysis normalizes pH and electrolytes. Pediatr Nephrol. 2003;18(11):1177–83.
26. Goldstein S. Continuous renal replacement therapy: mechanism of clearance, fluid removal, indications and outcomes. Curr Opin Pediatr. 2011;23(2):181–5.
27. Peng Y, Yuan Z, Li H. Removal of inflammatory cytokines and endotoxin by veno-venous continuous renal replacement therapy for burned patients with sepsis. Burns. 2005;31(5):623–8.
28. Bellomo R, Tipping P, Boyce N. Continuous veno-venous hemofiltration with dialysis removes cytokines from the circulation of septic patients. Crit Care Med. 1993;21(4):522–6.
29. Zhongheng Z, Xiao X, Hongyang Z. Intensive- vs less-intensive-dose continuous renal replacement therapy for the intensive care unit-related acute kidney injury: a meta-analysis and systematic review. J Crit Care. 2010;25(4):595–600.
30. Bellomo R, Cass A, Cole L, Finfer S, Gallagher M, Lo S, et al. Intensity of continuous renal-replacement therapy in critically ill patients. N Engl J Med. 2009;361(17):1627–38.
31. Palevsky P, Zhang J, O'Connor T, Chertow G, Crowley S, Choudhury D, et al. Intensity of renal support in critically ill patients with acute kidney injury. N Engl J Med. 2008;359(1):7–20.
32. Stoves J, Goode NP, Visvanathan R, Jones CH, Shires M, Will EJ, et al. The bradykinin response and early hypotension at the introduction of continuous renal replacement therapy in the intensive care unit. Artif Organs. 2001;25(12):1009–13.
33. Davenport A, Will EJ, Davison AM. Hyperlactataemia and metabolic acidosis during haemofiltration using lactate-buffered fluids. Nephron. 1991;59(3):461–5.
34. Zimmerman D, Cotman P, Ting R, Karanicolas S, Tobe SW. Continuous veno-venous haemodialysis with a novel bicarbonate dialysis solution: prospective cross-over comparison with a lactate buffered solution. Nephrol Dial Transplant. 1999;14(10):2387–91.
35. Barenbrock M, Hausberg M, Matzkies F, de la Motte S, Schaefer RM. Effects of bicarbonate- and lactate-buffered replacement fluids on cardiovascular outcome in CVVH patients. Kidney Int. 2000;58(4):1751–7.
36. Santiago M, Lpez-Herce J, Urbano J, Belln J, del Castillo J, Carrillo A. Hypophosphatemia and phosphate supplementation during continuous renal replacement therapy in children. Kidney Int. 2009;75(3):312–6.
37. Ringe H, Varnholt V, Zimmering M, Luck W, Gratopp A, Knig K, et al. Continuous veno-venous single-pass albumin hemodiafiltration in children with acute liver failure. Pediatr Crit Care Med. 2011;12(3):257–64.
38. Brophy P, Somers MJG, Baum M, Symons J, McAfee N, Fortenberry J, et al. Multi-centre evaluation of anticoagulation in patients receiving continuous renal replacement therapy (CRRT). Nephrol Dial Transplant. 2005;20(7):1416–21.
39. Kutsogiannis D, Gibney RTN, Stollery D, Gao J. Regional citrate versus systemic heparin anticoagulation for continuous renal replacement in critically ill patients. Kidney Int. 2005;67(6):2361–7.
40. Hetzel G, Schmitz M, Wissing H, Ries W, Schott G, Heering P, et al. Regional citrate versus systemic heparin for anticoagulation in critically ill patients on continuous venovenous haemofiltration: a prospective randomized multicentre trial. Nephrol Dial Transplant. 2011;26(1):232–9.
41. Werner HA, Herbertson MJ, Seear MD. Functional characteristics of pediatric veno-venous hemofiltration. Crit Care Med. 1994;22(2):320–5.
42. Ronco C, Bellomo R, Homel P, Brendolan A, Dan M, Piccinni P, et al. Effects of different doses in continuous veno-venous haemofiltration on outcomes of acute renal failure: a prospective randomised trial. Lancet. 2000;356(9223):26–30.

43. Schiffl H. The dark side of high-intensity renal replacement therapy of acute kidney injury in critically ill patients. Int Urol Nephrol. 2010;42(2):435–40.
44. Parakininkas D, Greenbaum L. Comparison of solute clearance in three modes of continuous renal replacement therapy. Pediatr Crit Care Med. 2004;5(3):269–74.
45. Spinale JM, Laskin BL, Sondheimer N, Swartz SJ, Goldstein SL. High-dose continuous renal replacement therapy for neonatal hyperammonemia. Pediatr Nephrol. 2013;28(6):983–6.
46. Bunchman T, Ferris M. Management of toxic ingestions with the use of renal replacement therapy. Pediatr Nephrol. 2011;26(4):535–41.
47. Kim Z, Goldfarb DS. Continuous renal replacement therapy does not have a clear role in the treatment of poisoning. Nephron Clin Pract. 2010;115(1):c1–6.
48. Goebel J, Ananth M, Lewy JE. Hemodiafiltration for vancomycin overdose in a neonate with end-stage renal failure. Pediatr Nephrol. 1999;13(5):423–5.
49. Yildiz TS, Toprak DG, Arisoy ES, Solak M, Md KT. Continuous venovenous hemodiafiltration to treat controlled-release carbamazepine overdose in a pediatric patient. Pediatr Anesth. 2006;16(11):1176–8.
50. Gunja N. Decontamination and enhanced elimination in sustained-release potassium chloride poisoning. Emerg Med Australas. 2011;23(6):769–72.
51. Milne C, Petros A. The use of haemofiltration for severe iron overdose. Arch Dis Child. 2010;95(6):482–3.
52. Ziółkowska H, Kisiel A, Leszczyńska B, Bilska K, Jankowska K, Kuźma Mroczkowska E, et al. Continuous veno-venous hemodiafiltration in methotrexate intoxication.
53. Uchino S, Kellum JA, Bellomo R, Doig GS, Morimatsu H, Morgera S, et al. Acute renal failure in critically ill patients. JAMA. 2005;294(7):813–8.
54. Payen D, de-Pont A, Sakr Y, Spies C, Reinhart K, Vincent J. A positive fluid balance is associated with a worse outcome in patients with acute renal failure. Crit Care. 2008;12(3):R74–R.
55. Ostermann M, Chang R. Correlation between parameters at initiation of renal replacement therapy and outcome in patients with acute kidney injury. Crit Care. 2009;13(6):R175–R.
56. Sutherland S, Zappitelli M, Alexander S, Chua A, Brophy P, Bunchman T, et al. Fluid overload and mortality in children receiving continuous renal replacement therapy: the prospective pediatric continuous renal replacement therapy registry. Am J Kidney Dis. 2010;55(2):316–25.
57. Askenazi DJ, Goldstein SL, Koralkar R, Fortenberry J, Baum M, Hackbarth R, et al. Continuous renal replacement therapy for children ≤10 kg: a report from the prospective pediatric continuous renal replacement therapy registry. J Pediatr. 2013;162(3):587–92.e3.
58. Hayes L, Oster R, Tofil N, Tolwani A. Outcomes of critically ill children requiring continuous renal replacement therapy. J Crit Care. 2009;24(3):394–400.
59. Fernndez C, Lpez-Herce J, Flores J, Galaviz D, Ruprez M, Brandstrup K, et al. Prognosis in critically ill children requiring continuous renal replacement therapy. Pediatr Nephrol. 2005;20(10):1473–7.
60. Meyer R, Brophy P, Bunchman T, Annich G, Maxvold N, Mottes T, et al. Survival and renal function in pediatric patients following extracorporeal life support with hemofiltration. Pediatr Crit Care Med. 2001;2(3):238–42.
61. Paden M, Warshaw B, Heard M, Fortenberry J. Recovery of renal function and survival after continuous renal replacement therapy during extracorporeal membrane oxygenation. Pediatr Crit Care Med. 2011;12(2):153–8.
62. Mammen C, Al Abbas A, Skippen P, Nadel H, Levine D, Collet JP, et al. Long-term risk of CKD in children surviving episodes of acute kidney injury in the intensive care unit: a prospective cohort study. Am J Kidney Dis. 2012;59(4):523–30.
63. Askenazi DJ, Feig DI, Graham NM, Hui-Stickle S, Goldstein SL. 3–5 year longitudinal follow-up of pediatric patients after acute renal failure. Kidney Int. 2006;69(1):184–9.

19 Drug Dosing in Continuous Renal Replacement Therapy (CRRT)

Helen C. Gallagher and Patrick T. Murray

19.1 Introduction

In intensive care medicine, both intermittent and continuous renal replacement therapies (CRRTs) are frequently used in the treatment of acute kidney injury (AKI). CRRT is considered superior to intermittent haemodialysis (IHD) in maintaining haemodynamic stability and also provides better volume, electrolyte and acid–base control [1]. As such, it has become the technique of choice for dealing with AKI in the intensive care unit (ICU). Critically ill patients with AKI who require CRRT comprise a very heterogeneous population, often with severe sepsis and/or multiple organ dysfunction [2]. Therefore, they frequently require complex drug therapy, and it is essential that drug dosing is appropriately prescribed and adjusted so as to be clinically safe and effective in optimising clinical outcomes. A prospective observational study across 23 countries suggested that up to 60 % of patients with AKI die during their hospital stay, despite considerable progress in critical care medicine and in CRRT technologies [3]. There is little doubt that inaccuracies in medication dosing contribute to the continued poor outcomes in this patient population.

Correct dosing of drugs in patients undergoing CRRT is extremely challenging, since it is necessary to consider both extracorporeal drug removal by the CRRT process itself and pharmacokinetic perturbations caused by organ dysfunction, sepsis and/or other aspects of critical illness. A further consideration is that the clinical situation in these patients is dynamic and may change rapidly. Thus, pharmacokinetic parameters observed in end-stage renal disease (ESRD) patients are not generalisable to ICU patients undergoing CRRT [4].

There is some robust evidence to guide dosing of individual drugs in CRRT, particularly antimicrobials, since sepsis is one of the main causes of AKI. However, wide variation exists in the type of CRRT technique, clinical setting and patient factors, all of which make generalisation difficult. Well-designed pharmacokinetic studies in critically ill patients receiving CRRT are relatively rare, and dosing guidelines are usually not included in the manufacturers' product labelling [5]. While there are multiple published dosing recommendations that are widely used, in reality these have not been adequately validated in prospective studies to see if their implementation either increases the attainment of target therapeutic serum concentrations of drugs or, more importantly, improves patient outcomes [6–8].

The aims of this review are to discuss the general principles determining whether a dose adjustment is necessary during CRRT and to provide some practical guidance enabling clinicians to avoid ineffective drug dosing in this setting.

19.2 CRRT Techniques and Methods of Drug Removal

CRRT began with continuous arteriovenous haemofiltration (CAVH) more than 50 years ago [9], in which arterial blood pressure drove blood flow through a haemofilter, and gravity controlled the fluid removal (ultrafiltration) rate. CRRT has since evolved to include more modalities, purpose-built pumps (for 'veno-venous' modalities) and associated technologies. The most commonly used modern-day CRRT therapies include pump-driven continuous venovenous modalities: haemofiltration (CVVH), continuous venovenous haemodialysis (CVVHD) and continuous venovenous haemodiafiltration (CVVHDF; Fig. 19.1). Continuous arteriovenous haemodialysis (CAVHD) and continuous arteriovenous

P. T. Murray (✉)
School of Medicine, University College Dublin, Dublin, Ireland
e-mail: patrick.murray@ucd.ie

H. C. Gallagher
School of Medicine & Conway Institute of Biomolecular and Biomedical Research, University College Dublin, Belfield, Dublin, Ireland

A. K. Singh et al. (eds.), *Core Concepts in Dialysis and Continuous Therapies,* DOI 10.1007/978-1-4899-7657-4_19

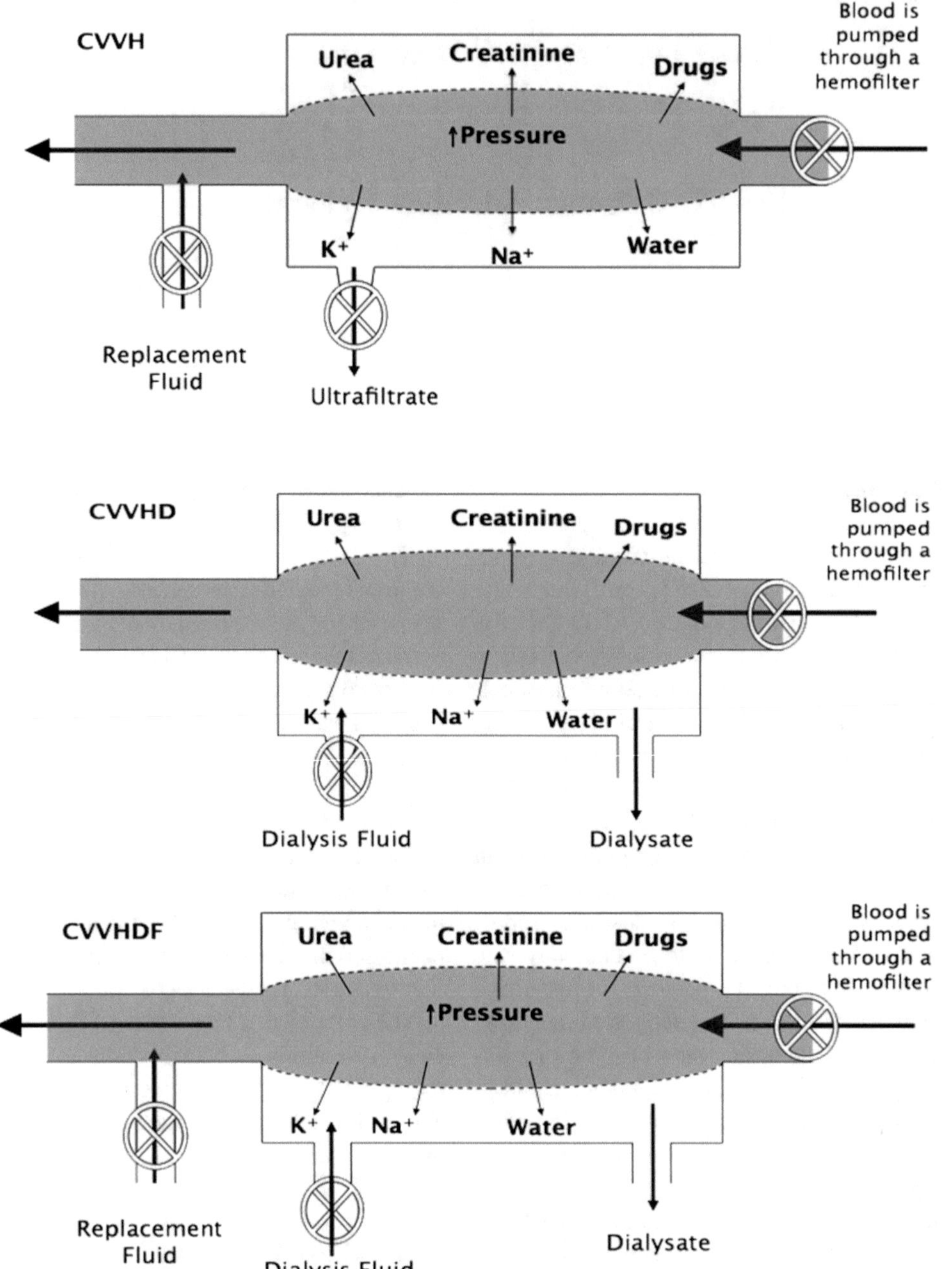

Fig. 19.1 Schematic representation of the most commonly employed continuous renal replacement therapies: Continuous venovenous haemofiltration *(CVVH)*; continuous venovenous haemodialysis *(CVVHD)* and continuous venovenous haemodiafiltration *(CVVHDF)*; and the mechanisms by which they drive the extracorporeal clearance of drugs. All three modalities involve the pumping of blood through a haemofilter *(hatched line)*. In CVVH, plasma water is forced through the membrane via a pressure gradient and solutes, including drugs, move via convective forces. In CVVHD, solutes move by diffusion into the dialysate, which runs countercurrent to blood flow to maximise the diffusion gradient. In CVVHDF, both diffusion and convection combine to remove solutes. In CVVHD and CVVHDF, large amounts of replacement fluids are administered either after (as illustrated above) or before the haemofilter to maintain desired fluid balance and to replace lost electrolytes and bicarbonate

haemodiafiltration (CAVHDF) are employed only rarely. More details are provided in Chap. 15.

The primary modes of solute removal during CRRT are convection, diffusion and combinations thereof (Table 19.1; Fig. 19.1). In continuous haemofiltraton (CAVH and CVVH), convection dominates, with solutes (including drugs) being carried along or 'dragged' with plasma water that is pushed through the membrane via a pressure gradient. In continuous

Table 19.1 Clearance mechanisms for continuous renal replacement modalities

Modality	Clearance mechanism		Key factors influencing drug removal
	Convection	Diffusion	
Intermittent haemodialysis	+	++++	Blood flow rate
Continuous arteriovenous haemodiafiltration	+++	+++	Ultrafiltration and dialysate flow rates
Continuous venovenous haemodiafiltration	+++	+++	Ultrafiltration and dialysate flow rates
Continuous arteriovenous haemofiltration	++++	–	Ultrafiltration rate
Continuous venovenous haemofiltration	++++	–	Ultrafiltration rate
Continuous venovenous haemodialysis	+	++++	Dialysate flow rate
Continuous arteriovenous haemodialysis	+	++++	Dialysate flow rate

haemodialysis (CAVHD and CVVHD), drug removal occurs by diffusion into the drug-free dialysate (running countercurrent to blood flow, to maximise diffusion gradient) and convection is less important, since the ultrafiltration rate is much lower than in CAVH/CVVH. Generally, in CAVHD and CVVHD, ultrafiltration rates are set for the sole purpose of achieving desired fluid and weight loss. In continuous haemofiltration (CAVH or CVVH) or in continuous haemodiafiltraton (CAVHDF or CVVHDF), ultrafiltration volumes are increased so that they exceed desired fluid-weight loss and large amounts of replacement fluids are administered before or after the haemofilter to maintain desired fluid balance and to replace lost electrolytes and bicarbonate. The use of haemofiltration with replacement fluid enhances solute clearance by convection. In general, the calculated 'dose' of CRRT is estimated as the hourly effluent flow rate divided by the body weight, and there is general consensus on the minimum, adequate prescribed dose required to improve survival [10–12].

Drug–membrane interactions also impact solute removal in CRRT, and some drugs are eliminated by binding to the membrane rather than passing through it. The Gibbs–Donnan equilibrium is one important determinant of membrane interactions for charged drugs [13]. Proteins such as albumin, which are sequestered on the blood side of a membrane, render that membrane negatively charged, resulting in an asymmetric distribution of permeant charged drugs. Cationic drugs, such as aminoglycosides and levofloxacin, will filter somewhat less readily than one would expect from the unbound fraction, whereas the opposite is true for anionic drugs such as ceftazidime and cefotaxime [14]. However, the clinical relevance of this phenomenon is unclear.

Adsorption is the other major source of drug–membrane interaction, with the extent of adsorption depending on both membrane and drug properties. Hydrophobic membranes, such as synthetic sulphonated polyacrylonitrile and polymethylmethacrylate membranes, are highly adsorptive, whereas cellulose triacetate is much less adsorptive and unsulphonated polyacrylonitrile and polysulphone lie somewhere in between [15]. Since adsorption is generally saturable early on, its influence on drug removal reflects the frequency of filter changes, and when filter changes occur on an average every 24–48 h or more with modern CRRT, the influence of adsorption on drug concentration is generally relatively minor. That said, there is a paucity of information describing adsorptive capacity of filters for most drugs and drug dosing guidelines tend not to consider adsorption to filters as a confounder.

19.3 Factors Influencing Extracorporeal Drug Removal

Drug removal during CRRT depends on the physicochemical properties and pharmacokinetic behaviour of that drug, the CRRT technique used, and other physical and patient factors including membrane selection, effluent flow rate and systemic pH.

Since only the fraction of the drug present in plasma is available for clearance by endogenous or extracorporeal routes, drugs with a high volume of distribution (V_d) are, overall, less likely to be cleared by CRRT than drugs with a small V_d, since their proportion contained in the plasma compartment at any given time is low relative to the total body load of the drug. However, an important distinction exists between IHD and CRRT with respect to the potential extracorporeal clearance of large V_d drugs. In IHD, drugs with a large V_d that are rapidly cleared from the plasma will quickly have their levels restored as drugs are released from tissue stores between dialysis treatments, resulting in a post-treatment 'rebound' in their plasma concentrations. By contrast, the slow, uninterrupted nature of CRRT allows continuous redistribution of the drug from tissue to blood. This means that the impact of V_d is reduced overall in CRRT and that for drugs with a high V_d, although CRRT has less effect on plasma concentration acutely than IHD, there is greater potential to clear drugs with higher V_d that are simply not practically removable with IHD [10].

Importantly, V_d values in critically ill patients typically differ substantially from standard reported values and there is a wide degree of both inter- and intra-patient variability, caused by factors such as lower protein binding in critical illness (discussed below), higher V_d of water soluble drugs, etc. For example, the V_d of aminoglycosides increases by approximately 25 % in critically ill patients, whereas penicillins and cephalosporins, vancomycin and metronidazole are relatively unaffected [16].

Unlike in conventional dialysis, the high-flux membranes used in CRRT generally have large pores allowing passage of molecules of up to 20,000–30,000 Da (Fig. 19.1). Since most drugs have molecular weights of less than 500 Da, and very few exceed 1500 Da, these membranes do not present a filtration barrier to drugs, such that the concentration of drug in the filtrate usually reflects the unbound plasma concentration of that drug [17]. This means that convection is independent of drug molecular weight, and haemofiltration is a superior modality for the removal of large solutes (drugs). Even large molecules such as vancomycin (1448 Da) and teicoplanin (1878 Da) are efficiently removed by haemofiltration. The capacity of a drug/solute to pass through a membrane by convection is mathematically expressed as the sieving coefficient, which is the ratio between the drug/solute concentration in the ultrafiltrate (C_{uf}) and the plasma (C_p):

$$S_c = C_{uf} / C_p$$

A sieving coefficient of 1 indicates that a drug/solute is removed in the same concentration as in the plasma, while a sieving coefficient of zero represents no drug/solute removal. In view of the large pore sizes used in CRRT, one of the major determinants of sieving coefficient is the extent of plasma protein binding by drugs (PB), as evidenced by the excellent correlation between S_c and the free fraction of drug (1-PB or f_u). However, in clinical studies a wide variation in S_c is noted [18]. Critically ill patients often have reduced serum albumin levels, and this may increase the unbound fraction of a drug to such an extent that toxic effects may ensue even though total serum levels remain constant, as demonstrated for phenytoin and ceftriaxone [19, 20]. However, removal by CRRT will be higher when the unbound fraction is increased by critical illness or by renal failure [21]. Notably renal failure also decreases binding of drugs to albumin independently of serum albumin level, a phenomenon that is thought to reflect displacement by 'uremic solutes'. Conversely, patients with hypoalbuminemia often have increased expression of acid α1 glycoprotein, which may actually decrease the unbound fraction of some basic drugs. There is also a wide inter-person variability in plasma protein binding, even among healthy volunteers.

Furthermore, in convective haemofiltration CRRT systems, the positioning of the replacement fluids has an important effect on solute clearance [22]. In the case of vancomycin, the sieving coefficient increased by up to 25 % as the proportion of replacement fluid given post-filter versus pre-filter was increased [23]. This occurs because pre-filter replacement fluid dilutes the blood that passes through the haemofilter and, therefore, decreases drug clearance. In clinical practice, the pre-filter or post-filter placement of fluid tends to differ in line with locally agreed protocols. Pre-filter fluid replacement is primarily intended to avoid haemoconcentration and decrease filter clotting, and it is thought that routine variation in this placement may account for many of the differences in S_c and drug clearance rates that have been reported in the literature [24].

In continuous dialysis (CAVHD and CVVHD), drug removal occurs by diffusion down a concentration gradient into the drug-free dialysate, and this equilibration depends on molecular weight as well on membrane flux properties, surface area and both blood and dialysate flow rates. The ability of a drug to diffuse through the filter membrane is expressed as the saturation coefficient S_d:

$$S_d = C_d / C_p$$

where C_d is the concentration of drug in the dialysate outflow.

The ratio between the dialysate flow rate (Q_d) and blood flow rate (Q_b) determines the time available for diffusion to occur and this especially determines the elimination of larger drugs, such as vancomycin, which require more time to saturate the dialysate because of their lower motion in solution compared to small solutes. In general, since the dialysate flow rate is usually relatively low compared to blood flow, small solutes have adequate time to saturate the dialysate. This means that, similar to S_c during haemofiltration modalities, protein binding becomes the major determinant of S_d in CVVHD and CAVHD and, for these smaller solutes, S_d will approach the free fraction (1-PB). For larger solutes, however, S_d is usually considerably smaller than 1-PB and this difference widens with higher Q_d values and with smaller membrane surface areas [7].

Overall, extracorporeal drug clearance in CRRT with continuous dialysis depends on S_d, Q_d and the relative diffusive mass transfer coefficient, K_{drel}, which accounts for the effect of a drug's molecular weight on its diffusive removal [17].

$$Cl_{HD} = S_d \times Q_d \times K_{drel}$$

Multiple studies indicate that at the same dialysate/ultrafiltrate flow rates, dialysis-based therapies will always have inferior drug/solute clearance to convective therapies and this difference becomes larger as the flow rates and molecular weight of the solute increases.

In haemodiafiltration, both convection and diffusion combine to eliminate drugs. These two processes may interact to reduce each other's efficiency of extracorporeal drug clearance, so that simple addition of convective and diffusive clearances tends to overestimate the total extracorporeal clearance [25]. For example, pre-filter haemofiltration replacement fluid dilutes inflow solutes and decreases diffusion. However, in comparison to CVVH, CVVHDF with equivalent effluent flow rates does result in a larger drug clearance [26].

19.4 Clinical Importance of Extracorporeal Drug Clearance: Contribution of Renal Clearance to Total Body Clearance

Total body clearance of a drug reflects the sum of clearances from different sites, and may include renal (Cl_R), hepatic and other metabolic processes, in addition to removal by extracorporeal devices. It is the contribution of renal clearance to total body clearance that primarily determines the extent of pharmacokinetic changes in renal failure and the requirement for dose adjustment in either IHD or CRRT. If the renal clearance of a drug is less than 25–30% of total body clearance, then impaired renal function does not usually have a clinically significant effect on drug clearance and drug removal by CRRT is less likely to necessitate dosing adjustment. The fractional extracorporeal clearance may be expressed as:

$$Fr_{EC} = Cl_{EC} / (Cl_{EC} + Cl_{NR} + Cl_R)$$

where Cl_{EC} represents extracorporeal clearance, Cl_R represents residual renal clearance and Cl_{NR} represents non-renal clearance. Thus, extracorporeal clearance is not usually clinically significant for drugs with low Cl_{EC} due either to low filtration or dialysis flow rates, or to high protein binding, as seen for amphotericin B, which is extensively protein bound [27]. It is also usually negligible for drugs with a high Cl_{NR} due to predominant hepatic clearance. The impact of residual renal function can be significant for some drugs, as demonstrated for meropenem [28]. Moreover, in early sepsis, hyperdynamic circulation may, paradoxically, result in higher renal clearances. Finally, in critical illness dynamic events such as the development of hepatic injury/failure can increase the extent to which CRRT contributes to total body clearance [6].

19.5 Practical Approaches to Adjusting Drug Dosing in CRRT

The critically ill patient with AKI is at obvious risk of drug accumulation and drug overdose, and dose reduction strategies tend to dominate prescribing strategies accordingly. However, modern CRRT methodologies also put these patients at risk of underdosing, which in itself may be life threatening, especially for antimicrobials [29, 30]. Moreover, inappropriate underdosing of antibiotics may be contributing to the increasing rate of antibiotic resistance, which is most prominent and dangerous in ICU patients [31]. Thus, an expert, holistic approach to dosage adjustment in patients with AKI undergoing CRRT is required. There is evidence that interprofessional co-operation between ICU pharmacists and physicians is of particular benefit, with a recent study indicating that antimicrobial dose adjustments performed by pharmacists reduced the length of ICU stay and resulted in fewer adverse drug reactions in septic patients receiving CRRT [32].

19.5.1 Consulting Pre-existing Resources

Perhaps the easiest and most obvious approach to dosage adjustment is to use available CRRT clearance data to estimate starting doses in individual patients. The problem is that high-quality data in critically ill patients is rare, and that which is available may not be generalisable across different CRRT prescriptions and/or clinical scenarios. Most publications on individual drugs in CRRT are case reports or small case series, rather than prospective, well-powered trials, and most do not satisfy quality criteria such as those laid out by the Acute Dialysis Quality Initiative (ADQI) [5, 33]. Furthermore, recent technological advances in CRRT, in particular higher dose rates and improved filters, mean that much of the previously published literature on drug disposition in CRRT is outdated. This could lead to the ineffective and potentially dangerous underdosing of drugs, including antibiotics [10].

There are several reference texts and resources that physicians and pharmacists typically consult when seeking dosing guidelines in renal impairment including *Drug Prescribing in Renal Failure (2007)* [34], *Martindale: The Complete Drug Reference* [35], *the British National Formulary* [36], *AHFS Drug Information* [37] and the online resource Micromedex [38]. Somewhat surprisingly, these resources differ as to the categorisation of renal impairment and the required dosing adjustments for individual drugs, and it is therefore advisable not to rely on one resource [39, 40]. They also generally provide very little information on dosage adjustment in the specialist realm of CRRT. A more recent textbook: *Renal Pharmacotherapy: Dosage Adjustment of Medications Eliminated by the Kidney* [41] includes some limited guidelines on CRRT, as well as references to the primary literature to inform clinical practice.

There have been several excellent review articles in this area, particularly in the field of antimicrobial dosing in CRRT, which tabulate relevant clinical trial data [5, 42–44]. However, these require constant updating, and often the descriptions of CRRT techniques and pharmacokinetic measurements in the original studies are far from complete, making extrapolations difficult [45]. In Table 19.2, we provide references to up-to-date antimicrobial drug data from clinical studies of CRRT within the past 3 years.

Table 19.2 Clinical studies of antimicrobial pharmacokinetics in patients receiving continuous renal replacement therapy (CRRT), published from 2012-date

Drug	Number of patients on CRRT	CRRT modality	Year of publication	Authors	Reference number(s)
Amikacin	5	CVVHDF	2012	D'Arcy et al.	[62]
Amphotericin B	8	CVVHDF	2013	Malone et al.	[63]
Anidulafungin	12	CVVHDF	2014	Aguilar et al.	[64]
Caspofungin	15	CVVH/CVVHD	2013	Weiler et al.	[65]
Ciprofloxacin	6	CVVHDF	2012	Roberts et al.	[66]
Colistin	3	CVVHDF	2012	Markou et al.	[67]
Daptomycin	6	CVVHD/CVVHDF	2012	Falcone et al.	[68]
Daptomycin	9	CVVHDF	2012	Wenisch et al.	[69]
Daptomycin	7	CVVHDF	2013	Preiswerk et al.	[70]
Daptomycin	9	CVVHDF	2013	Corti et al.	[71]
Ertapenem	8	CVVHD/CVVHDF	2014	Eyler et al.	[72]
Gentamicin	7	CVVH	2012	Petejova et al.	[73]
Imipenem	16	CVVHD	2013	Afshartous et al.	[74]
Meropenem	17	CVVHDF	2012	Roberts et al.	[66]
Meropenem	10	CVVHD	2013	Afshartous et al.	[74]
Piperacillin-tazobactam	42	CVVHD/CVVHDF	2012	Bauer et al.	[75]
Piperacillin-tazobactam	7	CVVHDF	2012	Roberts et al.	[66]
Piperacillin-tazobactam	16	CVVH	2014	Asin-Prieto et al.	[76]
Piperacillin-tazobactam	10	CVVHDF	2014	Varghese et al.	[77]
Vancomycin	40	CVVHD	2012	Wilson and Berns	[30]
Vancomycin	10	CVVHDF	2012	Roberts et al.	[66]
Vancomycin	32	CVVH/CVVHDF	2013	Beumier et al.	[78]
Vancomycin	85	CVVH/CVVHDF	2013	Covajes et al. and Udy et al.	[79, 80]
Vancomycin	4	CVVH	2013	Paciullo et al.	[81]

CVVH continuous venovenous haemofiltration; *CVVHD* continuous venovenous haemodialysis; *CVVHDF* continuous venovenous haemodiafiltration. Notably, many of the published reports are from small case series and/or retrospective studies

19.5.2 Adjusting Drug Dosage Based on Estimated Total Creatinine Clearance

For most drugs, CRRT clearance measurements are not available from any pre-existing resource and must be estimated. Notably, CRRT is much less uniform than conventional IHD and this renders drug dosing much less predictable and manageable. There are several possible approaches to this, and there is no consensus view on an optimal strategy. Overall, these estimates require clinical teams to conduct accurate research and interpret relevant pharmacokinetic data, which in itself is a skill that is often underdeveloped in clinical training programs.

One such method is to calculate total creatinine clearance based on residual Cl_R and expected or measured Cl_{EC} and devise a dose based on total Cl_{CR}, using maintenance dosing guidelines for Cl_{CR}, which are provided by many manufacturers [46]. Using this technique, Cl_{EC} will approximate either Q_f or Q_d, depending on the CRRT modality used, based on the principle that effluent flow rate equals creatinine clearance [47]. Most drugs will fall in the 20–25 ml/min range, but this may increase to 25–50 ml/min with higher effluent volumes in modern CRRT protocols. Since CRRT is often started somewhat earlier in the course of an illness than prior practice, residual renal function can also be significant in clearing some drugs [48].

This method will perform well for many drugs and, aside from estimation of creatinine clearance, is not reliant on individualised pharmacokinetic knowledge, such as V_d, Cl_{NR} or the extent of protein binding. Importantly, since it combines an individual patient's extracorporeal creatinine clearance and residual renal clearance to estimate drug clearance and dosing, maintenance doses could theoretically be adjusted if, and when, loss or recovery of residual renal function occurs. However, this would be reliant on regular measurement of residual function, which is not always practicable once a patient has commenced CRRT. A disadvantage to this approach is that it assumes free glomerular filtration and does not account for either tubular reabsorption or secretion. For example, since CRRT does not replace tubular function, drugs with high reabsorption, such as fluconazole, may actually be cleared more extensively in a patient undergoing CRRT, thereby necessitating higher doses than anticipated on the basis of a Cl_{CR} calculation [49]. The opposite is true when tubular secretion predominates, and clinicians are at risk of overdosing by relying on Cl_{CR} values. This is seen for many commonly used beta-lactam antibiotics. For example, while benzylpenicillin is largely cleared renally, only 10% of renal clearance involves glomerular filtration, while up to 90% is accounted for by tubular secretion, and this phenomenon can result in overdosing in CRRT [29].

19.5.3 Adjusting Drug Dosage Based on the Anuric Dose

An alternative approach is to start from the anuric (GFR <10 ml/min) dose and/or dosing interval and adapt the dose and/or dosing interval based on the expected Fr_{EC} [50]:

$$\text{Maintenance dose} = \text{anuric dose} / (1 - Fr_{EC})$$

And/or

$$\text{Dosing interval} = \text{anuric dosing interval} \times (1 - Fr_{EC})$$

An assumption with this approach is that the dose given to anuric patients achieves pharmacokinetic targets, such as optimal killing in the case of antimicrobials. This is not always the case, as demonstrated for moxifloxacin [43].

19.5.4 Adjusting Drug Dosage Based on Normal Clearance, Non-renal Clearance, Effluent Rate and Sieving Coefficient

Kroh [16] suggested predicting a dose suitable for CRRT by starting with the normal adult dose, and reducing it on the basis of normal total clearance, non-renal clearance and extracorporeal clearance, with extracorporeal clearance being calculated based on effluent rate and sieving coefficient [16]:

$$\text{Dose} = \text{Dose}_{\text{norm}} \times \left(Cl_{NR} + [Q_{\text{eff}} \times S_c]\right) / Cl_{\text{norm}}$$

The same authors suggested that for nontoxic drugs it is better to ensure adequate dosing by increasing doses by approximately 30% over these estimates. Although good correlations between calculated doses and measured kinetic data have been obtained using this method, it is not always clear how the extrarenal clearance fraction of a drug is derived. Usually, non-renal clearance is estimated from population pharmacokinetic studies in normal patients, and this sometimes results in an overestimation of actual non-renal clearance for antibiotics such as imipenem and vancomycin, whose non-renal clearance is significantly reduced in AKI [8, 13].

19.5.5 Adjusting Drug Dosage Based on Therapeutic Drug Monitoring

Since all prediction models have limitations, therapeutic drug monitoring (TDM) of plasma drug concentration is preferred for drugs with a low therapeutic index such as aminoglycosides. However, very few drugs have reliable (FDA/EMA-approved) TDM assays with acceptable turnaround times to make them clinically useful in adjusting CRRT dosages in a timely manner. TDM measures total body clearance, in which CRRT is only one contributor, and it therefore facilitates adjustments due to changes in CRRT dose or to other clinical factors such as liver disease.

Usually, when TDM is employed the required dose *(D)* is calculated to achieve the desired peak plasma concentration (C_{peak}) from a measured trough concentration (C_{actual}) as follows:

$$D = \left(C_{\text{peak}} - C_{\text{actual}}\right) \times Vd \times \text{Body Weight}$$

19.5.6 Adjusting Drug Dosage Based on Clinical Effect

Dosing based on obvious clinical effect may be a possibility for certain drugs, such as anti-hypertensives, analgesics and sedatives, in patients undergoing CRRT. However, there are many drugs for which this pharmacodynamic approach is not possible for drug dosing in the ICU setting.

19.6 General Principles of Dosage Adaptation for Antimicrobials During CRRT

The requirement for dose adjustment of antimicrobials depends not only on the pharmacokinetic considerations described above, notably CRRT-mediated drug clearance, but also on the pharmacodynamic behaviour of that drug. For antibiotics that exhibit time-dependent killing, such as the beta-lactam antibiotics, maintaining steady state plasma concentrations above the minimum inhibitory concentration (MIC) for a significant percentage of the dosing interval is crucial for efficacy. This typically requires frequent dosing and the recommended target drug concentration usually corresponds to the upper limit of the MIC range for susceptibility [42]. It is usually safer to shorten the maintenance dosing interval, rather than using large doses for time-dependent antibiotics in CRRT patients.

For other antibiotics, such as aminoglycosides, concentration-dependent killing prevails and the attainment of a high peak plasma concentration is most important for antimicrobial efficacy. But this must be balanced against the avoidance of toxicity, which reflects combined plasma levels over the whole dosing interval. Since aminoglycosides have low plasma protein binding and undergo mainly renal elimination they are subject to extensive extracorporeal clearance during CRRT. This means that CRRT may actually facilitate more frequent dosing of aminoglycosides with narrow therapeutic indices, since it helps to decrease plasma concentrations to low troughs, thereby decreasing the risk of adverse effects.

Overall, the choice of an initial loading dose (if any) of an antimicrobial drug should be primarily based on the known V_d of a drug, and this may change due to critical illness, renal failure or both, but generally not due to the CRRT process itself. Antimicrobial maintenance doses are largely determined by clearance, which includes both CRRT and non-CRRT mediated clearance.

19.7 Other Drugs Affected by CRRT

In comparison to antimicrobials, there is very little information on how CRRT affects the disposition of other drug classes. Drugs affecting haemodynamic stability, such as antihypertensives, inotropes or vasopressors, can be readily dose adjusted on the basis of haemodynamic measurements in ICU. However, for drugs such as anticonvulsants where serum levels are critical, but there is no outward clinical effect that can predict efficacy, clinicians should be aware of potential underdosing due to extracorporeal clearance, as seen for topiramate [51] and phenytoin [52]. For anticonvulsants such as valproate that are extensively albumin-bound, hypoalbuminemia may result in a large free fraction that is cleared readily by CRRT, leading to sub-therapeutic plasma levels [53]. Where possible, TDM should be conducted for anticonvulsants if the patient is at high risk of seizure activity and this is certainly routine practice for anticonvulsant drugs with unusual pharmacokinetics, such as phenytoin. The anticipated requirement for reduced doses of the renally eliminated direct thrombin inhibitor bivalirudin in patients with severe renal dysfunction has also been documented, but a higher dose is required following the initiation of IHD or CRRT to compensate for extracorporeal removal of bivalirudin [54].

19.8 Special Considerations: Hybrid RRTs

Extended intermittent or 'hybrid' RRT technologies are gaining popularity in the ICU setting and are considered technically less challenging than continuous therapies, since they generally use equipment designed for patients with chronic renal failure [55, 56]. They may also reduce the requirement for anticoagulation and avoid the considerable infection risks associated with frequent accessing of the CRRT circuit to facilitate changes in fluid bags. Patients on nocturnal hybrid or extended dialysis therapies are also more available for other diagnostic tests and interventions, minimising disruption to other aspects of their care. Hybrid therapies generally use higher dialysate flow rates and shorter treatment periods than CRRT, typically in the region of 8–12 h/day. Variants include sustained low-efficiency dialysis (SLED), sustained low-efficiency daily diafiltration (SLEDDf) and 'pulse' high-volume haemofiltration. These hybrid technologies are also of use in treating intoxications, such as lithium, as they have fewer complications than charcoal perfusion and are sometimes employed sequentially after standard dialysis to prevent post-dialytic 'rebound' [57].

There are multiple variants of hybrid RRT and very few pharmacokinetic studies have been published to aid drug dosing in patients undergoing hybrid RRT or extended dialysis, although recently these reports have become more numerous [58–60].

19.9 Special Populations: Paediatric Considerations

AKI is much more common than chronic renal failure in the paediatric population. However, like adult patients, children with AKI requiring CRRT often have multiple comorbidities requiring drug therapy (reviewed in 61). In calculating the dose and impact of CRRT in children, it should be borne in mind that although children have lower rates of blood flow than adults, they also have a much smaller volume of distribution due to their smaller size. Also, usually adult-sized membranes are employed in paediatric CRRT, meaning that the smaller total blood volume of a child is exposed to the same large filter surface area as an adult undergoing CRRT. Thus, even drugs with a low extracorporeal clearance in adults may be removed quite extensively in children. Conversely, in children, the volume of distribution for water-soluble drugs is larger than adults per unit of body weight because extracellular fluid volume and the quantity/quality of plasma proteins change significantly in the first few years of life. Overall this means that the management of drug therapy in children is not necessarily informed by reviewing adult data. Anecdotal evidence suggests that many paediatricians use the anuric dose, extrapolate from IHD doses or simply prescribe the full dose when prescribing for children on CRRT [61]. It is important that future studies of drug disposition during CRRT include children, as this would allow for more specific recommendations for drug dosing in paediatric patients.

19.10 Conclusions

CRRT and extended dialysis technologies are now widely used to support critically ill patients with AKI. Although it is clear that the CRRT can be life saving and that it offers improved haemodynamic stability with optimal fluid balance control, it may also have deleterious effects by altering the clearance of essential drugs. Drug doses used in IHD cannot reliably be applied directly to ICU patients receiving CRRT, and pharmacokinetic handling of drugs, including essential antimicrobials, is very different in these patients than in those with normal renal function. As a consequence, patients undergoing CRRT are at high risk of under-dosing and therapeutic failure.

Overall, the quality of pharmacokinetic studies on drug dosing in CRRT is, at best, moderate and many of the published reports are small case series. Because of the numerous variations in CRRT technologies, it is rare for physicians to be able to consult pre-existing dosing guidelines that are relevant to both the clinical condition of an individual patient and the CRRT modality being used. Well-powered and well-designed prospective studies are urgently required so that more reliable data can be generated, especially for the newer hybrid technologies. When there is no suitable pre-existing data available, several methods can be employed to estimate suitable CRRT drug doses, the simplest of which is based on estimating total creatinine clearance. However, it is important to remember that disease-related pharmacokinetic variability is often more important in the ICU patient than CRRT itself in altering drug disposition. An individualised and inter-professional team approach to drug dosing should be adopted in ICU patients undergoing CRRT, and clinical judgement should remain paramount.

References

1. Davenport A, Will EJ, Davidson AM. Improved cardiovascular stability during continuous modes of renal replacement therapy in critically ill patients with acute hepatic and renal failure. Crit Care Med. 1993;21(3):328–38.
2. Uchino S, Bellomo R, Morimatsu H, Morgera S, Schetz M, Tan I, et al. Continuous renal replacement therapy: a worldwide practice survey. The beginning and ending supportive therapy for the kidney (B.E.S.T. kidney) investigators. Intensive Care Med. 2007;33(9):1563–70.
3. Uchino S, Kellum JA, Bellomo R, Doig GS, Morimatsu H, Morgera S, et al. Acute renal failure in critically ill patients: a multinational, multicenter study. JAMA. 2005;294(7):813–8.
4. Mueller BA, Scarim SK, Macias WL. Comparison of imipenem pharmacokinetics in patients with acute or chronic renal failure treated with continuous hemofiltration. Am J Kidney Dis. 1993;21(2):172–9.
5. Vaara S, Pettila V, Kaukonen KM. Quality of pharmacokinetic studies in critically ill patients receiving continuous renal replacement therapy. Acta Anaesthesiol Scand. 2012;56(2):147–57.
6. Schetz M. Drug dosing in continuous renal replacement therapy: general rules. Curr Opin Crit Care. 2007;13(6):645–51.
7. Reetze-Bonorden P, Bohler J, Keller E. Drug dosage in patients during continuous renal replacement therapy. Pharmacokinetic and therapeutic considerations. Clin Pharmacokinet. 1993;24(5):362–79.
8. Matzke GR, Aronoff GR, Atkinson AJ Jr, Bennett WM, Decker BS, Eckardt KU, et al. Drug dosing consideration in patients with acute and chronic kidney disease-a clinical update from Kidney Disease: improving Global Outcomes (KDIGO). Kidney Int. 2011;80(11):1122–37.
9. Scribner BH, Caner JE, Buri R, Quinton W. The technique of continuous hemodialysis. Trans Am Soc Artif Intern Organs. 1960;10–11(6):88–103.
10. Mueller BA, Pasko DA, Sowinski KM. Higher renal replacement therapy dose delivery influences on drug therapy. Artif Organs. 2003;27(9):808–14.
11. Bellomo R, Cass A, Cole L, Finfer S, Gallagher M, Lo S, et al. Intensity of continuous renal-replacement therapy in critically ill patients. N Engl J Med. 2009;361(17):1627–38.
12. Palevsky PM, Zhang JH, O'Connor TZ, Chertow GM, Crowley ST, Choudhury D, et al. Intensity of renal support in critically ill patients with acute kidney injury. N Engl J Med. 2008;359(1):7–20.
13. Bugge JF. Pharmacokinetics and drug dosing adjustments during continuous venovenous hemofiltration or hemodiafiltration in critically ill patients. Acta Anaesthesiol Scand. 2001;45(8):929–34.
14. Tian Q, Gomersall CD, Wong A, Leung P, Choi G, Joynt GM, et al. Effect of drug concentration on adsorption of levofloxacin by polyacrylonitrile haemofilters. Int J Antimicrob Agents. 2006;28(2):147–50.
15. Clark WR, Hamburger RJ, Lysaght MJ. Effect of membrane composition and structure on solute removal and biocompatibility in hemodialysis. Kidney Int. 1999;56(6):2005–15.
16. Kroh UF. Drug administration in critically ill patients with acute renal failure. New Horiz. 1995;3(4):748–59.
17. Vincent HH, Vos MC, Akcahuseyin E, Goessens WH, van Duyl WA, Schalekamp MA. Drug clearance by continuous haemodiafiltration. Analysis of sieving coefficients and mass transfer coefficients of diffusion. Blood Purif. 1993;11(2):99–107.
18. Bouman CS, van Kan HJ, Koopmans RP, Korevaar JC, Schultz MJ, Vroom MB. Discrepancies between observed and predicted continuous venovenous hemofiltration removal of antimicrobial agents in critically ill patients and the effects on dosing. Intensive Care Med. 2006;32(12):2013–9.
19. Driscoll DF, McMahon M, Blackburn GL, Bistrian BR. Phenytoin toxicity in a critically ill, hypoalbuminemic patient with normal serum drug concentrations. Crit Care Med. 1988;16(12):1248–9.
20. Joynt GM, Lipman J, Gomersall CD, Young RJ, Wong EL, Gin T. The pharmacokinetics of once-daily dosing of ceftriaxone in critically ill patients. J Antimicrob Chemother. 2001;47(4):421–9.
21. Churchwell MD, Pasko DA, Smoyer WE, Mueller BA. Enhanced clearance of highly protein-bound drugs by albumin-supplemented dialysate during modeled continuous hemodialysis. Nephrol Dial Transplant. 2009;24(1):231–8.
22. De Pont AC, Bouman CS, Bakhtiari K, Schaap MC, Nieuwland R, Sturk A, et al. Predilution versus postdilution during continuous venovenous hemofiltration: a comparison of circuit thrombogenesis. ASAIO J. 2006;52(4):416–22.
23. Uchino S, Cole L, Morimatsu H, Goldsmith D, Bellomo R. Clearance of vancomycin during high-volume haemofiltration: impact of pre-dilution. Intensive Care Med. 2002;28(11):1664–7.
24. Churchwell MD, Mueller BA. Drug dosing during continuous renal replacement therapy. Semin Dial. 2009;22(2):185–8.
25. Brunet S, Leblanc M, Geadah D, Parent D, Courteau S, Cardinal J. Diffusive and convective solute clearances during continuous renal replacement therapy at various dialysate and ultrafiltration flow rates. Am J Kidney Dis. 1999;34(3):486–92.
26. Troyanov S, Cardinal J, Geadah D, Parent D, Courteau S, Caron S, et al. Solute clearances during continuous venovenous haemofil-

tration at various ultrafiltration flow rates using multiflow-100 and HF1000 filters. Nephrol Dial Transplant. 2003;18(5):961–6.
27. Bellmann R, Egger P, Gritsch W, Bellmann-Weiler R, Joannidis M, Kaneider N, et al. Amphotericin B lipid formulations in critically ill patients on continuous veno-venous haemofiltration. J Antimicrob Chemother. 2003;51(3):671–81.
28. Isla A, Maynar J, Sanchez-Izquierdo JA, Gascon AR, Arzuaga A, Corral E, et al. Meropenem and continuous renal replacement therapy: in vitro permeability of 2 continuous renal replacement therapy membranes and influence of patient renal function on the pharmacokinetics in critically ill patients. J Clin Pharmacol. 2005;45(11):1294–304.
29. Seyler L, Cotton F, Taccone FS, De Backer D, Macours P, Vincent JL, et al. Recommended beta-lactam regimens are inadequate in septic patients treated with continuous renal replacement therapy. Crit Care. 2011;15(3):R137.
30. Wilson FP, Berns JS. Vancomycin levels are frequently subtherapeutic during continuous venovenous hemodialysis (CVVHD). Clin Nephrol. 2012;77(4):329–31.
31. Roberts JA, Kruger P, Paterson DL, Lipman J. Antibiotic resistance—what's dosing got to do with it? Crit Care Med. 2008;36(8):2433–40.
32. Jiang SP, Zhu ZY, Ma KF, Zheng X, Lu XY. Impact of pharmacist antimicrobial dosing adjustments in septic patients on continuous renal replacement therapy in an intensive care unit. Scand J Infect Dis. 2013;45(12):891–9.
33. Gibney RT, Kimmel PL, Lazarus M. The Acute Dialysis Quality Initiative—part I: definitions and reporting of CRRT techniques. Adv Ren Replace Ther. 2002;9(4):252–4.
34. Aronoff G. Drug prescribing in renal failure. Philadelphia: ACP Press; 2007.
35. Sweetman SC, editor. Martindale: the complete drug reference. London: Pharmaceutical Press.
36. Joint Formulary Committee. British National Formulary. London: Pharmaceutical Press; 2014.
37. McEvoy GK, Snow ED, editors. AHFS: drug information. Bethseda: American Society of Health-Systems Pharmacists; 2014.
38. Micromedex Healthcare Series [Internet database]. Greenwood Village: Thomson Micromedex. Updated periodically; 2015.
39. Vidal L, Shavit M, Fraser A, Paul M, Leibovici L. Systematic comparison of four sources of drug information regarding adjustment of dose for renal function. BMJ. 2005;331(7511):263.
40. Khanal A, Castelino RL, Peterson GM, Jose MD. Dose adjustment guidelines for medications in patients with renal impairment: how consistent are drug information sources? Intern Med J. 2014;44(1):77–85.
41. Golightly LK, Teitelbaum I, Kiser TH, Levin DA, Barber GR, Jones MA, et al. Renal pharmacotherapy: dosage adjustment of medications eliminated by the kidneys. New York: Springer; 2013.
42. Trotman RL, Williamson JC, Shoemaker DM, Salzer WL. Antibiotic dosing in critically ill adult patients receiving continuous renal replacement therapy. Clin Infect Dis. 2005;41(8):1159–66.
43. Choi G, Gomersall CD, Tian Q, Joynt GM, Freebairn R, Lipman J. Principles of antibacterial dosing in continuous renal replacement therapy. Crit Care Med. 2009;37(7):2268–82.
44. Fissell WH. Antimicrobial dosing in acute renal replacement. Adv Chronic Kidney Dis. 2013;20(1):85–93.
45. Li AM, Gomersall CD, Choi G, Tian Q, Joynt GM, Lipman J. A systematic review of antibiotic dosing regimens for septic patients receiving continuous renal replacement therapy: do current studies supply sufficient data? J Antimicrob Chemother. 2009;64(5):929–37.
46. Bohler J, Donauer J, Keller F. Pharmacokinetic principles during continuous renal replacement therapy: drugs and dosage. Kidney Int Suppl. 1999;72:S24–8.
47. Connor MJ Jr, Salem C, Bauer SR, Hofmann CL, Groszek J, Butler R, et al. Therapeutic drug monitoring of piperacillin-tazobactam using spent dialysate effluent in patients receiving continuous venovenous hemodialysis. Antimicrob Agents Chemother. 2011;55(2):557–60.
48. Kroh UF, Lennartz H, Edwards DJ, Stoeckel K. Pharmacokinetics of ceftriaxone in patients undergoing continuous veno-venous hemofiltration. J Clin Pharmacol. 1996;36(12):1114–9.
49. Bergner R, Hoffmann M, Riedel KD, Mikus G, Henrich DM, Haefeli WE, et al. Fluconazole dosing in continuous veno-venous haemofiltration (CVVHF): need for a high daily dose of 800 mg. Nephrol Dial Transplant. 2006;21(4):1019–23.
50. Schetz M, Ferdinande P, Van den Berghe G, Verwaest C, Lauwers P. Pharmacokinetics of continuous renal replacement therapy. Intensive Care Med. 1995;21(7):612–20.
51. Browning L, Parker D Jr, Liu-DeRyke X, Shah A, Coplin WM, Rhoney DH. Possible removal of topiramate by continuous renal replacement therapy. J Neurol Sci. 2010;288(1–2):186–9.
52. Oltrogge KM, Peppard WJ, Saleh M, Regner KR, Herrmann DJ. Phenytoin removal by continuous venovenous hemofiltration. Ann Pharmacother. 2013;47(9):1218–22.
53. De Maat MM, van Leeuwen HJ, Edelbroek PM. High unbound fraction of valproic acid in a hypoalbuminemic critically ill patient on renal replacement therapy. Ann Pharmacother. 2011;45(3):e18.
54. Tsu LV, Dager WE. Bivalirudin dosing adjustments for reduced renal function with or without hemodialysis in the management of heparin-induced thrombocytopenia. Ann Pharmacother. 2011;45(10):1185–92.
55. Fliser D, Kielstein JT. Technology Insight: treatment of renal failure in the intensive care unit with extended dialysis. Nat Clin Pract Nephrol. 2006;2(1):32–9.
56. Kielstein JT, Schiffer M, Hafer C. Back to the future: extended dialysis for treatment of acute kidney injury in the intensive care unit. J Nephrol. 2010;23(5):494–501.
57. Kielstein JT, Woywodt A, Schumann G, Haller H, Fliser D. Efficiency of high-flux hemodialysis in the treatment of valproic acid intoxication. J Toxicol Clin Toxicol. 2003;41(6):873–6.
58. Bogard KN, Peterson NT, Plumb TJ, Erwin MW, Fuller PD, Olsen KM. Antibiotic dosing during sustained low-efficiency dialysis: special considerations in adult critically ill patients. Crit Care Med. 2011;39(3):560–70.
59. Czock D, Husig-Linde C, Langhoff A, Schopke T, Hafer C, de Groot K, et al. Pharmacokinetics of moxifloxacin and levofloxacin in intensive care unit patients who have acute renal failure and undergo extended daily dialysis. Clin J Am Soc Nephrol. 2006;1(6):1263–8.
60. Lorenzen JM, Broll M, Kaever V, Burhenne H, Hafer C, Clajus C, et al. Pharmacokinetics of ampicillin/sulbactam in critically ill patients with acute kidney injury undergoing extended dialysis. Clin J Am Soc Nephrol. 2012;7(3):385–90.
61. Veltri MA, Neu AM, Fivush BA, Parekh RS, Furth SL. Drug dosing during intermittent hemodialysis and continuous renal replacement therapy: special considerations in pediatric patients. Paediatr Drugs. 2004;6(1):45–65.
62. D'Arcy DM, Casey E, Gowing CM, Donnelly MB, Corrigan OI. An open prospective study of amikacin pharmacokinetics in critically ill patients during treatment with continuous venovenous haemodiafiltration. BMC Pharmacol Toxicol. 2012;13(1):14
63. Malone ME, Corrigan OI, Kavanagh PV, Gowing C, Donnelly M, D'Arcy DM. Pharmacokinetics of amphotericin B lipid complex in critically ill patients undergoing continuous venovenous haemodiafiltration. Int J Antimicrob Agents. 2013;42(4):335–42.
64. Aguilar G, Azanza JR, Carbonell JA, Ferrando C, Badenes R, Parra MA, et al. Anidulafungin dosing in critically ill patients with continuous venovenous haemodiafiltration. J Antimicrob Chemother. 2014;69(6):1620–3.
65. Weiler S, Seger C, Pfisterer H, Stienecke E, Stippler F, Welte R, et al. Pharmacokinetics of caspofungin in critically ill patients on continuous renal replacement therapy. Antimicrob Agents Chemother. 2013;57(8):4053–7.
66. Roberts DM, Roberts JA, Roberts MS, Liu X, Nair P, Cole L, et al. Variability of antibiotic concentrations in critically ill patients

receiving continuous renal replacement therapy: a multicentre pharmacokinetic study. Crit Care Med. 2012;40(5):1523–8.
67. Markou N, Fousteri M, Markantonis SL, Zidianakis B, Hroni D, Boutzouka E, et al. Colistin pharmacokinetics in intensive care unit patients on continuous venovenous haemodiafiltration: an observational study. J Antimicrob Chemother. 2012;67(10):2459–62.
68. Falcone M, Russo A, Cassetta MI, Lappa A, Tritapepe L, Fallani S, et al. Daptomycin serum levels in critical patients undergoing continuous renal replacement. J Chemother. 2012;24(5):253–6.
69. Wenisch JM, Meyer B, Fuhrmann V, Saria K, Zuba C, Dittrich P, et al. Multiple-dose pharmacokinetics of daptomycin during continuous venovenous haemodiafiltration. J Antimicrob Chemother. 2012;67(4):977–83.
70. Preiswerk B, Rudiger A, Fehr J, Corti N. Experience with daptomycin daily dosing in ICU patients undergoing continuous renal replacement therapy. Infection. 2013;41(2):553–7.
71. Corti N, Rudiger A, Chiesa A, Marti I, Jetter A, Rentsch K, et al. Pharmacokinetics of daily daptomycin in critically ill patients undergoing continuous renal replacement therapy. Chemotherapy. 2013;59(2):143–51.
72. Eyler RF, Vilay AM, Nader AM, Heung M, Pleva M, Sowinski KM, et al. Pharmacokinetics of ertapenem in critically ill patients receiving continuous venovenous hemodialysis or hemodiafiltration. Antimicrob Agents Chemother. 2014;58(3):1320–6.
73. Petejova N, Zahalkova J, Duricova J, Kacirova I, Brozmanova H, Urbanek K, et al. Gentamicin pharmacokinetics during continuous venovenous hemofiltration in critically ill septic patients. J Chemother. 2012;24(2):107–12.
74. Afshartous D, Bauer SR, Connor MJ, Aduroja OA, Amde M, Salem C, et al. Pharmacokinetics and pharmacodynamics of imipenem and meropenem in critically ill patients treated with continuous venovenous hemodialysis. Am J Kidney Dis. 2013;63(1):170–1.
75. Bauer SR, Salem C, Connor MJ Jr, Groszek J, Taylor ME, Wei P, et al. Pharmacokinetics and pharmacodynamics of piperacillin-tazobactam in 42 patients treated with concomitant CRRT. Clin J Am Soc Nephrol. 2012;7(3):452–7.
76. Asin-Prieto E, Rodriguez-Gascon A, Troconiz IF, Soraluce A, Maynar J, Sanchez-Izquierdo JA, et al. Population pharmacokinetics of piperacillin and tazobactam in critically ill patients undergoing continuous renal replacement therapy: application to pharmacokinetic/pharmacodynamic analysis. J Antimicrob Chemother. 2014;69(1):180–9.
77. Varghese JM, Jarrett P, Boots RJ, Kirkpatrick CM, Lipman J, Roberts JA. Pharmacokinetics of piperacillin and tazobactam in plasma and subcutaneous interstitial fluid in critically ill patients receiving continuous venovenous haemodiafiltration. Int J Antimicrob Agents. 2014;43(4):343–8.
78. Beumier M, Roberts JA, Kabtouri H, Hites M, Cotton F, Wolff F, et al. A new regimen for continuous infusion of vancomycin during continuous renal replacement therapy. J Antimicrob Chemother. 2013;68(12):2859–65.
79. Covajes C, Scolletta S, Penaccini L, Ocampos-Martinez E, Abdelhadii A, Beumier M, et al. Continuous infusion of vancomycin in septic patients receiving continuous renal replacement therapy. Int J Antimicrob Agents. 2013;41(3):261–6.
80. Udy AA, Covajes C, Taccone FS, Jacobs F, Vincent JL, Lipman J, et al. Can population pharmacokinetic modelling guide vancomycin dosing during continuous renal replacement therapy in critically ill patients? Int J Antimicrob Agents. 2013;41(6):564–8.
81. Paciullo CA, Harned KC, Davis GA, Connor MJ Jr, Winstead PS. Vancomycin clearance in high-volume venovenous hemofiltration. Ann Pharmacother. 2013;47(3):e14.

Part IV

Other Therapies

20 Therapeutic Plasmapheresis

Claire Kennedy and Colm C. Magee

20.1 Introduction and Definitions

Apheresis is an umbrella term used to describe selective removal of a blood component such as plasma (plasmapheresis) or blood cells (hemapheresis or cytapheresis). The process typically involves extracorporeal separation of the blood into component parts, removal of the desired component, and return of the remainder to the patient (special fluids to replace those removed are also returned).

Plasmapheresis may be performed in healthy donors for the purpose of blood product manufacture. It may also be performed with therapeutic intent, whereby a pathogenic substance is removed from the patient's plasma and replaced with pathogen-free plasma or other replacement fluid (therapeutic plasma exchange (TPE) or therapeutic plasmapheresis). This chapter will focus on TPE.

During TPE, the patient's venous blood is directed through either an extracorporeal centrifuge or a selectively permeable membrane, where plasma separation and removal occur (Fig. 20.1). Certain pathogenic substances, such as immune complexes, antibodies, complement components, and cryoglobulins, are removed with the plasma. It is thought that TPE offers a further degree of immunomodulation because of alterations in cytokine production and modulation of T lymphocyte populations [1, 2].

Replacement fluids, of which there are several choices, ensure that the patient does not develop intravascular volume depletion during the process of TPE (Fig. 20.1). Replacement has a dilutional effect on the patient's plasma. Thus, an exchange of 1–1.5 times the plasma volume will reduce plasma concentrations of the molecule by approximately 60–70%.

The usual target substances in TPE, such as immunoglobulins and cryoglobulins, have a high molecular weight. These substances equilibrate slowly between the intravascular and extravascular spaces; therefore, substance removal during a single plasma exchange is essentially limited to that which is in the intravascular space (Fig. 20.2). Equilibration occurs slowly after TPE, so repeated plasma exchanges separated by 24–48 h are usually required to substantially deplete the substance in question. In addition, production of the pathogenic substance must be rapidly halted, often by concurrent cytotoxic therapy.

20.2 Theoretical Background

TPE was traditionally performed by centrifugation. A spinning centrifuge separates the elements of whole blood on the basis of specific gravity (Fig. 20.3). Red blood cells settle to the bottom, with less dense elements such as white blood cells and platelets overlying the red cell layer. Plasma settles at the top, from where it can be selectively removed.

It is becoming increasingly popular to perform TPE using a membrane plasma separation (MPS) technique. This method uses a highly permeable, biocompatible membrane. The membrane pore size enables selective sieving of plasma constituents, while retaining cells and platelets. Membranes with pore sizes 0.1–0.6 μm are typically used. This achieves a sieving coefficient of over 0.95 for the plasma constituents, while retaining essentially all cellular elements.

Standard hemodialysis equipment is used, making it easily accessible to most larger hospitals (additional training of dialysis staff is required). The machine is set to isolated ultrafiltration mode, which generates a negative transmembrane pressure and facilitates plasma crossing the membrane.

Several important principles apply to MPS systems to ensure efficiency. The rate of plasma removal must be limited to ensure the hematocrit (Hct) does not rise excessively along the length of the filter, leading to deposition of cells

C. C. Magee (✉) · C. Kennedy
Department of Nephrology, Beaumont Hospital, Beaumont Road, Dublin 9, Dublin, Ireland
e-mail: colmmagee@beaumont.ie

C. Kennedy
e-mail: kennedyclaire@gmail.com

A. K. Singh et al. (eds.), *Core Concepts in Dialysis and Continuous Therapies*, DOI 10.1007/978-1-4899-7657-4_20

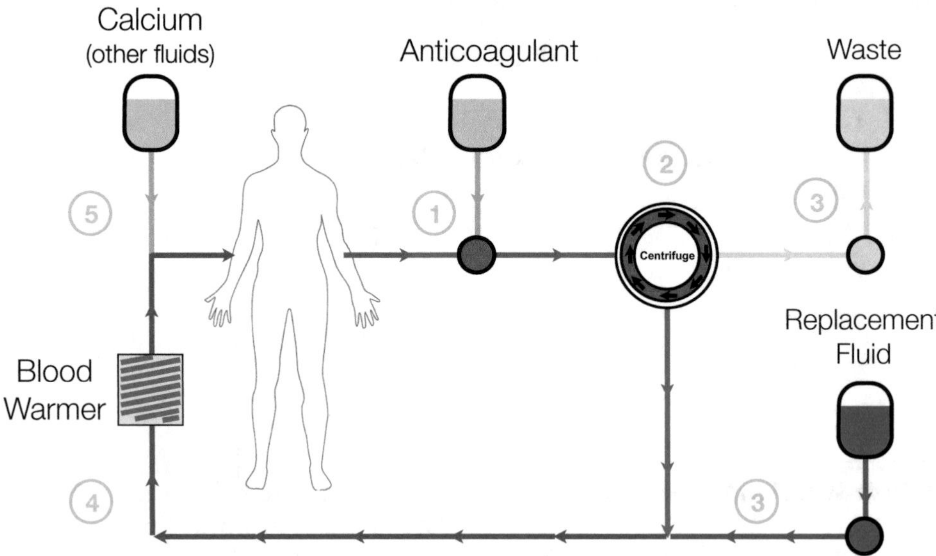

Fig. 20.1 Therapeutic plasmapheresis circuit. (Courtesy of Dr. P. Yenson, clinical assistant professor, University of British Columbia, and clinical hematologist, Vancouver General Hospital)

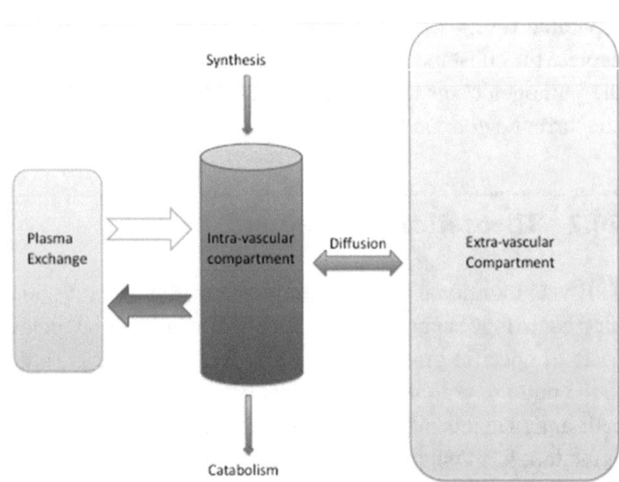

Fig. 20.2 Distribution and flow of target substances

Fig. 20.3 The constituents of whole blood, with their respective specific gravities, as they separate out following centrifugation

Plasma	• 1.025 – 1.029
Platelets	• 1.04
Lymphocytes	• 1.07
Granulocytes	• 1.087 – 1.092
Erythrocytes	• 1.093 – 1.096

on the membrane. The transmembrane pressure must also be limited to avoid red cell lysis and plugging of the pores.

20.3 Prescription

The prescription of each TPE procedure is tailored to the estimated patient plasma volume, the disease in question, and the individual clinical circumstances of the case. The number and frequency of exchanges must be planned, as well as the volumes of plasma to be removed and replaced. In addition, the type of replacement fluid, the anticoagulation dose and the calcium replacement should be carefully prescribed.

20.3.1 Volume

The plasma volume of an individual can be estimated by the following formula:

$$\text{Estimated plasma volume} \\ = 0.07 \times \text{weight}(\text{kg}) \times (1 - \text{hematocrit})$$

A standard single TPE procedure exchanges 1 to 1.5 times the plasma volume. Plasma exchange volumes in excess of this may remove slightly more of the substance in question but are avoided because of the adverse effects. Larger exchange volumes are very time-consuming, often poorly tolerated and increase blood product and anticoagulant exposure.

If a patient is significantly anemic, blood transfusion may be required pre-TPE to avoid hemodynamic instability.

20.3.2 Frequency and Duration

In general, TPE is continued until there is (a) return of the pathogenic antibody to near-normal levels and/or (b) improvement/stabilization of the patient's clinical status. If production rates of the pathogenic substance are modest, five separate TPE procedures within 7–10 days will remove approximately 85–90 % of the total body burden [3]. For example, approximately 45 % of immunoglobulin G (IgG) is intravascular; exchanging 1.25 times plasma volume will remove 32 % of total body IgG. Equilibration between intra- and extravascular compartments occurs within about 24 h of TPE. Therefore, approximately five plasma exchanges, on alternate days, are required to remove 85 % of IgG (assuming no more synthesis). In the case of IgM, approximately 75 % is intravascular, so a small number of exchanges will substantially reduce overall levels.

Exceptionally aggressive diseases, such as anti-GBM disease and hemolytic uremic syndrome (HUS)-TTP, usually require daily TPE in the initial stages of management [4]. The duration of TPE will depend on the individual disease and the clinical response to therapy (see later).

20.3.3 Replacement Fluids

To avoid intravascular volume depletion and hypotension, plasma is typically replaced with one, or combinations, of the following fluids: albumin, normal saline, and fresh frozen plasma.

Albumin, which exerts oncotic activity, is the replacement fluid of choice in most diseases [4]. It is typically administered as a 5 % solution. Although pooled from multiple donors, the risk of it transmitting viral infections is considered to be very low. It also carries little risk of anaphylactic reactions. However, it will cause a depletional coagulopathy, especially after multiple exchanges. Albumin is expensive and so saline can be used in combination with albumin replacement to help contain cost.

Saline alone as a replacement fluid is avoided, except in hyperviscosity syndrome, as it does not provide sufficient oncotic pressure to maintain hemodynamic stability. When used in combination with albumin, it should be limited to 40 % of the replacement fluid. In this setting, albumin and saline are administered alternately, with the majority of the albumin given in the latter stages of the exchange to ensure hemodynamic stability.

Plasma is the replacement fluid of choice in HUS-TTP syndromes [4]. In situations where there is increased bleeding risk, plasma is used in small volumes towards the end of the exchange to replace coagulation factors lost during the exchange. It is not usually used in other settings as it has a higher rate of adverse effects including allergic reactions, transfusion-related acute lung injury (TRALI), citrate-related complications, and, potentially, viral transmission.

20.3.4 Anticoagulation

Anticoagulation is required during TPE to avoid extracorporeal clotting and blood loss. Centrifugal devices usually use citrate as the anticoagulant, whereas MPS systems use heparin [5]. Citrate chelates ionized calcium, thereby blocking calcium-dependent clotting factor reactions. If heparin is used, a loading dose of 5000 units is typically administered with maintenance of approximately 1000 units per hour. This may need adjustment in extremes of body size or Hct [6].

20.3.5 Calcium

Hypocalcemia can occur for several reasons: calcium bound to albumin and other plasma proteins is removed (along with these proteins), there is a dilutional effect with administration of albumin/saline, and citrate (if administered) binds to, and inactivates, ionized calcium. To avoid complications of hypocalcemia (see below), oral or intravenous calcium is routinely administered in most centers. Non-randomized trial evidence supports the routine supplementation of the return fluid with calcium gluconate. The trial group that received constant calcium gluconate infusion (10 ml of 10 % calcium gluconate per liter of return fluid) had less symptomatic hypocalcemia than those that received no calcium or intermittent small boluses [7].

Intraprocedural measurement of ionized calcium is performed if the patient is symptomatic or at particular risk of citrate toxicity, such as sedated patients or those with other electrolyte abnormalities. Of note, patients with severe liver failure cannot metabolize citrate and are therefore at high risk of citrate toxicity. Ionized calcium levels should be measured every 30 min, with appropriate calcium replacement, in this setting.

20.3.6 Fibrinogen

Where most non-immunoglobulin proteins recover to almost normal levels within 48 h after TPE, fibrinogen recovery can vary depending on production levels. If intensive TPE is required, fibrinogen levels should be monitored. If depleted, and the patient is at risk of bleeding, FFP may be required towards the end of the exchange to correct fibrinogen levels. Some centers also give "pure" fibrinogen if bleeding is a major concern, for example, TPE immediately before a kidney transplant.

20.4 Vascular Access

Reliable, large-bore venous access is necessary to perform TPE. Peripheral venous access can support some TPE techniques, such as centrifugation-based systems with a low blood flow (100 ml/min). However, peripheral access becomes increasingly difficult after multiple venepunctures.

A wide-bore central venous catheter (CVC) may be required for the duration of TPE. If the duration of TPE is thought to be short (i.e., days), a temporary CVC may suffice. Several days of intensive TPE may lead to a depletion coagulopathy; therefore, CVC removal must be perfomed very carefully in this setting. Longer duration TPE necessitates insertion of a tunneled CVC with careful confirmation of position.

If long-term maintenance TPE is anticipated (this is rare), an arteriovenous fistula (AVF) or graft (AVG) can be fashioned to avoid the complications of long-term CVC use—namely catheter-related sepsis and central venous stenosis and thrombosis [8]. This practice stems from the large body of evidence in the hemodialysis population favoring AVF/AVG use over CVC use in the long term [9].

Table 20.1 Indications for TPE based on American Society for Apheresis categories, 2013 [4]

Category I	*Category II*
AIDP/Guillain–Barré syndrome	Acute disseminated encephalomyelitis
Hyperviscosity syndrome	Cold agglutinin disease
TTP	Catastrophic antiphospholipid syndrome
Severe ANCA-associated vasculitis	Lambert–Eaton myasthenic syndrome
Anti-GBM disease	Neuromyelitis optica, acute
Myasthenia gravis, severe	Hematopoietic cell transplantation
Severe cryoglobulinemia	Familial hypercholesterolemia
Atypical HUS (factor H related)	
Organ transplantation (specific situations; see text)	
Category III	*Category IV*
Hypertriglyceridemic pancreatitis	Active rheumatoid arthritis
Aplastic anemia	Lupus nephritis
Henoch–Schönlein purpura	Schizophrenia
Chronic progressive multiple sclerosis	Inclusion body myositis
Paraneoplastic neurologic syndromes	Amyotrophic lateral sclerosis
Idiopathic dilated cardiomyopathy	Systemic amyloidosis
	Psoriasis

TPE therapeutic plasma exchange, *AIDP* acute inflammatory demyelinating polyneuropathy, *TTP* thrombotic thrombocytopenic purpura, *ANCA* anti-neutrophil cytoplasmic antibody, *GBM* glomerular basement membrane, *HUS* hemolytic uremic syndrome

20.5 Indications

As TPE is an expensive and labor-intensive therapy, certain criteria must be met for it to be considered an appropriate therapy for a given disease. A substantial percentage of the pathogenic substance must be present in the vascular as opposed to the extravascular space. As the pathogen is usually thought to be an IgG or IgM molecule, this will usually be the case. It also should be large enough (molecular weight 15,000 Da) to rule out removal by dialysis or other cheaper purification techniques. The substance should be acutely toxic and resistant to other treatment modalities.

Pathogen removal by TPE is best suited to those pathogens with relatively long half-lives to provide a benefit over endogenous elimination [3]. IgG, for example, has a half-life of approximately 21 days and a molecular weight of over 150,000 Da. Medications which reduce autoantibody (or other pathogen) production are used in combination with TPE to ensure that rapid discontinuation of antibody production, as well as removal of circulating pathogenic antibody, occurs.

Previous international reports have identified that the majority of TPE procedures are performed for neurological and hematological conditions [10, 11]. The numerous indications for TPE are slowly evolving as pharmacological advances are made and TPE processes are refined and rationalized [10].

The American Society for Apheresis has divided the indications for TPE into four categories on the basis of the level of peer-reviewed evidence for efficacy [4]. The list of indications now contains 78 diseases and is updated at regular intervals. These guidelines provide a framework for clinical practice with succinct evidence-based synopses for each disorder [4].

Category I conditions are those disorders for which TPE is standard first-line therapy, alone or in conjunction with other treatments. Category II disorders are those in which TPE is acceptable second-line therapy, alone or in conjunction with other treatments. Category III disorders are those in which TPE is inadequately tested and therefore not an established therapy. Category IV disorders are those in which TPE has been shown to be ineffective or harmful. A selection of these indications can be seen in Table 20.1.

20.5.1 Renal Disorders

The pathogenic antibody in anti-glomerular basement membrane (GBM) disease is directed against the α3 chain of type IV collagen, which is present in abundance in the alveolar and glomerular basement membranes. This aggressive disease typically presents with a rapidly progressive glomerulonephritis (RPGN) and/or diffuse alveolar hemorrhage. Because of the disease rarity and its fulminant clinical course, there have been few randomized controlled trials (RCTs) to help guide practice. A small RCT ($n=17$) demonstrated benefit in terms of patient and renal outcomes with TPE, cyclophosphamide, and steroid (vs. cyclophosphamide and steroid alone; [12]). Observational data concur [13].

TPE is performed every 1–2 days for 2–3 weeks. Further TPE may be required if the disease remains clinically active or the anti-GBM titer remains elevated [14]. About 1.0–1.5 times the plasma volume is exchanged, using albumin and saline as replacement fluids. If there is diffuse alveolar hemorrhage, or a renal biopsy has been performed, plasma should be given as replacement fluid towards the end of TPE to help normalize coagulation. Recovery to dialysis independence is unlikely in those who require dialysis at presentation [15]; therefore, TPE is usually not performed in this situation unless the patient has intercurrent DAH.

TPE is also employed in the management of anti-neutrophil cytoplasmic antibody (ANCA)-associated vasculitis (AAV) in certain situations. Early, small-scale RCT evidence suggested that TPE was beneficial in patients with dialysis dependence [16]. Although the subsequent MEPEX trial had shortcomings, it also supported the use of TPE in patients with AAV and severe renal involvement (serum creatinine over 500 µmol/l; [17]). Longer term (median 3.95 years) follow-up of the MEPEX trial found that almost two thirds had either died or developed end-stage renal disease (the composite primary outcome), with no significant difference between the groups that received or did not receive TPE [18].

TPE is used in the initial management of AAV in the setting of dual antibody positivity (anti-GBM and ANCA), although RCT evidence is lacking [19]. Similarly, observational data support the use of TPE in AAV with diffuse alveolar hemorrhage [20]. TPE prescription in AAV is typically 1–1.5 times plasma volume exchanges, using albumin and saline as replacement fluids (with some plasma replacement in the setting of diffuse alveolar hemorrhage or recent renal biopsy; [4]). PEXIVAS, a large RCT, is underway and will hopefully further clarify the role of TPE in AAV [21].

The role of TPE as an adjunctive therapy in myeloma light-chain cast nephropathy is somewhat controversial. Standard treatment consists of intravenous fluids, steroids, and chemotherapy. A small RCT showed improved renal and patient survival in those with myeloma, renal failure, and significant Bence Jones proteinuria treated with adjunctive TPE [22]. A retrospective study similarly supported early adjunctive TPE in patients with biopsy-confirmed cast nephropathy [23]. The largest RCT did not reproduce these findings, although inclusion criteria were different and included patients with renal failure from causes other than cast nephropathy [24]. In our opinion, rapid diagnosis of acute cast nephropathy and rapid administration of fluids and chemotherapy are much more important than adding TPE.

Removal of toxic light chains by specialized hemodialysis is also an attractive therapeutic concept. Extended dialysis with a large-pore membrane (high cutoff hemodialysis) may be a beneficial adjunctive therapy but its role has not yet been clarified [25]. RCTs are underway—see also Chap. 10.

There is compelling RCT evidence for the use of TPE, with plasma as replacement fluid, in the treatment of certain HUS-TTP syndromes [26, 27]. In TTP, ADAMTS-13, a protease that cleaves von Willebrand factor, is deficient or dysfunctional due to inhibitory autoantibody action. Replacement plasma, as well as the "usual" antibody removal by TPE, helps to restore normal ADAMTS-13 levels and activity. The exact pathogenesis of HUS-TTP is unknown, although there is often a trigger such as a specific infection or drug. The exact mechanism of action of TPE in this setting is therefore unclear, although there is strong clinical evidence for its use.

In severe forms of HUS-TTP, TPE is initially performed daily (rarely, twice daily if life-threatening disease present), using platelet count and plasma lactate dehydrogenase as markers of disease activity [4]. The target for therapy is a platelet count greater than 150,000/µl for 2–3 days. At this point, treatment is often tapered before discontinuation, although there is no specific evidence to guide this practice. In many centers, ADAMTS13 levels are being used to assist in the diagnosis and management of cases of HUS-TTP. Note that levels should be sent *before* the first TPE and that initiation of TPE should *not* be delayed, pending results of the ADAMTS13 assay.

There is a general consensus that TPE has a therapeutic role in severe, active cryoglobulinemia, such as progressive renal failure or advancing neuropathy. All solutions and equipment should be pre-warmed to avoid precipitation of the cryoglobulins. Blood warmers and warming blankets are also useful. More selective filtration techniques, such as double filtration plasmapheresis (DFPP; see later), can reduce the need for replacement fluid. During *cryofiltration*, separated plasma is cooled. This leads to aggregation (and therefore increased size) of the cryoglobulins, which enables more efficient secondary filtration and return of autologous plasma.

There are several indications for TPE in renal transplantation. In the pre-transplant setting, it can be used to remove anti-HLA or anti-ABO blood group antibodies which are directed against donor antigens [28, 29]. This prevents the occurrence of hyperacute rejection, which would destroy the transplanted kidney within hours of transplant surgery. Typically, several immunosuppressive drugs are started around the time of the first TPE session. Low-dose intravenous immunoglobulin (IVIg) is often given after each TPE session. Some centers also prescribe "prophylactic" TPE after the transplant surgery to prevent a large rebound in antibodies, which might cause severe acute antibody-mediated rejection. In the peri-transplant period, it is very important to avoid depletion of clotting factors, as this will increase the risk of perioperative bleeding. Good results have been reported from specialist centers [30]. Importantly, if plasma is prescribed as part of the replacement for a patient undergoing ABI-incompatible transplantation, the plasma must not contain ABO antibodies against the donor kidney. Thus, an ABO-O patient receiving an ABO-A kidney would receive ABO-A plasma (but ABO-O blood).

In the posttransplant setting, TPE is often used (with variable success) to treat early recurrent focal segmental glomerulosclerosis (FSGS; [31]). Acute antibody-mediated rejection can occur at any time after transplant. In the early posttransplant period, it is sometimes seen after transplantation across HLA or ABO incompatibilities (as described above). It may occur later, often associated with nonadherence. Treatment typically involves TPE and increased immunosuppression; the rationale for TPE being that it quickly removes the pathogenic anti-HLA or anti-ABO antibodies [32]. The role, if any, of TPE in *chronic* antibody-mediated rejection remains to be defined.

20.5.2 Neurological Disorders

TPE is used in the management of a variety of antibody-mediated neurological conditions (Table 20.1). There is a large body of RCT evidence to support its use in Guillain–Barré syndrome if independent walking is impaired [33, 34]. This disease is associated with antibodies directed against gangliosides on the outer membrane of Schwann cells and/or axons. TPE (of 1–1.5 times plasma volume) is typically performed on alternate days for 10–14 days. Close monitoring, ideally in an intensive care setting, must be given to volume shifts in those patients with autonomic involvement.

The major antibody of interest in myasthenia gravis is directed against the acetylcholine receptor on the postsynaptic surface of the motor end plate (anti-acetylcholine receptor). TPE is used in a variety of acute situations—as initial management in severe disease, perioperatively to optimize muscle function, and during myasthenic crises. It can also be used as adjunctive therapy during the chronic phase of the disease [4, 35].

Anti-N-methyl D-aspartate (NMDA) receptor encephalitis, first described in 2005, is an autoimmune encephalitis which is often paraneoplastic. It presents with prominent psychiatric changes, dyskinesia, memory disturbance, and language dysfunction. Diagnosis is confirmed by identifying antibodies to the NR1 subunit of the NMDA receptor in serum or cerebrospinal fluid. Anti-NMDA receptor encephalitis is currently considered under the umbrella term "paraneoplastic neurological syndromes" and graded category III in the American Society for Apheresis guidelines. Observational evidence in favor of TPE (alone or in combination with steroid and intravenous immunoglobulin) as first-line therapy is mounting [36, 37]. It should be noted that TPE may be challenging in this setting, especially if the patient is agitated or has autonomic instability.

Small-scale RCT evidence supports the use of TPE in the management of chronic inflammatory demyelinating polyneuropathy ([38]). TPE has been used with positive outcomes in the management of acute disseminated encephalomyelitis, Lambert–Eaton myasthenic syndrome, and neuromyelitis optica, although RCT evidence is lacking.

20.5.3 Hematological Disorders

There is a strong evidence base supporting TPE in symptomatic hyperviscosity—typically in Waldenstrom macroglobulinemia, but also occasionally seen in multiple myeloma [39]. TPE does not specifically treat the underlying condition; therefore, it is usually performed in conjunction with chemotherapy. TPE-mediated removal of immunoglobulin improves the microcirculation of the vital organs [4]. Hyperviscosity is typically IgM related but can also occur with IgA and IgG disease, in which case a more intensive TPE regime may be required as a larger amount of these is extravascular. Importantly, replacement fluid in this setting should be normal saline alone.

20.5.4 Poisoning and Drug Overdose

TPE is theoretically useful for eliminating drugs/toxins that are highly protein-bound with a small volume of distribution (Vd). It has been used in a variety of poisonings, but the body of evidence is essentially anecdotal. There are conflicting data regarding the survival benefit with TPE in cases of amatoxin-containing mushroom ingestion. Because of the lack of clear evidence, the role of TPE in poisoning should ideally be limited to research protocols or life-threatening cases which have not responded to conventional therapy.

20.5.5 Selective Techniques/Experimental Uses

More refined plasmapheresis techniques have been developed to enable very selective substance removal and therefore minimize nonspecific depletion of plasma proteins. Such techniques also avoid or minimize the need for replacement fluids, which in turn reduces adverse effects and cost. However, these techniques are not widely available in some countries, often for financial reasons.

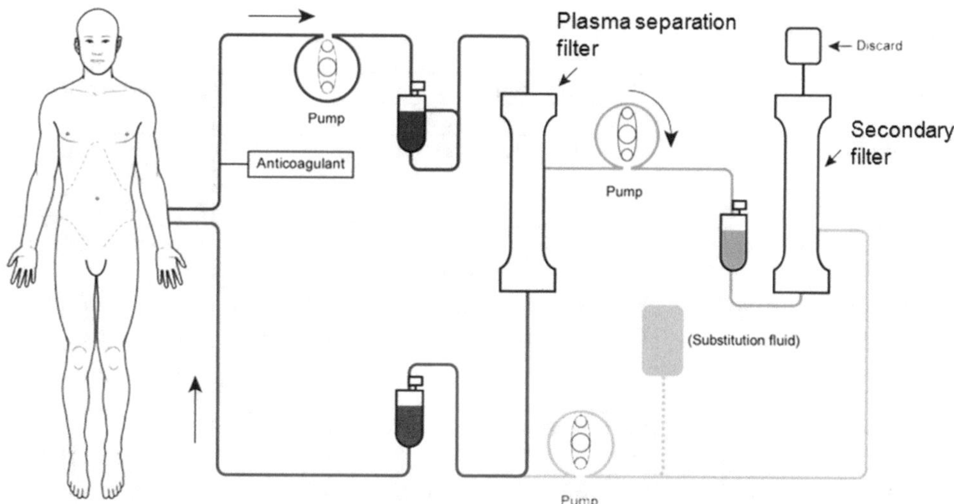

Fig. 20.4 Double filtration plasmapheresis circuit. (© 2011 Mina Hur, Hee-Won Moon, Seog-Woon Kwon. Originally published in *Understanding the Complexities of Kidney Transplantation*, ISBN 978-953-307-819-9, under CC BY-NC-SA 3.0 license. http://dx.doi.org/10.5772/20514)

Double filtration plasmapheresis (DFPP), or cascade filtration, applies a second filter (a plasma fractionator), with a smaller pore size, to separated plasma (Fig. 20.4). DFPP has been successfully used, mostly in European and Asian centers, in hyperviscosity syndrome and antibody-incompatible transplantation [40–42]. In the latter setting, it has the advantages of causing less depletion of clotting factors in the perioperative period (which would increase the risk of bleeding); higher volumes of plasma exchange may also be tolerated [42]. DFPP is occasionally employed in familial hypercholesterolaemia where large low-density lipoprotein (LDL) particles are retained and eliminated from plasma [43]. At ambient temperature, cryogels can form and occlude the pore structure of the second filter resulting in decreased selectivity of the filter and increased removal of high-density lipoprotein. To avoid this problem, a heating system that maintains the plasma at 38 °C can be incorporated. This process is referred to as *lipidfiltration*.

DFPP has been used with considerable success in dry age-related macular degeneration [44]. In this setting, certain substances with a high molecular weight (e.g., fibronectin, LDL cholesterol), which are associated with the disease, are selectively removed [4]. The removal of these substances improves blood microcirculation by reducing plasma viscosity and red cell aggregation. The use of DFPP to alter blood flow is termed *rheopheresis*.

Immunoadsorption (IA) is a modified form of plasmapheresis in which immunoglobulins or other proteins are removed from the plasma after passing it through a column. IA may be specific, where a single antibody of interest is removed, or nonspecific, where all antibodies are removed. Some IA columns become saturated with antibody binding and therefore treat a fixed plasma volume only. Others can be regenerated and treat unlimited volumes of plasma.

Selective IA, which removes antibodies directed towards a specific antigen, has been pioneered in Sweden. Such systems have worked effectively in ABO-incompatible organ transplantation [45]. In this setting, the IA column contains bound synthetic blood group A or B antigen. One single-use column selectively removes over 90 % of the target antibodies. When anti-A and anti-B are to be removed, two columns can be placed in series. The advantage, of course, is minimal removal of clotting factors and other plasma proteins. The disadvantage is the high cost of these columns. Selective removal of HLA antibodies has proven more difficult to develop. One problem here is that a given patient may have antibodies against many different antigens of the donor, thus multiple columns or columns with multiple specificities would be required to remove these antibodies.

Extracorporeal photopheresis (ECP) involves extracorporeal treatment of the buffy coat with a photoactive compound (psoralen) and exposure to ultraviolet A light prior to returning it to the patient. This is an established treatment for erythrodermic cutaneous T cell lymphoma [46] and an experimental treatment for other conditions including graft-versus-host disease after allogeneic hematopoietic cell transplantation.

20.6 Complications

Complications related to central venous access are not insignificant and include damage to surrounding structures, infections, venous stenosis, and thrombosis.

There are several other potential complications of TPE—some related to the procedure itself and others to the blood products and drugs used (Table 20.2). Most adverse effects are mild and do not prevent completion of TPE. With technique improvement over the years, the rate of adverse events has fallen substantially [47].

Aside from hypotension, complications are seen more frequently with plasma (rather than albumin) replacement [48,

Table 20.2 Prevention and treatment of TPE-related complications

	Complication	Prevention	Treatment
Vascular access	Infection	Standard precautions	Judicious antibiotic use
		Careful line maintenance	
Procedure	Hypotension	Hold antihypertensives before TPE	Trendelenburg position
			Saline bolus
			Reduce blood flow rate
	Electrolyte disturbance	Monitor daily	Replace electrolytes as required
		Calcium co-prescription	
	Depletional coagulopathy	Partial FFP replacement if intense TPE required	FFP administration
Blood product	Allergic reaction	Emergency drugs and equipment at the ready	Antihistamine
			Corticosteroid
			Adrenaline
	TRALI	Unpredictable; minimize blood product exposure	Oxygen
			Consideration ITU

TPE therapeutic plasma exchange, *TRALI* transfusion-related acute lung injury, *FFP* fresh frozen plasma, *ITU* intensive therapy unit

49]. Serious complications, including death, are extremely uncommon [50, 51], but are, again, more common in those receiving plasma replacement [52].

The main reported causes of death are cardiac arrhythmia, anaphylaxis, fatal thrombosis, and TRALI associated with plasma replacement. TRALI is a rare complication of blood product administration caused by passive transfusion of leukocyte antibodies leading to non-cardiogenic pulmonary edema.

Allergic reactions to plasma range from mild urticaria to fatal laryngospasm. Clinical features include fever, urticaria, wheezing, and hypotension [53]; treatment involves acetaminophen, antihistamines, steroids, and adrenaline depending on the severity. Following a mild allergic reaction, the patient should receive acetaminophen and antihistamines +/− steroids before subsequent TPE procedures. A more severe allergic reaction may warrant continuous antihistamine infusion during subsequent TPE procedures.

Hypotension occurs because approximately 200 ml of the patient's blood is extracorporeal at any given time and non-plasma replacement fluids have a lower oncotic pressure than plasma [48]. It usually responds to Trendelenburg positioning, saline boluses, and/or slowing of the procedure rate. In general, antihypertensive drugs should not be given shortly before TPE. The blood pressure should be checked every 15 min during TPE and with any change in clinical status. More serious causes of hypotension include hypokalemia- or hypocalcemia-related cardiac arrhythmias, acute coronary syndromes, anaphylactoid reactions, or hemorrhage. These should be excluded with clinical examination and appropriate investigations. If hypotension does not respond to a moderate saline bolus, the TPE should be discontinued to enable urgent patient evaluation.

Electrolyte disturbances are relatively common in TPE and require appropriate prevention and treatment. Dilutional hypokalemia can occur with albumin/saline replacement. As discussed above, hypocalcemia can occur for several reasons. Early symptoms include perioral and peripheral paresthesia. The patient should be encouraged to report these symptoms if they occur. Severe hypocalcemia can cause continuous muscle contraction and QT interval prolongation, which can progress to tetany (and potentially life-threatening laryngospasm) and cardiac arrhythmias, respectively. Citrate also chelates magnesium but the role of magnesium supplementation is unclear.

TPE is nonselective, leading to loss of physiologic plasma components. Plasma exchange with non-plasma replacement fluid causes a *depletion coagulopathy*, particularly of factors I, II, and X [54]. The coagulopathy is mild and transient immediately post exchange. However, reductions in coagulation factors, especially fibrinogen, occur when multiple exchanges are performed within a short period of time [55]. Despite reduced coagulation factor levels, the incidence of clinically significant bleeding appears to be low [56].

That said, caution is advised in patients with additional risk factors for hemorrhage, such as recent renal biopsy or diffuse alveolar hemorrhage. In these patients, the general consensus is that plasma is substituted for some (usually 500–1000 ml) of the standard replacement fluid and administered towards the end of the exchange (earlier administration would cause unnecessary exposure to blood products that would be partially removed later in the exchange; [4]). Similar practice may also be observed in patients who require intensive, daily TPE to avoid a severe depletional coagulopathy [4].

TPE predictably causes a *depletional hypogammaglobulinemia*. It is unclear whether this actually translates to an increased rate of opportunistic infections, as many patients who require intensive TPE will also require aggressive immunosuppression [57, 58]. There is no RCT evidence to guide immunoglobulin replacement in this setting. Some experts advocate replacement with single-dose IVIg (100–400 mg/kg) if IgG levels fall below 500 mg/dl and a systemic infection occurs. Ideally, this would be given after the course of TPE is completed.

Table 20.3 Drugs that may be removed during TPE

Drug
Aspirin
Gentamicin
Levothyroxine
Ceftriaxone
Verapamil
Diltiazem

Careful drug level (or action) monitoring should be performed where possible

There is a theoretical risk of viral transmission when plasma replacement is used. Hepatitis B vaccination should be considered if exposure to large volumes of plasma is predicted.

Careful attention to *administration of medications* is warranted in patients undergoing TPE. It is difficult to predict drug removal by TPE and pharmacokinetic studies are few [59]. Where possible, drugs should be given after TPE and, if appropriate, drug levels (or effects) should be frequently monitored. Drug removal by TPE depends on drug characteristics such as Vd, half-life, and protein binding. Those with a low Vd and/or high protein binding are more likely to be removed. This has been harnessed with (varying) success in cases of intentional and unintentional overdose with drugs including vincristine, verapamil, and diltiazem [59]. Of particular interest are the immunosuppressive agents that are often used in conjunction with TPE. Whole-blood levels of prednisolone and the calcineurin inhibitors have been shown to be essentially unaffected by TPE [59, 60]. Cyclophosphamide and azathioprine have low protein binding rates and are therefore thought to be not appreciably removed during TPE [59]. Basiliximab is significantly removed [61]. Removal rates of rituximab are unclear bur are likely to be high. Several commonly used drugs are variably removed in the available published reports (Table 20.3). Again, it is prudent to give all drugs—where possible—after the TPE session, rather than before.

Removal of plasma cholinesterase, involved in the metabolism of certain drugs including some muscle relaxants, can have important clinical implications [62]. Angiotensin-converting enzyme inhibitors (ACEi) should be discontinued prior to TPE. This is based on an observation that patients receiving an ACEi during TPE with albumin replacement experienced a higher rate of certain symptoms (flushing, hypotension, and abdominal cramping; [63]). The precise mechanism is not well understood although may relate to inhibition of kinin metabolism [3].

20.7 TPE in Special Patient Populations

20.7.1 Pediatric

A number of challenges exist when therapeutic plasmapheresis is used in the pediatric setting. The pediatric evidence base is small; therefore, practice is often extrapolated from the adult experience. The main technical issue is the large extracorporeal volume (ECV), relative to the child's intravascular volume. Adapted circuitry, with smaller circuit volume, can allow for safe TPE in small children, including infants [64]. Ideally, ECV should not exceed 10% of total blood volume in children to avoid significant hypovolemia.

At the start of TPE, whole blood enters the circuit and the priming saline is diverted to the effluent bag. If the priming volume exceeds 10% of total blood volume, the priming saline (or other fluid of choice depending on the clinical situation) should be infused into the child at the start of TPE rather than diverting. Red cell priming may be required in hemodynamically unstable children or those weighing less than 15 kg, to avoid a clinically significant drop in circulating blood volume. At the end of the procedure, the circuit should be "rinsed back" only if the child can tolerate the positive net volume shift that this creates.

Central venous access is required in small children, as peripheral veins will not accommodate large needles. Adverse events are more common in children [65]. Continuous calcium infusion and regular monitoring of ionized calcium levels should be undertaken if the child is unable to report symptoms of hypocalcemia.

Despite the above issues, TPE has been used in a wide variety of pediatric conditions. Renal indications include AAV, anti-GBM disease, atypical HUS, and posttransplant FSGS [66].

20.7.2 Pregnancy

Correct patient positioning is critical in later pregnancy to avoid aortocaval compression and associated hypotension. Appropriate adjustments should be made to allow for the relative changes in plasma volume during pregnancy.

20.7.3 Intensive Care Unit

TPE can be safely performed in critically unwell patients. The patient should be adequately resuscitated using standard treatment including vasopressors. Increased vasopressor doses may be required during TPE. Continuous cardiac monitoring is recommended. Ionized calcium levels should be monitored during the procedure, as the patient is unlikely to be able to report symptoms.

If a patient is volume overloaded, standard measures (diuretics/dialysis), and not TPE, should be used for volume removal. TPE may not be well tolerated immediately post hemodialysis because of hypovolemia; therefore, if both procedures are required in a given day, TPE should generally be performed first. Performing dialysis after TPE has the added advantage of correcting any remaining electrolyte abnormalities.

20.8 Conclusions and Future Direction

In conclusion, TPE is currently an important part of therapy for a wide range of immune-mediated diseases. That said, there is a paucity of RCT evidence to guide its use, even in conditions where it is considered standard of care. The future of TPE is likely to involve more selective techniques, which will offer a more refined therapy with fewer adverse effects. There are several ongoing clinical trials evaluating the role of TPE in a variety of diseases and we eagerly await the results of these.

20.9 Examples of TPE in Clinical Practice

20.9.1 Case 1

A 40-year-old male is referred with rapidly rising creatinine and hemoptysis. His lab values are significant for creatinine 4.8 mg/dl, Hct 25.0, and anti-GBM 114 units/ml. The renal biopsy shows a severe crescentic glomerulonephritis, involving approximately 70% of glomeruli. The diagnosis is anti-GBM disease with renal and lung involvement. He is started on cyclophosphamide and steroids. He weighs 80 kg. What TPE regimen would you prescribe?

An aggressive TPE regimen is required here, as the patient could develop end-stage renal disease and/or fatal pulmonary hemorrhage. A typical regimen would be 1.0–1.5 plasma volumes daily for 10–14 days. After this period, further TPE can be prescribed depending on the anti-GBM titre and the clinical status of the patient.

$$\text{Estimated plasma volume} = 0.07 \times \text{weight}(\text{kg}) \times (1 - \text{hematocrit})$$

So, 1 plasma volume is $0.07 \times 80 \times 0.75 = 4.2$ l

1.3 plasma volumes is 5.5 L (an easy number to prescribe). So the prescription would be:

1. Remove 5.5 L
2. Replace with 3.0 L of 5% albumin, 2.0 L of normal saline, and 0.5 L of FFP[1]
3. Premedicate with oral calcium
4. Premedicate with oral acetaminophen and oral diphenhydramine if any concern about allergic reaction to FFP
5. Give 55 ml of 10% calcium gluconate IV over the TPE session[2]

20.9.2 Case 2

A 30-year-old female is referred with TTP. She has altered mental status and lab values are significant for Hct 24.0, platelets 24×10^9/l, and LDH 3420 units/ml. She weighs 74 kg. What TPE regimen would you prescribe?

An aggressive TPE regimen is required here, as this is a life-threatening disease. A typical regimen would be 1.5 plasma volumes daily for 10–14 days. After this period, further TPE can be prescribed depending on the platelet count, plasma LDH, and the clinical status of the patient.

$$\text{Estimated plasma volume} = 0.07 \times \text{weight}(\text{kg}) \times (1 - \text{hematocrit})$$

So, 1 plasma volume is $0.07 \times 74 \times 0.76 = 3.9$ L

1.5 plasma volumes is 5.9 L (easier to round up to 6 L). So the prescription would be:

1. Remove 6.0 L
2. Replace with 6.0 L of FFP[3]
3. Premedicate with oral calcium
4. Premedicate with oral acetaminophen and oral diphenhydramine if any concern about allergic reaction to FFP
5. Give 60 ml of 10% calcium gluconate IV over the TPE session and further IV boluses of 10 ml of 10% calcium gluconate if ionized calcium < 0.9 mmol/l (check ionized calcium every hour during TPE)

20.9.3 Key Points

- TPE is an extracorporeal therapy that involves removal of pathogen-containing plasma and replacement with pathogen-free fluid
- Prescription is individualized to the patient and the disease
- Indications are divided into four categories depending on the strength of supporting evidence for the role of TPE
- Minor adverse effects are common; serious ones are rare

[1] FFP is given because of the renal biopsy and the hemoptysis. If bleeding is a major concern, then more FFP and less normal saline could be prescribed.

[2] If the patient received more FFP, more IV calcium gluconate may be required.Note: if DFPP were used, the prescription would simply ask for removal of 5.5 L plasma and replacement with small amounts of 5% albumin (as a small amount is removed). FFP and/or fibrinogen would only be given if there were laboratory evidence of a coagulopathy.

[3] FFP is given because it is therapeutic here.

References

1. Shariatmadar S, Nassiri M, Vincek V. Effect of plasma exchange on cytokines measured by multianalyte bead array in thrombotic thrombocytopenic purpura. Am J Hematol. 2005;79(2):83–8. PubMed PMID: 15929111.
2. Goto H, Matsuo H, Nakane S, Izumoto H, Fukudome T, Kambara C, et al. Plasmapheresis affects T helper type-1/T helper type-2 balance of circulating peripheral lymphocytes. Ther Apher. 2001;5(6):494–6. PubMed PMID: 11800088.
3. Kaplan AA. Therapeutic plasma exchange: core curriculum 2008. Am J Kidney Dis. 2008;52(6):1180–96. PubMed PMID: 18562061.
4. Schwartz J, Winters JL, Padmanabhan A, Balogun RA, Delaney M, Linenberger ML, et al. Guidelines on the use of therapeutic apheresis in clinical practice-evidence-based approach from the Writing Committee of the American Society for Apheresis: the sixth special issue. J Clin Apher. 2013;28(3):145–284. PubMed PMID: 23868759.
5. Gerhardt RE, Ntoso KA, Koethe JD, Lodge S, Wolf CJ. Acute plasma separation with hemodialysis equipment. J Am Soc Nephrol. 1992;2(9):1455–8. PubMed PMID: 1627768.
6. Frasca GM, Buscaroli A, Borgnino LC, Vangelista A. Optimization of heparin anticoagulation during membrane plasma separation. Int J Artif Organs. 1988;11(4):313–6. PubMed PMID: 3410572.
7. Weinstein R. Prevention of citrate reactions during therapeutic plasma exchange by constant infusion of calcium gluconate with the return fluid. J Clin Apher. 1996;11(4):204–10. PubMed PMID: 8986866.
8. Okafor C, Kalantarinia K. Vascular access considerations for therapeutic apheresis procedures. Semin Dial. 2012;25(2):140–4. PubMed PMID: 22176495.
9. Vascular Access Work G. Clinical practice guidelines for vascular access. Am J Kidney Dis. 2006;48(Suppl 1):S176–247. PubMed PMID: 16813989.
10. Rock G, Clark B, Sutton D, Cag C. The Canadian apheresis registry. Transfus Apher Sci. 2003;29(2):167–77. PubMed PMID: 12941357.
11. Malchesky PS, Skibinski CI. Summary of results of 1991 ASFA apheresis survey. American Society for Apheresis. J Clin Apher. 1993;8(2):96–101. PubMed PMID: 8226712.
12. Johnson JP, Moore J Jr, Austin HA 3rd, Balow JE, Antonovych TT, Wilson CB. Therapy of anti-glomerular basement membrane antibody disease: analysis of prognostic significance of clinical, pathologic and treatment factors. Medicine (Baltimore). 1985;64(4):219–27. PubMed PMID: 3892220.
13. Cui Z, Zhao J, Jia XY, Zhu SN, Jin QZ, Cheng XY, et al. Anti-glomerular basement membrane disease: outcomes of different therapeutic regimens in a large single-center Chinese cohort study. Medicine (Baltimore). 2011;90(5):303–11. PubMed PMID: 21862934.
14. Simpson IJ, Doak PB, Williams LC, Blacklock HA, Hill RS, Teague CA, et al. Plasma exchange in Goodpasture's syndrome. Am J Nephrol. 1982;2(6):301–11. PubMed PMID: 6762091.
15. Levy JB, Turner AN, Rees AJ, Pusey CD. Long-term outcome of anti-glomerular basement membrane antibody disease treated with plasma exchange and immunosuppression. Ann Intern Med. 2001;134(11):1033–42. PubMed PMID: 11388816.
16. Pusey CD, Rees AJ, Evans DJ, Peters DK, Lockwood CM. Plasma exchange in focal necrotizing glomerulonephritis without anti-GBM antibodies. Kidney Int. 1991;40(4):757–63. PubMed PMID: 1745027.
17. Jayne DR, Gaskin G, Rasmussen N, Abramowicz D, Ferrario F, Guillevin L, et al. Randomized trial of plasma exchange or high-dosage methylprednisolone as adjunctive therapy for severe renal vasculitis. J Am Soc Nephrol. 2007;18(7):2180–8. PubMed PMID: 17582159.
18. Walsh M, Casian A, Flossmann O, Westman K, Hoglund P, Pusey C, et al. Long-term follow-up of patients with severe ANCA-associated vasculitis comparing plasma exchange to intravenous methylprednisolone treatment is unclear. Kidney Int. 2013;84(2):397–402. PubMed PMID: 23615499.
19. Levy JB, Hammad T, Coulthart A, Dougan T, Pusey CD. Clinical features and outcome of patients with both ANCA and anti-GBM antibodies. Kidney Int. 2004;66(4):1535–40. PubMed PMID: 15458448.
20. Klemmer PJ, Chalermskulrat W, Reif MS, Hogan SL, Henke DC, Falk RJ. Plasmapheresis therapy for diffuse alveolar hemorrhage in patients with small-vessel vasculitis. Am J Kidney Dis. 2003;42(6):1149–53. PubMed PMID: 14655185.
21. Walsh M, Merkel PA, Peh CA, Szpirt W, Guillevin L, Pusey CD, et al. Plasma exchange and glucocorticoid dosing in the treatment of anti-neutrophil cytoplasm antibody associated vasculitis (PEXIVAS): protocol for a randomized controlled trial. Trials. 2013;14:73. PubMed PMID: 23497590.
22. Zucchelli P, Pasquali S, Cagnoli L, Ferrari G. Controlled plasma exchange trial in acute renal failure due to multiple myeloma. Kidney Int. 1988;33(6):1175–80. PubMed PMID: 3043077.
23. Leung N, Gertz MA, Zeldenrust SR, Rajkumar SV, Dispenzieri A, Fervenza FC, et al. Improvement of cast nephropathy with plasma exchange depends on the diagnosis and on reduction of serum free light chains. Kidney Int. 2008;73(11):1282–8. PubMed PMID: 18385667.
24. Clark WF, Stewart AK, Rock GA, Sternbach M, Sutton DM, Barrett BJ, et al. Plasma exchange when myeloma presents as acute renal failure: a randomized, controlled trial. Ann Intern Med. 2005;143(11):777–84. PubMed PMID: 16330788.
25. Hutchison CA, Bradwell AR, Cook M, Basnayake K, Basu S, Harding S, et al. Treatment of acute renal failure secondary to multiple myeloma with chemotherapy and extended high cut-off hemodialysis. Clin J Am Soc Nephrol. 2009;4(4):745–54. PubMed PMID: 19339414.
26. Rock GA, Shumak KH, Buskard NA, Blanchette VS, Kelton JG, Nair RC, et al. Comparison of plasma exchange with plasma infusion in the treatment of thrombotic thrombocytopenic purpura. Canadian Apheresis Study Group. N Engl J Med. 1991;325(6):393–7. PubMed PMID: 2062330.
27. Bell WR, Braine HG, Ness PM, Kickler TS. Improved survival in thrombotic thrombocytopenic purpura-hemolytic uremic syndrome. Clinical experience in 108 patients. N Engl J Med. 1991;325(6):398–403. PubMed PMID: 2062331.
28. Montgomery RA, Locke JE, King KE, Segev DL, Warren DS, Kraus ES, et al. ABO incompatible renal transplantation: a paradigm ready for broad implementation. Transplantation. 2009;87(8):1246–55. PubMed PMID: 19384174.
29. Stegall MD, Gloor J, Winters JL, Moore SB, Degoey S. A comparison of plasmapheresis versus high-dose IVIG desensitization in renal allograft recipients with high levels of donor specific alloantibody. Am J Transplant. 2006;6(2):346–51. PubMed PMID: 16426319.
30. Montgomery RA, Lonze BE, King KE, Kraus ES, Kucirka LM, Locke JE, et al. Desensitization in HLA-incompatible kidney recipients and survival. N Engl J Med. 2011;365(4):318–26. PubMed PMID: 21793744.
31. Artero ML, Sharma R, Savin VJ, Vincenti F. Plasmapheresis reduces proteinuria and serum capacity to injure glomeruli in patients with recurrent focal glomerulosclerosis. Am J Kidney Dis. 1994;23(4):574–81. PubMed PMID: 8154495.
32. Rocha PN, Butterly DW, Greenberg A, Reddan DN, Tuttle-Newhall J, Collins BH, et al. Beneficial effect of plasmapheresis and intravenous immunoglobulin on renal allograft survival of patients

with acute humoral rejection. Transplantation. 2003;75(9):1490–5. PubMed PMID: 12792502.
33. Efficiency of plasma exchange in Guillain-Barre syndrome. Role of replacement fluids. French Cooperative Group on plasma exchange in Guillain-Barre syndrome. Ann Neurol. 1987;22(6):753–61. PubMed PMID: 2893583.
34. Plasma exchange in Guillain-Barre syndrome. One-year follow-up. French Cooperative Group on plasma exchange in Guillain-Barre Syndrome. Ann Neurol. 1992;32(1):94–7. PubMed PMID: 1642477.
35. Cortese I, Chaudhry V, So YT, Cantor F, Cornblath DR, Rae-Grant A. Evidence-based guideline update: plasmapheresis in neurologic disorders: report of the therapeutics and technology assessment subcommittee of the American Academy of Neurology. Neurology. 2011;76(3):294–300. PubMed PMID: 21242498.
36. Pham HP, Daniel-Johnson JA, Stotler BA, Stephens H, Schwartz J. Therapeutic plasma exchange for the treatment of anti-NMDA receptor encephalitis. J Clin Apher. 2011;26(6):320–5. PubMed PMID: 21898576.
37. Titulaer MJ, McCracken L, Gabilondo I, Armangue T, Glaser C, Iizuka T, et al. Treatment and prognostic factors for long-term outcome in patients with anti-NMDA receptor encephalitis: an observational cohort study. Lancet Neurol. 2013;12(2):157–65. PubMed PMID: 23290630.
38. Hahn AF, Bolton CF, Pillay N, Chalk C, Benstead T, Bril V, et al. Plasma-exchange therapy in chronic inflammatory demyelinating polyneuropathy. A double-blind, sham-controlled, cross-over study. Brain. 1996;119(Pt 4):1055–66. PubMed PMID: 8813270.
39. Drew MJ. Plasmapheresis in the dysproteinemias. Ther Apher. 2002;6(1):45–52. PubMed PMID: 11886576.
40. Tanabe K. Double-filtration plasmapheresis. Transplantation. 2007;84(12 Suppl):S30–2. PubMed PMID: 18162985.
41. Nakaji S, Yamamoto T. Membranes for therapeutic apheresis. Ther Apher. 2002;6(4):267–70. PubMed PMID: 12164795.
42. Higgins R, Lowe D, Hathaway M, Lam FT, Kashi H, Tan LC, et al. Double filtration plasmapheresis in antibody-incompatible kidney transplantation. Ther Apher Dial. 2010;14(4):392–9. PubMed PMID: 20649760.
43. Geiss HC, Parhofer KG, Donner MG, Schwandt P. Low density lipoprotein apheresis by membrane differential filtration (cascade filtration). Ther Apher. 1999;3(3):199–202. PubMed PMID: 10427615.
44. Brunner R, Widder RA, Walter P, Luke C, Godehardt E, Bartz-Schmidt KU, et al. Influence of membrane differential filtration on the natural course of age-related macular degeneration: a randomized trial. Retina. 2000;20(5):483–91. PubMed PMID: 11039423.
45. Genberg H, Kumlien G, Wennberg L, Tyden G. Long-term results of ABO-incompatible kidney transplantation with antigen-specific immunoadsorption and rituximab. Transplantation. 2007;84(12 Suppl):S44–7. PubMed PMID: 18162990.
46. Edelson R, Berger C, Gasparro F, Jegasothy B, Heald P, Wintroub B, et al. Treatment of cutaneous T-cell lymphoma by extracorporeal photochemotherapy. Preliminary results. N Engl J Med. 1987;316(6):297–303. PubMed PMID: 3543674.
47. Korach JM, Guillevin L, Petitpas D, Berger P, Chillet P. Apheresis registry in France: indications, techniques, and complications. French Registry Study Group. Ther Apher. 2000;4(3):207–10. PubMed PMID: 10910021.
48. Shemin D, Briggs D, Greenan M. Complications of therapeutic plasma exchange: a prospective study of 1727 procedures. J Clin Apher. 2007;22(5):270–6. PubMed PMID: 17722046.
49. Bambauer R, Jutzler GA, Albrecht D, Keller HE, Kohler M. Indications of plasmapheresis and selection of different substitution solutions. Biomater Artif Cells Artif Organs. 1989;17(1):9–26. PubMed PMID: 2775871.
50. Mokrzycki MH, Kaplan AA. Therapeutic plasma exchange: complications and management. Am J Kidney Dis. 1994;23(6):817–27. PubMed PMID: 8203364.
51. Kaplan A. Complications of apheresis. Semin Dial. 2012;25(2):152–8. PubMed PMID: 22321209.
52. Huestis DW. Risks and safety practices in hemapheresis procedures. Arch Pathol Lab Med. 1989;113(3):273–8. PubMed PMID: 2645853.
53. Reutter JC, Sanders KF, Brecher ME, Jones HG, Bandarenko N. Incidence of allergic reactions with fresh frozen plasma or cryo-supernatant plasma in the treatment of thrombotic thrombocytopenic purpura. J Clin Apher. 2001;16(3):134–8. PubMed PMID: 11746540.
54. Chirnside A, Urbaniak SJ, Prowse CV, Keller AJ. Coagulation abnormalities following intensive plasma exchange on the cell separator. II. Effects on factors I, II, V, VII, VIII, IX, X and antithrombin III. Br J Haematol. 1981;48(4):627–34. PubMed PMID: 6791676.
55. Grgicevic D. Influence of long-term plasmapheresis on blood coagulation. Ric Clin Lab. 1983;13(1):21–31. PubMed PMID: 6407088.
56. Lin SM, Yeh JH, Lee CC, Chiu HC. Clearance of fibrinogen and von Willebrand factor in serial double-filtration plasmapheresis. J Clin Apher. 2003;18(2):67–70. PubMed PMID: 12874818.
57. Wing EJ, Bruns FJ, Fraley DS, Segel DP, Adler S. Infectious complications with plasmapheresis in rapidly progressive glomerulonephritis. JAMA. 1980;244(21):2423–6. PubMed PMID: 7431570.
58. Pohl MA, Lan SP, Berl T. Plasmapheresis does not increase the risk for infection in immunosuppressed patients with severe lupus nephritis. The Lupus Nephritis Collaborative Study Group. Ann Intern Med. 1991;114(11):924–9. PubMed PMID: 2024858.
59. Ibrahim RB, Liu C, Cronin SM, Murphy BC, Cha R, Swerdlow P, et al. Drug removal by plasmapheresis: an evidence-based review. Pharmacotherapy. 2007;27(11):1529–49. PubMed PMID: 17963462.
60. Hale GA, Reece DE, Munn RK, Kniska AB, Phillips GL. Blood tacrolimus concentrations in bone marrow transplant patients undergoing plasmapheresis. Bone Marrow Transplant. 2000;25(4):449–51. PubMed PMID: 10723590.
61. Okechukwu CN, Meier-Kriesche HU, Armstrong D, Campbell D, Gerbeau C, Kaplan B. Removal of basiliximab by plasmapheresis. Am J Kidney Dis. 2001;37(1):E11. PubMed PMID: 11136200.
62. Naik B, Hirshhorn S, Dharnidharka VR. Prolonged neuromuscular block due to cholinesterase depletion by plasmapheresis. J Clin Anesth. 2002;14(5):381–4. PubMed PMID: 12208445.
63. Owen HG, Brecher ME. Atypical reactions associated with use of angiotensin-converting enzyme inhibitors and apheresis. Transfusion. 1994;34(10):891–4. PubMed PMID: 7940662.
64. Kasprisin DO. Techniques, indications, and toxicity of therapeutic hemapheresis in children. J Clin Apher. 1989;5(1):21–4. PubMed PMID: 2777736.
65. Michon B, Moghrabi A, Winikoff R, Barrette S, Bernstein ML, Champagne J, et al. Complications of apheresis in children. Transfusion. 2007;47(10):1837–42. PubMed PMID: 17880609.
66. Hunt EA, Jain NG, Somers MJ. Apheresis therapy in children: an overview of key technical aspects and a review of experience in pediatric renal disease. J Clin Apher. 2013;28(1):36–47. PubMed PMID: 23420594.

21 High Cut Off Hemodialysis

Clara J. Day and Paul Cockwell

21.1 Introduction

Advances in dialysis membrane engineering have led to incremental developments in dialyzer technology towards the biological characteristics of the glomerular basement membrane (GBM) [1]. Some of these advances have been motivated by the principle that increased clearance of middle molecular weight (MW) molecules may be associated with better clinical outcomes [2]. Table 21.1 shows specific middle MW molecules that accumulate in kidney failure. Molecules with a MW in excess of 20 kDa are above the threshold for effective clearance by standard high-flux hemodialysis (HF-HD); however, some uremic toxins have a MW below that of albumin (65 kDa) and could be targeted by an appropriately engineered dialysis membrane.

High Cut Off HD (HCO-HD) uses a dialysis membrane that has a cut off for protein permeability that is close to the GBM and has the highest clearance of middle MW molecules of any dialyzer. It is defined by a significant sieving coefficient (SC) from blood for proteins up to the MW of albumin; this represents a major development in dialyzer technology. Figure 21.1 shows a high-magnification photomicrograph of an HCO membrane compared to a standard HF-HD membrane.

Over the past decade, HCO-HD has been evaluated for patients with the following clinical indications:

- Removal of pro-inflammatory cytokines associated with sepsis syndrome
- Diseases where acute kidney injury (AKI) is caused by a specific nephrotoxin (e.g., myeloma and rhabdomyolysis) of a MW that is preferentially removed by the membrane
- Uremic toxin removal in end-stage kidney disease (ESKD) in a chronic dialysis prescription.

While HCO-HD has not yet entered mainstream clinical practice, a growing clinical evidence base supports both the safety and (in part) the efficacy of this modality. Furthermore, HCO-HD provides a rationale for next-generation dialyzers that have high permeability but a more precise MW cut off. This addresses an important limitation of HCO-HD: albumin loss of a magnitude that precludes use of the modality in a long-term chronic HD prescription.

21.2 The Permeability Characteristics of a Dialysis Membrane

Pore size and pore size distribution are the two main permeability characteristics of a dialyzer membrane that distinguish between different groups of dialyzers. The potential of a molecule of a given MW to pass through a dialysis membrane is defined by these characteristics. The other membrane features that influence molecule clearance include the material used for the dialyzer membrane, which may produce different absorption and absorption characteristics for any given protein [3] and the thickness of the dialysis membrane.

The permeability of a dialysis membrane for a molecule of a defined MW can be quantified by the SC. Marker solutes are used to define the SC; this approach has been described in detail elsewhere [4, 5]. The most widely used molecule for characterization of the properties of a dialyzer is dextran, a linear carbohydrate chain available at different MW fractions. The relationship between the size of any given dextran chain and a protein of the same MW equivalence can be calculated from the radius of the dextran-coiled chain [3].

The SC for any molecule will have a value of between 0 and 1; 0 refers to no permeability and 1 refers to full

P. Cockwell (✉)
Department of Renal Medicine, Queen Elizabeth Hospital Birmingham, Mindelsohn Way, Birmingham, B15 2WB, UK
e-mail: paul.cockwell@uhb.nhs.uk

C. J. Day
Department of Renal Medicine, Queen Elizabeth Hospital Birmingham Mindelsohn Way, Birmingham, C15 2EB, UK
e-mail: clara.day@uhb.nhs.uk

A. K. Singh et al. (eds.), *Core Concepts in Dialysis and Continuous Therapies*, DOI 10.1007/978-1-4899-7657-4_21

Table 21.1 Selected uremic toxins, MW, and increased concentrations in ESKD

Molecule	MW (kDa)	Fold increase concentration in ESKD (max)
β2M	11.8	50
Cystatin C	13.3	12
κLC	22.5	30
IL-6	24.5	25
TNF-α	26	31
IL-1β	32	11
λLC	45	30

MW molecular weight, *kDa* kilodaltons, *ESKD* end-stage kidney disease, *max* maximum, *β2M* beta-2 microglobulin, *κLC* kappa light chain, *IL-6* interleukin 6, *TNF-α* tumor necrosis factor-alpha, *IL-1β* interleukin-1 beta, *λLC* lambda light chain

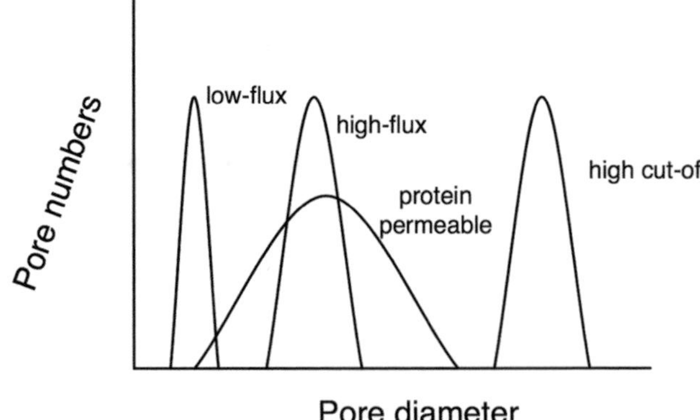

Fig. 21.2 Conceptualization of the relationship between pore size (diameter) and pore numbers for each of the major dialyzer groups

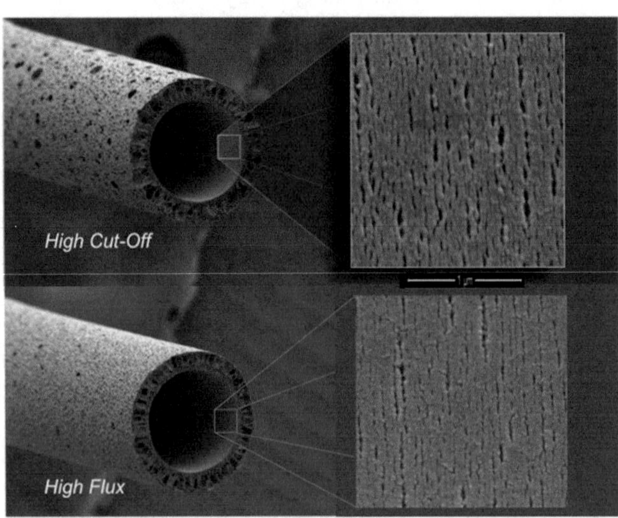

Fig. 21.1 A high-powered photomicrograph of (**a**) a *high cut off* hemodialysis (HCO-HD) membrane and (**b**) a standard *high-flux* hemodialysis (HF-HD) membrane. Note the differences in size of the pores and pore size distribution between the two dialyzers. (Courtesy of Baxter–Gambro)

permeability. Full permeability indicates that a molecule of a given MW will redistribute from blood into dialysate so that the concentration of that molecule is the same on each side of the dialyzer membrane. The permeability of a single dialysis membrane to molecules of a range of MW can be depicted visually by a sieving curve [6].

The SC of the dialysis membrane is used to categorize a dialyzer as: (i) low-flux (LF), (ii) HF, (iii) protein-permeable (PP), or (iv) HCO. A useful system for linking the membrane-specific characteristics to the dialyzer class has recently been proposed [7]. This system conceptualizes the permeability of a membrane based on the utilization of two thresholds: (i) the molecular weight cut off (MWCO); and (ii) the molecular weight retention onset (MWRO). The MWCO refers to the highest MW for which the SC of the membrane is at least 0.1; the MWRO refers to the lowest MW for which the SC of the membrane is at least 0.9. Figure 21.2 is a schematic of the relationship between dialyzer pore size and the efficacy of a dialyzer in each of the four major dialysis categories, Fig. 21.3 shows the sieving curve of each dialyzer group, and Fig. 21.4 shows how the MWCO and the MWRO of each dialyzer category relates to the pore size and pore distribution.

21.3 The Distinction Between HCO and Other Dialyzer Groups

The characteristics of different dialyzer groups are shown in Table 21.2. The in vitro figures are derived from experiments using dextran molecules of different MWs [7]. These characteristics change when blood is in contact with the dialyzer such that in vivo the SC curve moves to the left. In summary: (i) An LF dialyzer has low permeability to water and an SC that does not allow the clearance of β2-microglobulin (β2M; MW); (ii) an HF dialyzer has high permeability to water, a high SC for β2M (0.7–0.8) and very little albumin loss when used in an HD mode; (iii) a PP dialyzer has high permeability to water, a very high SC for β2M, and low albumin loss; (iv) an HCO dialyzer has very high water permeability and an SC of 1.0 for β2M and up to 0.2 for albumin. For HF, PP, and HCO dialyzer groups, there is demonstrable stratified clearance of molecules of MW between β2M and albumin.

When a HF, PP, or HCO dialyzer is used in HD mode, there is a component of convective clearance (ultrafiltration; water movement across the dialysis membrane) because of internal filtration across the membrane; this is a complex process that has been best modeled for HF-HD by using radio-labeled albumin [8]. The distinction between HF and PP dialysis becomes less clear when a HF membrane uses convective transfer though a hemodiafiltration (HDF) component; with high-convective transfer, the albumin leak that occurs with HF-HDF can be equivalent to that seen with PP dialysis [9, 10]. Recognizing the impact of convective clear-

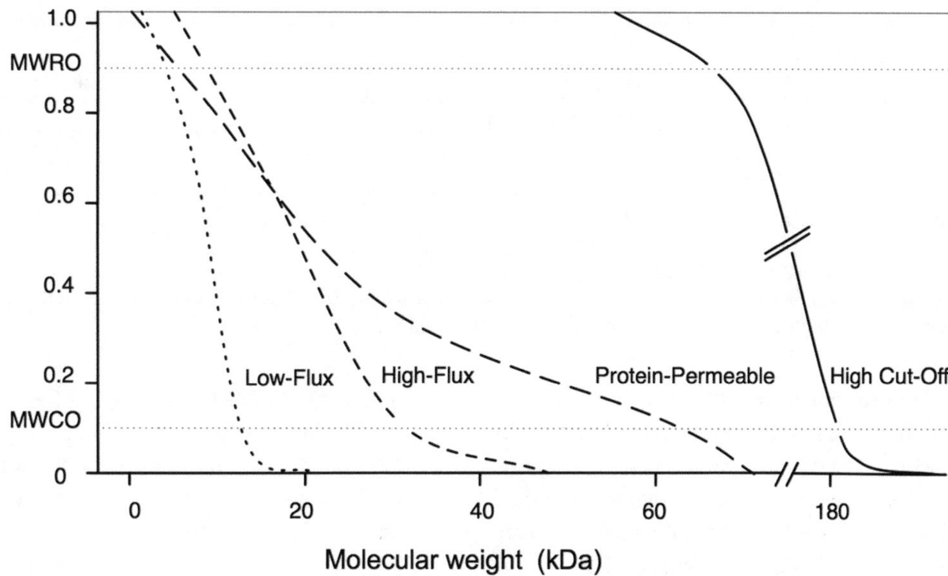

Fig. 21.3 Sieving curves for each of the major dialyzer group; based on in vitro studies with dextran. In vivo, the curves move to the *left* and the in vivo thresholds for *MWCO* and *MWRO* are less than those seen in vitro. *MWCO* molecular weight cut off, *MWRO* molecular weight retention onset

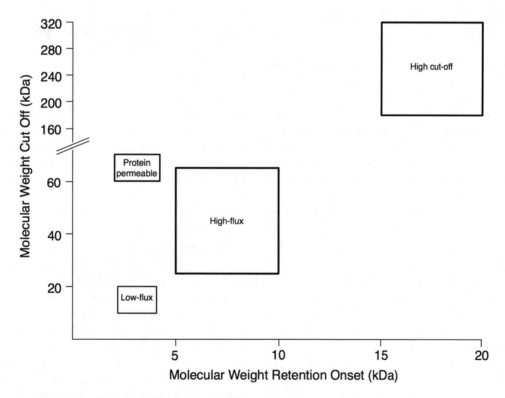

Fig. 21.4 The relationship between MWCO and MWRO for each of the major dialyzer groups has been shown. Note the distinct features of each dialyzer type, which form the basis of a classification system that identifies the HCO dialysis membrane as having characteristics distinct from *high-flux* and *protein-permeable* dialyzers. *MWCO* molecular weight cut off, *MWRO* molecular weight retention onset, HCO *high cut off*

ance across the dialysis membrane is important when considering the use of a dialyzer in clinical practice.

The three major classes of solutes that are removed by dialysis membranes and are classified as uremic molecules or toxins are: (i) small water-soluble molecules, such as creatinine and urea, that are removed by all dialyzer membranes; (ii) protein-bound solutes, that when free are of a MW similar to small soluble-water molecules (e.g., homocysteine);

Table 21.2 Characteristics of membrane by type: MWCO and MWRO in vitro defined by dextran sieving; sieving coefficients in vivo at QD 500 ml/min and QB 250 ml/min

Dialyzer type	MWCO (kDa)	MWRO (kDa)	Sieving coefficient			H_2O permeability	Albumin loss (g)
			Urea	β2M	Albumin		
LF	10–20	2–4	1	<0.1	<0.01	10–20	0
HF	25–65	5–10	1	0.8	<0.01	200–400	<0.5
PP	60–70	2–4	1	0.9	0.02	50–500	6
HCO	170–320	15–20	1	1.0	0.2	1100	9–28

Albumin loss over a conventional dialysis session, in vivo

MWCO molecular weight cut off, *MWRO* molecular weight retention onset, Q_D dialysis fluid flow rate, Q_B blood flow rate, *g* grams, *β2M* Beta-2 microglobulin, *LF* low-flux, *HF* high-flux, *PP* protein-permeable, *HCO* high cut off

(iii) free middle MW molecules up to the MW of albumin of which β2 M (MW 11.8 kDa) is the best characterized. Molecules within these groups both accumulate with loss of kidney function, and may be involved in the pathophysiological pathways that are associated with the poor clinical outcomes seen in patients with kidney failure (see Table 21.1 for examples). The European Uremic Toxin (EUTox) working group has produced detailed reviews of uremic toxins [2, 11–13].

21.4 The High Cut Off 1100 Dialysis Membrane

The HCO 1100 dialysis membrane is the only dialysis membrane that fulfils the criteria of classification for HCO dialysis. The membrane is produced by Baxter–Gambro and the name is derived from a membrane water permeability of 1100 ml/(m²/h/mmHg) for 0.9 % sodium chloride at body temperature and with a blood flow (QB) of 100–500 ml/min. The pore size radius for the HCO 1100 membrane is 8–12 nm; this compares to a typical dialyzer pore size radius of 2–3 nm for a LF membrane, 3.5–5.5 nm for a HF membrane, and 5–6 nm for a PP membrane [7]. The first HCO dialyzer used in man (HCO 1100 dialyzer) had a small (1.1 m^2) surface area. Subsequently, a large surface area (2.1 m^2) dialyzer (Theralite™) has been produced and is being used in clinical practice. The MWCO for the HCO 1100 membrane when used in vivo is around 50 kDa; however, the distribution of pores beyond this MWCO means that there is a loss of albumin that has been quantified as up to 20 g for a single HCO 1100 dialyzer used for 4 h [14].

The use of HCO-HD has been evaluated to date in the following clinical settings:

1. The treatment of patients with AKI associated with sepsis syndrome. In this setting, the dialyzer was effective at removing pro-inflammatory cytokines and improving cellular immune responses. However, these observations have not translated into clinical studies that have shown that HCO-HD improves clinical outcomes.
2. The removal of disease-specific nephrotoxins:
   i. The dialyzer was repurposed for assessment of the removal of immunoglobulin light chains (LC) in patients with MM and severe AKI. The large majority of clinical treatments with the dialyzer to date have been made for this indication; two randomized controlled trials of the utility of HCO-HD are in process and should be reporting soon.
   ii. Myoglobin removal in AKI secondary to rhabdomyolysis.
   iii. In short-term studies in patients with ESKD receiving chronic HD; these studies have focused on inflammation.

21.5 The Use of HCO-HD in Patients with Sepsis Syndrome

Pro-inflammatory cytokines, including tumor necrosis factor-alpha (TNF-α) and interleukin-6 (IL)-6, have an important role in the poor clinical outcomes sustained by patients with sepsis syndrome [15]. These cytokines are both a consequence of the underlying illness and are associated with aberrant immune responses triggered by the illness. Furthermore, the kidneys differentially clear many of the pro-inflammatory cytokines that are produced in sepsis syndrome; therefore, the development of AKI can lead to the accumulation of these molecules.

HDF can remove some cytokines that are involved in systemic sepsis; however, many of the molecules that are associated with sepsis syndrome are of a MW not effectively removed by conventional HDF. For example, Heering et al. were not able to show a decrease in levels of TNF-α over 24 h of hemofiltration delivered through a conventional HF dialysis membrane [16]. Shortly after this study, the utility of enhanced targeting of larger MW cytokines by dialysis was demonstrated by Kline et al.; they used a canine model of sepsis syndrome and showed that large pore compared to standard HD was associated with better left ventricular contractility and other indices of better cardiac function [17].

The limitation of conventional HD and HF for the removal of inflammatory mediators in sepsis syndrome provided impetus for the development of the HCO 1100 dialysis membrane. Preclinical and clinical studies were performed to quantify the utility of the dialyzer in sepsis syndrome and AKI. Studies on blood, from normal humans (300 ml/volun-

Table 21.3 Studies in patients with sepsis syndrome and acute kidney injury (AKI) with the HCO 1100 dialyzer

Type	Ref. No. (yr)	Patient No.	Design	Primary outcome	Result
Phase I/II	[20] (2003)	28	Randomization to either HCO-hemofiltration or HF-hemofiltration, then alternating treatments	PMN phagocytic activity	Decrease in phagocytosis during HCO treatment compared to HF treatment. Filtrate from HCO treatments induced phagocytosis, filtrate from HF did not
Phase I/II	[22] (2004)	24	Random allocation to continuous CVVH or CVVHD	Cytokine levels IL-1, IL-1rα, IL-1β, IL-6, TNF-α	High clearances of cytokines up to but not including TNFα for both modalities. Increased clearance of IL-1rα with CVVHD. A significant decline for some cytokines from baseline levels. More albumin loss with CVVHD
Phase I/II	[23] (2006)	30	Randomized 2:1 intervention/control	Norephenipherine dose	Decrease in adjusted norephenephrine dose by HCO-HD compared to HF-HD
Phase I	[24] (2007)	10	Double-blind crossover	Change in IL-6 at 4 h	Reduction in IL-6 levels by HCO-HD by 30.3 versus 1.1 % for HF-HD

HCO high cut off; *PMN* polymorphonuclear; *Ref* reference; *no* number, *HF* high-flux, *IL-1* Interleukin-1, *IL-1rα* interleukin-1 alpha, *IL-1β* interleukin-1 beta, *IL-6* interleukin-6, *TNF-α* tumor necrosis factor-alpha, *IL-6* interleukin-6, *CVVHD* continuous venovenous hemodialfiltration, *HD* hemodialysis

teer), treated with lipopolysaccharide and using an extracorporeal system incorporating the HCO 1100 dialyzer, showed that pro-inflammatory cytokines could be removed. Clinically relevant SCs were demonstrated for five cytokines (IL-1β, IL-6, IL-10, IL-8, and TNF-α) with MWs ranging from 11.1 to 51 kDa [18]. The SC for albumin in this study was 0.1.

A subsequent ex vivo study, using a membrane prototype with higher clearances than the HCO 1100 and quantifying the clearance of creatinine kinase (MW 80 kDa) and IgG (MW 160 kDa), assessed the albumin loss in HDF as well as HD. Using this membrane in HDF mode led to three times the albumin loss sustained in HD mode [19].

21.6 Clinical Studies in Sepsis

Morgera et al. studied the impact of the dialysis modality on peripheral blood mononuclear (PBMN) cell phagocytosis [20]. Twenty-eight patients with sepsis syndrome and AKI were randomized to receive 12-h cycles of hemofiltration using HCO 1100 or a conventional HF dialyzer. They showed that the high phagocytosis rates present in these patients were decreased significantly by the use of an HCO dialysis membrane; the conventional HF dialyzer had no effect on phagocytosis rates. They explored a mechanistic basis for this finding and showed that ultrafiltrate from HCO dialysis produced significant induction of phagocytosis; there was no equivalent effect when using ultrafiltrate from patients treated with conventional hemofiltration. As phagocytosis in the acute phase of sepsis syndrome may be aberrant (excess) [21], these data provided evidence that HCO treatment may contribute to the restoration of an appropriate physiological response in patients with sepsis syndrome.

Morgera et al. then proceeded to study the impact of the HCO 1100 dialyzer on cytokine levels in vivo. In comparison to CVVH and continuous venovenous hemodialfiltration (CVVHDF) with conventional HF dialyzers, they showed very high clearances of IL-6 and IL-1rα. Using HCO 1100 in an HDF mode led to more cytokine clearance; however, there were higher albumin losses in vivo with HCO-HD, consistent with the observations in the ex vivo model [22].

To assess the impact of HCO-HD on a clinical parameter, Morgera et al. performed a pilot randomised control trial (RCT) enrolling 30 patients with sepsis and severe AKI and patients and randomizing in a 2:1 ratio to HCO-HD or HF hemofiltration for 48 h [23]. They compared the effect of the treatment on norepinephrine dose and found a significantly decreased requirement for norepinephrine in the HCO-HD group. They also found that HCO-HD was associated with decreased levels of circulating cytokines compared to conventional hemofiltration.

In a subsequent trial of ten patients with sepsis syndrome and severe AKI, Haase et al. showed a decrease in a range of cytokines (IL-6, IL-8, IL-10, and IL-18) after a single intermittent 4-h dialysis treatment carried out with a single HCO 1100 dialyzer compared with standard HF-HD [24]. This study reported albumin loss of 7.7 g with HCO-HD compared to 1 g with standard HF-HD.

The studies are summarized in Table 21.3

21.7 The Current Status of HCO-HD in Sepsis Syndrome

The four studies that are outlined earlier and summarized in the table were the focus of a narrative review by Haase et al. published in 2007 [25]. The review was based on a formal search strategy of the then available published literature (phase 1b/2a studies). Haase et al. outlined significant limitations in all these studies which included: (i) they were all single center; (ii) the studies were not well controlled; (iii) they had significant inter-study variability in design.

The authors recommended proceeding to larger, multicenter, randomized controlled trials. However, further clinical trials with HCO dialysis in the setting of sepsis syndrome and AKI are unlikely. While the biological evidence for HCO-HD is supportive, properly designed multicenter phase 2 and phase 3 studies are expensive and most interventions of this type do not translate into studies that are fully evaluated for efficacy in routine clinical practice.

21.8 Multiple Myeloma and the Rationale for Extracorporeal Light Chain Removal

The major focus for developing an evidence base for a routine clinical use for HCO-HD is in the management of patients with myeloma kidney (cast nephropathy) and severe AKI. Almost 50 % of patients with MM have an estimated glomerular filtration rate (eGFR) of < 60 ml/min/1.73 m^2 and up to 10 % of all patients have severe AKI requiring dialysis treatment [26]. Around 90 % of the AKI associated with MM is caused by direct toxicity of excess clonal immunoglobulin LC that is produced as a consequence of the underlying tumor [27, 28]. This excess clonal LC causes the classical renal lesion of cast nephropathy (myeloma kidney).

Overall outcomes for patients with MM are improving, with a median survival now in excess of 4 years [29, 30]. Patients with severe AKI requiring dialysis treatment have very poor outcomes, however, with a median survival of less than 1 year [31, 32]. These poor outcomes are associated with failure to recover independent kidney function in the large majority of cases reported to date; patients who do recover independent kidney function have better long-term outcomes [33].

The poor outcomes sustained by patients with severe AKI and MM and a direct pathogenic link with a circulating nephrotoxic protein (Ig LC) provide a rational for assessing the efficacy of extracorporeal removal of LC. Until 2005, the focus was on clinical trials of the utility of plasma exchange (PEX) for LC removal. Early studies indicated a possible benefit associated with PEX, although these studies were small and poorly designed [34, 35]. Subsequently, the largest randomized controlled trial showed no benefit of treatment by PEX compared to standard care [36]. In this study, 104 patients with MM and severe AKI were randomized to receive 5–7 PEX treatments or no PEX. There was no difference in outcome for patients between the two groups for all clinical outcomes including independence of dialysis or kidney function at 6 months.

Subsequent open-label studies utilizing PEX have shown a higher proportion of patients recovering independent kidney function than has been historically reported; the likelihood of renal recovery is dependent on a rapid decrease in serum LC levels in the first 3 weeks after commencement of therapy [37, 38]. These results should be approached with caution, as they reported outcomes from patients who also received novel chemotherapy agents, in particular the proteasome inhibitor bortezomib, in combination with dexamethasone [39]. These regimes are associated with faster and deeper anti-tumor responses in patients with MM than traditional chemotherapy regimes [40].

From 2007, there has been an increasing body of evidence supporting the use of HCO-HD as a more effective modality than PEX for extracorporeal removal of LC. The utility of the therapy is based on two principles. First, the two isotypes of immunoglobulin LCs are of a MW that can be removed effectively by HCO-HD: κLC is a monomeric molecule with a MW of 22.5 kDa; λLC, a dimeric molecule with a MW of 45 kDa. Second, PEX is a short treatment, and while it will effectively remove intravascular LC, as proteins of the MW of LC are redistributed in all extracellular compartments, and around 85 % of the proteins are in the extravascular compartment [41], a short treatment (PEX) will have a limited impact on overall intravascular LC levels.

Figure 21.5 shows the relationship between the production and distribution of LC, and the main routes of removal. With normal kidney function, the half-life of κLC is around 2-h and λLC is 4 h. With severe AKI and anuria, the main route of clearance is through the reticuloendothelial system (mononuclear phagocyte system); this is a far slower clearance route, the half-life of both isotypes of LC in this setting is around 4 days.

There is disequilibrium between extravascular and intravascular clearance [42], and on discontinuation of extracorporeal therapy there is redistribution of extravascular LC into the intravascular compartment [43]. This can be addressed, in part, by extended HCO-HD. The efficacy of HCO-HD for LC removal in MM and AKI has been modeled theoretically for treatment times of up to 72 h [44]; HCO-HD treatment sessions are being used in clinical practice for times of up to 8 h [14].

A direct comparison of the efficacy of HCO-HD to PEX requires an understanding of the effect of the chemotherapy regime on the impact of the extracorporeal therapy. For example, with no renal clearance and chemotherapy delivering a tumor kill rate of 2 % a day, 8 h of daily HCO-HD treatment with two HCO 1100 dialyzers in series will decrease the starting LC load by 83 %; daily PEX remove around 9 % over the same period of time [44].

21.9 The Clearance of Immunoglobulin Light Chains by HCO-HD

Using two HCO 1100 dialyzers in series produce clearances of both isotypes of LC of around 40 ml/min. Serum λLC levels decrease more than κLC levels for an equivalent dialysis

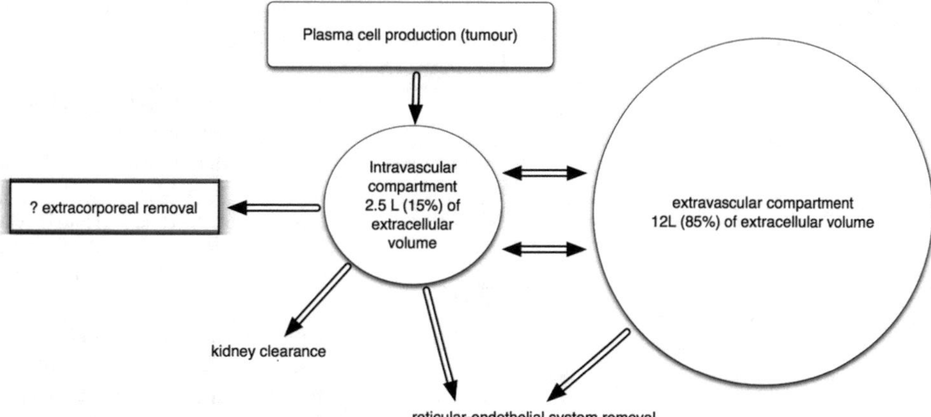

Fig. 21.5 The basis for targeting the intravascular compartment with extended extracorporeal removal. Eighty-five percent of extracellular fluid is extravascular and light chains (*LC*) redistribute into all extracellular fluid. The contribution of extracorporeal removal to *LC* depletion is dependent on at least three other variables: (i) tumor load and the impact of chemotherapy; (ii) kidney clearance; and (iii) reticuloendothelial system clearance

dose; this reflects higher resistance to the inter-compartmental transfer of λLC leading to a higher measurable decrease in serum λLC compared to serum κLC at a given extracorporeal clearance rate [14]. There is reduced clearance of each isotype with time; this stabilizes at 3 h for κFLCs but continues throughout the dialysis session for λLC, probably as a consequence of protein blunting [45]. Protein blunting refers to the phenomenon of larger MW molecules, close to the MW cut off of the dialyzer membrane, accumulating at the membrane surface; these increased local levels then lead to increased clearance. Replacing the dialyzer(s) results in a significant increase in the sustained clearance rates of λFLC but not κFLC, [14] further emphasizing the enhanced effect of protein blunting on molecules approaching the MW cut off of the membrane.

After an initial proof of principle study, [44] that included detailed modeling of LC clearance, subsequent open label studies reported excellent outcomes for patients receiving HCO-HD, with recovery rates from dialysis-dependent AKI higher than those previously reported [33, 46–54]. These studies are summarized in Table 21.4.

However, these data from these open label studies are confounded by at least two factors:

i. Centers that use HCO-HD may be more focused on the management of cast nephropathy; the length of time to starting HCO-HD and the experience of the center in dealing with the emergency are important outcome confounders [50].
ii. Current chemotherapy regimes are associated with a very high tumor response rate compared to historic chemotherapy regimes.

An additional consideration is that some patients have polymers of LC that are above an MW that can be removed by the HCO dialyzer [55]; the MW of the polymers will also be above that of a size that is freely filtered by the glomerulus and will not contribute to the development of cast nephropathy.

21.10 Current Considerations for the Use of HCO-HD in Patients with MM

The published literature till date mainly reports on the efficacy of the 1.1 m^2 HCO 1100 dialyzer. There are large differences between the studies in the delivered dialysis dose that patients received; the studies variably reported the use of one dialyzer or two dialyzers in series and the length of time of any single dialysis session varied from 4–8 h.

The data from uncontrolled studies do not report an increased rate of complications over the number anticipated for standard dialysis treatments. In particular, there have been no reports of increased infective or thrombotic complications; although there has been no direct comparative data with standard dialysis regimes to date, so caution should be applied until the randomized controlled trials report.

In 2011, Baxter–Gambro introduced a 2.1 m^2 dialyzer called Theralite™ into clinical practice. This dialyzer clears around 80 % of the LC cleared by two HCO 1100 dialyzers in series. The difference in clearances is mainly due to internal filtration in the second dialyzer, providing an increased convective dose with this prescription. Experiments performed with a single 1.1 m^2 HCO dialyzer showed that using a formal convective component (HCO-HDF) will lead to a loss of albumin of 50 % more than that seen with HCO-HD [14].

Table 21.4 Published studies of high cut off hemodialysis in patients with multiple myeloma and severe acute kidney injury (four patients or more)

First author	Ref no	Year published	Number treated	% recovery renal function (no)	Comments
Hutchison	44	2007	5	60 (3)	Includes detailed modeling of light chain removal by HCO-HD and plasma exchange prescription
Kleeberg	46	2009	4	Not reported	Patients with κLC myeloma only. Narrative report on kinetics of removal
Hutchison	33	2009	19	68 (13)	Includes five patients previously reported. Recovery of kidney function associated with better long-term outcomes. Largest single-center report (with Heyne 2011)
Peters	47	2011	5	60 (3)	
Heyne	48	2011	19	74 (14)	Largest single-center report (with Hutchison 2009)
Martin Reyes	49	2011	6	50 (3)	Uses Theralite as the standard of care
Hutchison	50	2011	67	63 (42)	Includes patients from Hutchison (2009) and Heyne (2011). Renal recovery was independently associated with the time to commencement of treatment
Sinisalo	51	2012	7	86 (6)	Theralite and bortezomib chemotherapy
Borrego-Hinojossa	52	2013	5	80 (4)	
Khalafallah	53	2013	4	75 (3)	Bortezomib, thalidomide, and dexamethasone chemotherapy
Tan	54	2014	6	50 (3)	

Ref reference, *no* number, *HCO-HD* high cut off hemodialysis, *κLC* kappa light chain

21.11 Chemotherapy Clearance

If HCO-HD is being used, then the timing of the chemotherapy prescription should be considered. A recent in vitro study assessed the clearance of chemotherapy drugs used in clinical practice for myeloma by HCO-HD [56]. Drug levels were assayed up to 12 min after injection, and up to this point of time there was significant clearance of chemotherapy by HCO-HD.

If HCO-HD remains a long-term option for the treatment of patients with MM and AKI, then this area will require further study to ensure that disease responses are not being compromised by drug clearance across the membrane. Caution should be exercised in transposing the results of this in vitro study to clinical practice, where drugs in use in routine clinical care are usually given orally or (in the case of bortezomib) by subcutaneous injection.

21.12 Randomized Controlled Trials of HCO-HD in Patients with MM

Two randomized controlled trials are now in process. The first study "European Trial of Free Light Chain Removal by Extended Haemodialysis in Cast Nephropathy" (EuLITE) has finished recruitment and results should be reported shortly [57]. The second study "Multiple Myeloma and Renal Failure Due to Myeloma Cast Nephropathy" (MYRE) is in progress and the protocol for the study can be reviewed at http://clinicaltrials.gov/ct2/show/NCT01208818. EuLITE and MYRE are using bortezomib- and dexamethasone-based regimens; EuLITE used two HCO 1100 dialyzers in series and MYRE is using Theralite™. An important part of both studies is to report on the safety and efficacy of bortezomib-based chemotherapy in dialysis-dependent AKI. The HCO-HD dialysis intervention for both these studies is intensive; for example, EuLITE involved dialysis treatment or chemotherapy daily for the first 12 days and then alternate-day dialysis through to 3 weeks if the patient remained dialysis dependent. Each dialysis session for patients in the HCO-HD treatment arm lasted 8 h.

21.13 Myoglobin Clearance by HCO-HD

Rhabdomyolysis is an important cause of AKI, due to cast nephropathy associated with myoglobinuria. The first published use of the HCO 1100 dialyzer for this indication was reported in a patient with multifactorial rhabdomyolysis [58]. The patient was initially treated with conventional CVVH and then converted to HCO dialysis treatment. The myoglobin level in the ultrafiltrate of the HCO dialysis was over five times that seen with a standard high-flux dialyzer, with a calculated SC for myoglobin by HCO-HD of around 0.7.

These data have been confirmed by subsequent case reports. The largest series published to date [59] showed that using the dialyzer in both conventional and sustained low-efficiency daily dialysis protocols provided clearances of myoglobin up to twentyfold those seen in patients treated with conventional HF-HD. Subsequent modeling studies have confirmed the potential for increased clearance of myoglobin by HCO-HD [60].

It is highly unlikely that an adequately powered randomized controlled trial will be performed to assess the utility HCO-HD for this indication. However, the good single-center results that are reported indicate that HCO-HD may be an option in clinical practice.

21.14 The Theoretical Basis for Uremic Toxin Removal by HCO-HD in a Chronic Dialysis Prescription

Low and middle MW molecules may contribute to the poor clinical outcomes seen in patients with ESKD [2] by effecting both immune function and vascular biology. Chronic inflammation may be an important component of the adverse morbidity and mortality seen and is linked to the accelerated development of vascular disease [61, 62]. Using a dialyzer with increased capability for removal of those uremic toxins which are thought to contribute to the inflammation and vascular injury in ESKD might improve clinical outcomes.

When dialyzers with different sieving coefficients are compared, the dialyzer with the higher clearance can lead to measurable decreases in inflammatory molecules. For example:

i. Changing the dialysis prescription in ESRF from LF-HD to HF-HD led to decreased concentrations of some molecules associated with poor outcomes in people with kidney disease [63].
ii. When super-flux dialysis was used over a 6-month-treatment period, advanced glycation end-product (AGE) peptides, pentosidine levels and protein bound pentosidine were lower in patient with and without diabetes compared to HF-HD [64].

Using HF-HD as a standard of care provides an MWCO of >0.1 for molecules of 15–20 kDa [65]. This can be extended to 20–25 kDa by use of an HF dialyzer in HDF mode [65, 66]. However, many of the middle MW molecules that accumulate as a consequence of renal failure are too big for significant removal by HF-HDF or protein permeable dialysis (PPD) (see Table 21.1) [2].

HCO-HD will directly remove molecules up to and including the MW of albumin. Increasing the removal of free uremic solutes may also lead to enhanced removal of protein-bound molecules, variably carried by albumin and other larger serum proteins. As the free (unbound) molecule is removed, there is solute shift from the bound to unbound state as a lower concentration of the unbound molecule leads to increased dissociation of the bound molecule. For homocysteine, which has a low MW and is cleared by all dialysis modalities but is heavily bound to plasma protein, the use of PPD, compared to HF-HD in a chronic dialysis prescription, led to a decrease in serum homocysteine levels of one third from baseline after 12 weeks [10].

More recent studies have reinforced the differential effect of the dialysis modality on the clearance of protein-bound uremic toxins, for example, pre-dilution HDF has an effect on the levels of bound p-cresol but not bound homocysteine when compared to HF-HD [66]. While some of the clearance of bound molecules is due to dissociation of bound from unbound molecules, a significant component of the loss is due to the direct leakage of albumin across the dialysis membrane. This is an important consideration. Understanding the levels of albumin loss that are both clinically acceptable and without adverse effects is an important challenge for dialysis researchers. A major limitation of HCO-HD is a high albumin leak; this has restricted the use of the dialyzer in patients with ESKD to short exploratory studies.

21.15 What Is the Impact of Albumin Leak on the Pathophysiology of ESRF?

The clinical impact of albumin loss across a dialysis membrane is unknown [45]. Although a low serum albumin level is associated with worse survival in patients with ESKD [67], this may only represent a surrogate biomarker as albumin is a negative acute phase reactant; hypo-albuminaemia in ESKD is predominantly secondary to decreased production of albumin as a consequence of malnutrition and inflammation, which is common in patients with ESKD [68, 69]. Furthermore, patients with ESKD have increased levels of modified (e.g., oxidized) albumin; modified albumin fractions may be associated with adverse clinical outcomes. Consequently, it is possible that some albumin loss associated with dialysis may be desirable, as a fraction of removed albumin will be modified and will be replaced by fresh albumin synthesis. However, the loss of albumin associated with HCO may be too high for use in long-term dialysis, particularly in patients who have suppressed baseline liver synthesis of albumin and therefore will not produce an appropriate response to hypo-albuminaemia sustained as a consequence of HCO-HD.

21.16 HCO-HD in a Chronic Dialysis Prescription

While the albumin-loss associated with HCO-HD may be too high for use in a long-term chronic dialysis prescription, there have been short-term treatment studies that have assessed the impact of HCO-HD. In single center open label studies of up to 6 weeks with all dialysis delivered by HCO dialysis or 12 weeks with alternate HCO dialysis,

Table 21.5 Published studies in HCO-HD in patients with end-stage kidney disease

Type	Ref no	Patient no	Design	Primary outcome	Result
Phase I	[70] (2009)	8	Randomized double blind cross-over	β2 M	Significantly lower β2 M post-dialysis concentrations and clearance by HCO-HD vs. HF-HD
Phase I/II	[71] (2012)	19	Randomized double blind cross-over	Co-primary: feasibility and inflammation	Tolerable over 2 weeks of study period; possible increase in adverse (but not serious adverse) events. Decrease in inflammatory markers but no decrease in inflammatory monocyte subsets

HCO-HD high cut off hemodialysis, *Ref* reference, *no* number, *β2 M* beta-2 microglobulin, *HF-HD* high-flux hemodialysis

no apparent increased incidence of major adverse events were noted. However, only two studies have been reported in peer-reviewed journals to date; these are summarized in Table 21.5 [70, 71].

In the best designed study to date [71], there appeared to be more adverse events below the level of major/serious adverse events in the HCO group; these comprised dizziness or low blood pressure. While the authors did not identify an association with dialysis treatment, the large amount of albumin lost on dialysis and associated changes in intravascular volume status could provide an explanation for this finding.

Fiedler et al. used a randomized double blind cross-over study to examine the impact of 2 weeks of treatment with HCO-HD in 19 chronic hemodialysis patients with evidence of chronic inflammation as a consequence of elevation of the levels of C-reactive protein (CRP) [71]. They found that HCO-HD cleared large quantities of pro-inflammatory cytokines. However, over this period there was no decrease in the pre-dialysis cytokine levels. They also measured the numbers of circulating activated monocytes (defined by the presence of CD14 and CD16 on the cell surface) and found modest reductions in the numbers of these cells indicating an immune-modulatory effect in these studies.

The study of Fiedler et al. reinforced the impact of HCO-HD on albumin levels. They showed a 50-fold increase in albumin loss across the HCO membrane compared to an HF dialysis membrane; a 5-h HCO-HD treatment led to the loss of approximately 9 g of albumin in total. There was no clinical indication for supplementing albumin during the course of this study. These losses are consistent with the findings of studies of HCO-HD for FLC removal in multiple myeloma, where in some prescriptions 40 g of albumin are required as supplementation for extended (8 h) dialysis sessions using two HCO 1100 dialyzers in series [57].

21.17 Conclusions

High cut off HD is one of the major advances in dialysis technology over the past two decades. Clinical studies in patients have shown biological effects in sepsis syndrome, multiple myeloma and AKI, and ESKD. However, there is no level 1 evidence to date for any indication; pilot studies carried out in AKI and MM show that the use of the dialyzer is associated with rates of renal recovery at least twice that being reported by historic studies. The major limitation associated with HCO-HD is albumin loss; this is related to the pore distribution of the membrane. Next-generation dialyzers should deliver dialysis targeting the same molecules as HCO-HD but with decreased albumin loss; this will provide greater utility, particularly in the setting of ESKD and chronic dialysis prescriptions.

References

1. Davenport A. Membrane designs and composition for hemodialysis, hemofiltration and hemodialfiltration: past, present and future. Minerva Urol Nefrol. 2010;62(1):29–40.
2. Vanholder R, De Smet R, Glorieux G, Argilés A, Baurmeister U, Brunet P, et al. Review on uremic toxins: classification, concentration, and interindividual variability. Kidney Int. 2003;63(5):1934–43.
3. Leypoldt JK, Cheung AK. Characterization of molecular transport in artificial kidneys. Artif Organs. 1996;20(5):381–9.
4. Hwang K-J, Sz P-Y. Effect of membrane pore size on the performance of cross-flow microfiltration of BSA/dextran mixtures. J Membr Sci. 2011;378(1):272–9.
5. Bakhshayeshi M, Zhou H, Olsen C, Yuan W, Zydney AL. Understanding dextran retention data for hollow fiber ultrafiltration membranes. J Membr Sci. 2011;385:243–50.
6. Leypoldt JK, Frigon RP, Henderson LW. Dextran sieving coefficients of hemofiltration membranes. Trans Am Soc Artif Intern Organs. 1983;29:678–83.
7. Boschetti-de-Fierro A, Voigt M, Storr M, Krause B. Extended characterization of a new class of membranes for blood purification: the high cut-off membranes. Int J Artif Organs. 2013;36(7):455–63.
8. Ronco C, Brendolan A, Feriani M, Milan M, Conz P, Lupi A, et al. A new scintigraphic method to characterize ultrafiltration in hollow fiber dialyzers. Kidney Int. 1992;41(5):1383–93.
9. Samtleben W, Dengler C, Reinhardt B, Nothdurft A, Lemke HD. Comparison of the new polyethersulfone high-flux membrane DIAPES HF800 with conventional high-flux membranes during on-line haemodiafiltration. Nephrol Dial Transplant. 2003;18(11):2382–6.
10. Galli F, Benedetti S, Buoncristiani U, Piroddi M, Conte C, Canestrari F, et al. The effect of pmma-based protein-leaking dialyzers on plasma homocysteine levels. Kidney Int. 2003;64(2):748–55.
11. Vanholder R, Meert N, Schepers E, Glorieux G, Argiles A, Brunet P, et al. Review on uraemic solutes ii—variability in reported concentrations: causes and consequences. Nephrol Dial Transplant. 2007;22(11):3115–21.

12. Cohen G, Glorieux G, Thornalley P, Schepers E, Meert N, Jankowski J, et al. Review on uraemic toxins III: recommendations for handling uraemic retention solutes in vitro—towards a standardized approach for research on uraemia. Nephrol Dial Transplant. 2007;22(12):3381–90.
13. Vanholder R, Abou-Deif O, Argiles A, Baurmeister U, Beige J, Brouckaert P, et al. The role of eutox in uremic toxin research. Semin Dial. 2009;22(4):323–8.
14. Hutchison CA, Harding S, Mead G, Goehl H, Storr M, Bradwell A, Cockwell P. Serum free-light chain removal by high cutoff hemodialysis: optimizing removal and supportive care. Artif Organs. 2008;32(12):910–7.
15. Pinsky MR, Vincent JL, Deviere J, Alegre M, Kahn RJ, Dupont E. Serum cytokine levels in human septic shock. Relation to multiple-system organ failure and mortality. Chest. 1993;103(2):565–75.
16. Heering P, Morgera S, Schmitz FJ, Schmitz G, Willers R, Schultheiss HP, et al. Cytokine removal and cardiovascular hemodynamics in septic patients with continuous venovenous hemofiltration. Intensive Care Med. 1997;23(3):288–96.
17. Kline JA, Gordon BE, Williams C, Blumenthal S, Watts JA, Diaz-Buxo J. Large-pore hemodialysis in acute endotoxin shock. Crit Care Med. 1999;27(3):588–96.
18. Uchino S, Bellomo R, Goldsmith D, Davenport P, Cole L, Baldwin I, et al. Super high flux hemofiltration: a new technique for cytokine removal. Intensive Care Med. 2002;28(5):651–5.
19. Morgera S, Klonower D, Rocktäschel J, Haase M, Priem F, Ziemer S, et al. TNF-alpha elimination with high cut-off haemofilters: a feasible clinical modality for septic patients? Nephrol Dial Transplant. 2003;18(7):1361–9.
20. Morgera S, Haase M, Rocktäschel J, Böhler T, von Heymann C, Vargas-Hein O, et al. High permeability haemofiltration improves peripheral blood mononuclear cell proliferation in septic patients with acute renal failure. Nephrol Dial Transplant. 2003;18(12):2570–6.
21. Bosmann M, Ward PA. The inflammatory response in sepsis. Trends Immunol. 2013;34(3):129–36.
22. Morgera S, Slowinski T, Melzer C, Sobottke V, Vargas-Hein O, Volk T, et al. Renal replacement therapy with high-cutoff hemofilters: impact of convection and diffusion on cytokine clearances and protein status. Am J Kidney Dis. 2004;43(3):444–53.
23. Morgera S, Haase M, Kuss T, Vargas-Hein O, Zuckermann-Becker H, Melzer C, et al. Pilot study on the effects of high cutoff hemofiltration on the need for norepinephrine in septic patients with acute renal failure. Crit Care Med. 2006;34(8):2099–104.
24. Haase M, Bellomo R, Baldwin I, Haase-Fielitz A, Fealy N, Davenport P, et al. Hemodialysis membrane with a high-molecular-weight cutoff and cytokine levels in sepsis complicated by acute renal failure: a phase 1 randomized trial. Am J Kidney Dis. 2007;50(2):296–304.
25. Haase M, Bellomo R, Morgera S, Baldwin I, Boyce N. High cut-off point membranes in septic acute renal failure: a systematic review. Int J Artif Organs. 2007;30(12):1031–41.
26. Dimopoulos MA, Delimpasi S, Katodritou E, Vassou A, Kyrtsonis MC, Repousis P, et al. Significant improvement in the survival of patients with multiple myeloma presenting with severe renal impairment after the introduction of novel agents. Ann Oncol. 2014;25(1):195–200.
27. Stringer S, Basnayake K, Hutchison C, Cockwell P. Recent advances in the pathogenesis and management of cast nephropathy (myeloma kidney). Bone Marrow Res 2011, 493697.
28. Basnayake K, Stringer SJ, Hutchison CA, Cockwell P. The biology of immunoglobulin free light chains and kidney injury. Kidney Int. 2011;79(12):1289–301.
29. Kumar SK, Rajkumar SV, Dispenzieri A, Lacy MQ, Hayman SR, Buadi FK, et al. Improved survival in multiple myeloma and the impact of novel therapies. Blood. 2008;111(5):2516–20.
30. Ludwig H, Beksac M, Blade J, Boccadoro M, Cavenagh J, Cavo M, et al. Current multiple myeloma treatment strategies with novel agents: a european perspective. Oncologist. 2010;15(1):6–25.
31. Haynes RJ, Read S, Collins GP, Darby SC, Winearls CG. Presentation and survival of patients with severe acute kidney injury and multiple myeloma: a 20-year experience from a single centre. Nephrol Dial Transplant. 2010;25(2):419–26.
32. Tsakiris DJ, Stel VS, Finne P, Fraser E, Heaf J, de Meester J, et al. Incidence and outcome of patients starting renal replacement therapy for end-stage renal disease due to multiple myeloma or light-chain deposit disease: an ERA-EDTA registry study. Nephrol Dial Transplant. 2010;25(4):1200–6.
33. Hutchison CA, Bradwell AR, Cook M, Basnayake K, Basu S, Harding S, et al. Treatment of acute renal failure secondary to multiple myeloma with chemotherapy and extended high cut-off hemodialysis. Clin J Am Soc Nephrol. 2009;4(4):745–54.
34. Zucchelli P, Pasquali S, Cagnoli L, Ferrari G. Controlled plasma exchange trial in acute renal failure due to multiple myeloma. Kidney Int. 1988;33(6):1175–80.
35. Johnson WJ, Kyle RA, Pineda AA, O'Brien PC, Holley KE. Treatment of renal failure associated with multiple myeloma. Plasmapheresis, hemodialysis, and chemotherapy. Arch Intern Med. 1990;150(4):863–9.
36. Clark WF, Stewart AK, Rock GA, Sternbach M, Sutton DM, Barrett BJ, et al. Plasma exchange when myeloma presents as acute renal failure: a randomized, controlled trial. Ann Intern Med. 2005;143(11):777–84.
37. Leung N, Gertz MA, Zeldenrust SR, Rajkumar SV, Dispenzieri A, Fervenza FC, et al. Improvement of cast nephropathy with plasma exchange depends on the diagnosis and on reduction of serum free light chains. Kidney Int. 2008;73(11):1282–8.
38. Burnette BL, Leung N, Rajkumar SV. Renal improvement in myeloma with bortezomib plus plasma exchange. N Engl J Med. 2011;364(24):2365–6.
39. Kastritis E, Terpos E, Dimopoulos MA. Current treatments for renal failure due to multiple myeloma. Expert Opin Pharmacother. 2013;14(11):1477–95.
40. Popat R, Joel S, Oakervee H, Cavenagh J. Bortezomib for multiple myeloma. Expert Opin Pharmacother. 2006;7(10):1337–46.
41. Takagi K, Kin K, Itoh Y, Enomoto H, Kawai T. Human alpha 1-microglobulin levels in various body fluids. J Clin Pathol. 1980;33(8):786–91.
42. Ward RA, Greene T, Hartmann B, Samtleben W. Resistance to intercompartmental mass transfer limits beta2-microglobulin removal by post-dilution hemodiafiltration. Kidney Int. 2006;69(8):1431–7.
43. Cserti C, Haspel R, Stowell C, Dzik W. Light-chain removal by plasmapheresis in myeloma-associated renal failure. Transfusion. 2007;47(3):511–4.
44. Hutchison CA, Cockwell P, Reid S, Chandler K, Mead GP, Harrison J, et al. Efficient removal of immunoglobulin free light chains by hemodialysis for multiple myeloma: in vitro and in vivo studies. J Am Soc Nephrol. 2007;18(3):886–95.
45. Ward RA. Protein-leaking membranes for hemodialysis: a new class of membranes in search of an application? J Am Soc Nephrol. 2005;16(8):2421–30.
46. Kleeberg L, Morgera S, Jakob C, Hocher B, Schneider M, Peters H, et al. Novel renal replacement strategies for the elimination of serum free light chains in patients with kappa light chain nephropathy. Eur J Med Res. 2009;14:47–54.
47. Peters NO, Laurain E, Cridlig J, Hulin C, Cao-Huu T, Frimat L. Impact of free light chain hemodialysis in myeloma cast nephropathy: a case-control study. Hemodial Int. 2011;15(4):538–45.
48. Heyne N, Denecke B, Guthoff M, Oehrlein K, Kanz L, Haring HU, Weisel KC. Extracorporeal light chain elimination: high cut-off (HCO) hemodialysis parallel to chemotherapy allows for a high proportion of renal recovery in multiple myeloma pa-

tients with dialysis-dependent acute kidney injury. Ann Hematol 2011;91:729–35.
49. Martin-Reyes G, Toledo-Rojas R, Torres-de Rueda A, Sola-Moyano E, Blanca-Martos L, Fuentes-Sanchez L, et al. Haemodialysis using high cut-off dialysers for treating acute renal failure in multiple myeloma. Nefrologia. 2012;32(1):35–43.
50. Hutchison CA, Heyne N, Airia P, Schindler R, Zickler D, Cook M, et al. Immunoglobulin free light chain levels and recovery from myeloma kidney on treatment with chemotherapy and high cut-off haemodialysis. Nephrol Dial Transplant. 2012;27(10):3823–8.
51. Sinisalo M, Silvennoinen R, Wirta O. High cut-off hemodialysis and bortezomib-based therapy to rescue kidneys in myeloma-dependent cast nephropathy. Am J Hematology. 2012;87(6):640.
52. Borrego-Hinojosa J, Perez-Del Barrio MP, Biechy-Baldan MD, Merino-Garcia E, Sanchez-Perales MC, Garcia-Cortes MJ, et al. Treatment by long haemodialysis sessions with high cut-off filters in myeloma cast nephropathy: our experience. Nefrologia. 2013;33(4):515–23.
53. Khalafallah AA, Loi SW, Love S, Mohamed M, Mace R, Khalil R, et al. Early application of high cut-off haemodialysis for de-novo myeloma nephropathy is associated with long-term dialysis-independency and renal recovery. Mediterr J Hematol Infect Dis. 2013;5(1):e2013007.
54. Tan J, Lam-Po-Tang M, Hutchison CA, de Zoysa JR. Extended high cut-off haemodialysis for myeloma cast nephropathy in auckland, 2008–2012. Nephrology (Carlton). 2014;19(7):432–5.
55. Harding S, Provot F, Beuscart JB, Cook M, Bradwell AR, Stringer S, et al. Aggregated serum free light chains may prevent adequate removal by high cut-off haemodialysis. Nephrol Dial Transplant. 2011;26(4):1438.
56. Krieter DH, Devine E, Wanner C, Storr M, Krause B, Lemke HD. Clearance of drugs for multiple myeloma therapy during in vitro high-cutoff hemodialysis. Artif Organs 2014;38:888–93.
57. Hutchison CA, Cook M, Heyne N, Weisel K, Billingham L, Bradwell A, Cockwell P. European trial of free light chain removal by extended haemodialysis in cast nephropathy (eulite): a randomised control trial. Trials. 2008;9:55.
58. Naka T, Jones D, Baldwin I, Fealy N, Bates S, Goehl H, et al. Myoglobin clearance by super high-flux hemofiltration in a case of severe rhabdomyolysis: a case report. Crit Care. 2005;9(2):R90.
59. Heyne N, Guthoff M, Krieger J, Haap M, Häring HU. High cut-off renal replacement therapy for removal of myoglobin in severe rhabdomyolysis and acute kidney injury: a case series. Nephron Clin Pract. 2012;121(3–4):c159–64.
60. Keir R, Evans ND, Hutchison CA, Vigano MR, Stella A, Fabbrini P, et al. Kinetic modelling of haemodialysis removal of myoglobin in rhabdomyolysis patients. Comput Methods Programs Biomed. 2014;114(3):e29–38.
61. Ritz E. Atherosclerosis in dialyzed patients. Blood Purif. 2004;22(1):28–37.
62. Barreto DV, Barreto FC, Liabeuf S, Temmar M, Lemke HD, Tribouilloy C, et al. Plasma interleukin-6 is independently associated with mortality in both hemodialysis and pre-dialysis patients with chronic kidney disease. Kidney Int. 2010;77(6):550–6.
63. Lonnemann G, Novick D, Rubinstein M, Passlick-Deetjen J, Lang D, Dinarello CA. A switch to high-flux helixone membranes reverses suppressed interferon-gamma production in patients on low-flux dialysis. Blood Purif. 2003;21(3):225–31.
64. Stein G, Franke S, Mahiout A, Schneider S, Sperschneider H, Borst S, Vienken J. Influence of dialysis modalities on serum AGE levels in end-stage renal disease patients. Nephrol Dial Transplant. 2001;16(5):999–1008.
65. Maduell F, Navarro V, Cruz MC, Torregrosa E, Garcia D, Simon V, Ferrero JA. Osteocalcin and myoglobin removal in on-line hemodiafiltration versus low-and high-flux hemodialysis. Am J Kidney Dis. 2002;40(3):582–9.
66. Meert N, Eloot S, Schepers E, Lemke HD, Dhondt A, Glorieux G, et al. Comparison of removal capacity of two consecutive generations of high-flux dialysers during different treatment modalities. Nephrol Dial Transplant. 2011;26(8):2624–30.
67. Honda H, Qureshi AR, Heimbürger O, Barany P, Wang K, Pecoits-Filho R, et al. Serum albumin, c-reactive protein, interleukin 6, and fetuin a as predictors of malnutrition, cardiovascular disease, and mortality in patients with ESRD. Am J Kidney Dis. 2006;47(1):139–48.
68. Kaysen GA, Dubin JA, Müller HG, Mitch WE, Rosales LM, Levin NW. Relationships among inflammation nutrition and physiologic mechanisms establishing albumin levels in hemodialysis patients. Kidney Int. 2002;61(6):2240–9.
69. Haller C. Hypoalbuminemia in renal failure: pathogenesis and therapeutic considerations. Kidney Blood Press Res. 2005;28(5–6):307–10.
70. Lee D, Haase M, Haase-Fielitz A, Paizis K, Goehl H, Bellomo R. A pilot, randomized, double-blind, cross-over study of high cut-off versus high-flux dialysis membranes. Blood Purif. 2009;28(4):365–72.
71. Fiedler R, Neugebauer F, Ulrich C, Wienke A, Gromann C, Storr M, et al. Randomized controlled pilot study of 2 weeks' treatment with high cutoff membrane for hemodialysis patients with elevated c-reactive protein. Artif Organs. 2012;36(10):886–93.

Sorbents, Hemoperfusion Devices

22

James F. Winchester, Nikolas B. Harbord and Elliot Charen

22.1 Introduction

This chapter will outline the use of sorbents in relation to toxicology, nephrology, and immunology and the newer field of cytokine removal in various disease (inflammatory) states, and also the potential for removing viruses from the blood stream. (Ad)sorbents are defined as particles or structures which adsorb or bind ions, molecules, or drugs and chemicals, loosely or tightly, by physical forces and remove them from solution. Hemoperfusion is defined as passage of blood over sorbents contained in a device (usually cylindrical), almost always requiring anticoagulation with agents such as heparin. The application of sorbents in medicine has spanned many decades; examples include oral activated charcoal in poisoning and hemoperfusion for uremia, poisoning, hepatic encephalopathy, sepsis, and acute lung injury. Sorbent technology forms a basic component in the development of the wearable artificial kidney [1] (See Chap. 14). Other available techniques include exposure of sorbents to dialysis fluid, or the exposure of plasma generated by plasma filtration, in the process of coupled plasma filtration adsorption (CPFA; [2, 3]). These methods will be discussed briefly.

22.2 Oral Sorbents

Table 22.1 gives the common oral sorbents used in management of poisoning (usually by multiple-dose activated charcoal administration; MDAC) and renal disease. An exciting possibility is the adsorption of dietary advanced glycosylation end products by sevelamer and its potential to slow the progression of diabetic nephropathy [4].

J. F. Winchester (✉) · N. B. Harbord · E. Charen
Department of Medicine and Division of Nephrology and Hypertension, Mount Sinai Beth Israel/Icahn School of Medicine at Mount Sinai, New York, NY, USA
e-mail: jwinches@bethisraelny.org

22.3 Hemoperfusion

Hemoperfusion (Table 22.2, Fig. 22.1) devices are available in most developed countries, but the shelf life of around 2 years in most instances may render them unavailable locally as was recently found in New York [5, 6]. Cost may be a consideration for single or repeat use, as most devices cost around US$500 or higher. Data from the 2012 report of the American Association of Poison Control Centers shows that MDAC and alkalinization treatments far outnumber treatments by hemodialysis (2324), and these in turn far outnumber treatments using hemoperfusion (61) [7]. Table 22.3 lists common drugs for which hemoperfusion has been used. Some drugs and chemicals removed with high flux dialysis (compared to reports of cuprophane dialyzers in the past) can be removed at rates equal to or exceeding that of hemoperfusion devices [8, 9]. A review of the recent literature on extracorporeal treatment in poisoning (EXTRIP) has focused on a critical appraisal of the efficiency of both dialysis and hemoperfusion [10]. Hemoperfusion can be performed in conjunction with dialysis, in dialysis patients or in multiple drug intoxications complicated by acidosis or hypothermia (Fig. 22.2). For a detailed description of hemoperfusion devices in intoxication see Ghannoum et al. [11].

22.4 Indications for and Side Effects of Hemoperfusion in Poisoning

The clinical condition of the patient is the primary indicator for hemoperfusion in poisoning, with deep coma induced by central nervous system depressants being paramount. However agents that have delayed effects, such as paraquat, demand immediate treatment within 24 h. Thrombocytopenia is the main hematologic side effect, but since the charcoal devices use particles coated with a polymer membrane, thrombocytopenia may be relatively minor (15 % fall in platelet count). Other effects such as leukopenia, hypocalcemia, and hypoglycemia have been reported. Physical

A. K. Singh et al. (eds.), *Core Concepts in Dialysis and Continuous Therapies*, DOI 10.1007/978-1-4899-7657-4_22

Table 22.1 Oral sorbents

Sorbent	Use	Manufacturer	Side effects	Cost	Current use
Activated charcoal	Drugs and chemicals	Many	None	+	Yes in poisoning
Aluminum hydroxide	Pi binder	Many	Bone disease, encephalopathy	+	No
Calcium Carbonate	Pi binder	Many	Hypercalcemia, calcification	+	Yes
Calcium acetate	Pi binder	Many	Hypercalcemia, calcification, possible enhanced aluminum absorption	+	Yes
Sevelamer	Pi binder	Sanofi	Gastrointestinal	++	Yes
	Cholesterol binder				No
	Binds AGEs				Under investigation
Lanthanum Carbonate	Pi binder	Shire	Gastrointestinal	+++	Yes
Polynuclear iron hydroxide	Pi binder	Fresenius Medical Care	Adsorbs vitamin D	+++	Yes
Ferric citrate	Pi binder, Fe donor	Keryx Biopharmaceuticals, USA	Gastrointestinal	+++	Yes
AST-120 spherical activated charcoal	Indoxyl sulfate, p-cresol sulfate	Kureha Corporation, Japan	Gastrointestinal	++	Under investigation
Sodium polystyrene sulfonate	Potassium, lithium	Covis Pharmaceutical, USA	Volume overload, intestinal necrosis	++	Yes
ZS-9, zirconium silicate	Potassium	ZS Pharma, USA	Unknown	?	Under investigation

Pi inorganic phosphate, *AGEs* advanced glycosylation end products
(?) unavailable

Table 22.2 Current hemoperfusion devices for treatment of intoxications or hepatic encephalopathy

Device	Use	Manufacturer	Substrate	Side effects
MARS	Hepatic encephalopathy	Gambro, USA	Activated charcoal/anionic substances, cholestyramine, anion exchange resin, and serum albumin	No reduction in platelets
Adsorba	Drug removal	Gambro, Sweden	Activated carbon particles	Reduction in platelets
Hemosorba	Drug removal	Asahi Medical, Japan	Activated carbon particles	Reduction in platelets
Prometheus	Hepatic encephalopathy	Fresenius, Germany	Plasma filtration exposed to adsorption columns	Reduction in platelets
Toraymyxin	Endotoxin and cytokine removal	Toray Industries, Japan	Polymyxin-B immobilized on polystyrene fibers	Reduction in platelets
HA 289, HA 330	Drug removal	Jafron Medical, Guandong, China	Neutral microporous polymer resin beads	Unavailable

MARS molecular adsorbents recirculating system

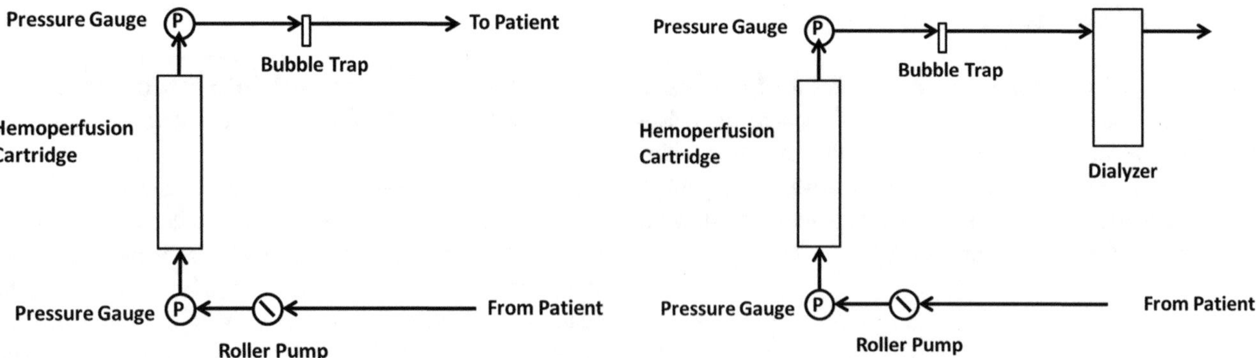

Fig. 22.1 Circuit diagram for hemoperfusion alone

Fig. 22.2 Circuit diagram for hemoperfusion combined with hemodialysis

Table 22.3 Drugs and chemicals removed with hemoperfusion. (Adapted from [12])

Analgesics	Acetaminophen, aspirin, colchicine, d-propoxyphene, methylsalicylate, phenylbutazone, salicylic acid
Anticancer	(Adriamycin), carmustine, chloroquine, doxorubicin, (5-flurouracil), (methotrexate)
Antidepressants	(amitryptiline), (imipramine), (tricyclics), bupropion
Antimicrobials	Ampicillin, clindamycin, chloramphenicol, dapsone, gentamicin, isoniazid, thiabendazole
Barbiturates	Amobarbital, butabarbital, hexabarbital, pentobarbital, phenobarbital, quinalbital, secobarbital, thiopental, vinalbital
Cardiovascular	Digoxin, diltiazem, (disopyramide), flecainide, metoprolol, n-acetylprocainamide, procainamide, quinidine
Plant/animal toxins	Amanitin, *Averrhoa carambola* (star fruit), chlordane, demeton sulfoxide, dimethoate, diquat, methylparathion, nitrostigmine, (organophosphates), parathion, paraquat, phalloidin, polychlorinated biphenyls
Sedatives	Carbromal, carbamazepine, chloral hydrate, (clozapine),(diazepam), diphenhydramine, ethchlorvynol, glutethimide, meprobamate, methaqualone, methsuximide, methyprylon, promazine, promethazine, quetiapine, (valproate)
Solvents/gases	Carbon tetrachloride, ethylene oxide, trichloroethane, xylene
Miscellaneous	Aminophylline, cimetidine, (phencyclidine), phenols, (podophyllin), theophylline, thyroxine, (aluminum)#, (iron)#, 2,4-dinitrophenol

() not well removed, ()# removed with chelating agent

factors influencing drug removal include volume of distribution (which renders hemoperfusion unlikely to be effective in tricyclic drug poisoning) [13], protein binding, and water solubility.

22.5 Immunoadsorption

Antibodies attached to resins or inert particles can remove antigens from blood or other solution (e.g., plasma from plasmapheresis). Hemoperfusion over anti- DNA antibodies attached to particles was tried in the treatment of systemic lupus erythematosus [14], while removal of preformed human leukocyte antigen (HLA) antibodies by staphylococcal A protein column was used before transplantation [15]. The latter technique has been supplanted by plasmapheresis and administration of intravenous immunoglobulin G (IVIG) [16].

Recently, several novel devices for removing immune products by exposure to antigens, antibodies, or chemical ligands have become available, mostly in Europe or Japan. These devices are outlined in Table 22.4. Randomized controlled studies have not been published for any of these devices, but several small series have demonstrated their potential in a variety of disease states. Two devices are direct hemoperfusion devices, and the rest have plasma separation components (Fig. 22.3). The Toraymyxin device has also been shown to be associated with a serial reduction in anti-CADM-140/MDA5 antibody in amyopathic dermatomyositis with prevention of lung injury [17].

22.6 Hemoperfusion in Uremia

In the quest to remove molecules greater than those removed with conventional or high flux dialysis, the addition of charcoal [38, 39] or resin [40, 41] hemoperfusion in line with dialyzers has undergone clinical trials. It has been demonstrated that "middle molecules," β2-microglobulin (12 kDa) and molecules up to ~65 kDa (the molecular weight of albumin) including cytokines and small proteins can be removed more readily than high flux dialysis. No commercial products are available in the USA for uremia, but the Lixelle device is available in Japan, Europe, and recently approved in USA (Table 22.5) for the treatment of β2-microglobulin-related amyloidosis. The significant extra cost of sorbent hemoperfusion devices in this setting may hinder further development

22.7 Cytokine Adsorption

Our understanding of the systemic inflammatory response syndrome (SIRS) and sepsis has advanced considerably over the past two decades, generating a great deal of interest in removing proinflammatory cytokines from plasma in a nonspecific manner [44]. Continuous hemodiafiltration techniques [45] and hemoperfusion devices have been studied in this regard. The perceived need has generated the construction of several devices varying in content and mechanism of adsorption. Such devices are outlined in Table 22.5.

The most studied devices are Lixelle, MATISSE, Toraymyxin, and CytoSorb, approved in Japan or Europe for the treatment of sepsis.

22.8 Virus Adsorption

Adsorption to cell surfaces is the first step in viral invasion and replication. Adsorption of viruses to nonorganic surfaces has been used to concentrate viruses for use in vaccine production, isolation from blood, or other solutions, and in prevention of viruses entering the potable water table. An extension of the physicochemical process has been applied to the removal of hepatitis C virus in a human trial in India, using a lectin-based adsorbent attached to the dialysate surface of

Table 22.4 Hemoperfusion or plasma perfusion devices for immunoadsorption

Device	Manufacturer	Substrate	Selectivity	Diseases treated	Reference
CF-X	Ube Industries, Ichihara, Japan	Cellulose beads-hexamethyl diisocyanate	Anti-DNA antibody, pemphigus antibody	SLE, pemphigus	[18, 19]
Coraffin	Affina, Germany	Plasmapheresis-derived plasma exposed to Sepharose-CL beads-2 linear peptide ligands	Autoantibodies to Beta-1 adrenergic receptor	Dilated cardiomyopathy	[20]
DNA 230	Jafron Medical, Guangdong, China	Neutral microporous polymer resin	Anti-DNA antibody?	SLE	Not available
Globaffin	Fresenius-Affina Medical Care, Bad Homburg, Germany	Plasmapheresis-derived plasma exposed to Sepharose-CL beads-peptide ligands	IgG, IgA, IgM	RA, SLE, Transplant rejection, Goodpasture, and others	[21]
GlucosorbABO	Glycorex Transplantation, Lund, Sweden	Plasmapheresis-derived plasma exposed to Sepharose linked A or B blood group antigen	A and B blood group antibodies	Transplantation	[22–24]
Ig-Therasorb	Baxter, Munich, Germany	Plasmapheresis-derived plasma exposed to Sepharose-sheep anti-human Ig	IgG, IgA, IgM	Goodpasture disease, SLE, acquired hemophilia A	[25]
Immunosorba	Fresenius Medical Care, Bad Homburg, Germany	Plasmapheresis-derived plasma exposed to Sepharose-Protein A	IgG, IgA, IgM	ANCA positive vasculitis, FSGS	[26, 27]
Immusorba-TR350	Asahi Medical, Japan	Plasmapheresis-derived plasma exposed to Polyvinyl alcohol-Tryptophan	Fibrinogen, immunoglobulins, others	Myasthenia gravis, Guillain Barre, dilated cardiomyopathy, multiple sclerosis	[28–31]
Immusorba-PH 350	Asahi Medical, Japan	Plasmapheresis-derived plasma exposed to Polyvinyl alcohol-Phenylalanine	Fibrinogen, immunoglobulins, anti-acetylcholine antibodies	Myasthenia gravis, Guillain Barre, SLE, RA	[32]
Miro	Fresenius Medical Care, Bad Homburg, Germany	Polyacrylate-C1q-ligand	C1q-CIC, C1q antibodies, antiphospholipid antibodies, fibrinogen	SLE	[33, 34]
Prosorba	Fresenius Medical Care, Bad Homburg, Germany	Silica-Protein-A	IgG, IgA, IgM	FSGS, Henoch-Schönlein, vasculitis, SLE, RA	[35]
Selesorb	Kaneka, Japan	Dextran sulfate	Anti-ds DNA antibodies, lipids, fibrinogen, immunoglobulins, cryoglobulins	SLE	[36, 37]

SLE systemic lupus erythematosus, *RA* rheumatoid arthritis, *FSGS* focal segmental glomerulosclerosis, *IgG* immunoglobulin G, *IgA* immunoglobulin A, *IgM* immunoglobulin M, *Anti-ds DNA* anti-double stranded deoxyribonucleic acid, *CIC* circulating immune complexes
(?) possible mechanism (proprietary information)

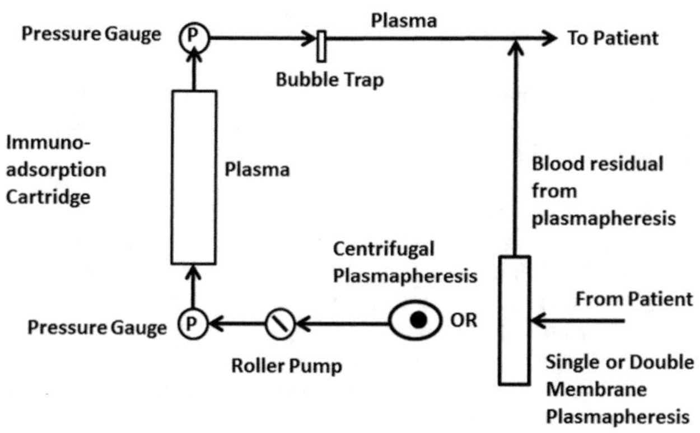

Fig. 22.3 Circuit diagram for immunadsorption of plasma derived from centrifugal plasmapheresis or plasma derived from membrane plasmapheresis

a modified hollow fiber dialyzer [46]. The device has also been demonstrated to remove cancer cell exosomes in vitro [47]. The Planova device has been used to remove scrapie virus from biological solutions (Table 22.6) [48].

22.9 Conclusion

The use of sorbents in medicine offers clinicians the ability to remove a variety of substances from the body and in turn modify the course of a disease or condition. Oral sorbents are commonly used in the treatment of poisoning, as with MDAC, or the treatment of mineral derangements, as with phosphate binders or cation binders. Hemoperfusion can be combined with plasma filtration to provide removal of protein-bound substances in the treatment of hepatic encephalopathy or employed in the treatment of drug intoxications or poisonings. Immunoadsorption employs the specificity of the antigen and antibody binding to reduce specific antibody titers in advance of organ transplantation or to improve immune-mediated diseases. Finally, cytokine and virion

Table 22.5 Cytokine/Endotoxin Adsorption Devices

Substance removed	Device	Manufacturer	Substrate	Method	Availability
Cytokines	CPFA	Bellco, Mirandola, Italy	Hydrophobic resin after plasma filtration	Adsorption	Europe
Cytokines	CTR-001	Kaneka Medical Products, Osaka, Japan	Cellulose beads	Adsorption	Japan
Cytokines	CYT-860	Toray Industries, Inc, Tokyo, Japan	Polystyrene-based fibers	Adsorption	Japan [42]
Cytokines, β[beta]2-Microglobulin	CytoSorb	CytoSorbents Inc, Princeton Junction, NJ, USA	Polystyrene divinylbenzene copolymer beads	Adsorption	Europe [43]
Cytokines, β[beta]2-Microglobulin	Lixelle	Kaneka Medical Products, Osaka, Japan	Cellulose beads-hexadecyl ligand	Adsorption	Japan, Europe, USA
Endotoxin	LPS adsorber	Alteco Medical, Sweden	Polypeptide bound to porous polyethylene discs	Adsorption	Europe
Endotoxin	MATISSE	Fresenius, Germany	Albumin bound to polymethacrylate beads	Adsorption	Europe
Cytokines	MPCF-X	Ube Industries, Ichihara, Japan	Cellulose beads	Adsorption	Japan
Endotoxin, cytokines	oXiris	Gambro-Hospal, France	Acrylonitrile membrane grafted with polyethyeneimine/heparin	Adsorption Convection	Europe
Cytokines, endotoxin	Toraymyxin	Toray Industries, Japan	Polymyxin B bound to polypropylene-polystyrene fibers	Adsorption	Europe
Cytokines	HA 280, HA330	Jafron Medical, Guandong, China	Neutral microporous polymer resin	Adsorption	China

Table 22.6 Virus adsorbers

Substance removed	Device	Manufacturer	Substrate	Method	Availability
Hepatitis C virus, circulating cancer exosomes, Ebola virus[a]	Hemopurifier	Aethlon Medical, San Diego, CA, USA	Modified hollow fiber dialyzer	Adsorption	Under investigation
Unnamed virus	Planova 15N, 20N, 35N	Asahi KASEI, Tokyo, Japan	Hollow fiber devices	Adsorption?	Under investigation
Unnamed virus	Planova BioEX	Asahi KASEI, Tokyo, Japan	Hollow fiber devices	Adsorption?	Under investigation

[a] Oral presentation Helmut Geiger, M.D., Goethe University, Frankfurt am Main, Germany, American Society of Nephrology, Philadelphia, PA, November 2014

(?) possible mechanism of action

adsorption have the potential to modify the systemic inflammatory response and treat viral infection.

Disclosures Dr. Winchester was previously employed as chief medical officer of RenalTech International, USA, before it was renamed Cytosorbents, Inc. He holds stock and stock options in Cytosorbents, Inc.

Dr. Harbord and Dr. Charen have no disclosures.

References

1. Davenport A, Ronco C, Gura V. From wearable ultrafiltration device to wearable artificial kidney. Contrib Nephrol. 2011;171:237–42.
2. Formica M, Inguaggiato P, Bainotti S, Wratten ML. Coupled plasma filtration adsorption. Contrib Nephrol. 2007;156:405–10.
3. Bellomo R, Honoré PM, Matson J, Ronco C, Winchester J. Extracorporeal blood treatment (EBT) methods in SIRS/Sepsis. Int J Artif Organs. 2005;28:450–8.
4. Uribarri J. Personal communication. 2014.
5. Shalkham AS, Kirrane BM, Hoffman RS, Goldfarb DS, Nelson LS. The availability and use of charcoal hemoperfusion in the treatment of poisoned patients. Am J Kidney Dis. 2006;48:239–41.
6. Holubek WJ, Hoffman RS, Goldfarb DS, Nelson LS. Use of hemodialysis and hemoperfusion in poisoned patients. Kidney Int. 2008;74(10):1327–34.
7. Mowry JB, Spyker DA, Cantilena LR Jr, Bailey JE, Ford M. 2012 Annual Report of the American Association of Poison Control Centers' National Poison Data System (NPDS): 30th Annual Report. Clin Toxicol (Phila). 2013;51:949–1229.
8. Palmer BF. Effectiveness of hemodialysis in the extracorporeal therapy of phenobarbital overdose. Am J Kidney Dis. 2000;36:640–3.
9. Mactier R, Laliberté M, Mardini J, Ghannoum M, Lavergne V, Gosselin S, Hoffman RS, Nolin TD, EXTRIP Workgroup. Extracorporeal treatment for barbiturate poisoning: recommendations From the EXTRIP workgroup. Am J Kidney Dis. 2014;64:347–58.
10. Lavergne V, Nolin TD, Hoffman RS, Roberts D, Gosselin S, Goldfarb DS, Kielstein JT, Mactier R, Maclaren R, Mowry JB, Bunchman TE, Juurlink D, Megarbane B, Anseeuw K, Winchester JF, Dargan PI, Liu KD, Hoegberg LC, Li Y, Calello DP, Burdmann EA, Yates C, Laliberté M, Decker BS, Mello-Da-Silva CA, Lavonas E, Ghannoum M. The EXTRIP (EXtracorporeal TReatments In Poisoning) workgroup: guideline methodology. Clin Toxicol (Phila). 2012;50:403–13.
11. Ghannoum M, Bouchard J, Nolin TD, Ouellet G, Roberts DM. Hemoperfusion for the treatment of poisoning: technology, determinants of poison clearance, and application in clinical practice. Semin Dial. 2014;27:350–61.
12. Winchester JF, Harbord NB, Charen E, Ghannoum M. Use of dialysis and hemoperfusion, in treatment of poisoning. In: Daugirdas JT, Blake PG, Todd SI, editors. Handbook of dialysis. 5th edn. Philadelphia: Lippincott Willliams & Wilkins; 2015. p. 368–90.
13. Yates C, Galvao T, Sowinski KM, Mardini K, Botnaru T, Gosselin S, Hoffman RS, Nolin TD, Lavergne V, Ghannoum M, EXTRIP Workgroup. Extracorporeal treatment for tricyclic antidepressant poisoning: recommendations from the EXTRIP Workgroup. Semin Dial. 2014;27:381–9.
14. Terman DS, Stewart I, Robinette J, Carr R, Harbeck R. Specific removal of DNA antibodies in vivo with an extracorporeal immunoadsorbent. Clin Exp Immunol. 1976;24:231–7.
15. Alarabi AA, Wikström B, Backman U, Danielson BG, Tufvesson G, Sjöberg O. Pretransplantation immunoadsorption therapy in patients immunized with human lymphocyte antigen: effect of treatment and three years' clinical follow-up of grafts. Artif Organs. 1993;17:702–7.
16. Keven K, Sengul S, Celebi ZK, Tuzuner A, Yalcin F, Duman T, Tutkak H. Kidney transplantation in immunologically high-risk patients. Transplant Proc. 2013;45:919–22.
17. Teruya A, Kawamura K, Ichikado K, Sato S, Yasuda Y, Yoshioka M. Successful polymyxin B hemoperfusion treatment associated with serial reduction of serum anti-CADM-140/MDA5 antibody levels in rapidly progressive interstitial lung disease with amyopathic dermatomyositis. Chest. 2013;144:1934–6.
18. Stummvoll GH, Schmaldienst S, Smolen JS, Derfler K, Biesenbach P. Lupus nephritis: prolonged immunoadsorption (IAS) reduces proteinuria and stabilizes global disease activity. Nephrol Dial Transpl. 2012;27:618–26.
19. Herrero-González JE, Brauns O, Egner R, Rönspeck W, Mascaró JM Jr, Jonkman MF, Zillikens D, Sitaru C. Immunoadsorption against two distinct epitopes on human type XVII collagen abolishes dermal-epidermal separation induced in vitro by autoantibodies from pemphigoid gestationis patients. Eur J Immunol. 2006;36:1039–48.
20. Dandel M, Wallukat G, Englert A, Hetzer R. Immunoadsorption therapy for dilated cardiomyopathy and pulmonary arterial hypertension. Atheroscler Suppl. 2013;14:203–11.
21. Rönspeck W, Brinckmann R, Egner R, Gebauer F, Winkler D, Jekow P, Wallukat G, Müller J, Kunze R. Peptide based adsorbers for therapeutic immunoadsorption. Ther Apher Dial. 2003;7:91–7.
22. Genberg H, Kumlien G, Wennberg L, Berg U, Tydén G. ABO-incompatible kidney transplantation using antigen-specific immunoadsorption and rituximab: a 3-year follow-up. Transplantation. 2008;85:1745–54.
23. Genberg H, Kumlien G, Wennberg L, Tyden G. The efficacy of antigen-specific immunoadsorption and rebound of anti-A/B antibodies in ABO-incompatible kidney transplantation. Nephrol Dial Transpl. 2011;26:2394–400.
24. Donauer J, Wilpert J, Geyer M, Schwertfeger E, Kirste G, Drognitz O, Walz G, Pisarski P. ABO-incompatible kidney transplantation using antigen-specific immunoadsorption and rituximab: a single center experience. Xenotransplantation. 2006;13:108–10.
25. Braun N, Gutenberger S, Erley CM, Risler T. Immunoglobulin and circulating immune complex kinetics during immunoadsorption onto protein A sepharose. Transfus Sci. 1998;19 Suppl:25–31.
26. Koch M1, Kohnle M, Trapp R. A case report of successful long-term relapse control by protein-a immunoadsorption in an immunosuppressive-treated patient with end-stage renal disease due to Wegener's granulomatosis. Ther Apher Dial. 2009;13:150–6.
27. Kandus A, Ponikvar R, Buturović-Ponikvar J, Bren AF, Oblak M, Mlinšek G, Kmetec A, Arnol M. Plasmapheresis and immunoadsorption for treatment and prophylaxis of recurrent focal segmental glomerulosclerosis in adult recipients of deceased donor renal grafts. Ther Apher Dial. 2013;17:438–43.
28. Sawada K, Malchesky PS, Koo AP, Mitsumoto H. Myasthenia gravis therapy: immunoadsorbent may eliminate need for plasma products. Cleve Clin J Med. 1993;60:60–4.
29. Jiménez C1, Rosenow F, Grieb P, Haupt WF, Borberg H. Adsorption therapy with tryptophan-conjugated polyvinyl alcohol gels in 10 patients with acute Guillain-Barré syndrome. Transfus Sci. 1993;14:9–11.
30. Ikeda U, Kasai H, Izawa A, Koyama J, Yazaki Y, Takahashi M, Higuchi M, Koh CS, Yamamoto K. Immunoadsorption therapy for patients with dilated cardiomyopathy and heart failure. Curr Cardiol Rev. 2008;4:219–22.
31. Koziolek MJ, Tampe D, Bähr M, Dihazi H, Jung K, Fitzner D, Klingel R, Müller GA, Kitze B. Immunoadsorption therapy in patients with multiple sclerosis with steroid-refractory optical neuritis. J Neuroinflammation. 2012;9:80–9.
32. Fadul JEM, Danielson BG, Wistron B. Reduction of plasma fibrinogen, immunoglobulin G, and immunoglobulin M concentrations

by immunoadsorption therapy with tryptophan and phenylalanine adsorbents. Artif Org. 1996;20:986–90.
33. Pfueller B, Wolbart K, Bruns A, Burmester GR, Hiepe F. Successful treatment of patients with systemic lupus erythematosus by immunoadsorption with a C1q column: a pilot study. Arthritis Rheum. 2001;44:1962–3.
34. Hiepe F, Pfüller B, Wolbart K, Bruns A, Leinenbach HP, Hepper M, Schössler W, Otto V. C1q: a multifunctional ligand for a new immunoadsorption treatment. Ther Apher. 1999;3:246–51.
35. Felson DT, LaValley MP, Baldassare AR, Block JA, Caldwell JR, Cannon GW, Deal C, Evans S, Fleischmann R, Gendreau RM, Harris ER, Matteson EL, Roth SH, Schumacher HR, Weisman MH, Furst DE. The Prosorba column for treatment of refractory rheumatoid arthritis: a randomized double-blind, sham-controlled trial. Arthritis Rheum. 1999;42:2153–9.
36. Stefanutti C, Di Giacomo S, Mareri M, De Lorenzo F, D'Alessandri G, Angelico F, Bucci A, Musca A, Mammarella A. Immunoadsorption apheresis (Selesorb) in the treatment of chronic hepatitis C virus-related type 2 mixed cryoglobulinemia. Transfus Apher Sci. 2003;28:207–14.
37. Matsuki Y1, Suzuki K, Kawakami M, Ishizuka T, Hidaka T, Nakamura H. Adsorption of anaphylatoxins from the plasma of systemic lupus erythematosus patients using dextran sulfate cellulose columns. J Clin Apher. 1998;13:108–13.
38. Chang TM, Malave N. The development and first clinical use of semipermeable microcapsules (artificial cells) as a compact artificial kidney. Trans Am Soc Artif Intern Organs. 1970;16:141–8.
39. Winchester JF, Ratcliffe JG, Carlyle E, Kennedy AC. Solute, amino acid, and hormone changes with coated charcoal hemoperfusion in uremia. Kidney Int. 1978;14:74–81.
40. Yamamoto Y, Hirawa N, Yamaguchi S, Ogawa N, Takeda H, Shibuya K, Kawahara K, Kojima H, Dobashi Y, Fujita M, Azusima K, Miyazaki N, Kobayashi M, Kobayashi C, Fujiwara A, Yuto J, Saka S, Yatsu K, Toya Y, Yasuda G, Ohnishi T, Umemura S. Long-term efficacy and safety of the small-sized β2-microglobulin adsorption column for dialysis-related amyloidosis. Ther Apher Dial. 2011;15:466–74.
41. Winchester JF, Silberzweig J, Ronco C, Kuntsevich V, Levine D, Parker T, Kellum JA, Salsberg JA, Quartararo P, Levin NW. Sorbents in acute renal failure and end stage renal disease: middle molecule and cytokine removal. Blood Purif. 2004;22:73–7.
42. Kobe Y, Oda S, Matsuda K, Nakamura M, Hirasawa H. Direct hemoperfusion with a cytokine-adsorbing device for the treatment of persistent or severe hypercytokinemia: a pilot study. Blood Purif. 2007;25:446–53.
43. Hetz H, Berger R, Recknagel P, Steltzer H. Septic shock secondary to β[beta]-hemolytic streptococcus-induced necrotizing fasciitis treated with a novel cytokine adsorption therapy. Int J Artif Organs. 2014;37:422–6.
44. Atan R, Crosbie DC, Bellomo R. Techniques of extracorporeal cytokine removal: a systematic review of human studies. Ren Fail. 2013;35:1061–70.
45. Haase M, Bellomo R, Baldwin I, Haase-Fielitz A, Fealy N, Davenport P, Morgera S, Goehl H, Storr M, Boyce N, Neumayer HH. Hemodialysis membrane with a high-molecular-weight cutoff and cytokine levels in sepsis complicated by acute renal failure: a phase 1 randomized trial. Am J Kidney Dis. 2007;50:296–304.
46. Tullis RH, Duffin RP, Ichim TE, Joyce JA, Levin NW. Modeling hepatitis C virus therapies combining drugs and lectin affinity plasmapheresis. Blood Purif. 2010;29:210–5.
47. Ichim TE, Zhong Z, Kaushal S, Zheng X, Ren X, Hao X, Joyce JA, Hanley HH, Riordan NH, Koropatnick J, Bogin V, Minev BR, Min WP, Tullis RH. Exosomes as a tumor immune escape mechanism: possible therapeutic implications. J Transl Med. 2008;6:37.
48. Tateishi J, Kitamoto T, Mohri S, Satoh S, Sato T, Shepherd A, Macnaughton MR. Scrapie removal using Planova virus removal filters. Biologicals. 2000;29:17–25.

Hemodiafiltration

23

Jonathan Wong, Sivakumar Sridharan, Roger Greenwood and Ken Farrington

23.1 A Brief History

Conventional hemodialysis (HD) was developed for the treatment of patients with end-stage kidney disease as a predominantly diffusive process, deploying "tight" membranes, initially cuprophane-based, with small pore size (low flux), and with low hydraulic permeability characteristics. Dialyzers were arranged in a flat-plate configuration. Use of an effluent pump in the dialysis fluid circuit provided the capacity for low-volume ultrafiltration. Use of this technology provided good clearance of small solutes, such as urea, and was effective in correcting electrolyte, acid–base, and fluid imbalances. Removal of larger molecular weight solutes was poor, however. The concept that accumulation of such solutes (middle molecules) may be toxic and contribute to conditions, such as uremic peripheral neuropathy, led to the notion of the "square meter-hour" hypothesis [1], with long dialysis sessions posited as the only means of middle molecule removal. The development of new classes of dialyzer membranes with increased pore size (high flux) and higher hydraulic permeability, most frequently configured in a more robust hollow fiber array, allowed improved diffusive clearance of middle molecules and also increased the capacity for their convective removal [2].

These technological developments provided the possibility of providing a blood purification method based solely on the use of convection hemofiltration (HF) (Fig. 23.1). HD and HF have different clearance profiles. HD provides good clearance of small solutes but poor clearance of middle molecules; HF provides better clearance of these larger solutes but poor small-solute clearance [3]. Deficient small-solute clearance precludes the use of HF as an intermittent maintenance therapy for patients with end-stage kidney disease. It has found a major use though in continuous mode as a treatment for patients with acute kidney injury in critical care settings.

Combining these modalities HD and HF as hemodiafiltration (HDF) allowed the best characteristics of both to be utilized. The first reported use of HDF was carried out by Leber and coworkers in Giessen, Germany [4]. They treated six patients over 6 months and reported higher clearances of small and larger solutes with HDF compared to either HD or HF alone. They also suggested that patients treated with HDF were able to tolerate higher amounts of fluid removal. They considered HDF a method of choice to shorten dialysis time. Subsequently, Wizemann et al. from the same group demonstrated the efficiency and hemodynamic tolerance of ultrashort HDF (2 h thrice weekly) [5], though later their enthusiasm was dampened by longer-term studies showing high inter-dialytic weight gains, a greater requirement for antihypertensive drugs, and higher hospitalization rates in these subjects [6].

The recognition of dialysis-related amyloidosis as a serious complication of low-flux HD due to the accumulation of large uremic toxins or "middle molecules" prompted urgent efforts to find ways to improve their removal and implement HDF on a wider scale. ß2-microglobulin is implicated in dialysis-related amyloid and with a molecular weight of 11,800 Da, it is considered a representative of middle molecules and the most extensively studied [7]. Adequate clearance of this surrogate marker of middle molecules is considered an important goal of HDF.

The development of membrane technology that produced membranes with better diffusive characteristics for middle molecules and with higher hydraulic permeability enhanced the amount of convective transport that could be achieved in a single session [8]. Improvements in the volumetric control of ultrafiltration to allow safe and accurate removal of high volumes of hemofiltrate were further important steps [9, 10].

The biggest hurdle to the development of HDF as a routine maintenance therapy was the availability of a suitable fluid that could be used for both dialysis and substitution. The major issues related to the composition, quality, and cost of the fluid. These fluids needed to be sterile and

K. Farrington (✉) · J. Wong · S. Sridharan · R. Greenwood
Department of Renal Medicine, Lister Hospital, Corey Mills Lane, Stevenage, Hertfordshire, UK
e-mail: ken.farrington@nhs.net

A. K. Singh et al. (eds.), *Core Concepts in Dialysis and Continuous Therapies*, DOI 10.1007/978-1-4899-7657-4_23

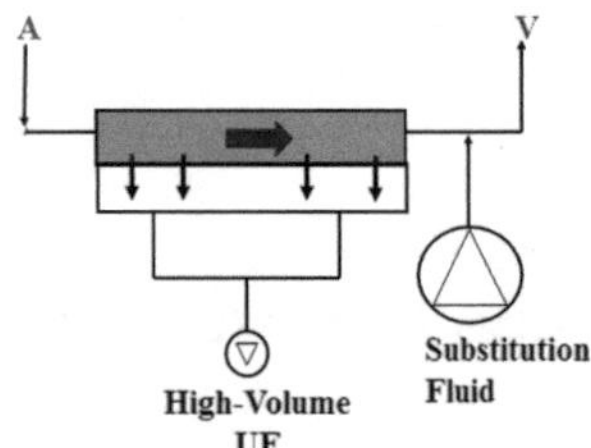

Fig. 23.1 Schematic diagram of a hemofiltration circuit—the volume of fluid ultrafiltered from the patient is replenished by an equal amount of substitution fluid infused intravenously minus the desired fluid volume removal

non-pyrogenic. The use of manufactured bagged fluids with these characteristics for substitution made the cost of the treatment prohibitive for routine maintenance therapy. The solution came in 1978 when Henderson and colleagues produced large amounts of intravenous grade solution from standard dialysate by cold filtration [11]. In the same year, they also published a method for "On-line" preparation of substitution fluid which had the potential to reduce significantly the costs associated with HDF therapy [12]. This development could be considered the birth certificate of online HDF, the beginning of a new era in the development of the HDF modality.

23.2 Technical Aspects of HDF

23.2.1 Characteristics of HDF

Solute removal during HD occurs principally by two mechanisms: diffusion and convection. Diffusion refers to the movement of solutes from an area of high concentration to low concentration along an electrochemical gradient. During HD, this is achieved by running fresh dialysis solution countercurrent to blood flowing on the other side of a semipermeable membrane. Small molecules such as urea are efficiently removed by diffusion, but larger molecules are poorly cleared by this process. In convection, solutes dissolved in fluid are moved across a semipermeable membrane in response to a transmembrane pressure gradient, a process known as solvent drag. Middle-sized molecules such ß2-microglobulin and myogloblin are more efficiently removed by this process (Table 23.1).

Convection occurs independently of solute concentration gradients across the membrane and is determined by the ultrafiltered volume and the porosity of the membrane, which is characterized by the sieving coefficient. The sieving coefficient of a given solute for a given membrane is defined as a ratio of the solute concentration in the ultrafiltrate and the solute concentration of the plasma [13].

A small amount of convection occurs in high-flux HD due to the pressure drop across the dialyzer membrane resulting in around 4–8 l of internal filtration per treatment session. However, high-flux HD is not regarded as a form of convective therapy since minimum effective convective volume of at least 20% of the total blood volume processed must be achieved to be classified as such [14]. Additionally, the convective process during high-flux HD is not controllable, variable, and difficult to measure [15]. HF is a purely convective modality which is effective at removing larger molecular weight solutes, but small-solute clearance is limited by the ultrafiltration volume. By adding a diffusive component—hemodiafiltration, this further enhances the capability of small-solute removal compared with HF.

23.2.2 Types of HDF

Prior to the development of online HDF, different techniques have been used to deliver HDF historically. This section describes some of the relevant HDF techniques and the schematic representations of these circuits are shown in Fig. 23.2.

Table 23.1 Comparison of average clearance rates in hemodiafiltration (HDF) and high-flux hemodialysis (HFHD). (From Spalding et al. [56]; used with permission)

		HDF	HFHD	*P*
Urea	Diffusive	256.6 ± 50.7	239.5 ± 52.6	0.167
	Convective	13.9 ± 7.2	2.10 ± 1.50	< 0.001
	Total	270.5 ± 53.1	241.5 ± 52.9	0.027
Phosphate	Diffusive	147.2 ± 35.2	142.9 ± 30.3	0.739
	Convective	17.3 ± 11.7	2.3 ± 1.4	< 0.001
	Total	164.4 ± 33.1	145.3 ± 30.9	0.041
β2M	Diffusive	49.6 ± 31.4	38.5 ± 19.6	0.252
	Convective	63.2 ± 20.9	6.7 ± 2.6	< 0.001
	Total	112.8 ± 27.8	45.2 ± 19.7	< 0.001
Myoglobulin	Diffusive	25.9 ± 44.6	12.5 ± 18.8	0.817
	Convective	76.5 ± 24.7	7.9 ± 3.0	< 0.001
	Total	102.4 ± 37.4	20.4 ± 18.6	< 0.001

HDF hemodiafiltration, *HFHD* high-flux hemodialysis

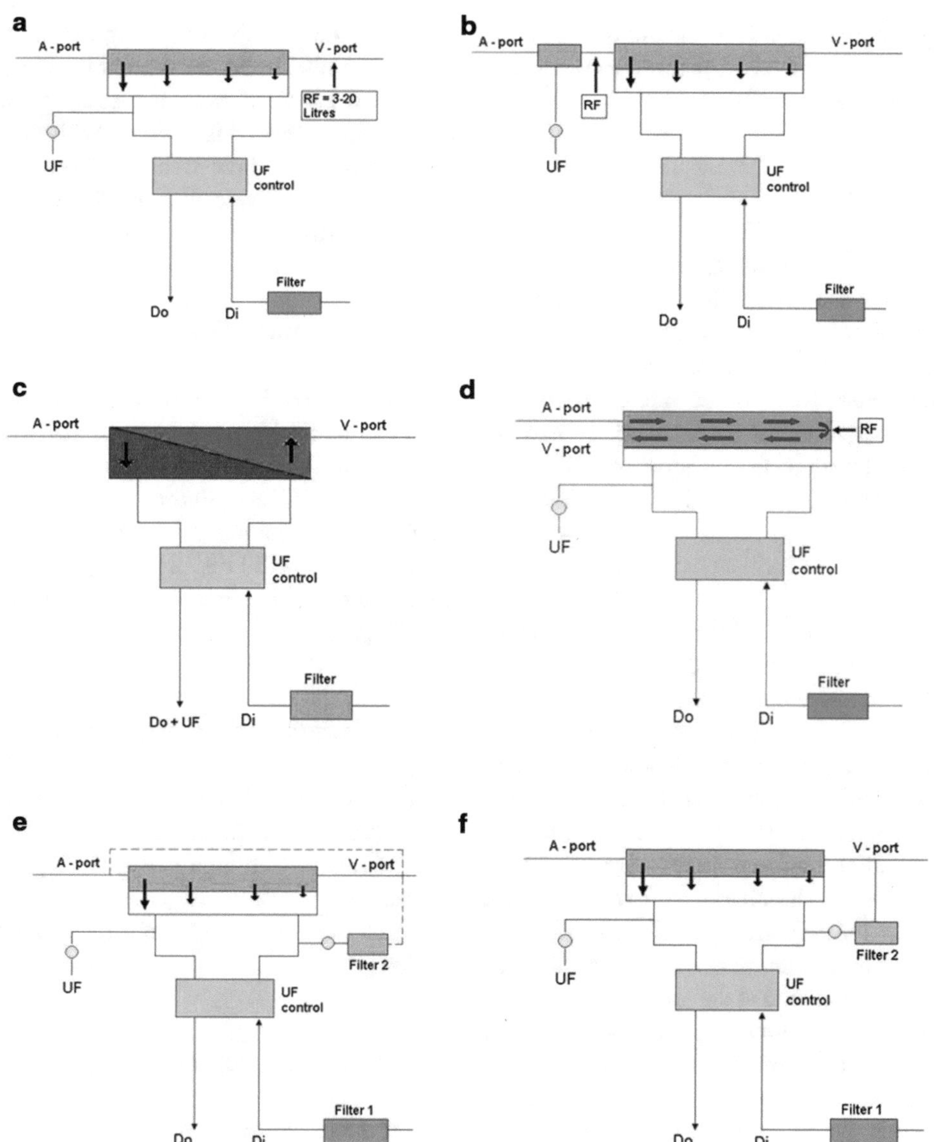

Fig. 23.2 HDF Techniques. **a** Classic HDF, **b** paired filtration HDF, **c** internal HDF, **d** mid-dilution HDF, **e** online HDF (pre-dilution), **f** online HDF (post-dilution); *A*—port=arterial port; *V*—port=venous port; *UF*=ultrafiltration; *Di*=dialysate inlet line; *Do*=dialysate outlet line; *RF*=replacement fluid

23.2.3 Classic HDF

This technique involves giving substitution fluid usually in the range of 9–12 l, which is typically given through the venous port. The substitution fluid is contained in separate commercial bags. It is essential to have an ultrafiltration control system in the equipment and a reinfusion pump for administration of the substitution fluid. Depending on the volume of replacement fluid, this type of HDF is termed soft HDF (3–6 l) or hard HDF (> 15 l).

23.2.4 Paired Filtration HDF

In this technique, two filters are placed in series. The first filter removes fluid and solutes through convection and the second is a dialyzer where diffusion is used to clear solutes. Replacement fluid is administered in between the two filters. This technique is used to minimize the overlap between convection and diffusion within a single filter, thereby increasing the efficiency of each of these processes. A modification of this technique, termed online hemodiafiltration with endogenous reinfusion (HFR), utilizes the ultrafiltrate from the filter and purifies it through adsorption and subsequently uses it as replacement fluid.

23.2.5 Internal HDF

In high-flux HD, a small degree of convection occurs within the dialyzer. This is due to variation in transmembrane pressures between the arterial port, where fluid movement from blood to dialysis fluid is favored and the venous port, where the reverse pertains. This form of "internal HDF" can be enhanced by various methods: by reducing the internal diameter of the fibers, by applying a constriction to the fiber bundle, or by obstructing the dialysate flow in the dialysate compartment [16].

Online HDF

The various forms of HDF described above have now largely been superseded by online hemodiafiltration (OL-HDF) primarily due to its lower cost and the ability to generate large quantities of dialysate water of high purity. In this technique, dialysis fluid is sequentially passed through a series of filters to obtain ultrapure water. This is then reconstituted with the desired balance of acid and bicarbonate concentrate to produce substitution fluid and infused directly into the blood compartment either before the arterial port (pre-dilution), after the venous port (post-dilution), or mid-dilution. Pre-dilution technique has the advantage of reducing shear stress in the filter by diluting the blood at the arterial port and has less risk of albumin leakage, but due to the dilution effect, the concentration gradient of small solutes between blood and the dialyzer is reduced resulting in less small-solute removal. Post-dilution, on the other hand, results in better removal of solutes and low–molecular-weight proteins but is associated with higher transmembrane pressures leading to the risk of albumin leakage and ultrafiltration failure due to clotting of fibers. Mid-dilution HDF is a technique that requires the use of a special filter with two longitudinal compartments in series. The blood flows through the arterial port into the first compartment where ultrafiltration occurs, resulting in hemoconcentration at the end of the compartment. However, instead of exiting the filter through a venous port, blood is directed to the second compartment in the direction opposite to that of the first compartment. Replacement fluid is infused between the first and second compartments so that the blood is diluted to the required volume at the beginning of the second compartment. Mid-dilution HDF may be able to overcome the difficulties of ultrafiltration failure due to hemoconcentration that occurs with post-dilution HDF without compromising middle-molecule removal [17].

It is essential to use "ultrapure" water as substitution fluid for HDF to be employed. Improvements in dialysate preparation and higher purity of the water with cold-sterilization techniques have enabled the adoption of OL-HDF by many centers worldwide. Moreover, many new pieces of dialysis equipment are fitted with necessary software and system controls to perform online HDF. With the exception of the USA, OL-HDF is now well established in routine clinical practice in most developed countries, particularly in Europe and Japan [18].

23.2.6 Technical Requirements of HDF

The use of HDF in clinical practice requires several technical and clinical conditions to be satisfied. These include suitable high-flux dialyzers coupled with specifically designed OL-HDF and European Community-certified HD machines, vascular access capable of delivering high blood flow rates (300–450 ml/min), and the availability of ultrapure water with appropriate water quality monitoring systems in place.

23.2.7 Choice of Hemodiafilter

To achieve high-volume HDF, it is necessary to use highly permeable hemodiafilters to optimize ultrafiltration flow. Hemodiafilters with high hydraulic ($K_{UF} \geq 50$ ml/h/mmHg) and solute permeability (K_0A urea > 600 and ß2-microglobulin > 60 ml/min) and a large surface area (1.5–2.1 m^2) are needed [19].

23.2.8 Production of Online Substitution Fluid

One of the greatest risks to patients during HD is the exposure to contaminated dialysis water. Due to the large ultrafiltration volume achieved HDF, fluid is replaced by diverting a proportion of the fresh dialysis water (mixed with the desired concentration of electrolytes) and infusing it directly into patient's blood. Water quality must therefore meet strict criteria as set by the European Best Practice Guidelines (EBPG) and Association for Advancement of Medical Instrumentation (AAMI) to avoid delivering any pyrogenic or inflammatory stimulus to the patient. Ultrapure water used for HDF must contain < 0.1 colony-forming units (CFU)/ml and < 0.03 endotoxin units (EU)/ml.

This is prepared by passing water that has been pretreated with micro-filters, softeners, and activated carbon through two reverse osmosis (RO) modules in series. RO refers to the process of forcing water through a semipermeable membrane producing purified water leaving behind dissolved solids and organic particles. Purified water from the RO module is further passed through a series of ultrafilters prior to infusion into the patient (Fig. 23.3). The ultrafilters are highly permeable to water and solutes up to a molecular weight of

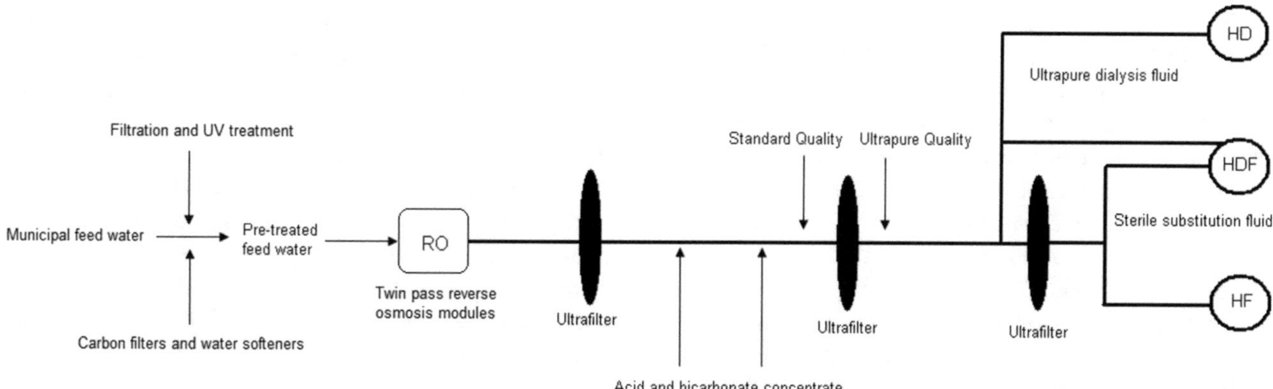

Fig. 23.3 Flow diagram of online fluid preparation. Following pretreatment with reverse osmosis, water is mixed with acid and bicarbonate concentrates and after ultrafiltration becomes ultrapure water used for hemodialysis and hemodiafiltration. Ultrapure dialysis fluid undergoes further filtration through a sterile quality controlled ultrafilter and converted to sterile substitution fluid used for hemofiltration and hemodiafiltration

30–40 kDa and act to prevent the passage of bacterial cells and large cell wall components [20].

Water quality must be regularly tested for microbiological and chemical purity. Maintenance of online systems is essential with adherence to regular disinfection protocols to prevent the buildup of biofilms in water distribution systems and areas of low flow in the fluid pathways of HD machines. Ultrafilters need to be replaced at regular intervals as specified by the manufacturer, and the final filter that is placed prior to infusion into the patient (used to convert ultrapure dialysis fluid to sterile substitution fluid) acts an additional safety feature to prevent the infusion of contaminated substitution fluid into patients [20].

23.2.9 Vascular Access

Patients treated with HDF require a good vascular access that is able to deliver at least 300 ml/min blood flow to facilitate the high ultrafiltration volume necessary to avoid increased transmembrane pressures which may cause alarms, reduce clearance, and cause potential clotting of the extracorporeal circuit. In situations of inadequate vascular access, poor blood flow rate, or conditions that increase blood viscosity (e.g., high hematocrit) pre-dilution or mixed dilution HDF may be preferred.

23.3 Clinical Outcomes

23.3.1 Mortality and Cardiovascular Outcome in HDF

The clinical superiority of HDF over conventional high-flux HD has been a matter of much intense debate. The recent publication of three large prospective randomized controlled trials—the Dutch Convective Transport Study (CONTRAST) study [21], the Turkish Online HDF study [22], and the Catalonian On-line Hemodiafiltration Survival Study (or Estudio de Supervivencia de Hemodiafiltración On-Line [ESHOL]) [23]—has helped bring more light to this matter. All three trials had a similar design: between 714 and 906 prevalent HD patients were randomized to receive post-dilution OL-HDF and matched against either low-flux HD [21] or high-flux HD [22, 23] and followed up for 2–3 years with death or cardiovascular events as their primary and secondary outcomes. The Dutch CONTRAST and Turkish OL-HDF study did not demonstrate any overall survival benefits in patients receiving OL-HDF, but the largest of the three randomized-controlled trials, the ESHOL study demonstrated a 30% lower risk of all-cause mortality (hazard ratio [HR], 0.70; 95% confidence interval [95% CI], 0.53–0.92; $P=0.01$) and 33% lower risk of cardiovascular mortality (HR 0.45, 95% CI, 0.21–0.96; $P=0.03$) in HDF patients compared to high-flux HD arm. However, the HDF group tended to be healthier (being younger), having less incidence of diabetes and catheter access. Although adjustments were made to account for these factors in the statistical analysis, they may still have caused a survival bias for patients receiving HDF.

All three randomized controlled trials were incorporated into two recent large meta-analyses comparing convective and diffusive therapies by Wang [24] and Nistor [25] comprising 3220 [24] to 4039 [25] patients. Both meta-analyses demonstrated no benefit in all-cause mortality, but Nistor et al. found that convective therapies (HDF, HF, and acetate-free biofiltration) were associated with a reduction in cardiovascular mortality (RR 0.87; 95% CI 0.72–1.05) [25]. Unfortunately, the limitation of both meta-analyses was that the majority of studies included were of suboptimal quality, underpowered, and had a high risk of bias in domains such as blinding, data completeness, or selective outcome reporting.

Overall, current literature does not definitely conclude the superiority of HDF over standard HD. However, it has been suggested that delivered dose of convective volume may be a possible explanation for improved survival with HDF observed in some studies. Delivered convective dose was not studied in both meta-analyses [26], but post hoc analysis of the CONTRAST study and the Turkish OL-HDF study suggested a survival benefit in patients that received convective volumes > 21.95 and 17.4 l respectively per session. Similarly, the ESHOL group found that HDF patients in the highest tertile of delivered convective volumes (> 25 l) had the greatest mortality risk reduction. This suggests that the possible prognostic benefit of HDF is mediated through better clearance of toxic middle molecules, though ß2-microglobulin increased significantly in both arms of the ESHOL Study. Unfortunately, residual kidney function (RKF), a critical determinant of ß2-microglobulin [27] was not measured. This finding mirrors that of the Turkish OL-HDF study, but the CONTRAST investigators did find ß2-microglobulin levels significantly lowered by HDF especially in those without RKF [28], though the comparator group used low-flux HD. It may therefore be that improved survival in HDF is mediated by mechanisms other than improved middle-molecule clearance or that ß2-microglobulin is not a good representative of toxic middle molecules.

Although all three randomized controlled trials demonstrated improved outcome in those with the highest achieved convective volume, cautious interpretation of this observation is required given the inherent problem with post hoc analysis and that no studies to date have randomized patients to different convective volumes. In addition, convective volume is dependent upon a good functioning access and session time. Therefore, patients with better vascular access and dialysis for longer hours are able to achieve higher convective volumes. Both of these characteristics may themselves confer a survival advantage [29]. The results of a fourth French prospective randomized controlled trial looking primarily at all-cause mortality, cardiovascular events, and intra-dialytic morbidity in elderly patients on HDF are currently awaited.

23.3.2 Middle-Molecule Clearance—HDF as a Substitute for Residual Kidney Function

Toxic middle molecules such as $ß_2$-microglobulin accumulate in kidney failure, and this molecule is an important predictor of mortality in patients with end-stage kidney disease [30, 31]. Maximizing removal of middle molecules was a major driving factor for the development of convective therapies such as HDF. Many studies demonstrated a reduction in predialysis $ß_2$-microglobulin levels after switching from low- or high-flux HD [32–36], a phenomenon which has also been confirmed in two recent meta-analyses [24, 25]. However, RKF is the most important determinant of $ß_2$-microglobulin levels and its presence supersedes any enhanced convective clearance by HDF [27, 28]. Data from the CONTRAST study demonstrated that reduction in $ß_2$-microglobulin levels with HDF was more pronounced in patients without RKF. Given the importance of RKF in improved clinical outcomes in dialysis patients [37, 38], possibly mediated via its effect on middle-molecule clearance [39, 40], it may be particularly important to employ the use of convective therapies such as HDF in those patients who have lost RKF and thus their native ability to clear toxic middle molecules.

23.3.3 Other Clinical Benefits of HDF

A whole host of other clinical benefits with HDF have been proposed including improved inflammatory and nutritional states, better bone mineral metabolism, lower incidence of intradialytic hypotension (IDH), and better anemia management. This is summarized in Table 23.1.

23.3.4 Anemia, Erythropoietin Resistance, and Inflammation

Anemia is hypothesized to be improved by HDF possibly due to improved removal of medium–large molecules that may inhibit erythropoiesis. There are a number of positive and negative trials in relation to this. These include the Turkish OL-HDF study which showed a reduction in erythropoietin dose in patients on HDF (Table 23.2). However, from the current literature, it is difficult to draw any firm conclusions on the beneficial effect of HDF in anemia management.

It has also been postulated that improvements in erythropoietin resistance may be due to enhanced clearance of uremic toxins which cause inflammation. Chronic inflammation is a common problem in the HD population. It is of prognostic importance and its pathogenesis is likely to be multifactorial but possibly related to the dialysis procedure such as exposure to contaminated dialysis fluid, membrane incompatibility, or intestinal bacterial translocation due to gut ischemia during dialysis.

A few studies have found that switching HD patients to ultrapure dialysate reduced erythropoietin requirements and reduced levels of inflammatory biomarkers such as C-reactive protein and IL-6 [41, 42], probably due to decreased endotoxin transfer from dialysis fluid. A number of observational studies demonstrated an improved inflammatory profile in HDF patients [33, 43, 44], but this effect may have been mediated through improved water quality. The Turkish OL-HDF and ESHOL study found no effect of HDF on inflammatory biomarkers as compared to high-flux HD; however, the CONTRAST study found that CRP and IL-6 increased

Table 23.2 Clinical trials on the effect of hemodiafiltration on various clinical outcomes

Study	Type of study	Number of patients	Modality	Anemia or EPO resistance	Nutrition	Inflammation	Bone metabolism	Intradialytic hypotension	Quality of life
Locatelli et al. 1996 [34]	RCT	380	Low-flux HD vs. high-flux HD vs. HDF	No difference	No difference	–	–	No difference	–
Maduell et al. 1999 [52]	Crossover	37	Switch from high-flux HD to HDF	Improved Hb	No difference	–	–	Better BP control allowing reduction in antihypertensives	–
Eiselt et al. 2000 [53]	RCT	10	Acetate-free biofiltration vs. low-flux HD	Improved	Improved	No difference	–	–	–
Wizemann et al. 2000 [32]	RCT	44	Low-flux HD vs. HDF	No difference	No difference	–	No difference	No difference	–
Ward et al. 2000 [35]	RCT	45	High-flux HD vs. HDF	No difference		–	–	–	No difference
Lin et al. 2001 [54]	RCT	67	High-flux HD vs. HDF	Improved	–	–	–	Improved	Improved
Vinhas et al. 2007 [55]	Prospective Observational	329	High-flux HD vs. HDF	No difference	No difference	No difference	No difference	–	–
Schiffll et al. 2007 [33]	Crossover	76	High-flux HD vs. HDF	Improved	Improved	No difference	Lower phosphate level	Improved	Improved
Panichi et al. 2008 [44]	Prospective Observational	757	Low-flux HD vs. high-flux HD vs. HDF	–	–	Improved—lower IL-6 but not CRP	–	–	–
Vilar et al. 2009 [43]	Retrospective Observational	858	High-flux HD vs. HDF	No difference	No difference	Improved—lower CRP	No difference	Improved	–
Locatelli et al. 2010 [46]	RCT	146	HF/HDF vs. low-flux HD	–	–	–	–	Improved	–
CONTRAST 2012 [21]	RCT	714	Low-flux HD vs. HDF	No difference	–	Improved [45]	Lower phosphate level	–	No effect
Turkish OL-HDF 2013 [22]	RCT	782	High-flux HD vs. HDF	Improved—lower EPO resistance	No difference	No difference	No difference	No difference	–
ESHOL 2013 [23]	RCT	906	High-flux HD vs. HDF	No difference	No difference	No difference	No difference	Improved	–

in patients treated with low-flux HD but remained stable in patients treated with HDF. The annual increase of CRP and IL-6 differed by 20 and 16 %, respectively ($p < 0.05$) between groups after adjustment for baseline variables. This observation could not be explained by differences in dialysis fluid quality since both arms were treated with ultrapure dialysate [45].

23.3.5 Mineral and Bone Metabolism

Phosphate has clearance profile similar to middle molecular weight molecules. Its clearance can be enhanced by adding a convective element to HD treatment. A number of studies have shown improved phosphate removal in HDF [21, 33], though others show no significant effect on serum phosphate levels [22, 23, 32].

In the CONTRAST study, slightly lower serum phosphate levels were obtained in the HDF group compared to its low-flux HD comparator. On the other hand the ESHOL and Turkish OL-HDF studies found no significant differences in calcium, phosphate, and parathyroid hormone levels (PTH) compared to the high-flux HD group.

23.3.6 Nutrition and Quality of Life

The majority of published studies do not demonstrate any significant improvements in nutritional status. In a small crossover trial, Schiffl et al. [33] showed that switching to HDF resulted in increases in dry body weight, mid-arm circumference, and serum albumin. The ESHOL investigators did not find significant improvement in nutritional state in terms of albumin and dry weight with HDF. Unfortunately, there have been few studies which have looked specifically at nutritional state (beyond weight and albumin). Further studies are needed in this area to determine whether convective therapies improve nutritional status in patients. Similarly, there is a paucity of studies looking at the effect of HDF on quality of life. In their meta-analysis, Wang et al. [24] reported only three trials which studied the effect of HDF on quality of life. Two studies reported no significant differences in physical symptoms domain scores between HDF and HD at 12 months. The CONTRAST study also found no differences in quality of life measured by the Kidney Disease Quality of Life Short Form at 2 years post-recruitment.

23.3.7 Hemodynamic Stability on HDF

IDH is a common complication of HD therapy and is associated with significant long-term harm possibly mediated by recurrent episodes of reduced myocardial blood flow resulting in episodes of cardiac ischemia. Reduction in episodes of IDH could improve quality of life and prognosis for HD patients. There are a large number of studies, including the ESHOL study which demonstrate improved hemodynamic stability with HDF compared to conventional and high-flux HD [33, 43, 46]. Convective modalities demonstrated fewer episodes of symptomatic hypotension in two large meta-analyses [24, 25]. The precise mechanisms of apparent improved hemodynamic stability are unknown but may be related to increased sodium delivery due to the large volume of substitution fluid infused, resulting in more rapid vascular refilling. Donauer et al. [47] found that the beneficial effects of improved hemodynamic stability in HDF compared to HD could be obliterated by cooling the dialysate, suggesting that cooling may be the main blood pressure stabilizing factor in HDF.

23.4 Indications and Conclusions

23.4.1 Indications for HDF

The large volume of conflicting data on the efficacy of HDF over standard HD poses difficult questions for clinical nephrologists. Should HDF be the preferred modality over standard HD? If so, in what circumstances should it be deployed?

Whether HDF alters long-term mortality and cardiovascular outcome remains to be fully resolved. However, there is increasing evidence that HDF is associated with better hemodynamic stability so there may be a specific benefit of this modality for patients who are at high risk of dialysis-related hypotension. IDH is associated with increased morbidity and mortality and may also contribute to more rapid decline in RKF [48]. Avoidance of this problem is important in maintaining RKF, improving quality of life, and improving long-term prognosis. In patients without RKF, HDF plays a greater role in middle-molecule removal and in maintaining an overall better inflammatory profile [45]. Anuric dialysis patients may represent a second target group who would specifically benefit from HDF.

23.4.2 Conclusion

HDF is an effective method of renal replacement therapy, and high-volume HDF may offer a survival advantage over conventional and high-flux HD. HDF appears to be safe, with no evidence of clinical harm to patients in any published studies so far. The long-term microbiological safety of online HDF has also been demonstrated [49]. The higher cost of HDF appear to be the only disadvantage over standard HD [50]. However, most modern dialysis machines are capable of delivering HDF and since ultrapure water is already required for high-flux HD, any extra expense may be marginal [51].

HDF makes sense physiologically since it utilizes the same process of convection which occurs in the natural kidney to achieve solute clearance (albeit at a lower rate). With mounting evidence supporting the efficacy of HDF in end-stage kidney disease, it is envisaged that there will be further widespread adoption of this form of renal replacement therapy in the future.

References

1. Babb AL, Popovich RP, Christopher TG, Scribner BH. The genesis of the square meter-hour hypothesis. Trans Am Soc Artif Intern Organs. 1971;17:81–91.
2. Henderson LW, Besarab A, Michaels A, Bluemle LW. Blood purification by ultrafiltration and fluid replacement (diafiltration). Hemodial Int. 2004;8(1):10–8.
3. Leypoldt JK. Solute fluxes in different treatment modalities. Nephrol Dial Transpl. 2000;15(Suppl 1):3–9.
4. Leber HW, Wizemann V, Goubeaud G, Rawer P, Schütterle G. Simultaneous hemofiltration/hemodialysis: an effective alternative to hemofiltration and conventional hemodialysis in the treatment of uremic patients. Clin Nephrol. 1978;9(3):115–21.
5. Wizemann V, Rawer P, Schütterle G. Ultrashort hemodiafiltration: long term efficiency and hemodynamic tolerance. Proc Eur Dial Transplant Assoc. 1983;19:175–81.
6. Wizemann V, Kramer W. Short-term dialysis—long-term complications. Ten years experience with short-duration renal replacement therapy. Blood Purif. 1987;5(4):193–201.
7. Tattersall J. Clearance of beta-2-microglobulin and middle molecules in hemodiafiltration. Contrib Nephrol. 2007;158:201–9.
8. Henderson LW. The birth of hemodiafiltration. Contrib Nephrol. 2007;158:1–8.
9. Roy T, Ahrenholz P, Falkenhagen D, Klinkmann H. Volumetrically controlled ultrafiltration. Current experiences and future prospects. Int J Artif Organs. 1982;5(3):131–5.
10. Ronco C, Fabris A, Feriani M, Chiaramonte S, Brendolan A, Bragantini L, et al. Technical and clinical evaluation of a new system for ultrafiltration control during hemodialysis. ASAIO Trans. 34(3):613–6.
11. Henderson LW, Beans E. Successful production of sterile pyrogen-free electrolyte solution by ultrafiltration. Kidney Int. 1978;14(5):522–5.
12. Henderson LW, Sanfelippo ML, Beans E. "On line" preparation of sterile pyrogen-free electrolyte solution. Trans Am Soc Artif Intern Organs. 1978;24:465–7.
13. Ronco C, Ghezzi PM, Brendolan A, Crepaldi C, La Greca G. The hemodialysis system: basic mechanisms of water and solute transport in extracorporeal renal replacement therapies. Nephrol Dial Transpl. 1998;13(Suppl 6):3–9.
14. Tattersall JE, Ward RA. Online hemodiafiltration: definition, dose quantification and safety revisited. Nephrol Dial Transpl. 2013;28(3):542–50.
15. van der Weerd NC, Penne EL, van den Dorpel MA, Grooteman MPC, Nube MJ, Bots ML, et al. Hemodiafiltration: promise for the future? Nephrol Dial Transpl. 2008;23(2):438–43.
16. Ronco C, Orlandini G, Brendolan A, Lupi A, La Greca G. Enhancement of convective transport by internal filtration in a modified experimental hemodialyzer: technical note. Kidney Int. 1998;54(3):979–85.
17. Krieter DH, Falkenhain S, Chalabi L, Collins G, Lemke H-D, Canaud B. Clinical cross-over comparison of mid-dilution hemodiafiltration using a novel dialyzer concept and post-dilution hemodiafiltration. Kidney Int. 2005;67(1):349–56.
18. Bowry S, Canaud B. Achieving high convective volumes in on-line hemodiafiltration. Blood Purif. 2013;35(Suppl 1):23–8.
19. Canaud B, Chenine L, Renaud S, Leray H. Optimal therapeutic conditions for online hemodiafiltration. Contrib Nephrol. 2011;168:28–38.
20. Ledebo I. On-line preparation of solutions for dialysis: practical aspects versus safety and regulations. J Am Soc Nephrol. 2002;13(Suppl 1):S78–83.
21. Grooteman MPC, van den Dorpel MA, Bots ML, Penne EL, van der Weerd NC, Mazairac AHA, et al. Effect of online hemodiafiltration on all-cause mortality and cardiovascular outcomes. J Am Soc Nephrol. 2012;23(6):1087–96.
22. Ok E, Asci G, Toz H, Ok ES, Kircelli F, Yilmaz M, et al. Mortality and cardiovascular events in online hemodiafiltration (OL-HDF) compared with high-flux dialysis: results from the Turkish OL-HDF Study. Nephrol Dial Transpl. 2013;28(1):192–202.
23. Maduell F, Moreso F, Pons M, Ramos R, Mora-Macià J, Carreras J, et al. High-efficiency postdilution online hemodiafiltration reduces all-cause mortality in hemodialysis patients. J Am Soc Nephrol. 2013;24(3):487–97.
24. Wang AY, Ninomiya T, Al-Kahwa A, Perkovic V, Gallagher MP, Hawley C, et al. Effect of hemodiafiltration or hemofiltration compared with hemodialysis on mortality and cardiovascular disease in chronic kidney failure: a systematic review and meta-analysis of randomized trials. Am J Kidney Dis. 2014;63(6):968–78.
25. Nistor I, Palmer SC, Craig JC, Saglimbene V, Vecchio M, Covic A, et al. Convective versus diffusive dialysis therapies for chronic kidney failure: an updated systematic review of randomized controlled trials. Am J Kidney Dis. 2014;63(6):954–67.
26. Susantitaphong P, Jaber BL. Understanding discordant meta-analyses of convective dialytic therapies for chronic kidney failure. Am J Kidney Dis. 2014;63(6):888–91.
27. Fry AC, Singh DK, Chandna SM, Farrington K. Relative importance of residual renal function and convection in determining beta-2-microglobulin levels in high-flux hemodialysis and on-line hemodiafiltration. Blood Purif. 2007;25(3):295–302.
28. Penne EL, van der Weerd NC, Blankestijn PJ, van den Dorpel MA, Grooteman MPC, Nubé MJ, et al. Role of residual kidney function and convective volume on change in beta2-microglobulin levels in hemodiafiltration patients. Clin J Am Soc Nephrol. 2010;5(1):80–6.
29. Farrington K, Davenport A. The ESHOL study: hemodiafiltration improves survival-but how? Kidney Int. 2013;83(6):979–81.
30. Cheung AK, Rocco MV, Yan G, Leypoldt JK, Levin NW, Greene T, et al. Serum beta-2 microglobulin levels predict mortality in dialysis patients: results of the HEMO study. J Am Soc Nephrol. 2006;17(2):546–55.
31. Okuno S, Ishimura E, Kohno K, Fujino-Katoh Y, Maeno Y, Yamakawa T, et al. Serum beta2-microglobulin level is a significant predictor of mortality in maintenance hemodialysis patients. Nephrol Dial Transplant. 2009;24(2):571–7.
32. Wizemann V, Lotz C, Techert F, Uthoff S. On-line hemodiafiltration versus low-flux hemodialysis. A prospective randomized study. Nephrol Dial Transpl. 2000;15(Suppl 1):43–8.
33. Schiffl H. Prospective randomized cross-over long-term comparison of online hemodiafiltration and ultrapure high-flux hemodialysis. Eur J Med Res. 2007;12(1):26–33.
34. Locatelli F, Mastrangelo F, Redaelli B, Ronco C, Marcelli D, La Greca G, et al. Effects of different membranes and dialysis technologies on patient treatment tolerance and nutritional parameters. The Italian cooperative dialysis study group. Kidney Int. 1996;50(4):1293–302.
35. Ward RA, Schmidt B, Hullin J, Hillebrand GF, Samtleben W. A comparison of on-line hemodiafiltration and high-flux hemodialysis: a prospective clinical study. J Am Soc Nephrol. 2000;11(12):2344–50.

36. Lornoy W, Becaus I, Billiouw JM, Sierens L, Van Malderen P, D'Haenens P. On-line hemodiafiltration. Remarkable removal of beta2-microglobulin. Long-term clinical observations. Nephrol Dial Transplant. 2000;15(Suppl 1):49–54.
37. Termorshuizen F, Dekker FW, van Manen JG, Korevaar JC, Boeschoten EW, Krediet RT. Relative contribution of residual renal function and different measures of adequacy to survival in hemodialysis patients: an analysis of the Netherlands Cooperative Study on the Adequacy of Dialysis (NECOSAD)-2. J Am Soc Nephrol. 2004;15(4):1061–70.
38. Vilar E, Wellsted D, Chandna SM, Greenwood RN, Farrington K. Residual renal function improves outcome in incremental hemodialysis despite reduced dialysis dose. Nephrol Dial Transplant. 2009;24(8):2502–10.
39. Babb AL, Ahmad S, Bergström J, Scribner BH. The middle molecule hypothesis in perspective. Am J Kidney Dis. 1981;1(1):46–50.
40. Bargman J, Golper T. The importance of residual renal function for patients on dialysis. Nephrol Dial Transpl. 2005;20:671–3.
41. Hsu P-Y, Lin C-L, Yu C-C, Chien C-C, Hsiau T-G, Sun T-H, et al. Ultrapure dialysate improves iron utilization and erythropoietin response in chronic hemodialysis patients-a prospective cross-over study. J Nephrol. 17(5):693–700.
42. Sitter T, Bergner A, Schiffl H. Dialysate related cytokine induction and response to recombinant human erythropoietin in hemodialysis patients. Nephrol Dial Transpl. 2000;15(8):1207–11.
43. Vilar E, Fry AC, Wellsted D, Tattersall JE, Greenwood RN, Farrington K. Long-term outcomes in online hemodiafiltration and high-flux hemodialysis: a comparative analysis. Clin J Am Soc Nephrol. 2009;4(12):1944–53.
44. Panichi V, Rizza GM, Paoletti S, Bigazzi R, Aloisi M, Barsotti G, et al. Chronic inflammation and mortality in hemodialysis: effect of different renal replacement therapies. Results from the RISCAVID study. Nephrol Dial Transpl. 2008;23(7):2337–43.
45. Den Hoedt CH, Bots ML, Grooteman MPC, van der Weerd NC, Mazairac AHA, Penne EL, et al. Online hemodiafiltration reduces systemic inflammation compared to low-flux hemodialysis. Kidney Int. 2014;86(2):423–32.
46. Locatelli F, Altieri P, Andrulli S, Bolasco P, Sau G, Pedrini LA, et al. Hemofiltration and hemodiafiltration reduce intradialytic hypotension in ESRD. J Am Soc Nephrol. 2010;21(10):1798–807.
47. Donauer J, Schweiger C, Rumberger B, Krumme B, Böhler J. Reduction of hypotensive side effects during online-hemodiafiltration and low temperature hemodialysis. Nephrol Dial Transpl. 2003;18(8):1616–22.
48. Jansen MAM, Hart AAM, Korevaar JC, Dekker FW, Boeschoten EW, Krediet RT. Predictors of the rate of decline of residual renal function in incident dialysis patients. Kidney Int. 2002;62(3):1046–53.
49. Penne EL, Visser L, van den Dorpel MA, van der Weerd NC, Mazairac AHA, van Jaarsveld BC, et al. Microbiological quality and quality control of purified water and ultrapure dialysis fluids for online hemodiafiltration in routine clinical practice. Kidney Int. 2009;76(6):665–72.
50. McBrien KA, Manns BJ. Hemodiafiltration: not effective or cost-effective compared with hemodialysis. Nephrol Dial Transplant. 2013;28(7):1630–3; discussion 1633.
51. Oates T, Cross J, Davenport A. Cost comparison of online hemodiafiltration with high-flux hemodialysis. J Nephrol. 25(2):192–7.
52. Maduell F, del Pozo C, Garcia H, Sanchez L, Hdez-Jaras J, Albero MD, et al. Change from conventional hemodiafiltration to on-line hemodiafiltration. Nephrol Dial Transpl. 1999;14(5):1202–7.
53. Eiselt J, Racek J, Opatrny K. The effect of hemodialysis and acetate-free biofiltration on anemia. Int J Artif Organs. 2000;23(3):173–80.
54. Lin CL, Huang CC, Chang CT, Wu MS, Hung CC, Chien CC, et al. Clinical improvement by increased frequency of on-line hemodialfiltration. Ren Fail. 2001;23(2):193–206.
55. Vinhas J, Vaz Á, Barreto C, Assunção J. Survival advantage of patients on hemodiafiltration is independent of dialysis dose and patient characteristics: data from a single centre. Port J Nephrol Hypert. 2007;21(4):287–92.
56. Spalding EM, Pandya P, Farrington K. Effect of high haematocrit on the efficiency of high-flux dialysis therapies. Nephron Clin Pract. 2008;110(2):c86–92.

Index

A. K. Singh et al. (eds.), *Core Concepts in Dialysis and Continuous Therapies,* DOI 10.1007/978-1-4899-7657-4

I

K

L

M